Clinical Gynecologic Endocrinology & Infertility

Third Edition

Clinical Gynecologic Endocrinology & Infertility

Third Edition

Leon Speroff
Robert H. Glass
Nathan G. Kase

WILLIAMS & WILKINS

Baltimore • London • Los Angeles • Sydney

Copyright 1983
Williams & Wilkins Co.
428 East Preston Street
Baltimore
Maryland 21202
USA

Made in the United States of America

First edition, 1973
Reprinted 1973, 1975, 1976, 1977

Second edition, 1978
Reprinted 1978, 1979, 1981, 1982

Third edition, 1983

Library of Congress Cataloging in Publication Data

Speroff, Leon.
  Clinical gynecologic endocrinology and infertility.

  Includes bibliographies and index.
1. Endocrine gynecology. 2. Infertility. I. Glass, Robert H.
II. Kase, Nathan G., 1930–   III. Title. [DNLM: 1.
Endocrine diseases. 2. Genital diseases, Female. 3. Sterility,
Female. WP 505 S749c]
RG159.S63 1983   618.1   82-23735
ISBN 0-683-07895-X

Design by Kayo Parsons-Korn and Don Moyer

Composed and printed at the Waverly Press, Inc.
Mt. Royal & Guilford Avenues
Baltimore, Maryland 21202 USA

    86 87 88 89   10 9 8 7 6 5

Preface

The years march inexorably onward. Progress and passage of time are marked by increasingly gray hair (not to mention diminishing amounts of hair) and the appearance of the third edition of our book. As we get older and time seems to move even faster, it feels like we are always in the process of writing the next edition.

This book is a formulation derived from our teaching and clinical activities. The basic form of the book is unchanged. We again review physiologic principles and then present our methods of clinical management which are based on a foundation of those principles. We continue to believe that an encyclopedic style burdens rather than informs.

Reproductive endocrinology is a field that changes rapidly. Clinical and laboratory research are quickly translated into improved patient management. Two therapeutic regimens which illustrate the point are the use of bromocriptine for amenorrhea and galactorrhea, and the mandatory addition of a progestational agent to an estrogen replacement program. The coming years will see greater clinical use of long-acting analogs of gonadotropin releasing hormone.

This book provides a compilation of up-to-date information, but the clinician must always be alert to changes and developments reported in the current literature. The book is dedicated to the improvement of patient care, and we hope that it will aid you to accomplish that goal.

Leon Speroff, M.D.
Cleveland, Ohio

Robert H. Glass, M.D.
San Francisco, California

Nathan G. Kase, M.D.
New York, New York

Contents

1 Hormone Biosynthesis, Metabolism, and Mechanism of Action

To begin a clinical book with a chapter on biochemistry only serves to emphasize that competent clinical judgment is founded upon a groundwork of basic knowledge. On the other hand, clinical practice does not require a technical and sophisticated proficiency in a basic science. *The purpose of this chapter, therefore, is not to present an intensive course in biochemistry, but rather to present a selective review of the most important principles of how hormones are formed and metabolized, and how hormones work.* This information is essential for the development of the physiological concepts to follow, and it is intended that certain details, which we all have difficulty remembering, will be available in this chapter for reference.

The classical definition of a hormone is a substance which travels from a special tissue, where it is released into the bloodstream, to distant responsive cells where the hormone exerts it characteristic effects. What was once thought of as a simple voyage is now appreciated as an odyssey which becomes more complex as new facets of the journey are unraveled in research laboratories throughout the world.

Indeed, the notion that hormones are products only of special tissues is being challenged. Complex hormones and hormone receptors have been discovered in primitive, unicellular organisms, suggesting that endocrine glands are a late development of evolution. The widespread capability of cells to make hormones explains the puzzling discoveries of hormones in strange places, such as gastrointestinal hormones in the brain, reproductive hormones in saliva and intestinal secretions, and the ability of cancers to unexpectedly make hormones. This pervasive idea may lead to significant conceptual changes. Meanwhile, let us follow an estradiol molecule throughout its career, and in so doing gain an overview of how hormones are formed, how hormones work, and how hormones are metabolized.

Estradiol begins its life span with its synthesis in a cell specially suited for this task. For this biosynthesis to take place, the proper enzyme capability must be present along with the proper precursors. In the human female the principal sources of estradiol are the granulosa cells of the developing follicle and the corpus luteum. These cells possess the ability to turn on steroidogenesis in response to specific stimuli. The stimulating agents are the gonadotropins, follicle-stimulating hormone (FSH) and luteinizing hormone (LH). The initial step in the process which will give rise to estradiol is the transmission of the message from the stimulating agents to the steroid-producing mechanisms within the cells.

Messages which stimulate steroidogenesis must be transmitted through the cell membrane. This is necessary because gonadotropins, being large glycopeptides, do not ordinarily enter cells, but must communicate with the cell by joining with specific receptors on the cell membrane. In so doing they activate a sequence of communication. A considerable amount of investigation has been devoted to determining the methods by which this communication takes place. E. M. Sutherland received the Nobel Prize in 1971 for proposing the concept of a second messenger.

Gonadotropin, the first messenger, activates an enzyme in the cell membrane called adenylate cyclase. This enzyme transmits the message by catalyzing the production of a second messenger within the cell, cyclic adenosine 3'5'-monophosphate (cyclic AMP). The message passes from LH to cyclic AMP, much like a baton in a relay race.

Cyclic AMP, the second messenger, initiates the process of steroidogenesis, leading to the synthesis and secretion of the hormone, estradiol. This notion of message transmission has grown more and more complex with the appreciation of new physiological concepts such as the heterogeneity of peptide hormones, the up and down regulation of cell membrane receptors, and the regulation of adenylate cyclase activity.

Secretion of estradiol into the bloodstream directly follows its synthesis. Once in the bloodstream, estradiol exists in two forms, bound and free. A majority of the hormone is bound to protein carriers, albumin and sex steroid hormone binding globulin. The purpose of this binding is not totally clear. The biologic activity of a hormone may be limited by binding in the blood, thereby avoiding extreme or sudden reactions. In addition, binding may prevent unduly rapid

2

metabolism, allowing the hormone to exist for the length of time necessary to ensure a biologic effect. This reservoir-like effect avoids peaks and valleys in hormone levels and allows a more steady state of hormone action.

The biologic and metabolic effects of a hormone are determined by a cell's ability to receive and retain the hormone. The estradiol which is not bound to a protein, but floating free in the bloodstream, readily enters cells by rapid diffusion. For estradiol to produce its effect, however, it must be grasped by a receptor within the cell. Only those cells which contain estradiol-specific receptors will respond to estradiol. The job of the receptor is to transport the hormone to the nucleus, allowing transmission of the hormone's message to the nuclear chromatin. The result is production of messenger RNA leading to protein synthesis and a cellular response characteristic of the hormone.

Once estradiol has accomplished its mission, it is probably released back into the bloodstream. It is possible that estradiol may perform its duty several times before being cleared from the circulation by metabolism. On the other hand, many molecules will be metabolized without ever having the chance to produce an effect. Unlike estradiol, other hormones, such as testosterone, are metabolized and altered within the cell in which an effect has been produced. In the latter case, a steroid is released into the bloodstream as an inactive compound. Clearance of steroids from the blood varies according to the structure of the molecule.

Cells which are capable of clearing estradiol from the circulation accomplish this by biochemical means (conversion to estrone and estriol, moderately effective and very weak estrogens, respectively) and conjugation to products which are water-soluble and excreted in the urine and bile (sulfo- and glucuro-conjugates).

Thus, a steroid hormone has a varied career packed into a short lifetime, and it is now appropriate to review the important segments of this life span in greater detail.

Nomenclature

All steroid hormones are of basically similar structure with relatively minor chemical differences leading to striking alterations in biologic activity. The basic structure is the perhydrocyclopentanephenanthrene molecule. It is composed of three 6-carbon rings and one 5-carbon ring. One ring is benzene, two rings naphthalene, and three rings phenanthrene; add a cyclopentane (5-carbon ring) and you have the perhydrocyclopentanephenanthrene structure of the steroid nucleus.

The sex steroids are divided into three main groups according to the number of carbon atoms they possess. The 21-carbon series includes the corticoids and the progestins and the basic structure is the pregnane nucleus. The 19-carbon series includes all the androgens and is based on the androstane nucleus, whereas the estrogens are 18-carbon steroids based on the estrane nucleus.

21 – pregnane nucleus
corticoids
progestins

19 – androgens
androstane nucleus

18 – estrane nucleus
estrogens.

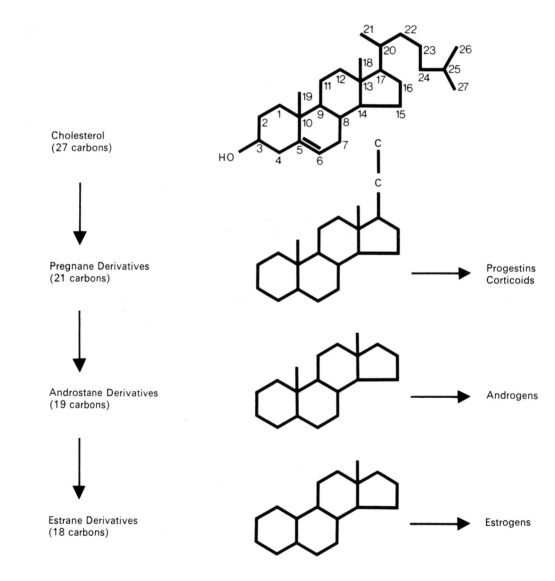

Cholesterol
(27 carbons)

Pregnane Derivatives
(21 carbons)

→ Progestins
Corticoids

Androstane Derivatives
(19 carbons)

→ Androgens

Estrane Derivatives
(18 carbons)

→ Estrogens

4

There are 6 centers of asymmetry on the basic ring structure, and there are 64 possible isomers. Almost all naturally occurring and active steroids are nearly flat, and substituents below and above the plane of the ring are designated alpha (α) (dotted line) and beta (β) (solid line), respectively. Changes in the position of only one substituent can lead to inactive isomers. For example, 17-epitestosterone is considerably weaker than testosterone, the only difference being a hydroxyl group in the α position at C-17 rather than in the β position.

Progesterone

Top View

Side View

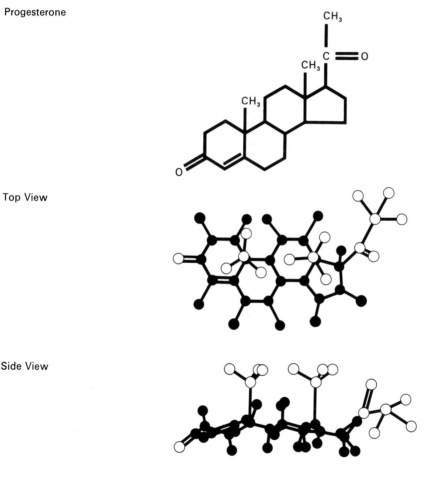

The convention of naming steroids uses the number of carbon atoms to designate the basic name (e.g. pregnane, androstane or estrane). The basic name is preceded by numbers which indicate the position of double bonds and the name is altered as follows to indicate 1, 2, or 3 double bonds: -ene, -diene, and -triene. Following the basic name, hydroxyl groups are indicated by the number of the carbon attachment, and 1, 2, or 3 hydroxyl groups are designated -ol, -diol, or -triol. Ketone groups are listed last with numbers of carbon attachments and 1, 2, or 3 groups designated -one, -dione, or -trione. Special designations include: dehydro, elimination of 2 hydrogens; deoxy, elimination of oxygen; nor, elimination of carbon; delta or Δ, location of double bond.

Estrone
1,3,5(10)-Estratriene-3β-o1-17-one

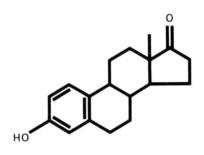

Testosterone
4-Androstene-17β-o1-3-one

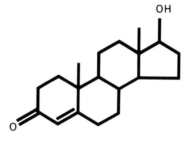

Progesterone
4-Pregnene-3,20-dione

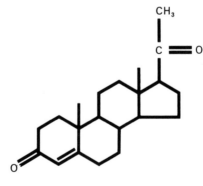

Steroidogenesis

The overall steroid biosynthesis pathway shown in the figure is based primarily on the pioneering work of K. J. Ryan and his co-workers. These pathways follow the fundamental pattern displayed by all steroid-producing endocrine organs. As a result, it should be no surprise that the normal human ovary produces all three classes of sex steroids: estrogens, progestins, and androgens. The importance of ovarian androgens is appreciated, not only as obligate precursors to estrogens, but also as clinically important secretory products. The ovary differs from the testis in its functional complement of critical enzymes and, hence, its distribution of secretory products. The ovary is distinguished from the adrenal gland in that it is deficient in 21-hydroxylase and 11β-hydroxylase enzymes. Glucocorticoids and mineralocorticoids, therefore, are not produced in normal ovarian tissue.

During steroidogenesis, the number of carbon atoms in cholesterol or any other steroid molecule can be reduced but never increased. The following reactions may take place:

1. Cleavage of a side chain (desmolase reaction).

2. Conversion of hydroxyl groups into ketones or ketones into hydroxyl groups (dehydrogenase reactions).

3. Addition of OH group (hydroxylation reaction).

4. Creation of double bonds (removal of hydrogen).

5. Addition of hydrogen to reduce double bonds (saturation).

Cholesterol is the basic building block in steroidogenesis. All steroid-producing organs except the placenta can synthesize cholesterol from acetate. Progestins, androgens, and estrogens, therefore, can be synthesized in situ in the various ovarian tissue compartments from the 2-carbon acetate molecule via cholesterol as the common steroid precursor. However, the major resource is blood cholesterol which enters the ovarian cells and can be inserted into the biosynthetic pathway, or stored in esterified form for later use. The cellular entry of cholesterol is mediated via a cell membrane receptor for low density lipoprotein (LDL)—the bloodstream carrier for cholesterol.

LDL receptors in ovarian tissue

Conversion of cholesterol to pregnenolone involves hydroxylation at the carbon 20 and 22 positions (20-hydroxylase and 22-hydroxylase enzymes), with subsequent cleavage of the side chain (20,22-desmolase). Conversion of cholesterol to pregnenolone takes place within the mitochondria. It is a rate-limiting step in the steroid pathway and is one of the principal effects of LH stimulation.

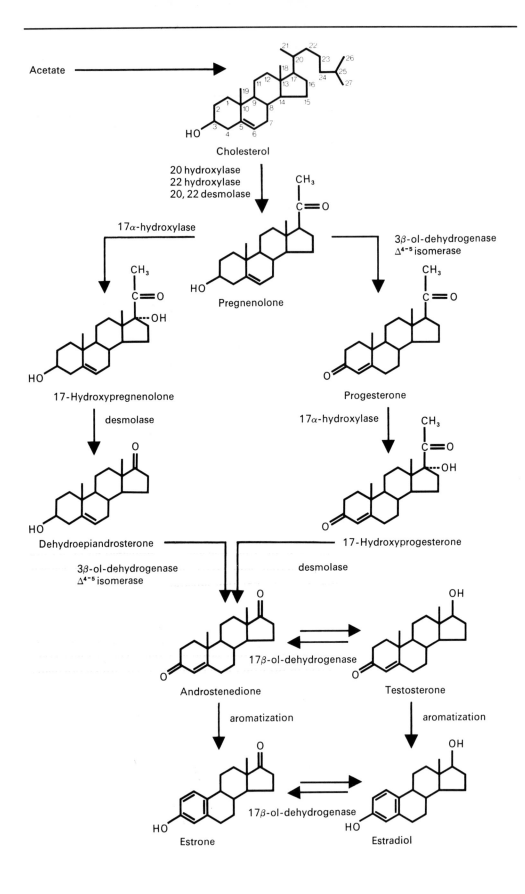

Acetate

Cholesterol

20 hydroxylase
22 hydroxylase
20, 22 desmolase

17α-hydroxylase

Pregnenolone

3β-ol-dehydrogenase
Δ⁴⁻⁵ isomerase

17-Hydroxypregnenolone

Progesterone

desmolase

17α-hydroxylase

Dehydroepiandrosterone

17-Hydroxyprogesterone

3β-ol-dehydrogenase
Δ⁴⁻⁵ isomerase

desmolase

Androstenedione

17β-ol-dehydrogenase

Testosterone

aromatization

aromatization

Estrone

17β-ol-dehydrogenase

Estradiol

It is important to note that once pregnenolone is formed further steroid synthesis in the ovary may proceed by one of two pathways, either via Δ^5-3β-hydroxysteroids or via the Δ^4-3-ketone pathway. The first (the Δ^5 pathway) proceeds by way of 17-hydroxypregnenolone and dehydroepiandrosterone (DHA) and the second (the Δ^4 pathway) via progesterone and 17α-hydroxyprogesterone.

The conversion of pregnenolone to progesterone involves two enzyme steps: the 3β-hydroxysteroid dehydrogenase and Δ^{4-5} isomerase reactions which convert the 3-hydroxyl group to a ketone and transfer the double bond from the 5–6 position to the 4–5 position. Once the Δ^{4-5} ketone is formed, progesterone is hydroxylated at the 17 position to form 17α-hydroxyprogesterone. 17α-Hydroxyprogesterone is the immediate precursor of the C-19 (19 carbons) series of androgens in this pathway. By peroxide formation at C-20, followed by epoxidation of the C-17, C-20 carbons, the side chain is split off forming androstenedione. The 17-ketone may be reduced to a 17β-hydroxyl to form testosterone by 17β-hydroxysteroid dehydrogenase. Both C-19 steroids (androstenedione and testosterone) are rapidly converted to corresponding C-18 phenolic steroid estrogens (estrone and estradiol) by microsomal enzymes in a process referred to as aromatization. This process includes hydroxylation of the angular 19-methyl group, followed by oxidation, loss of the 19-carbon as formaldehyde, and ring A aromatization (dehydrogenation).

As an alternative, pregnenolone may be directly converted to the Δ^5-3β-hydroxy C-19 steroid, DHA, by 17α-hydroxylation followed by desmolase cleavage of the side chain. With formation of the Δ^4-3-ketone, DHA is converted into androstenedione. It is thought that conversion of each of the Δ^5 compounds to their corresponding Δ^4 compounds can occur at any step; however, the principal pathways are via progesterone and DHA. Regardless of the precursor source, C-19 Δ^4-3-ketone substrates proceed to estrogens as noted above.

There is a midcycle increase in circulating levels of androstenedione and testosterone, probably arising from LH stimulation of ovarian stromal tissue. The stromal compartment of the ovary is derived from cells which originally comprised the thecal layer of developing follicles. This tissue responds to gonadotropins (LH and human chorionic gonadotropin (HCG)) with increased steroidogenesis. Postmenopausally, when only stromal tissue remains active, androstenedione and testosterone secretion are increased for a few years, until even this compartment of the ovary becomes atrophic.

The Two-Pathway Theory

According to the two-pathway theory, the selection of pathways is governed by the cell type involved. The Δ^4 pathway seems to be predominant in luteal tissue, whereas the Δ^5 pathway is characteristic of nonluteinized tissue. Thus the corpus luteum secretes mainly progesterone and estrogens via the Δ^4 pathway, whereas in the follicle, DHA and androstenedione serve as precursors for estrogens. Androgens are the principal secretory products in stromal tissue.

The Δ^5 pathway in nonluteinized tissue avoids preliminary synthesis of progesterone as a precursor to estradiol. The predominance of estrogen prior to ovulation is then explained on a morphological basis. Limitation of vascularization within the follicular thecal layer ensures that estrogen is the major secretory product. The implication is that the progesterone synthesized by granulosa cells during the pre-ovulatory period serves as a precursor for estrogen synthesis in the theca. The absence of vascularization in the granulosa layer until after ovulation requires progesterone to diffuse toward the theca, where it can be utilized for estrogen production. In the corpus luteum where vascularization and luteinization of the granulosa layer have been achieved, both estrogen and progesterone are major secretory products via the Δ^4 pathway.

This theory implies that, following follicular atresia, the thecal layer loses its ability to aromatize androgens, hence its designation as a new cell type, the stromal tissue, which secretes androgens. The two-pathway mechanism is not favored currently. Instead, the two-cell system is thought to be a more accurate explanation of ovarian steroidogenesis.

The Two-Cell System

The two-cell system is a logical explanation of the events involved in ovarian follicular steroidogenesis and development. (1–5) This explanation brings together recent information on the site of specific steroid production, along with the appearance and importance of hormone receptors. The following facts are important:

1. FSH receptors are present on the granulosa cells.

2. FSH receptors are induced by FSH itself.

3. LH receptors are present on the thecal cells and initially absent on the granulosa cells, but, as the follicle grows, FSH induces the appearance of LH receptors on the granulosa cells.

4. FSH induces aromatase enzyme activity in granulosa cells.

5. Granulosa cells contain estrogen and testosterone-specific receptors.

6. Estrogen enhances FSH activity.

10

The above facts combine into the two-cell system to explain the sequence of events in ovarian follicular growth and development. The initial change from a primordial follicle is independent of hormones, and the stimulus governing this initial step in growth is unknown. Continued growth, however, depends upon FSH stimulation. As the granulosa responds to FSH, growth is associated with an increase in FSH receptors, a specific effect of FSH itself, but an action which is enhanced very significantly by estradiol. The theca cells are characterized by steroidogenic activity in response to LH, specifically resulting in androgen production. Aromatization of androgens to estrogens is a specific activity within the granulosa layer induced by FSH. Androgens produced in the theca layer, therefore, must diffuse into the granulosa layer. In the granulosa layer they are converted to estrogens, and the increasing level of estradiol in the peripheral circulation reflects release of the estrogen back toward the theca layer and into the blood vessels.

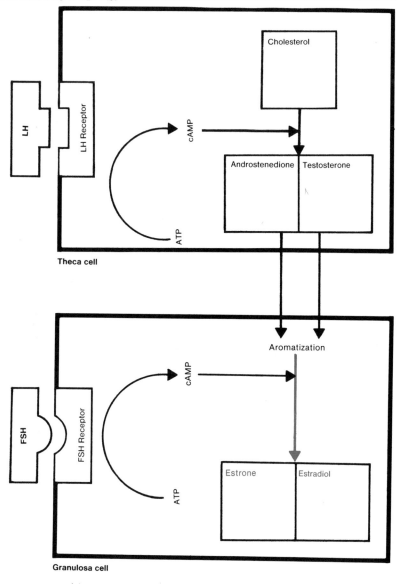

The estradiol produced by the cooperative effort of the two cells, theca and granulosa, plays an important role in enhancing the activity of FSH, thus promoting the growth and function of its own follicle. As the follicle approaches ovulation, LH receptors begin to appear on the granulosa layer, induced by FSH in another action enhanced by estradiol. After ovulation the dominance of the luteinized granulosa layer is dependent upon preovulatory induction of an adequate number of LH receptors and, therefore, dependent upon adequate FSH action. Prior to ovulation the granulosa layer is characterized by aromatization activity and conversion of the thecal androgens to estrogens, an FSH-mediated activity. After ovulation, the granulosa layer secretes progesterone and estrogens directly into the bloodstream, an LH-mediated activity.

early surge

Granulosa and thecal cells each have an androgen aromatase system which can be demonstrated in vitro. However, in vivo, the activity of the granulosa layer in the follicular phase is several hundred times greater than the in vitro activity of the thecal layer, and therefore the granulosa is the main biosynthetic source of estrogen in the growing, dominant follicle. (6) The rate of aromatization in the granulosa layer is directly related to the androgen substrate made available by the thecal cells. Hence, estrogen secretion by the follicle prior to ovulation is the result of combined LH and FSH stimulation of the two cell types, the theca and the granulosa.

Blood Transport of Steroids

While circulating in the blood a majority of the principal sex steroids, estradiol and testosterone, is bound to a β-globulin, a protein carrier, known as sex hormone binding globulin (SHBG). Another 10–40% is loosely bound to albumin, leaving only about 1% unbound and free. Transcortin, also called corticosterone binding globulin, is a plasma glycoprotein which binds cortisol, progesterone, deoxycorticosterone, corticosterone, and some of the other minor corticoid compounds. Normally about 75% of circulating cortisol is bound to transcortin, 15% is loosely bound to albumin, and 10% is unbound or free. Hyperthyroidism, pregnancy, and estrogen administration all increase SHBG levels, whereas corticoids, androgens, progestins, and growth hormone decrease SHBG.

The biologic effects of the major sex steroids are determined by the unbound portion, known as the free hormone. In other words, the active hormone is unbound and free while the bound hormone is inactive. This concept is not without controversy. The albumin-bound fraction of steroids may also be available for cellular action. Routine assays determine the total hormone concentration, bound plus free, and special steps are required to measure the active free level of testosterone, estradiol, and cortisol.

Estrogen Metabolism

Androgens are the common precursors of estrogens. 17β-Hydroxydehydrogenase activity converts androstenedione to testosterone which is not a major secretory product of the normal ovary. It is rapidly demethylated at the C-19 position and aromatized to estradiol, the major estrogen secreted by the human ovary. Estradiol also arises to a major degree from androstenedione via estrone, and estrone itself is secreted in significant daily amounts. Estriol is the peripheral metabolite of estrone and estradiol, and not a secretory product of the ovary. The formation of estriol is typical of general metabolic "detoxification," conversion of biologically active material to less active forms.

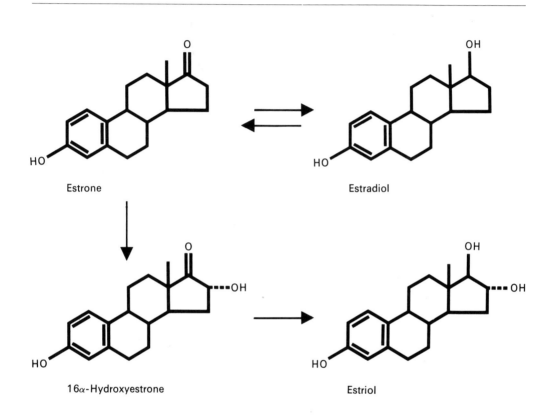

Estrone

Estradiol

16α-Hydroxyestrone

Estriol

The conversion of steroids in peripheral tissues is not always a form of inactivation. <u>Free androgens are peripherally converted to free estrogens</u>, for example, in skin and adipose cells. The work of Siiteri and MacDonald (7) showed that enough estrogen can be derived from circulating androgens to produce bleeding in the postmenopausal woman. In the female the adrenal gland remains the major source of circulating androgens, in particular androstenedione. In the male, almost all of the circulating estrogens are derived from peripheral conversion of androgens.

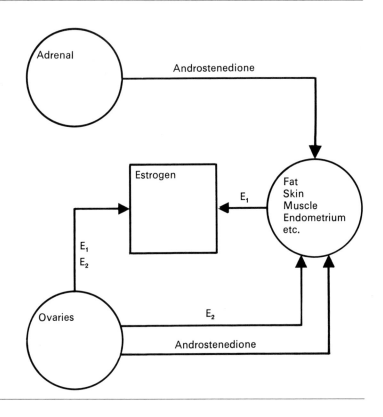

It can be seen, therefore, that the pattern of circulating steroids in the female is influenced by the activity of various processes outside the ovary. Because of the peripheral contribution to steroid levels, the term "secretion rate" is reserved for direct organ secretion, whereas "production rate" includes organ secretion plus peripheral contribution via conversion of precursors. The metabolic clearance rate (MCR) equals the volume of blood which is cleared of the hormone per unit of time. The blood production rate (PR) then equals the metabolic clearance rate multiplied by the concentration of the hormone in the blood.

$$MCR = Liters/Day$$

$$PR = MCR \times Concentration$$

$$PR = Liters/Day \times Amount/Liter = Amount/Day$$

In the normal nonpregnant female, estradiol is produced at the rate of 100–300 μg/day. The production of androstenedione is about 3 mg/day, and the peripheral conversion (about 1%) of androstenedione to estrone accounts for about 20–30% of the estrone produced per day. Since androstenedione is secreted in milligram amounts, even a small percent conversion to estrogens results in a significant contribution to estrogens which exist and function in microgram amounts. Thus the circulating estrogens in the female are the sum of direct ovarian secretion of estradiol and estrone, plus peripheral conversion of C-19 precursors.

Premenopausal Peripheral Conversion

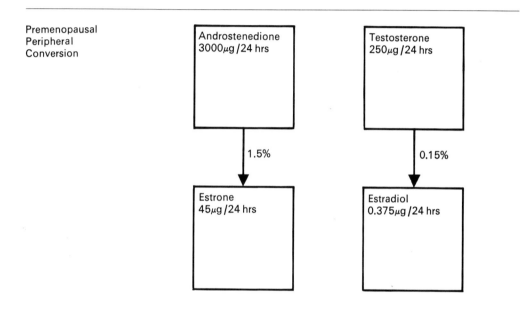

Progesterone Metabolism

Peripheral conversion of steroids to progesterone is not seen in the nonpregnant female, rather the production rate is a combination of secretion from the adrenal and the ovaries. Including the small contribution from the adrenal, the blood production rate of progesterone in the preovulatory phase is about 2–3 mg/day. During the luteal phase, production increases to 20–30 mg/day. The metabolic fate of progesterone, as expressed by its many excretion products, is more complex than estrogen. About 10–20% of progesterone is excreted as pregnanediol.

Pregnanediol glucuronide is present in the urine in concentrations less than 1 mg/day until ovulation. Postovulation pregnanediol excretion reaches a peak of 3–6 mg/day, which is maintained until 2 days prior to menses. The assay of pregnanediol in the urine now has limited use.

Newer methods utilizing binding proteins or antibodies to measure plasma levels of progesterone are more rapid, more sensitive, and more precise. In the preovulatory phase in adult females, in all prepubertal females, and in the normal male, the blood levels of progesterone are at the lower limits of assay sensitivity: less than 1 ng/ml. After ovulation, i.e., during the luteal phase, progesterone ranges from 5 to 20 ng/ml. In congenital adrenal hyperplasia, progesterone blood levels may be as high as 50 times above normal.

Pregnanetriol is the chief urinary metabolite of 17α-hydroxyprogesterone, and has clinical significance in the adrenogenital syndrome, where an enzyme defect results in accumulation of 17α-hydroxyprogesterone and increased excretion of pregnanetriol. The plasma or serum assay of 17α-hydroxyprogesterone is a more sensitive and accurate index of this enzyme deficiency. Normally the blood level of 17α-hydroxyprogesterone is less than 1 ng/ml, although after ovulation and during the luteal phase of a normal menstrual cycle, a peak of 2 ng/ml may be reached. In syndromes of adrenal hyperplasia, values may be 50–400 times normal.

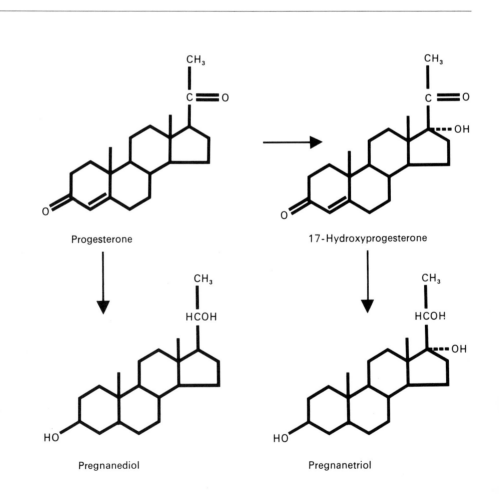

Progesterone

17-Hydroxyprogesterone

Pregnanediol

Pregnanetriol

Androgen Metabolism

The major androgen products of the ovary are dehydroepiandrosterone (DHA) and androstenedione which are secreted mainly by stromal tissue. With excessive accumulation of stromal tissue or in the presence of an androgen-producing tumor, testosterone becomes a significant secretory product. Occasionally, a nonfunctioning tumor may induce stromal proliferation and increased androgen production. The normal accumulation of stromal tissue at midcycle results in a rise in circulating levels of androstenedione and testosterone at the time of ovulation.

The adrenal cortex produces three groups of steroid hormones, the glucocorticoids, the mineralocorticoids, and the sex steroids. The sex steroids represent intermediate byproducts in the synthesis of glucocorticoids and mineralocorticoids, and excessive secretion of the sex steroids occurs only with neoplastic cells or in association with enzyme deficiencies. Under normal circumstances, adrenal gland production of the sex steroids is less significant than gonadal production of androgens and estrogens.

There is no circadian cycle in the major sex steroids in the female. However, short-term variations in the blood levels of testosterone require multiple sampling for absolutely accurate assessment. Although frequent sampling is necessary for a high degree of accuracy, a random sample is usually sufficient to determine whether a level is within a normal range.

The testosterone binding capacity is decreased by androgens. Hence, the binding capacity in men is lower than that in normal women; the binding globulin level in women with increased androgen production is also depressed. Androgenic effects are dependent upon the unbound fraction which can move freely from the vascular compartment into the target cells. Routine assays determine the total hormone concentration, bound plus free. Thus, a total testosterone concentration may be in the normal range in a woman who is hirsute or even virilized, but, since the binding globulin level is depressed by the androgen effects, the percent free and active testosterone is elevated. The need for a specific assay for the free portion of testosterone can be questioned since the very presence of hirsutism or virilism indicates increased androgen effects. In the face of hirsutism, one can reliably interpret a normal testosterone level as compatible with decreased binding capacity and increased active free testosterone. Both total and unbound testosterone are normal in only a few women with hirsutism. Here, the hirsutism most likely results from an increase in unbound levels of other androgens such as dihydrotestosterone and androstenediol. Hirsutism which, heretofore, has been regarded as idiopathic, may have a basis in unappreciated and excessive intracellular androgen effects or receptor variability. It should be emphasized that the degree of increased androgen in the circulation does not necessarily parallel the degree of hirsutism.

17

The production rate of testosterone in the normal female is 0.2–0.3 mg/day, and approximately 50% arises from peripheral conversion of androstenedione to testosterone, whereas 25% is secreted by the ovary and 25% by the adrenal.

Reduction of the Δ^4 unsaturation in testosterone is very significant, producing derivatives very different in their spatial configuration and activity. The 5β derivatives are not androgenic; however, the 5α derivative is extremely potent. Indeed, dihydrotestosterone (DHT), the 5α derivative, is the principal androgenic hormone in a variety of target tissues and is formed within the target tissue itself.

The majority of circulating DHT is derived from testosterone which enters a target cell and is converted by means of a 5α-reductase to DHT. The blood DHT is only about $\frac{1}{10}$ the level of circulating testosterone, and it is clear that testosterone is the major circulating androgen. In tissues sensitive to DHT (which include hair follicles), only DHT enters the nucleus to provide the androgen message. DHT also can perform androgenic actions within cells which do not possess the ability to convert testosterone to DHT. DHT may be reduced by a 3α-keto-reductase to a further metabolite, androstanediol, which is relatively inactive.

Not all androgen-sensitive tissues, however, require the prior conversion of testosterone to DHT. In the process of masculine differentiation, the development of the Wolffian duct structures (epididymis, the vas deferens, and the seminal vesicle) appears to be dependent upon testosterone as the intracellular mediator, whereas development of the urogenital sinus and urogenital tubercle into the male external genitalia, urethra, and prostate requires the conversion of testosterone to DHT.

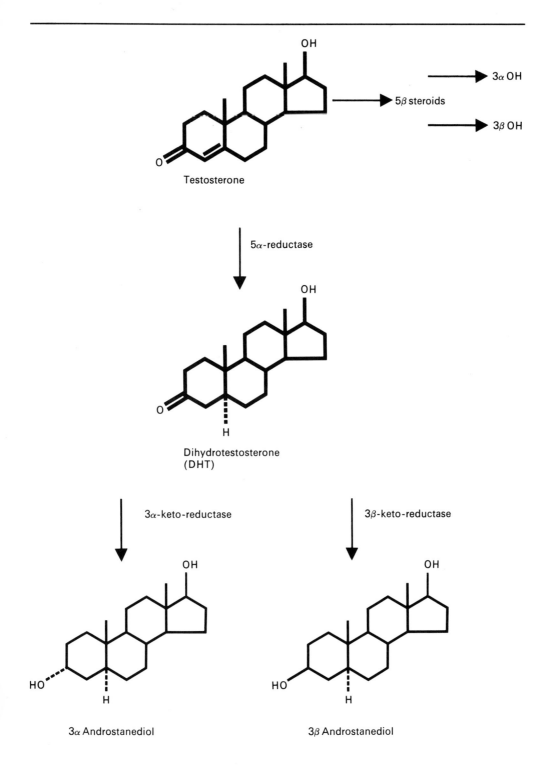

Testosterone

5β steroids

3α OH

3β OH

5α-reductase

Dihydrotestosterone
(DHT)

3α-keto-reductase

3β-keto-reductase

3α Androstanediol

3β Androstanediol

Excretion of Steroids

Active steroids and metabolites are excreted as sulfo- and glucuro-conjugates. Conjugation of a steroid generally reduces or eliminates the activity of a steroid. This is not completely true, however, since hydrolysis of the ester linkage may occur in target tissues and restore the active form. Furthermore, estrogen conjugates may have biologic activity, and it is known that sulfated conjugates are actively secreted and may serve as precursors. Ordinarily, however, conjugation by liver and intestinal mucosa is a step in deactivation preliminary to, and essential for, excretion into urine and bile.

Glucosiduronate

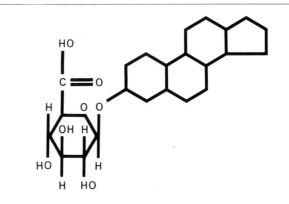

Sulfate

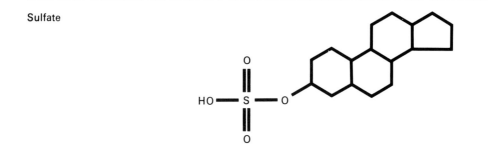

Cellular Mechanism of Action

Hormones circulate in extremely low concentrations and, in order to respond with specific and effective actions, target cells require the presence of special mechanisms. There are two types of hormone action at the cellular level. One mediates the action of tropic hormones (peptide and glycoprotein hormones) at the cell membrane level and involves adenylate cyclase activity. In contrast, the smaller steroid hormones enter cells readily, and the basic mechanism of action involves specific cytoplasm receptor molecules. It is the affinity and specificity of the receptors together with the large concentration of receptors in cells which allow a small amount of hormone to produce a biologic response.

Mechanism of Action for Steroid Hormones

The specificity of the reaction of tissues to steroid hormones is due to the presence of intracellular receptor proteins. (8, 9) Different types of tissues, such as liver, kidney, and uterus, respond in a similar manner. The mechanism includes: 1) diffusion across the cell membrane, 2) binding to cytoplasmic receptor protein and transfer of the hormone-receptor complex across the nuclear membrane to the nucleus, 3) binding of a hormone-receptor complex to nuclear DNA, 4) synthesis of messenger RNA (mRNA), 5) transport of the mRNA to the ribosomes, and, finally, 6) protein synthesis in the cytoplasm which results in specific cellular activity. Each of the major classes of steroid hormones, including estrogens, progestins, androgens, glucocorticoids, and mineralocorticoids, has been shown to act according to this general mechanism.

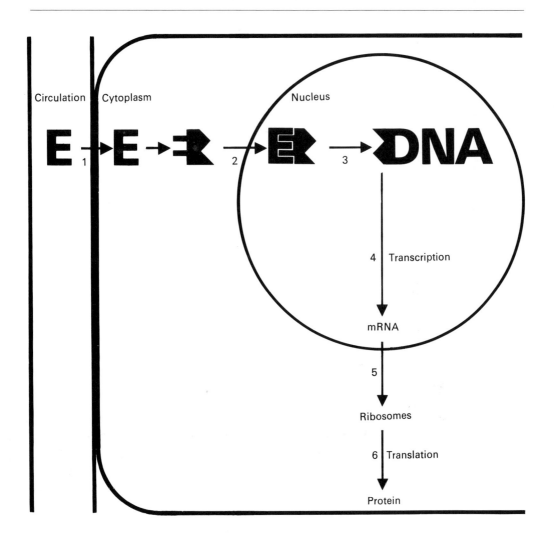

Steroid hormones are rapidly transported across the cell membrane by simple diffusion. The factors responsible for this transfer are unknown, but the concentration of free (unbound) hormone in the bloodstream seems to be an important and influential determinant of cellular function. Once within the cell, assuming the cell is responsive to the steroid hormone, the hormone is quickly bound by a protein receptor. It is still a somewhat theoretical concept that the receptor may exist in an inactive form and require activation prior to binding. This could serve as a reservoir of available receptor. Hormones which bind to receptors can also be called ligands, in that ligands are defined as molecules which bind to receptors and produce specific biologic responses.

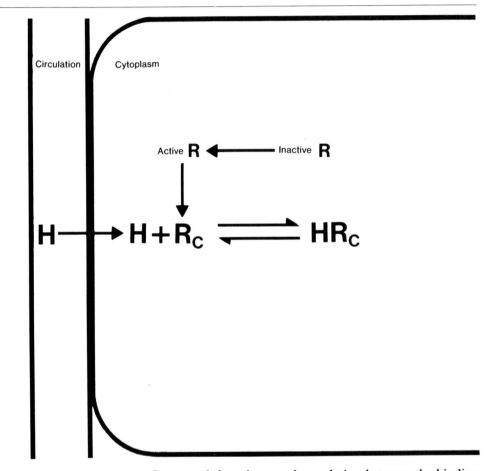

In general there is a good correlation between the binding affinity of a steroid hormone (H) for its cytoplasmic receptor (Rc) and the potency of the hormone. Regardless of the total number of receptors present, a given quantity of receptors must be bound to yield a given response. With increasing availability of hormone, there will be greater and faster formation of the hormone-receptor complexes, hence an increased response. Changes in hormone and receptor concentrations, therefore, affect dose-response (magnitude of response), the kinetics of the response, and the duration of the response.

22

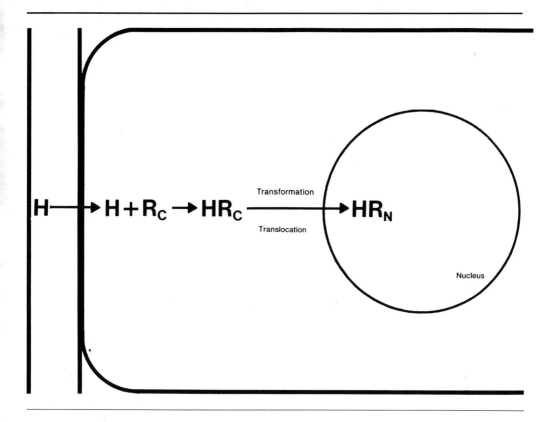

Characteristics of steroid hormone receptors include:

1. Large protein molecules (MW 50,000–300,000).

2. High affinity binding.

3. Limited capacity—saturable, and therefore sensitive to small changes in hormone concentrations.

4. High specificity.

5. Reversible binding.

The physiologic response to steroid hormones requires movement of the hormone and receptor into the nucleus to interact with DNA, leading to the production of messenger RNA (gene transcription). This movement is known as *translocation*. Exactly how the hormone-receptor complex enters the nucleus is unknown; it appears that the shape of the receptor, an elongated ellipsoid, is important in this process. In order for the complex to bind to the chromatin, it must undergo a conformational change revealing or producing a nuclear binding site. This latter process is called *transformation*, a change from an inactive to an active complex (HR_N).

23

Receptors can be separated according to their size and shape by ultracentrifugation and their migration through solutions of varying sucrose density. With estrogen receptors, transformation is associated with a change in sedimentation rate on sucrose gradients from 4S to 5S, smaller and larger molecules, respectively. The change may take place after translocation or during the relocation. In the cytoplasm, estrogen receptors exist in 4S forms and 8S forms. The larger 8S is probably a dimer storage form, while the 4S is the traditional, active receptor. Prolactin induces a shift from 4S to 8S; thus, during pregnancy, there is an accumulation in the breast of the 8S estrogen receptors. This variation is further confused by a description of two types of estrogen receptors. The traditional, active receptor is designated as Type I, while the Type II receptors, newly described, are smaller with low affinity. They do not translocate, and may be another storage form.

Once in the nucleus, the complex moves along the chromosome until the site for gene activation (DNA acceptor site) is encountered. The specific binding of the hormone-receptor complex with DNA results in RNA polymerase initiation of transcription. Transcription leads to translation, mRNA-mediated protein synthesis in the ribosomes. The principal action of steroid hormones is the regulation of intracellular protein synthesis by means of the receptor mechanism. In target tissues which respond to steroid hormones by growth (e.g. endometrium) nuclear binding and prolonged nuclear retention directly lead to increased DNA synthesis.

An important action of estrogen is its modification of its own and other steroid hormone activity by affecting receptor concentration. Estrogen increases target tissue responsiveness to itself and to progestins and androgens by increasing the concentration of its own receptor and that of the intracellular progestin and androgen receptors. This process is called *replenishment*. Progesterone and clomiphene, on the other hand, limit tissue response to estrogen by blocking the replenishment mechanism, thus decreasing over time the concentration of cytoplasmic estrogen receptors. Replenishment is very responsive to the available amount of steroid and receptors. Small amounts of receptor depletion and small amounts of steroid in the blood activate the mechanism.

There are differences among the various steroids in this basic mechanism of action. For example, the progesterone receptor is 7S in size and is tranformed to a smaller 5.5S form with nuclear relocation. It is a complex (a dimer) of two nonidentical subunits, one of which is keyed to specific nonhistone proteins in the chromatin and thus is responsible for finding the appropriate nuclear binding site, allowing the other subunit to bind directly to the DNA and initiate transcription. Androgens and progestins crossreact for their receptors, but probably do so only when present in pharmacologic concentrations.

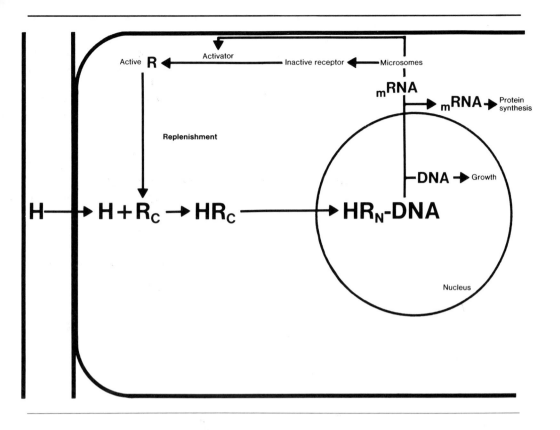

The mechanism is more complex for androgens. The cellular action of androgens can result from one of three possibilities:

1. From intracellular conversion of testosterone to dihydrotestosterone (DHT).

2. From testosterone itself.

3. From intracellular conversion of testosterone to estradiol (aromatization).

In those cells which respond only to DHT, only DHT will be found within the nucleus activating messenger RNA production. The cytoplasmic androgen receptor preferentially will bind DHT. Progestins not only compete for androgen receptors, but also compete for the metabolic utilization of the 5α-reductase enzyme. The dihydroprogesterone which is produced, in turn also competes with testosterone and DHT for the androgen receptor. A progestin, therefore, can act both as an antiandrogen and as an antiestrogen.

Tissues which exclusively operate via the testosterone pathway are the derivatives of the Woffian duct, whereas hair follicles and derivatives of the urogenital sinus require the conversion of testosterone to DHT. The hypothalamus actively converts androgens to estrogens, hence aromatization may be necessary for certain androgen feedback messages in the brain.

The syndrome of testicular feminization (androgen insensitivity) represents a congenital abnormality in the androgen intracellular mechanism. There is either a defect in receptor production or an abnormality in receptor function. In either event, there is a failure in nuclear binding of androgens.

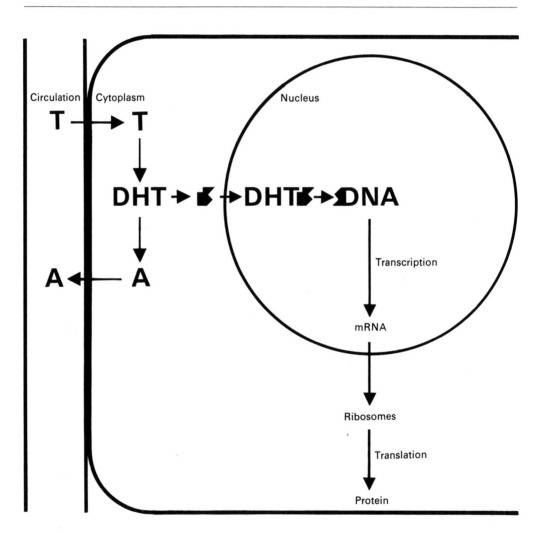

Biologic activity is maintained only while the nuclear site is occupied with the hormone-receptor complex. The dissociation rate of the hormone and its receptor as well as the half-life of the nuclear chromatin-bound complex are factors in the biologic response. One reason only small amounts of estrogen need be present in the circulation is the long half-life of the estrogen hormone-receptor complex. Indeed, a major factor in the potency differences among the various estrogens (estradiol, estrone, estriol) is the length of time the estrogen-receptor complex occupies the nucleus. The higher rate of dissociation with the weak estrogen (estriol) can be compensated for by continuous application to allow prolonged nuclear binding and activity. Cortisol and progesterone must circulate in large concentrations because their receptor complexes have short half-lives in the nucleus. Upon dissociation, hormone and receptor can be reutilized, a process called *recycling*.

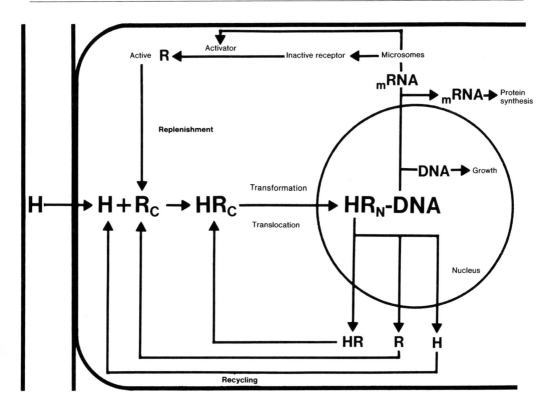

Therefore, there are four main determinants of biologic response and hormone activity:

1. Concentration of the free hormone in the circulation.

2. Concentration of cytoplasmic receptors.

3. The dissociation rate of the hormone-receptor complex.

4. The dissociation rate of the hormone-receptor complex bound to the chromatin.

Pharmacologic agents which interfere with steroid hormone action can do so in the following ways:

1. Inhibition of steroidogenesis, e.g. aminoglutethimide (in general—toxic agents).

2. Reduction in the intracellular availability of cytoplasmic receptors, e.g. irreversible covalent binding between the receptor and steroid derivatives (nothing available clinically).

3. Prevention of translocation of hormone-receptor complex into the nucleus; e.g. spironolactone.

4. Decrease in receptor concentrations, e.g. the antiestrogenic effect of progestins and clomiphene.

5. Inhibition of transcription, e.g. actinomycin D.

6. Inhibition of translation, e.g. cyclohexamide.

Mechanism of Action for Tropic Hormones

Tropic hormones include the releasing hormones originating in the hypothalamus, and a variety of peptides and glycoproteins released by the anterior pituitary gland. The specificity of the tropic hormone depends upon the presence of a receptor in the cell membrane of the target tissue. Tropic hormones do not enter the cell to stimulate physiological events but simply unite with a receptor on the surface of the cell. Union with the receptor activates the adenylate cyclase enzyme within the membrane wall leading to the conversion of adenosine 5'-triphosphate (ATP) within the cell to cyclic AMP. Specificity of action and/or intensity of stimulation may be altered by changes in the structure or concentration of the receptor at the cell wall binding site. In addition to changes in biological activity due to target cell alterations, changes in the molecular structure of the tropic hormone may interfere with cellular binding and physiologic activity.

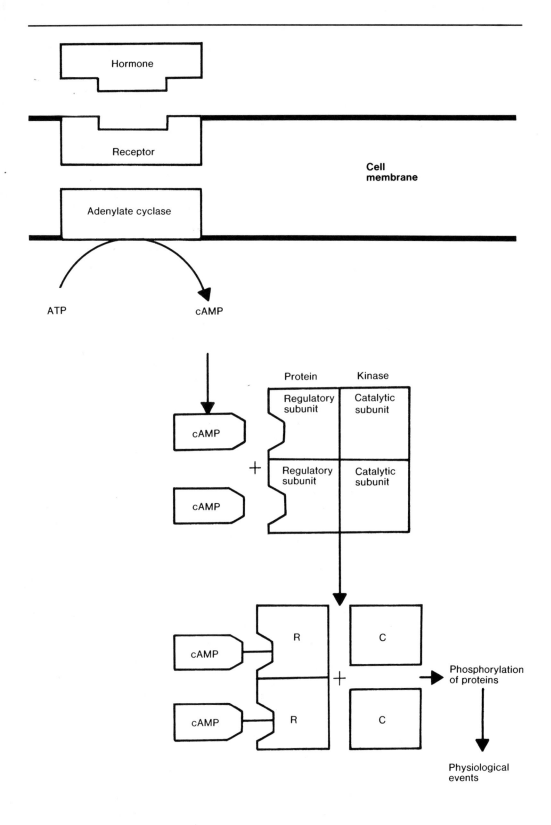

The cell's mechanism for sensing the low concentrations of circulating tropic hormone is to have an extremely large number of receptors but to require only a very small percentage (as little as 1%) to be occupied by the tropic hormone. The cyclic AMP (cAMP) released is specifically bound to a cytoplasm receptor protein, and this cAMP-receptor protein complex activates a protein kinase. The protein kinase is thought to be present in an inactive form as a tetramer, containing two regulatory subunits and two catalytic subunits. Binding of cAMP to the regulatory units releases the catalytic units, the regulatory units remaining as a dimer. The catalytic units catalyze the phosphorylation of cellular proteins such as enzymes and mitochondral, microsomal, and chromatin proteins. The physiological event follows this cAMP-mediated energy-producing event. cAMP is then degraded by the enzyme phosphodiesterase into the inactive compound 5'-AMP.

Acute responses such as increased steroidogenesis do not operate through gene transcription but rather through phosphorylation. Long-term effects of peptide hormones, such as differentiation and growth, do operate through nuclear activity, and cAMP may exert an effect on RNA polymerase activity (transcription) as well as on translation. Because LH can stimulate steroidogenesis without apparent changes in cAMP (at low hormone concentrations), it is possible that an independent pathway exists; i.e., a mechanism independent of cAMP. Mechanisms independent of cAMP could include ion flow, calcium distribution, and changes in phospholipid metabolism.

Prostaglandins have been implicated in the cAMP mechanism. Because prostaglandins stimulate adenylate cyclase activity and cAMP accumulation, a role is implied for prostaglandins in transmitting the message from the exterior cell wall to the interior cell wall and the adenylate cyclase enzyme. Despite the effect on adenylate cyclase, prostaglandins appear to be synthesized after the action of cAMP. This implies that tropic hormone stimulation of cAMP occurs first; cAMP then activates prostaglandin synthesis, and finally intracellular prostaglandin moves to the cell wall to facilitate the response to the tropic hormone.

In addition, prostaglandins and cGMP (cyclic guanosine 3'5'-monophosphate) may participate in an intracellular negative feedback mechanism governing the degree of, or direction of, cellular activity (e.g. the extent of steroidogenesis or shutting off of steroidogenesis after a peak of activity is reached). In other words, the level of cellular function may be determined by the interaction among prostaglandins, cAMP, and cGMP. Furthermore, the intracellular calcium concentration is a regulator of both cAMP and cGMP levels. This calcium flux is also an important intracellular mediator of response to hormones.

The biologic actions of calcium involve a regulator protein called calmodulin. Its structural and functional properties are similar to those of troponin C, the substance which binds calcium during muscle contractions, facilitating the interaction between actin and myosin. The calcium regulatory protein, calmodulin, serves as an intracellular calcium receptor, modifies calcium transport, the calcium regulation of cyclic nucleotide and glycogen metabolism, and such processes as secretion and cell motility. Thus, calmodulin serves a role analogous to that of troponin C, mediating calcium's actions in noncontractile tissues, and cAMP works together with calcium and calmodulin in the regulation of intracellular metabolic activity.

There are differences among the tropic hormones. Oxytocin, insulin, growth hormone, prolactin, and human placental lactogen (HPL) do not utilize the adenylate cyclase mechanism. The message of these hormones is somehow passed directly to nuclear and cytoplasmic metabolic sites. Gonadotropin releasing hormone (GnRH) is probably calcium dependent in its mechanism of action.

Modulation of the peptide hormone mechanism is an important biological system for enhancing or reducing target tissue response. This regulation of hormone action currently has three major components:

1. Heterogeneity of the hormone.

2. Up and down regulation of receptors.

3. Regulation of adenylate cyclase.

Heterogeneity

The preciseness of the chemical makeup of the tropic hormones is an essential element in determining the ability of the hormone to mate with its receptor. The glycopeptides (FSH, LH, TSH, and HCG) all share a common α chain, an identical structure containing between 89 and 92 amino acids. The β chains (or the β subunits) differ in both amino acid and carbohydrate content, conferring the specificity inherent in the relationship between hormones and their receptors. Therefore, the specific biological activity of a glycopeptide hormone is determined by the β subunit. The α and β subunits are linked by disulfide bonds.

β-HCG is the largest β subunit, containing a larger carbohydrate moiety and 145 to 150 amino acid residues including a unique carboxyl terminal tail piece of 28 to 30 amino acid groups. It is this unique part of the HCG structure which allows the production of highly specific antibodies and the utilization of highly specific radioimmunological assays.

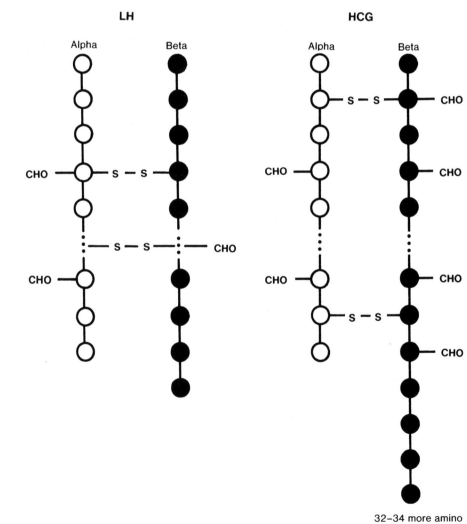

32–34 more amino acids than β-LH

32

The rate-limiting step in the synthesis of gonadotropins and TSH may be the availabity of β units, since excess α units can be found in blood and in tissue. The half-life of α-HCG is 6–8 minutes, that of whole HCG about 12 hours. Recent reports indicate that all human tissues make HCG as a whole molecule, but the placenta is different in having the ability to glycosylate the protein, thus reducing its rate of metabolism and giving it biological activity through a long half-life. The carbohydrate components are comprised of fructose, galactose, mannose, galactosamine, glucosamine, and sialic acid. Whereas the other sugars are necessary for hormonal function, sialic acid is the critical determinant of biological half-life.

Certain clinical conditions may be associated with alterations in the usual chemical structure of the glycopeptides, that interfere with the ability to bind to receptors and stimulate biological activity. A low estrogen environment in the pituitary gland, for example, favors the production of so-called big gonadotropins, gonadotropins with an increased carbohydrate component and, as a result, decreased biological activity.

Up and Down Regulation

Positive or negative modulation of receptors by homologous hormones is known as up and down regulation. (10) Little is known regarding the mechanism of up regulation, however hormones such as prolactin and GnRH can increase the cell membrane concentration of their own receptors. Theoretically, deactivation of the hormone-receptor complex could be accomplished by dissociation of the complex, or loss of receptors from the cell, either by shedding (externally) or by internalization of the receptors into the cell. It is the process of *internalization* which is the major biologic mechanism by which polypeptide hormones down regulate their own receptors and thus limit hormonal activity. As a general rule, an excess concentration of a tropic hormone such as LH or GnRH will stimulate the process of internalization, leading to a loss of receptors in the cell membrane and a decrease in biologic response.

It is believed that receptors are randomly inserted into the cell membrane after intracellular synthesis. The polypeptide receptor may be viewed as having two important sites, an external binding site which is specific for a polypeptide hormone, and an internal site which plays a role in the process of internalization. When the receptor is bound to a polypeptide hormone and when high concentrations of the hormone are present in the circulation, the hormone-receptor complex moves through the cell membrane in a process called *lateral migration.* Lateral migration carries the complex to a specialized region of the cell membrane, the coated pit. Lateral migration thus concentrates hormone-receptor complexes in the coated pit (clustering), allowing increased internalization of the complex via the special mechanism of receptor-mediated endocytosis. (11, 12) The time course for this process (minutes rather than seconds) is too slow to explain the immediate hormone-induced responses, but other cellular events may be mediated by this mechanism which circumvents the intracellular messenger, cAMP.

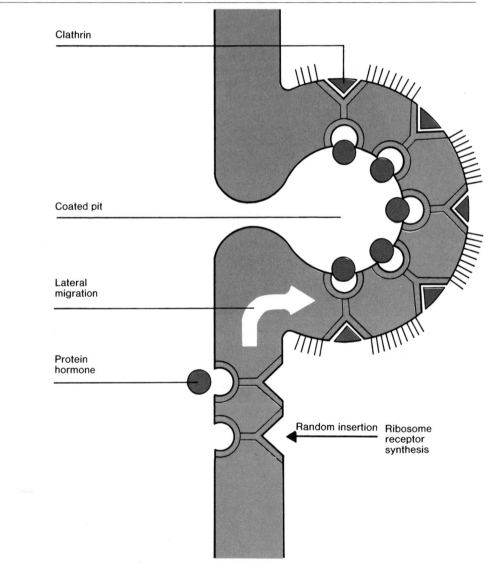

Clathrin

Coated pit

Lateral migration

Protein hormone

Random insertion   Ribosome receptor synthesis

The coated pit is a lipid vesicle hanging on a basket of specific proteins, called *clathrins*. The internal margin of the pit has a brush border, hence the name coated pit. The clathrin protein network may serve to localize the hormone-receptor complexes by binding to the internal binding site on the receptor.

When fully occupied, the coated pit invaginates, pinches off, and enters the cell as a coated vesicle also called a receptosome. The coated vesicle is delivered to the lysosomes where the structure then undergoes degradation, releasing the substance (e.g. a polypeptide hormone) and the receptor. The receptor may be recycled, i.e., it may be reinserted into the cell membrane and used again. On the other hand, the receptor and the hormone may be metabolized, thus decreasing that hormone's biologic activity. The internalized hormones may also mediate biologic response by influencing cellular organelles such as the Golgi apparatus, the endoplasmic reticulum, and even the nucleus.

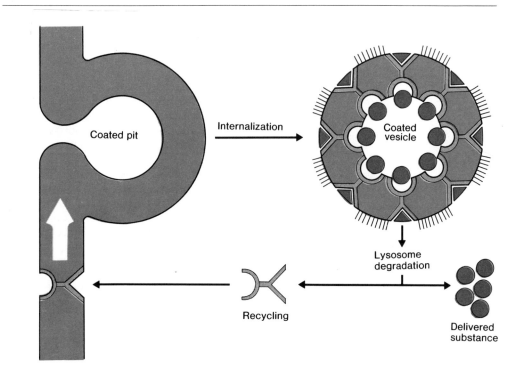

Besides down regulation of polypeptide hormone receptors, the process of internalization may be utilized for other cellular metabolic events, including the transfer into the cell of vital substances such as iron or vitamins. Hence, cell membrane receptors may be separated into two classes. (13).

The Class I receptors are randomly distributed in the cell membrane and transmit information to modify cell behavior. For these receptors, internalization is a method for down regulation by degradation in lysosomes. Because of this degradation, recycling is not a feature of this class of receptors. Hormones which utilize this category of receptors include: FSH, LH, HCG, GnRH, TSH, TRH, and insulin.

The Class II receptors are located in the coated pits and binding leads to internalization, thus providing the cell with required factors, or the removal of noxious agents from the biological fluid bathing the cell, or the transfer of substances through the cell. These receptors are spared from degradation and can be recycled. Examples of this category include: low density lipoproteins (LDL) which supply cholesterol to steroid-producing cells, cobalamin and transferrin which supply vitamin B_{12} and iron, respectively, and the uptake of immunoglobulins across the placenta to provide fetal immunity.

Class II receptors can be influenced by traditional hormones. For example, prolactin appears to be important for the operation of the LDL-cholesterol transport system in steroidogenic tissue. Malfunction of the system can lead to disease. A genetic defect in receptors for LDL can lead to a failure in internalization and hyperlipidemia. Autoantibodies to these receptors may compete with a hormone for binding to the receptor and result in specific diseases, e.g. myasthenia gravis with antibodies to acetylcholine receptors, Graves' disease with antibodies to TSH receptors, and asthma with antibodies to adrenergic receptors.

Regulation of Adenylate Cyclase

The biologic activity of a polypeptide hormone (such as FSH or LH) may be altered by the heterogeneity of the molecules, up and down regulation of the receptors and, finally, by modulation of the activity of the enzyme, adenylate cyclase.

In a useful concept of how this enzyme works, adenylate cyclase is considered to be composed of two protein units, a guanyl nucleotide regulatory unit and a catalytic unit. (14) The receptor and the nucleotide regulatory unit are structurally linked, but inactive until the hormone binds to the receptor. Upon binding, the complex of hormone, receptor, and nucleotide regulatory unit is activated leading to an uptake of guanosine 5'-triphosphate (GTP) by the regulatory unit. The activation and uptake of GTP result in an active enzyme which can convert ATP to cAMP. This result can be viewed as the outcome of the regulatory unit "coupling" with the catalytic unit, forming an intact complete enzyme. Enzyme activity can be further regulated by hydrolysis of the GTP to guanosine 5'-diphosphate (GDP) returning the enzyme to its inactive state.

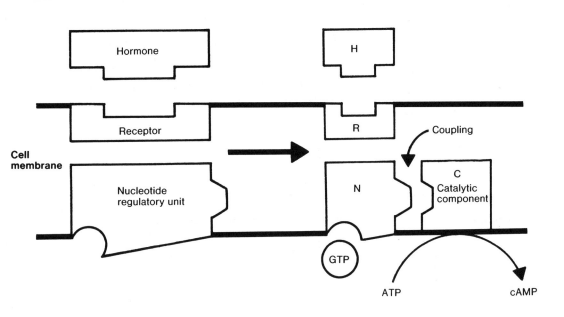

The ability of the hormone-receptor complex to work through a common messenger (cAMP) and produce contrasting actions (stimulation and inhibition) is thought to be due to the presence of both stimulatory nucleotide regulatory units and inhibitory nucleotide regulatory units. Thus, stimulating agents may work through specific stimulatory units.

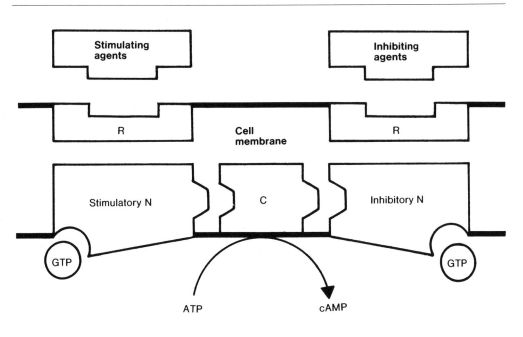

Another way to explain stimulating and inhibiting actions at the adenylate cyclase level focuses on the mechanism of coupling. LH stimulates steroidogenesis in the corpus luteum and works through the coupling of stimulatory regulatory units to the catalytic units of adenylate cyclase.

Both prostaglandin $F_{2\alpha}$ and GnRH are directly luteolytic, inhibiting luteal steroidogenesis through a mechanism which follows binding to specific receptors. This luteolytic action may be exerted via inhibitory regulatory units which lead to uncoupling with the catalytic units, thus interfering with gonadotropin action.

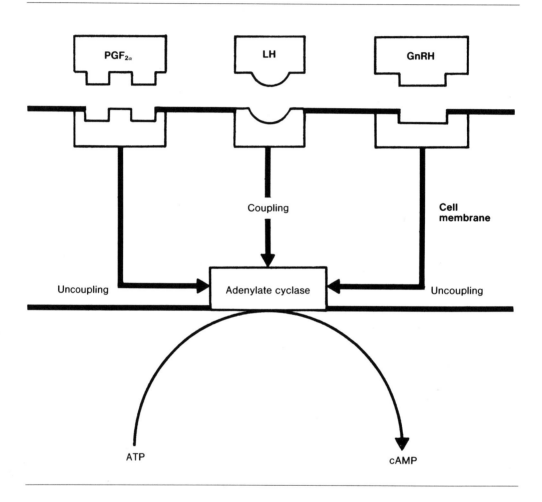

Increasing concentrations of tropic hormones, such as gonadotropins, are directly associated with desensitization of adenylate cyclase independently of the internalization of receptors. Desensitization is a rapid, acute change without loss of receptors in contrast to the slower process of internalization and true receptor loss. The desensitization process probably involves uncoupling, perhaps through hydrolysis of GTP, thus returning the active enzyme to its inactive state.

References

1. **Moon YS, Tsang BK, Simpson C, Armstrong DT,** 17-Estradiol biosynthesis in cultured granulosa and theca cells of human ovarian follicles: stimulation by follicle stimulating hormone, J Clin Endocrinol Metab 47:263, 1978.

2. **McNatty KP, Baird DT,** Relationship between follicle-stimulating hormone, androstenedione and oestradiol in human follicular fluid, J Endocrinol 76:527, 1978.

3. **Tsang BK, Moon YS, Simpson CW, Armstrong DT,** Androgen biosynthesis in human ovarian follicles: cellular source, gonadotropic control, and adenosine-3'5'-monophosphate mediation, J Clin Endocrinol Metab 48:153, 1979.

4. **McNatty KP, Makris A, DeGrazie C, Osathanoudh R, Ryan KJ,** The production of progesterone, androgens, and estrogens by granulosa cells, thecal tissue, and stromal tissue from human ovaries in vitro, J Clin Endocrinol Metab 49:687, 1979.

5. **Leung PCK, Armstrong DT,** Interactions of steroids and gonadotropins in the control of steroidogenesis in the ovarian follicle, Ann Rev Physiol 42:71, 1980.

6. **Hillier SG, Reichert LE Jr., Van Hall EV,** Control of preovulatory follicular estrogen biosynthesis in the human ovary, J Clin Endocrinol Metab 52:847, 1981.

7. **Siiteri PK, MacDonald PC,** Role of extraglandular estrogen in human endocrinology, in *Handbook of Physiology, Section 7, Endocrinology*, Geiger SR, Astwood EB, Greep RO, eds, American Physiology Society, Washington, DC, 1973, pp 615–629.

8. **Grady WW, Schader WT, O'Malley BW,** Activation, transformation, and subunit structure of steroid hormone receptors, Endocr Rev 3:141, 1982.

9. **Muldoon TG,** Regulation of steroid hormone receptor activity, Endocr Rev 1:339, 1980.

10. **Catt KJ, Harwood JP, Clayton RN, Davies TF, Chan V, Katikineni M, Nozu K, Dufau ML,** Regulation of peptide hormone receptors and gonadal steroidogenesis, Recent Prog Horm Res 36:557, 1980.

11. **Goldstein JL, Anderson RGW, Brown MS,** Coated pits, coated vesicles, and receptor-mediated endocytosis, Nature 279:679, 1979.

12. **King AC, Cuatrecasas P,** Peptide hormone-induced receptor mobility, aggregation, and internalization, N Engl J Med 305:77, 1981.

13.   **Kaplan J,** Polypeptide-binding membrane receptors: analysis and classification, Science 212:14, 1981.

14.   **Rodbell M,** The role of hormone receptors and GTP-regulatory proteins in membrane transduction, Nature 284:17, 1980.

2   Neuroendocrinology

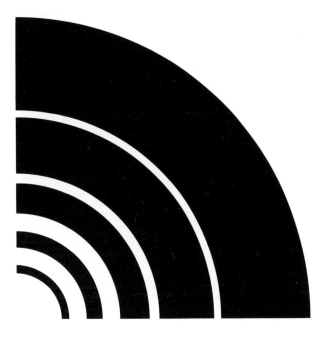

There are two major sites of action within the brain which are important in the regulation of reproductive function, the hypothalamus and the pituitary gland. In the past, the pituitary gland was viewed as the master gland. Then a new concept emerged, the concept of a transducer, in which the pituitary was relegated to the role of an orchestra, with the hypothalamus as the conductor, responding to both peripheral and central nervous system messages and exerting its influence by means of neurotransmitters transported to the pituitary by a portal vessel network. However, recent developments now indicate that the complex sequence of events known as the menstrual cycle is controlled by the sex steroids produced within the very follicle destined to ovulate. The hypothalamus and its direction are essential for the operation of the entire mechanism, but the fine tuning which leads to ovulation is brought about by steroid feedback on the anterior pituitary.

A full understanding of this feature of reproductive biology will benefit the clinician who faces problems in gynecologic endocrinology. With this understanding, the clinician can comprehend the hitherto mysterious, but significant, effects of stress, diet, exercise, and other diverse influences on the pituitary-gonadal axis. Furthermore, we will be prepared to make advantageous use of the numerous neuropharmacologic agents that are the dividends of neuroendocrine research. *To these ends, this chapter offers a review of the current status of reproductive neuroendocrinology.*

Hypothalamic-Hypophyseal Portal Circulation

In order to influence the anterior pituitary gland, the brain requires a means of transmission or connection between the two organ systems. A direct nervous connection does not exist. The blood supply of the anterior pituitary, however, originates in the capillaries which richly lace the median eminence area of the hypothalamus. The direction of the blood flow in this hypophyseal portal circulation is from the brain to the pituitary. Section of the neural stalk which interrupts this portal circulation leads to inactivity and atrophy of the gonads, along with a decrease in adrenal and thyroid activity to basal levels. With regeneration of the portal vessels, anterior pituitary function is restored. Thus, the anterior pituitary gland is under the influence of the hypothalamus by means of neurohormones released into this portal circulation. There also exists retrograde flow so that pituitary hormones can be delivered directly to the hypothalamus, but the importance of such pituitary feedback is not clear.

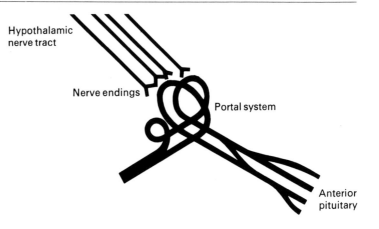

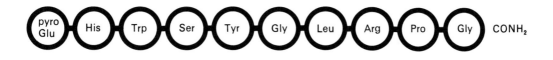

pyro Glu – His – Trp – Ser – Tyr – Gly – Leu – Arg – Pro – Gly   CONH$_2$

Neurohormone Concept

A considerable body of evidence has accumulated indicating that influence of the pituitary by the hypothalamus is achieved by materials secreted in the cells of the hypothalamus and transported to the pituitary by the portal vessel system. In addition to the stalk section experiments cited above, transplantation of the pituitary to ectopic sites (e.g. under the kidney capsule) results in failure of gonadal function. With retransplantation to an anatomic site under the median eminence, followed by regeneration of the portal system, normal pituitary function is regained. This retrieval of gonadotropic function is not accomplished if the pituitary is transplanted to other sites in the brain. Hence, there is something very special about the blood draining the basal hypothalamus. An exception to this overall pattern of positive influence is the control of prolactin secretion. Stalk section and transplantation cause release of prolactin from the anterior pituitary, implying a negative hypothalamic control. Furthermore, cultures of anterior pituitary tissue release prolactin in the absence of hypothalamic tissue or extracts.

Neuroendocrine agents originating in the hypothalamus have positive stimulatory impact on growth hormone, thyroid stimulating hormone (TSH), ACTH, as well as gonadotropins, and represent the individual neurohormones of the hypothalamus. The neurohormone which controls gonadotropins is called gonadotropin releasing hormone, GnRH. The neurohormone which controls prolactin is called prolactin inhibiting factor, and is probably dopamine. In addition to their effects on the pituitary, behavioral effects within the brain have been demonstrated for several of the releasing factors. Thyrotropin releasing hormone antagonizes the sedative action of a number of drugs and also has a direct antidepressant effect in humans. GnRH evokes mating behavior in male and female animals.

Initially, it was believed that there were two separate releasing hormones for follicle-stimulating hormone (FSH) and luteinizing hormone (LH). It is now apparent that there is a single neurohormone for both gonadotropins. Purified or synthesized GnRH stimulates both FSH and LH secretion. The divergent patterns of FSH and LH in response to a single GnRH are due to the modulating influences of the endocrine environment, specifically the feedback effects of steroids on the anterior pituitary gland.

43

The Hypothalamus and GnRH Secretion

The hypothalamus is the part of the diencephalon, at the base of the brain, which forms the floor of the third ventricle and part of its lateral walls. Within the hypothalamus are peptidergic neural cells which secrete the releasing and inhibiting hormones. These cells share the characteristics of both neurons and endocrine gland cells. They respond to signals in the bloodstream, as well as to neurotransmitters within the brain, in a process known as neurosecretion. In neurosecretion, a neurohormone or neurotransmitter is synthesized on the ribosomes in the cytoplasm of the neuron, packaged into a granule in the Golgi apparatus, and then transported by active axonal flow to the neuronal terminal for secretion into a blood vessel or across a synapse.

In primates, the primary network of GnRH cell bodies is located within the medial basal hypothalamus. Most of these can be seen within the arcuate nucleus where GnRH appears to be synthesized in GnRH neurons. (1) The delivery of GnRH to the portal circulation is via the axonal pathway, the GnRH tuberoinfundibular tract.

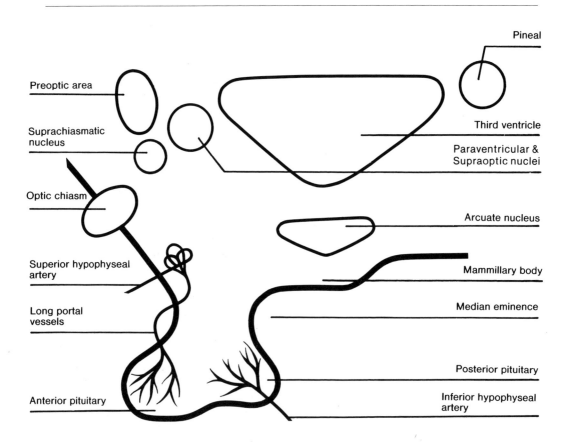

Fibers, identified with immunocytochemical techniques using antibodies to GnRH, can also be visualized in the posterior hypothalamus, descending into the posterior pituitary, and in the anterior hypothalamic area, projecting to sites within the limbic system. (1) However, lesions which interrupt GnRH neurons projecting to regions other than the median eminence do not affect gonadotropin release. Only lesions of the arcuate nucleus in the monkey lead to gonadal atrophy and amenorrhea. (2) Therefore, the arcuate nucleus may be viewed with the median eminence as a unit, the key locus within the hypothalamus for GnRH secretion.

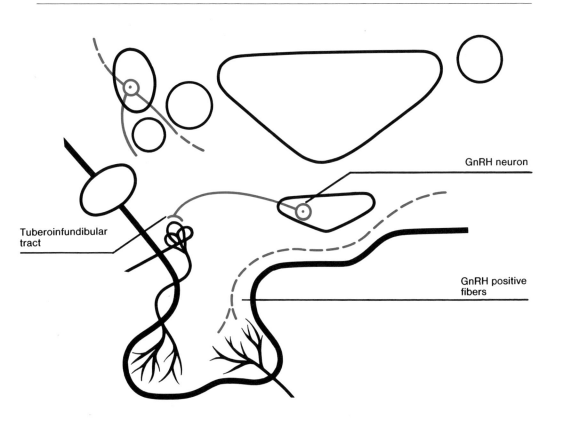

GnRH neuron

Tuberoinfundibular tract

GnRH positive fibers

GnRH Secretion

The half-life of GnRH is only a few minutes. Therefore, control of the reproductive cycle depends upon constant release of GnRH. This function, in turn, depends upon the complex and coordinated interrelationship among this releasing hormone, other neurohormones, the pituitary gonadotropins, and the gonadal steroids. The interplay among these substances is governed by feedback effects, both positive stimulatory and negative inhibitory. The long feedback loop refers to the feedback effects of circulating levels of target gland hormones, and this occurs both in the hypothalamus and the pituitary. The short feedback loop indicates a negative feedback of gonadotropins on pituitary secretion, presumably via inhibitory effects on GnRH in the hypothalamus. Ultrashort feedback refers to inhibition by the releasing hormone of its own synthesis. These signals as well as signals from higher centers in the central nervous system may modify GnRH secretion through an array of neutrotransmitters, primarily dopamine and norepinephrine, but also serotonin, melatonin, and endorphins.

Dopamine and norepinephrine are synthesized in the nerve terminals by decarboxylation of dihydroxyphenylalanine (DOPA), which in turn is synthesized by hydroxylation of tyrosine. Dopamine is the immediate precursor of norepinephrine, but dopamine itself may function as a key neurotransmitter in the hypothalamus and the pituitary.

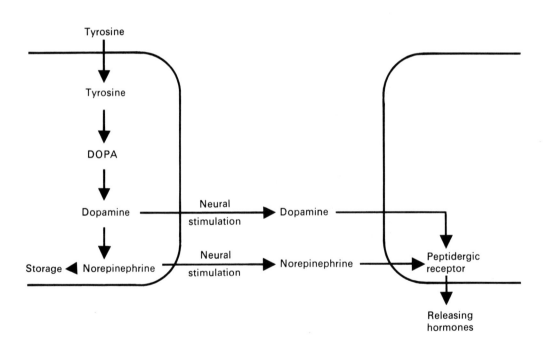

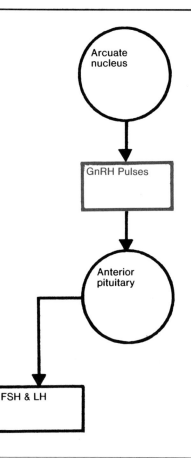

A most useful concept is to view the arcuate nucleus as the central component, releasing GnRH into the portal circulation in pulsatile fashion. In a classic series of experiments, it was demonstrated that normal gonadotropin secretion requires pulsatile GnRH discharge in a frequency and concentration within a critical range. (3)

Experimental manipulations have suggested that the critical range of GnRH pulsatile secretion is rather narrow. The administration (to monkeys) of 1 μg GnRH per minute for 6 minutes every hour (1 pulse per hour) produces a portal blood concentration about equal to the peak concentration of GnRH in human portal blood, about 2 ng/ml. Increasing the frequency to 2 and 5 pulses per hour extinguishes gonadotropic secretion. A similar decline in gonadotropin secretion is obtained by increasing the dose of GnRH. Decreasing the pulse frequency decreases LH secretion, but increases FSH secretion.

Like GnRH, gonadotropins are also secreted in pulsatile fashion. Initiation of the pulsatile pattern of gonadotropin secretion occurs just before puberty with night time increases in LH. After puberty, pulsatile secretion is maintained throughout the 24-hour period, but it varies in both amplitude and frequency. During the menstrual cycle maximum amplitude and frequency are reached at midcycle. The pulsatile secretion of gonadotropins is due to the pulsatile release of GnRH into the portal system. (4) In puberty, arcuate activity begins with a low frequency of GnRH release and proceeds through a cycle of acceleration of frequency, characterized by passage from total inactivity, to nocturnal activation, to the full adult pattern. The progressive changes in FSH and LH reflect this activation of GnRH pulsatile secretion.

Control of GnRH Pulses

Normal menstrual cycles require the maintenance of the pulsatile release of GnRH within a critical range. This pulsatile release is mediated by a catecholaminergic mechanism and can be modified by gonadal steroids and endorphins.

The Dopamine Tract. Cell bodies for dopamine synthesis can be found in the arcuate and periventricular nuclei. The dopamine tuberoinfundibular tract arises within the medial basal hypothalamus and projects to the median eminence.

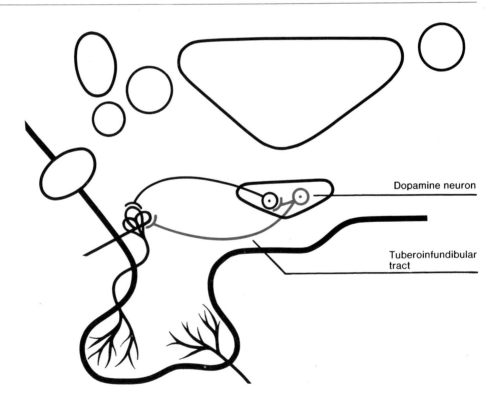

Dopamine neuron

Tuberoinfundibular tract

The administration of dopamine by intravenous infusion to men and women is associated with a suppression of circulating prolactin and gonadotropin levels. Dopamine does not exert a direct effect on LH secretion by the anterior pituitary, thus this effect is mediated through GnRH release in the hypothalamus. While the exact chemical nature of the prolactin inhibiting factor is still not known, evidence is rather overwhelming that dopamine is the hypothalamic inhibitor of prolactin secretion and is directly secreted into the portal blood, thus behaving like a neurohormone. Therefore, dopamine may directly suppress arcuate GnRH activity, and also be transported via the portal system to directly and specifically suppress pituitary prolactin secretion. Ergot derivatives, such as bromocriptine, used clinically to treat high prolactin levels, activate dopaminergic receptors and directly inhibit the secretion of prolactin in a fashion identical to dopamine.

The Norepinephrine Tract. Most of the cell bodies which synthesize norepinephrine are located in the mesencephalon and lower brainstem. These cells also synthesize serotonin. Axons for amine transport ascend into the medial forebrain bundle to terminate in various brain structures including the hypothalamus.

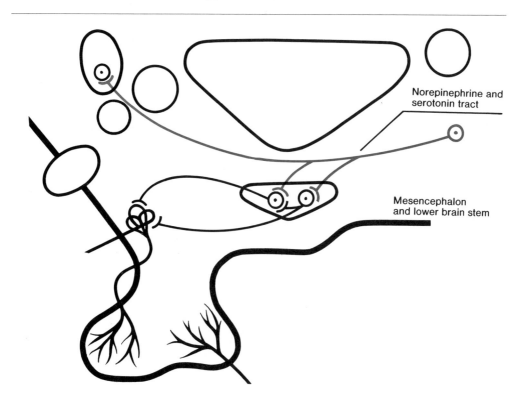

Norepinephrine and serotonin tract

Mesencephalon and lower brain stem

The current concept is that the biogenic catecholamines regulate GnRH pulsatile release into the tuberoinfundibular tract or into the portal blood system or at both sites. Norepinephrine is thought to exert stimulatory effects on GnRH, while dopamine and serotonin exert inhibitory effects. Little is known, however, about the role of serotonin.

The probable mode of action of catecholamines is to change the frequency of GnRH discharge. Thus, pharmacological or psychological factors that affect pituitary function probably do so by altering catecholamine synthesis or metabolism, and thus the pulsatile release of GnRH.

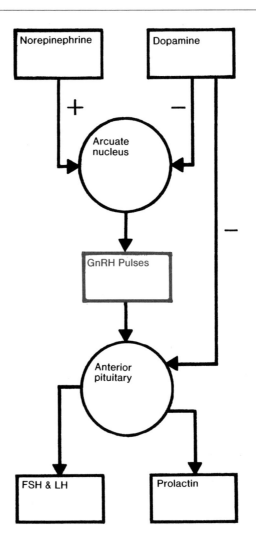

The following clinical observations illustrate the preceding physiologic mechanisms: Pseudocyesis, with high LH and prolactin secretion, can be explained by a lack of dopamine activity in the hypothalamus, thus luteal function and galactorrhea are maintained. Amenorrhea on a central basis can be due to a decrease in GnRH pulses below the critical frequency, caused, perhaps, by excessive dopamine in the hypothalamus. Marijuana use is associated with decreased gonadotropins and reproductive function. Because response to GnRH is not impaired, this inhibitory effect appears to be due to a decrease in GnRH pulsatile release in the hypothalamus. (5, 6).

Endogenous Opiates and the Endorphin Story

There are a large variety of brain peptides which may function as neurotransmitters. (7) Examples include the following:

Neurotensin. A brain peptide which is vasodilatory, alters pituitary hormone release, and lowers body temperature.

Substance P. A sensory transmitter of pain.

Cholecystokinin. An intestinal hormone which is found in the brain and may be involved in the regulation of behavior, satiety, and fluid intake.

Vasoactive Intestinal Polypeptide (VIP). High levels of this peptide are found in the cerebral cortex, and it is also found in the hypothalamus. VIP causes vasodilation, stimulates conversion of glycogen to glucose, enhances lipolysis and insulin secretion, stimulates pancreatic and intestinal secretion, and inhibits the production of gastric acid.

Thyroid Releasing Hormone (TRH). TRH is found in many areas of the brain. It elicits behavioral excitation and anorexia in animals, and may cause mood enhancement in humans.

Somatostatin. This hypothalamic peptide inhibits the release of growth hormone, prolactin, and TSH from the pituitary. It is also a typical gut-brain peptide, being found in neurons throughout the brain, stomach, intestine, and pancreas. It inhibits secretion of glucagon, insulin, and gastrin. It is also located in sensory neurons and may be a transmitter of pain sensation.

The Endorphins. The most fascinating peptide group is the ACTH-lipotropin family. (8) β-Lipotropin is a 91 amino acid molecule which was first isolated from the pituitary in 1964. Its function remained a mystery for over 10 years. ACTH and β-lipotropin share a high molecular weight common precursor called pro-opiomelanocortin.

Receptors for opioid compounds were first identified in 1973, and, by virtue of their existence, it was postulated that endogenous opioid compounds must exist and serve important physiological roles. Endorphin was a word coined to denote their morphine-like action and their endogenous origin in the brain.

Pro-opiomelanocortin is split into two fragments, an ACTH intermediate fragment and β-lipotropin. β-Lipotropin has no opioid activity, but is broken down in a series of steps to β-melanocyte stimulating hormone (β-MSH), enkephalin, and α-, γ-, and β-endorphins.

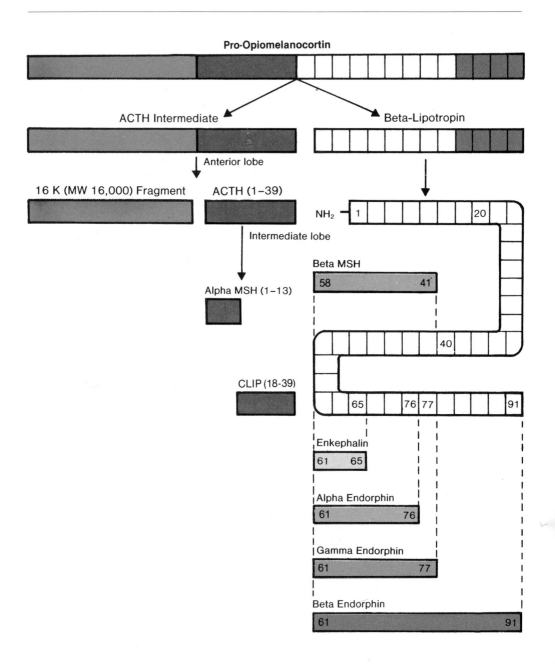

Enkephalin and the α- and γ-endorphins are as active as morphine on a molar basis, while β-endorphin is 5–10 times more potent. Localization of opioid receptors explains many of the pharmacological actions of the opiates. Opioid receptors and enkephalin are found in the nerve endings of sensory neurons, in the limbic system (site of euphoric emotions), in brainstem centers for reflexes such as respiration, and widely distributed in the brain and in the spinal cord.

In the adult pituitary gland, the major products are ACTH and β-lipotropin, with only small amounts of endorphin. Thus ACTH and β-lipotropin blood levels show similar courses and they are major secretion products of the anterior pituitary in response to stress and corticosteriods. In the intermediate lobe of the pituitary (which is prominent only during fetal life), ACTH is cleaved to CLIP (corticotropin-like intermediate lobe peptide) and β-MSH.

In the brain, the major products are the opiates, with little ACTH. In the hypothalamus the major product is β-endorphin in the region of the arcuate nucleus and the ventromedial nucleus. Therefore, the pituitary system is a system for secretion into the circulation while the hypothalamic system allows for distribution via axons to regulate other brain regions and the pituitary gland.

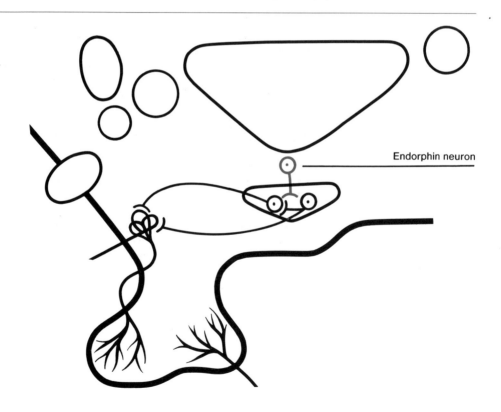

Endorphin neuron

The following facts are known about endogenous opiates: (9, 10)

1. Opioid compounds stimulate growth hormone, prolactin, and ACTH, and inhibit FSH, LH, and TSH.

2. Opiates have no direct action on the pituitary, nor do they alter the action of releasing hormones on the pituitary.

3. Opioid receptors have been localized on dopamine neurons in the brain.

4. Blockage of opioid receptors increases the frequency and amplitude of LH pulses.

Endogenous opiates appear to participate in the regulation of the pulsatile pattern of gonadotropin secretion by directly inhibiting GnRH neurons in the arcuate area, and they increase prolactin by inhibiting the dopamine neurons. Based on these findings it could be anticipated that increased opioid activity would be characteristic of hypothalamic, hypogonadotropic amenorrhea, and this has been reported. (11) Furthermore, decreased gonadotropin secretion and increased prolactin associated with exercise and stress may be mediated by endogenous opiates. The effect of opiates on GnRH appears to be a direct one, although there also may be an indirect effect via the norepinephrine system.

Catecholestrogens

Catecholestrogens have two faces, a catechol side and an estrogen side. The enzyme which converts estrogens to catecholamines is very rich in the hypothalamus, hence there are higher concentrations of catecholestrogens than estrone and estradiol in the hypothalamus and pituitary gland.

Because catecholestrogens have two faces, they have the potential for interacting with both catecholamine and estrogen-mediated systems. (12) To be specific, catecholestrogens may inhibit tyrosine hydroxylase (which would decrease catecholamines) and compete for catechol-*o*-methyltransferase (which would increase catecholamines). Since GnRH, estrogens, and catecholestrogens are located in similar sites, it is possible that catecholestrogens may serve to interact between catecholamines and GnRH secretion.

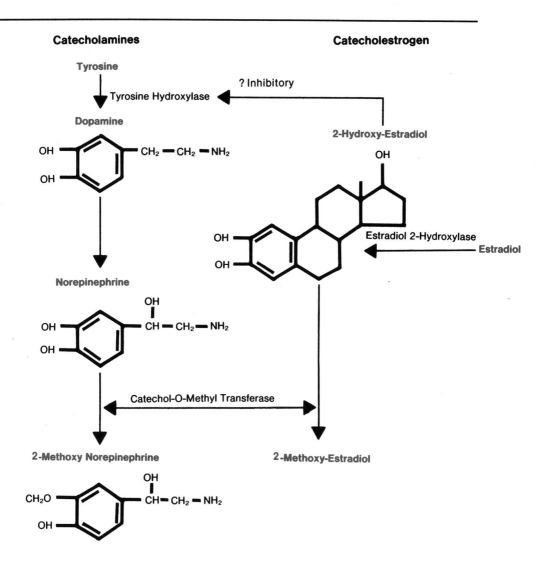

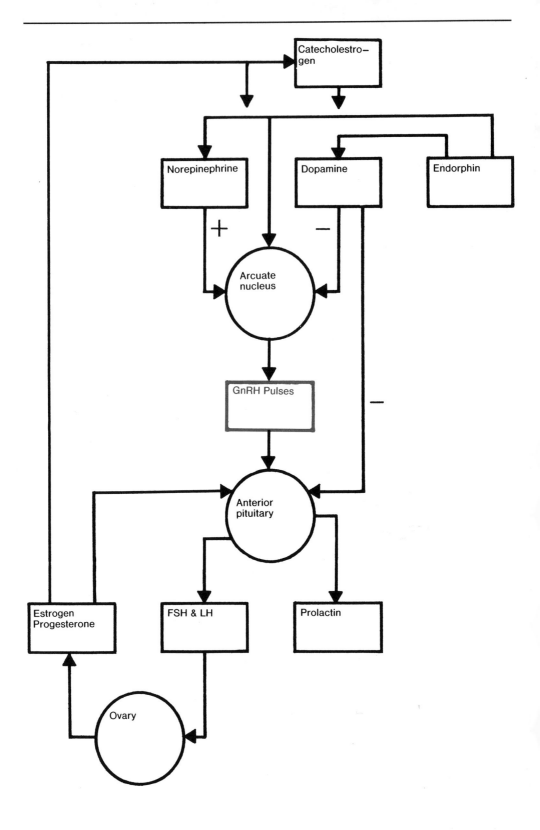

Summary: Control of GnRH Pulses

The key concept is that normal menstrual function requires GnRH pulsatile secretion in a critical range of frequency and concentration. Both normal physiology and pathophysiology of the menstrual cycle, at least in terms of central control, can be explained by mechanisms which affect the pulsatile secretion of GnRH. The pulses of GnRH appear to be directly under the influence of a dual catecholaminergic system: norepinephrine facilatory and dopamine inhibitory. In turn the catecholamine system can be influenced by endogenous opioid activity. The feedback effects of steroids may be mediated through this system via catecholsteroid messengers.

Tanycytes

A significant pathway for hypothalamic influence may be via the cerebrospinal fluid (CSF). Tanycytes are specialized ependymal cells whose ciliated cell bodies line the third ventricle over the median eminence. The cells terminate on portal vessels, and they can transport materials from ventricular CSF to the portal system, e.g. substances from the pineal gland, or vasopressin, or oxytocin. Tanycytes change morphologically in response to steroids, and exhibit morphological changes with the ovarian cycle.

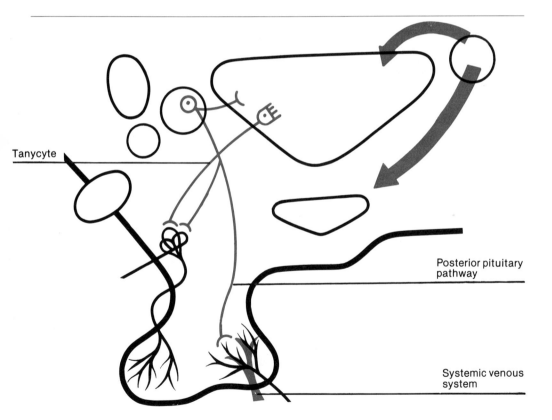

Tanycyte

Posterior pituitary pathway

Systemic venous system

The posterior pituitary is a direct prolongation of the hypothalamus via the pituitary stalk. Separate neurosecretory cells in both the supraoptic and paraventricular nuclei make vasopressin, oxytocin, and their transport peptide, neurophysin. (13) Both oxytocin and vasopressin consist of 9 amino acid residues. In the human, vasopressin contains arginine, unlike animals which have lysine vasopressin. The molecular weights of oxytocin and vasopressin are 1007 and 1084, respectively. The neurophysins are polypeptides with a molecular weight of about 10,000. There are two distinct neurophysins, estrogen-stimulated neurophysin known as neurophysin I, and nicotine-stimulated neurophysin, known as neurophysin II.

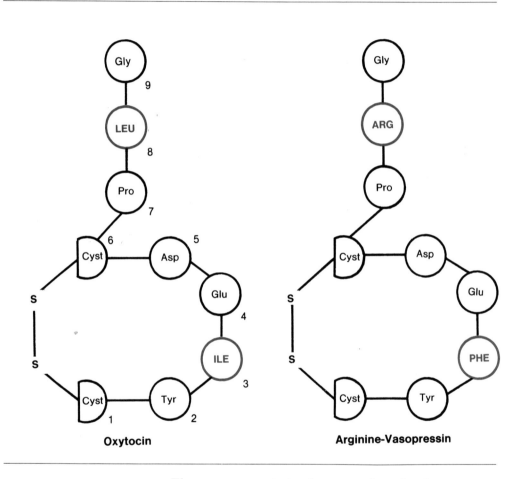

Oxytocin   Arginine-Vasopressin

The neurons secrete two large protein molecules, a precursor called pro-pressophysin which contains vasopressin and its neurophysin, and a precursor called pro-oxyphysin, which contains oxytocin and its neurophysin. (14) It is thought that neurophysin I is specifically related to oxytocin, and neurophysin II accompanies vasopressin. Because of this unique packaging, the hormones and their neurophysins are stored together and released at the same time into the circulation.

The posterior pituitary pathway is complex and not limited to the transmission of vasopressin and oxytocin to the posterior pituitary. These hormones are also secreted into the cerebrospinal fluid and directly into the portal system. Therefore, vasopressin and oxytocin can reach the anterior pituitary and influence, in the case of vasopressin, ACTH secretion, and in the case of oxytocin, gonadotropin secretion.

Neurophysin II is called nicotine neurophysin because the administration of nicotine or hemorrhage increases the circulating levels. Neurophysin I is called estrogen neurophysin because estrogen administration increases the levels in the peripheral blood, and peak levels of both neurophysin I and oxytocin are found at the time of the LH surge. (15) The rise in estrogen neurophysin begins 10 hours after the rise in estrogen, precedes that of the LH surge, and the elevation of neurophysin lasts longer than the LH surge. Because GnRH and oxytocin are competing substrates for hypothalamic degradation enzymes, it has been hypothesized that oxytocin in the portal blood at the midcycle may inhibit the metabolism of GnRH, thus increasing the amount of GnRH available. Furthermore, oxytocin may have direct actions on the pituitary, ovary, uterus, and Fallopian tube during ovulation.

Neurophysin-containing pathways have been traced from the hypothalamic nuclei to various centers in the brainstem and the spinal cord. In addition, behavioral studies suggest a role for vasopressin in learning and memory. Administration of vasopressin has been associated with improvement in memory in brain-damaged human subjects, and enhanced cognitive responses (learning and memory) in both young, normal individuals and depressed patients.

Both oxytocin and vasopressin circulate as the free peptides. The half-life of vasopressin is 3–6 minutes and that of oxytocin 5–17 minutes (a mean of 10 minutes). Three major stimuli for vasopressin secretion are changes in osmolality of the blood, alterations in blood volume, and psychogenic stimuli such as pain and fear. The osmoreceptors are located in the hypothalamus; the volume receptors are in the left atrium, aortic arch, and carotid sinus. Angiotensin II also produces a release of vasopressin, suggesting a link between the kidney and hypothalamus. Cortisol may modify the osmotic threshold for the release of vasopressin.

The release of oxytocin is so episodic that it is described as spurts. Ordinarily there are about 3 spurts every 10 minutes. Oxytocin is released during coitus, probably by the Ferguson reflex (vaginal and cervical stimulation), but also by olfactory, visual, and auditory pathways. Perhaps oxytocin has some role in muscle contractions during orgasm. In the male, release of oxytocin during coitus may contribute to sperm transport during ejaculation.

59

During pregnancy, maternal plasma oxytocin increases with gestational age, as do amniotic fluid levels. Fetal urine and meconium contain large amounts of oxytocin. During labor, maternal levels increase from the first stage to the second stage, but decline during the third stage. The major mechanism is thought to be the Ferguson reflex.

Umbilical artery levels of oxytocin are always higher than umbilical vein levels, except when oxytocin is administered. Since oxytocin readily crosses the placenta, it is likely that during normal labor fetal oxytocin crosses into the maternal compartment, and during oxytocin administration there is a reverse movement into the fetal compartment. It appears that fetal oxytocin plays the major role during the first stage of labor, while maternal oxytocin is significant during the second stage. (16)

Oxytocin is released in response to suckling, mediated through impulses generated at the nipple and transmitted via the 3rd, 4th, and 5th thoracic nerves to the spinal cord up to the hypothalamus. In addition to causing milk ejection, the reflex is responsible for the uterine contractions associated with breast feeding.

The Brain and Ovulation

The Classic Concept. Classic studies in a variety of rodents indicated the presence of feedback centers in the hypothalamus that responded to steroids with the release of GnRH. The release of GnRH was the result of the complex, but coordinated relationships among the neurohormones, the pituitary gonadotropins, and the gonadal steroids designated by the time-honored terms positive and negative feedback.

FSH levels were thought to be largely regulated by a negative inhibitory feedback relationship with estradiol. In the case of LH, there existed both a negative inhibitory feedback relationship with estradiol, and a positive stimulatory feedback with high levels of estradiol. The feedback centers were located in the hypothalamus, and they were called the tonic and cyclic centers. The tonic center controlled the day to day basal level of gonadotropins, and was responsive to the negative feedback effects of steroids. The cyclic center in the female brain was responsible for the midcycle surge of gonadotropins, a response mediated by the positive feedback of estrogen. Specifically, the midcycle surge of gonadotropins was thought to be due to an outpouring of GnRH in response to the positive feedback action of estradiol on the cyclic center of the hypothalamus.

This classic concept was not inaccurate. The problem was that the concept accurately described events in the rodent, but the mechanism is different in the primate.

The New Concept. In the primate, the "center" for the midcycle surge of gonadotropins has moved from the hypothalamus to the pituitary. Experiments in the monkey have clearly demonstrated that GnRH, originating in the hypothalamus, plays a permissive role. Its secretion in pulse-like bursts every hour is an important prerequisite for normal pituitary function, but the feedback responses regulating gonadotropin levels are controlled by ovarian follicle steroid feedback on the anterior pituitary cells.

The new concept is derived from experiments in which the medial basal hypothalamus (MBH) is either destroyed (3) or the hypothalamus is surgically separated from the pituitary. (17) In a typical experiment, lesion of the MBH by radiofrequency waves was followed by loss of LH levels as the source of GnRH was eliminated. (2) Administration of GnRH by an intravenous pump restored LH secretion. The administration of estradiol was then able to produce both negative and positive feedback responses, clearly actions that must be directly on the anterior pituitary because the hypothalamus was absent and GnRH was being administered in a steady and unchanging frequency and dose.

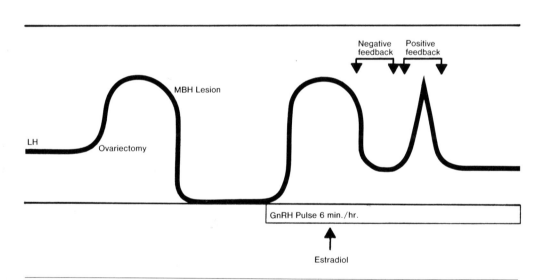

Administration of GnRH intravenously, as a bolus, produces an increase in blood levels of LH and FSH within 5 minutes, reaching a peak in about 20–25 minutes for LH and 45 minutes for FSH. Levels return to pretreatment values over several hours. When administered by constant infusion at submaximal doses, there is first a rapid rise with a peak at 30 minutes followed by a plateau or fall between 45 and 90 minutes, then a second and sustained increase at 225–240 minutes. This biphasic response suggests the presence of two functional pools of pituitary gonadotropins. (18) The readily releasable pool (secretion) produces the initial response, and the later response is dependent upon a second, reserve pool of stored gonadotropins.

Synthesis of gonadotropins takes place on the rough endoplasmic reticulum. The hormones are packaged into secretory granules by the Golgi cisternae of the Golgi apparatus, and then stored as secretory granules. Secretion requires migration (activation) of the mature secretory granule to the cell membrane where an alteration in membrane permeability results in extrusion of the secretory granules in a process which involves calcium and cyclic AMP changes in response to GnRH.

There are three principal positive actions of GnRH on gonadotropin elaboration:

1.   Synthesis and storage (the reserve pool) of gonadotropins.

2.   Activation, movement of gonadotropins from the reserve pool to a pool ready for direct secretion.

3.   Immediate release (direct secretion) of gonadotropins.

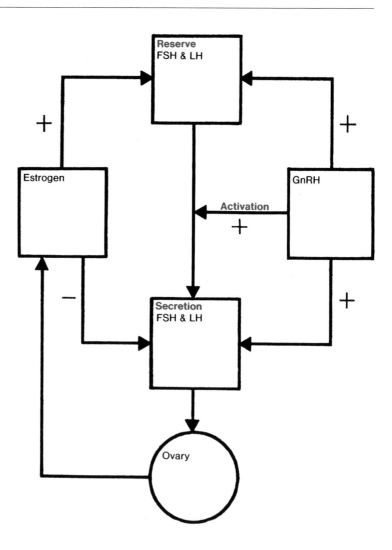

Secretion, synthesis, and storage change during the cycle. At the beginning of the cycle, when estrogen levels are low, both secretion and storage levels are low. With increasing levels of estradiol, a greater increase occurs in storage, with little change in secretion. Thus, in the early follicular phase, estrogen has a positive effect on the synthesis and storage response, building up a supply of gonadotropins in order to meet the requirements of the midcycle surge. Premature release of gonadotropins is prevented by a negative (inhibitory) action of estradiol on the pituitary secretory response to GnRH.

As the midcycle approaches, subsequent responses to GnRH are greater than initial responses, indicating that each response not only induces release of gonadotropins, but also activates the storage pool for the next response.

Because the midcycle surge of LH can be produced in the experimental monkey in the absence of a hypothalamus, and, in the face of unchanging GnRH, the ovulatory surge of LH is now thought to be a response to positive feedback action of estradiol on the anterior pituitary. When the estradiol level in the circulation reaches a critical concentration and this concentration is maintained for a critical time period, the inhibitory action on LH secretion changes to a stimulatory action. The mechanism of this steroid action is unknown, but experimental evidence suggests that the positive feedback action involves an increase in GnRH receptor concentration, while the negative feedback of estrogen operates through a different mechanism. (19)

What a logical mechanism! The midcycle surge must occur at the right time of the cycle to ovulate a ready and waiting mature follicle. What better way to achieve this extreme degree of coordination and timing than by the follicle itself, through the feedback effects of the sex steroids originating in the follicle destined to ovulate.

GnRH has been found to be increased in both peripheral blood of women and portal blood of monkeys at midcycle. While this increase may not be absolutely necessary (as demonstrated in the monkey experiments), it may contribute to the effectiveness of the surge. A small increase in endogeneous GnRH may be important in increasing activation of gonadotropins from the reserve to the readily releasable pool. On the other hand, at least one laboratory has indicated that an acute release of GnRH is in fact necessary for the ovulatory gonadotropin surge. (20)

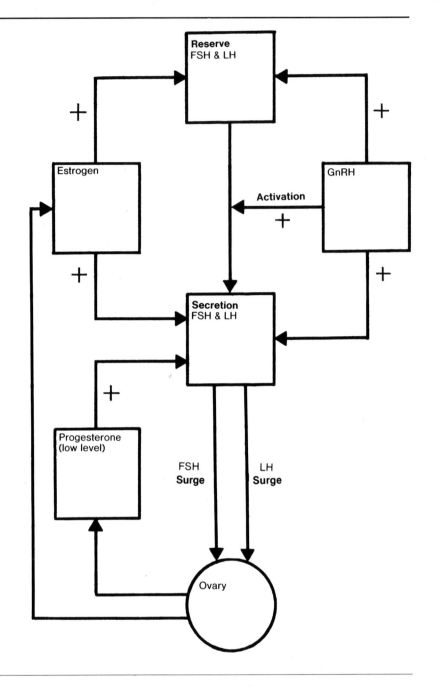

Another aspect of gonadotropin secretion appears to be growing in significance. A disparity exists between the quantity of LH measured during the midcycle surge as determined by radioimmunoassay and bioassay. More LH is secreted at midcycle in a molecular form with greater biological activity. (21) There is a well-established relationship between the activity and half-life of glycoprotein hormones and their content of sialic acid (see Chapter 1, under "Heterogeneity," of tropic hormones). Estrogen enhancement of sialic acid content is an additional method for maximizing the biologic effects of the midcycle surge.

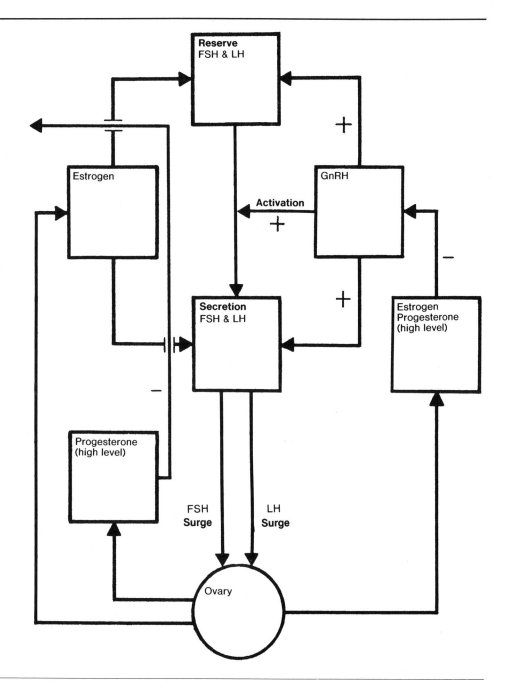

The purpose and mechanism for the midcycle surge of FSH have only recently been appreciated. A normal corpus luteum requires the induction of an adequate number of LH receptors on granulosa cells, a specific action of FSH. The midcycle surge of FSH, therefore, plays an important role in ensuring an adequate LH response and a normal corpus luteum. Emerging progesterone secretion, just prior to ovulation, is the key.

Progesterone, at low levels and in the presence of estrogen, augments the pituitary secretion of LH and elicits the FSH surge in response to GnRH. (22) As the rising levels of LH produce the morphologic change of luteinization in the ovulating follicle, the granulosa layer begins to secrete progesterone directly into the bloodstream. The process of luteinization is inhibited by the presence of the oocyte, and therefore, progesterone secretion is relatively suppressed ensuring that only low levels of progesterone reach the pituitary gland.

After ovulation, rapid and full luteinization is accompanied by a marked increase in progesterone levels, which, in the presence of estrogen, exercise a profound negative feedback action to suppress gonadotropin secretion. This action of progesterone takes place in two locations. First, there definitely is a central action to decrease GnRH. Progesterone fails to block estradiol-induced gonadotropin discharges in monkeys with hypothalamic lesions if pulsatile GnRH replacement is provided. (23) Therefore, high levels of progesterone inhibit ovulation at the hypothalamic level. In addition, the depressed gonadotropin levels associated with the luteal phase in the lesioned monkeys suggest that progesterone also can block estrogen-induced responses to GnRH (remember that progesterone will deplete target cells of estrogen receptors and thus block estrogen action). In contrast, the facilitory action of low levels of progesterone is exerted at the pituitary on the response to GnRH. (23)

Summary: Key Points in the New Concept

1. Pulsatile GnRH secretion must be within a critical range for frequency and concentration.

2. GnRH has only positive actions on the anterior pituitary: synthesis and storage, activation, and secretion of gonadotropins. The gonadotropins are secreted in a pulsatile fashion in response to the similar pulsatile release of GnRH.

3. Low levels of estrogen enhance FSH and LH synthesis and storage, have little effect on LH secretion, and inhibit FSH secretion.

4. High levels of estrogen induce the LH surge at midcycle, and high steady levels of estrogen lead to sustained elevated LH secretion.

5. Low levels of progesterone acting at the level of the pituitary gland enhance the LH response to GnRH and are responsible for the FSH surge at midcycle.

6. High levels of progesterone inhibit pituitary secretion of gonadotropins by inhibiting GnRH pulses at the level of the hypothalamus. In addition, high levels of progesterone may blunt pituitary response to GnRH by interfering with estrogen action through the depletion of estrogen receptors.

The Pineal Gland

The reproductive functions of the hypothalamus may also be under inhibitory control of the brain via the pineal gland. The pineal arises as an outgrowth of the roof of the third ventricle, but soon after birth it loses all afferent and efferent neural connections with the brain. Instead the parenchymal cells receive a new and unusual sympathetic innervation which allows the pineal gland to be an active neuroendocrine organ that responds to photic and hormonal stimuli and exhibits circadian rhythms. (24)

The neural pathway begins in the retina and passes through the inferior accessory optic tracts and the medial forebrain bundle to the upper cord. Preganglionic fibers terminate at the superior cervical ganglion, and postganglionic sympathetic nerves terminate directly on pineal cells. Interruption of this pathway gives the same effect as darkness, which is an increase in pineal biosynthetic activity.

Hydroxyindole-o-methyltransferase (HIOMT) is found mainly in pineal parenchymal cells, and its products, therefore, are essentially unique to the pineal. Norepinephrine stimulates tryptophan entry into the pineal cell and also adenylate cyclase activity in the membrane. The resulting increase in cyclic AMP leads to N-acetyltransferase activity, the rate-limiting step in melatonin synthesis. Thus, melatonin synthesis is controlled by norepinephrine stimulation of adenylate cyclase, and the norepinephrine is liberated by sympathetic stimulation due to the absence of light. HIOMT is also found in the retina where melatonin may serve to regulate the pigment in retinal cells.

The association of hyperplastic pineal tumors with decreased gonadal function, and destructive tumors with precocious puberty, suggested that the pineal is the source of gonadal inhibiting substances. However, pineal mechanisms cannot be absolutely essential for gonadal function. Normal reproductive function returns to the pinealectomized rat several weeks after pinealectomy, and blind women have normal fertility.

A rat in constant light develops a small pineal with decreased HIOMT and melatonin, while the ovarian weight increases. A rat in constant dark has the opposite result, increased pineal size, HIOMT, and melatonin, with decreased ovarian weight and pituitary function. A rhythm is established in pineal HIOMT activity by the presence or absence of light. Short days and long nights result in gonadal atrophy, and this may be a mechanism governing seasonal breeding. Possible roles in humans may be to give circadian rhythmicity to other functions such as temperature and sleep. In all vertebrates tested so far, there is a daily rhythm in melatonin secretion, high values during the dark and low during light.

The gonadal changes associated with melatonin are mediated via the hypothalamus and suggest a general suppressive effect on GnRH pulsatile secretion and reproductive function. In women, melatonin blood levels are highest in the prepubertal period, and they decrease with age. During the menstrual cycle, they are lowest at the time of the midcycle, ovulatory surge.

Melatonin is synthesized and secreted by the pineal gland and circulates in the blood like a classical hormone. It affects distant target organs, especially the neuroendocrine centers of the central nervous system. Whether melatonin is secreted primarily into the CSF or blood is still debated, most evidence, however, favors blood. From the CSF, melatonin may reach the hypothalamus by way of tanycyte transport.

Pineal activity can be viewed as the net balance between hormonal and neuronal mediated influences. The pineal contains receptors for the active sex hormones, estradiol, testosterone, dihydrotestosterone, progesterone and prolactin. Furthermore, the pineal converts testosterone and progesterone to the active 5α-reduced metabolites, and androgens are aromatized to estrogens. The pineal also appears to be unique in that a catecholamine neurotransmitter (norepinephrine), interacting with cell membrane receptors, stimulates cellular synthesis of estrogen and androgen receptors. In general, however, the sympathetic activity producing the circadian rhythm takes precedence over hormonal effects.

Despite a variety of suggestive leads, there is little evidence for a role of the pineal in humans. A possible influence of the pineal gland may be the synchronization of menstrual cycles noted among women who spend time together. A significant increase in synchronization of cycles among roommates and among closest friends occurred in the first 4 months of residency in a dormitory of a women's college. (25)

Gonadotropin Secretion through Fetal Life, Childhood and Puberty

Gonadotropin production has been documented throughout fetal life, during childhood, and into adult life. Remarkable levels of FSH and LH, similar to postmenopausal levels, can be measured in the fetus. GnRH is detectable in the hypothalamus by 10 weeks of gestation, and, by 10–13 weeks, FSH and LH are being produced in the pituitary. The peak concentrations of FSH and LH occur at about 20 weeks of intrauterine life. (26)

The increasing production rate of gonadotropins until mid-gestation reflects the growing ability of the hypothalamic-pituitary axis to perform at full capacity. Beginning at midgestation, there is an increasing sensitivity to inhibition by steroids and a resultant decrease in gonadotropin secretion. Full sensitivity to steroids is not reached until late in infancy. The rise in gonadotropins after birth reflects loss of the high levels of placental steroids. Thus, in the first year of life there is considerable follicular activity in the ovaries in contrast to later in childhood when gonadotropin secretion is suppressed.

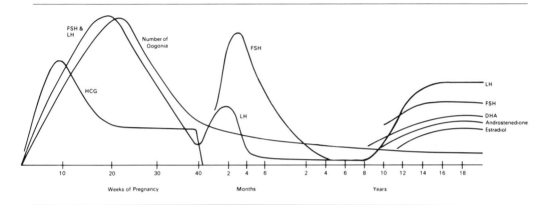

Testicular function in the fetus can be correlated with the fetal hormonal patterns. (26) Initial testosterone production and sexual differentiation are in response to the high fetal levels of HCG, whereas further testosterone production and differentiation appear to be maintained by the fetal pituitary gonadotropins. Decreased testosterone levels in late gestation probably reflect the decrease in gonadotropin levels. In the female, the peak of oogenesis and the onset of atresia coincide with peak production of pituitary gonadotropins by the fetus.

There is a sex difference in gonadotropin levels. There are higher FSH and LH levels in female fetuses. The lower male levels are probably due to the higher testosterone production. In infancy, the postnatal FSH rise is more marked and more sustained in females, while LH values are not as high. After the postnatal rise, gonadotropin levels reach a nadir during early childhood (2–3 years) and then rise slightly between 4 and 10 years. This childhood period is characterized by low levels of gonadotropins in the pituitary and in the blood, little response of the pituitary to GnRH, and maximum hypothalamic suppression.

The precise signal which initiates the events of puberty is unknown. In girls, the very first steroid to rise in the blood is dehydroepiandrosterone (DHA) beginning at 6–8 years of age, at the same time that FSH begins to increase. Estrogen levels, as well as LH, do not begin to rise until 10–12 years of age. If the onset of puberty is triggered by the first hormone to increase in the circulation, then a role for

69

adrenal steroids must be considered. However, there is no evidence to suggest that the adrenal steroids are necessary for the proper timing of puberty.

Puberty is associated with the development of episodic LH secretion associated with sleep. At the time of appearance of secondary sex characteristics, the mean LH levels are 2–4 times higher during sleep than during wakefulness, and the number of LH spurts correspond to the number of sleep cycles of rapid and nonrapid eye movements (REM and NREM). This pattern is not present before or after puberty, and is an early sign of changes taking place in the hypothalamus. This pattern can be detected in individuals who develop increasing and decreasing degrees of hypothalamic suppression (such as in individuals with worsening and improving anorexia nervosa). FSH levels plateau by mid-puberty while LH and estradiol levels continue to rise until late puberty.

The rise of gonadotropins at puberty is somewhat independent of the gonads in that the same response can be observed in patients with gonadal dysgenesis (who lack functional steroid-producing gonadal tissue). Adolescent girls with Turner's syndrome (45,X) also demonstrate augmented gonadotropin secretion during sleep. Thus, maturation at puberty must involve changes in the hypothalamus which are independent of ovarian steroids. (27)

The maturational change in the hypothalamus is followed by an orderly and predictable sequence of events. Increased GnRH secretion leads to increased pituitary responsiveness to GnRH, leading to increasing production and secretion of gonadotropins. Increased gonadotropins are responsible for follicular growth and development in the ovary and increased sex steroid levels. The rising estrogen may contribute to achieving an adult pattern of pulsatile GnRH secretion, finally leading to cyclic menstrual patterns.

The trend toward lowering of the menarcheal age and the period of acceleration of growth appears to have halted. In a 10-year prospective study of middle class contemporary American girls, the mean age of menarche was 12.83 with a range of 9.14–17.70. (28) The age of onset of puberty is variable and influenced by genetic factors, socioeconomic conditions, and general health. The earlier menarche in this decade when compared to past decades is undoubtedly due to improved nutrition and better health. It has been suggested that initiation of growth and menarche occur at a particular body weight (48 kg) and percent of body fat (17%). (29) It is thought that this relationship reflects a required stage of metabolism. Although the hypothesis of a critical weight is a helpful concept, the extreme variability in onset of menarche indicates that there is no particular age or size at which an individual girl should be expected to experience menarche.

70

In the female, the typical sequence of events is growth initiation, thelarche, pubarche, and finally menarche. This generally begins sometime between 8 and 14 years of age. The length of time involved in this evolution is usually 2–4 years. During this time span, puberty is said to occur. Individual variation in the order of appearance of this sequence is great. For example, growth of pubic hair and breast development are not always correlated.

If the systems are potentially responsive, what holds function in check until puberty? The hypothalamic-pituitary-gonadal system is operative prior to puberty, but extremely sensitive to steroids, and therefore suppressed. The changes at puberty are due to a gradually increasing gonadotropin secretion which takes place because of a decrease in the sensitivity of the hypothalamic centers to the negative-inhibitory action of gonadal steroids. This can be pictured as a slowly rising set point of decreased sensitivity, resulting in increasing GnRH pulsatile secretion, leading to increasing gonadotropin production and ovarian stimulation, and finally increasing estrogen levels. The reason that FSH is the first gonadotropin to rise at puberty is that arcuate activity begins with a low frequency of GnRH pulses. This is associated with a rise in FSH and little change in LH. With acceleration of frequency, FSH and LH reach adult levels.

Negative feedback of steroids cannot be the sole explanation for the low gonadotropin levels in children. Agonadal children show the same decline in gonadotropins from age 2 to 6 as do normal children. (30) This suggests an intrinsic CNS inhibitory mechanism independent of gonadal steroids. Therefore, the restraint of puberty can be viewed as the result of two forces:

1. A CNS inhibitory force, a mechanism suppressing GnRH pulsatile secretion.

2. A very sensitive negative feedback of gonadal steroids.

Agonadal children show a rise in gonadotropins at pubertal age following suppression to a nadir during childhood. Thus, the dominant mechanism must be a CNS inhibitory force. The initial maturational change in the hypothalamus would then be a decrease in this inhibitory influence. A possible mechanism would be prepubertal suppression of GnRH by opioid inhibition of GnRH neurons. A genetically determined maturational change in the hypothalamus at the time of puberty would lead to decreased opioid activity and increasing GnRH pulses.

The development of the positive feedback response to estrogens occurs later. This could explain the well-known finding of anovulation in the first months (as long as 18 months) of menstruation. There are frequent exceptions, however, and ovulation can occur even at the time of menarche.

71

The overall result of this change in the hypothalamus is the development of secondary sex characteristics, attainment of adult set point levels, and the ability to reproduce. Neoplastic and vascular disorders which alter hypothalamic sensitivity may reverse the prepubertal threshold restraint and lead to precocious puberty. If necessary, pituitary responsiveness to GnRH can differentiate between true idiopathic precocious puberty and precocity due to estrogen secretion from a tumor. Girls with estrogen secreting cysts or tumors have suppressed or prepubertal gonadotropin responses to GnRH while girls with true idiopathic precocious puberty have adult type LH responses. (31)

References

1. **Silverman AJ, Antunes JL, Ferin M, Zimmerman EA,** The distribution of LHRH in the hypothalamus of the rhesus monkey. Light microscopic studies using immunoperoxidase technique, Endocrinology 101:134, 1977.

2. **Nakai Y, Plant TM, Hess DL, Keogh EJ, Knobil E,** On the sites of the negative and positive feedback actions of estradiol in the control of gonadotropin secretion in the rhesus monkey, Endocrinology 102:1008, 1978.

3. **Knobil E,** The neuroendocrine control of the menstrual cycle, Recent Prog Horm Res 36:53, 1980.

4. **Santen RJ, Ruby EB,** Enhanced frequency and magnitude of episodic LH-releasing hormone discharge as a hypothalamic mechanism for increased LH secretion, J Clin Endocrinol Metab 48:315, 1979.

5. **Smith CG, Besch NF, Smith RG, Besch PK,** Effect of tetrahydrocannabinol on the hypothalamic-pituitary axis in the ovariectomized rhesus monkey, Fertil Steril 31:335, 1979.

6. **Asch RH, Smith CG, Siler-Khodr TM, Pauerstein CJ,** Effects of Δ^9-tetrahydrocannabinol during the follicular phase of the rhesus monkey (*Macaca mulatta*), J Clin Endocrinol Metab 52:50, 1981.

7. **Snyder SH,** Brain peptides as neurotransmitters, Science 209:976, 1980.

8. **Krieger DT, Liotta AS, Brownstein MJ, Zimmerman EA,** ACTH, β-lipotropin, and related peptides in brain, pituitary, and blood, Recent Prog Horm Res 36:277, 1980.

9. **Wilkes MM, Watkins WB, Stewart RD, Yen SSC,** Localization and quantitation of β-endorphin in human brain and pituitary, Neuroendocrinology 30:113, 1980.

10. **Robert JF, Quigley ME, Yen SSC,** Endogenous opiates modulate pulsatile luteinizing hormone release in humans, J Clin Endocrinol Metab 52:583, 1981.

11. **Quigley ME, Sheehan KL, Casper RF, Yen SSC,** Evidence for an increased dopaminergic and opioid activity in patients with hypothalamic hypogonadotropic amenorrhea, J Clin Endocrinol Metab 50:949, 1980.

12. **Fishman J, Norton B,** Brain catecholestrogens: formation and possible functions, Adv Biosci 15:123, 1975.

13. **Dierick K, Vandesdande F,** Immunocytochemical demonstration of separate vasopressin-neurophysin and oxytocin neurophysin neurons in the human hypothalamus, Cell Tissue Res 196:203, 1979.

14. **Brownstein MJ, Russell JT, Gainer H,** Synthesis, transport, and release of posterior pituitary hormones, Science 207:373, 1980.

15. **Amico JA, Seif SM, Robinson AG,** Elevation of oxytocin and the oxytocin-associated neurophysin in the plasma of normal women during midcycle, J. Clin Endocrinol Metab 53:1229, 1981.

16. **Dawood MY, Raghavan KS, Pociask C, Fuchs F,** Oxytocin during human pregnancy and parturition, Obstet Gynecol 51:138, 1978.

17. **Ferin M, Rosenblatt H, Carmel PW, Antunes JL, VandeWiele RL,** Estrogen-induced gonadotropin surges in female rhesus monkeys after pituitary stalk section, Endocrinology 104:50, 1979.

18. **Yen SSC, Lein A,** The apparent paradox of the negative and positive feedback control system on gonadotropin secretion, Am J Obstet Gynecol 126:942, 1976.

19. **Adams TE, Norman RL, Spies HG,** Gonadotropin-releasing hormone receptor binding and pituitary responsiveness in estradiol-primed monkeys, Science 213:1388, 1981.

20. **Marut EL, Williams RF, Cowan BD, Lynch A, Lerner SP, Hodgen GD,** Pulsatile pituitary gonadotropin secretion during maturation of the dominant follicle in monkeys: estrogen positive feedback enhances the biological activity of LH, Endocrinology 109:2270, 1981.

21. **Norman RL, Gliessman P, Lindstrom SA, Hill J, Spies HG,** Reinitiation of ovulatory cycles in pituitary-stalk-sectioned Rhesus macaques: evidence for a specific hypothalamic message for the preovulatory release of luteinizing hormone, Endocrinology 111:1874, 1982.

22. **Chang RJ, Jaffe RB,** Progesterone effects on gonadotropin release in women pretreated with estradiol, J Clin Endocrinol Metab 47:119, 1978.

23. **Wildt L, Hutchison JS, Marshall G, Pohl CR, Knobil E,** On the site of action of progesterone in the blockade of the estradiol-induced gonadotropin discharge in the rhesus monkey, Endocrinology 109:1293, 1981.

24. **Cardinali DP,** Melatonin. A mammalian pineal hormone, Endocr Rev 2:327, 1981.

25. **McClintock MK,** Menstrual synchrony and suppression, Nature 229:244, 1971.

26. **Ojeda SR, Andrews WW, Advis JP, White SS,** Recent advances in the endocrinology of puberty, Endocr Rev 1:228, 1980.

27. **Boyar RM, Ramsey J, Chapman J, Fevere M, Madden J, Marks JF,** Luteinizing hormone and follicle-stimulating hormone secretory dynamics in Turner's syndrome, J Clin Endocrinol Metab 47:1078, 1978.

28. **Zacharias L, Rand WM, Wurtman RJ,** A prospective study of sexual development and growth in American girls: the statistics of menarche, Obstet Gynecol Surv 31:325, 1976.

29. **Frisch RE,** Pubertal adipose tissue: is it necessary for normal sexual maturation? Evidence from the rat and human female, Fed Proc 39:2395, 1980.

30. **Conte FA, Grumbach MM, Kaplan SL, Reiter EO,** Correlation of luteinizing hormone-releasing factor, induced luteinizing hormone and follicle-stimulating hormone release from infancy to 19 years with the changing pattern of gonadotropin secretion in agonadal patients: relation to the restraining of puberty, J Clin Endocrinol Metab 50:163, 1980.

31. **Zipf WB, Kelch RP, Hopwood NJ, Spencer ML, Bacon GE,** Suppressed responsiveness to gonadotropin-releasing hormone in girls with unsustained isosexual precocity, J Pediatr 95:38, 1979.

3 Regulation of the Menstrual Cycle

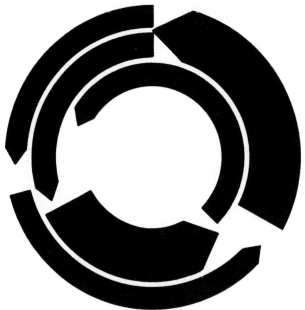

Diagnosis and management of abnormal menstrual function must be based upon an understanding of the physiologic mechanisms involved in the regulation of the normal cycle. Dynamic relationships exist between the pituitary and gonadal hormones which allow for the cyclic nature of normal reproductive processes. These hormonal changes are correlated with morphologic changes in the ovary, making the coordination of this system one of the most remarkable events in biology.

The menstrual cycle can be best described by dividing the cycle into three phases: the follicular phase, ovulation, and the luteal phase. *We will examine each of these phases, concentrating on the changes in ovarian and pituitary hormones, what governs the pattern of hormonal changes, and the effects of these hormones on the ovary, pituitary, and hypothalamus in regulating the menstrual cycle.*

Follicular Phase

During the follicular phase an orderly sequence of events takes place which ensures that the proper number of follicles is ready for ovulation. In the human ovary the end result of this follicular development is (usually) one surviving mature follicle. This process, which occurs over the space of 10–14 days, features a series of sequential actions of hormones on the follicle, leading the follicle destined to ovulate through a period of initial growth from a primordial follicle through the stages of the preantral, antral, and preovulatory follicle.

The Primordial Follicle

The primordial follicle consists of an oocyte, arrested in the diplotene stage of meiotic prophase, surrounded by a single layer of granulosa cells. Follicular growth is a process, best described by Peters as a continuum. (1) Until their numbers are exhausted, follicles begin to grow under all physiologic circumstances. Growth is not interrupted by pregnancy, ovulation, or periods of anovulation. Growth continues at all ages, including infancy and around the menopause.

The number of follicles which starts growing each cycle is probably dependent upon the size of the residual pool of inactive follicles. (1) Reducing the size of the pool (e.g. unilateral oophorectomy) causes the remaining follicles to redistribute their availability over time. The mechanism for determining which follicles or how many will develop during any one cycle is unknown. It is possible that the follicle which is singled out to play the leading role in a particular cycle is the beneficiary of a timely match of follicle "readiness" and appropriate tropic hormone stimulation. The first follicle able to respond to stimulation may achieve an early lead which it never relinquishes.

The initiation of follicular growth appears to be independent of gonadotropin stimulation. In the vast majority of instances this growth is limited and rapidly followed by atresia. The general pattern is interrupted at the beginning of the menstrual cycle when a group of follicles responds to a hormonal change and is propelled to further growth. The most important hormonal event at this time is a rise in the follicle-stimulating hormone (FSH). Indeed, follicular growth may have begun in the waning days of the previous luteal phase, when the regressing corpus luteum secretes diminishing amounts of steroids. The decline in luteal phase steroidogenesis allows the rise in FSH which rescues a group of follicles from atresia.

The Preantral Follicle

Once growth is initiated, the follicle progresses to the preantral stage as the oocyte enlarges and is surrounded by a membrane, the zona pellucida. The granulosa cells undergo a multilayer proliferation as the thecal layer begins to organize from the surrounding stroma. This growth is dependent upon gonadotropins and is correlated with increasing production of estrogen.

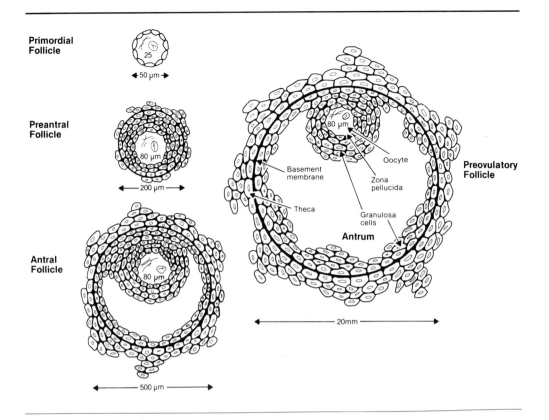

Primordial Follicle

25

←50 µm→

Preantral Follicle

80 µm

←200 µm→

Antral Follicle

80 µm

←500 µm→

80 µm

Oocyte

Basement membrane

Zona pellucida

Theca

Granulosa cells

Antrum

Preovulatory Follicle

←20mm→

The granulosa cells of the preantral follicle have the ability to synthesize all three classes of steroids; however, significantly more estrogens than either androgens or progestins are produced. An aromatase enzyme system acts to convert androgens to estrogens and appears to be a factor limiting ovarian estrogen production. Aromatization is induced or activated through the action of FSH. Specific receptors for FSH are present on preantral granulosa cells and, in the presence of FSH, the preantral follicle can aromatize limited amounts of androgen and generate its own estrogenic microenvironment. (2) Estrogen production is, therefore, also limited by FSH receptor content. The administration of FSH will raise the concentration of its own receptor on granulosa cells both in vivo and in vitro. (3) In addition, FSH combines with estrogen to exert a mitogenic action on granulosa cells to stimulate their proliferation. Together, FSH and estrogen promote a rapid accumulation of FSH receptors which reflects both an increase in the number of granulosa cells and a change in the receptor density of individual cells.

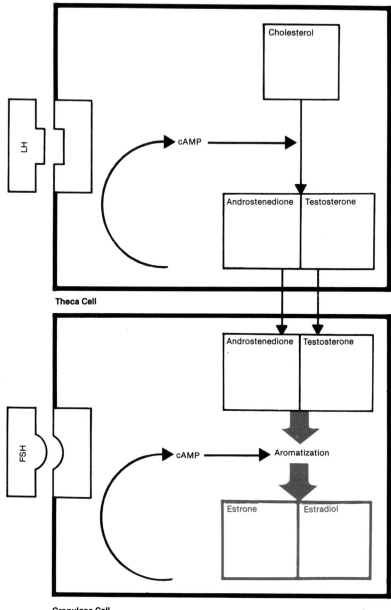

Theca Cell

Granulosa Cell

The role of androgens in early follicular development is complex. Specific androgen receptors have been identified in the cytoplasm of granulosa cells. Serving not only as substrate for FSH-induced aromatization, the androgens may also further enhance aromatase activity, an effect which can be blocked by preventing nuclear translocation of the androgen-receptor complex. (4, 5) When placed in an androgen-rich environment in vitro, however, preantral granulosa cells actually favor the conversion of androstenedione to more potent androgens rather than to estrogens. (6) Products include 5α-reduced androgens such as dihydrotestosterone and androstanedione. These androgens cannot be converted to estrogen, and in fact, may inhibit aromatase activity. (7)

The fate of the preantral follicle is in delicate balance. At low concentrations, androgens enhance their own aromatization and contribute to estrogen production. At higher levels, the limited capacity of aromatization is overwhelmed and the follicle becomes androgenic and ultimately atretic. Perhaps follicles will progress in development only if emerging when FSH is elevated and luteinizing hormone (LH) is low. Those follicles arising late in the luteal phase or early in a subsequent cycle would be favored by an environment in which aromatization in the granulosa cell can prevail. *The success of a follicle depends upon its ability to convert an androgen microenvironment to an estrogen microenvironment.*

Summary of events in the preantral follicle:

1. Initial follicular growth occurs independent of hormonal influence.

2. FSH stimulation propels follicles to the preantral stage.

3. FSH-induced aromatization of androgen in the granulosa results in the production of estrogen.

4. Together, FSH and estrogen increase the FSH receptor content of the follicle.

The Antral Follicle

Under the synergistic influence of estrogen and FSH there is an increase in the production of follicular fluid which accumulates in the intercellular spaces of the granulosa, eventually coalescing to form a cavity, as the follicle makes its gradual transition to the antral stage. The accumulation of follicular fluid provides a means whereby the oocyte and surrounding granulosa cells can be nurtured in a specific endocrine environment for each follicle.

FSH is detectable in follicular fluid when estrogen concentrations exceed those of androgens. Conversely, in the absence of FSH, androgens predominate. (8) LH is not normally present in follicular fluid until, or just, after the midcycle surge. If LH is prematurely elevated in plasma and antral fluid, mitotic activity in the granulosa decreases, degenerative changes ensue, and intrafollicular androgen levels rise. Therefore, the presence of estrogen and FSH in antral fluid is essential for sustained accumulation of granulosa cells and continued follicular growth. Antral follicles with the greatest rates of granulosa proliferation contain the highest estrogen concentrations, the lowest androgen/estrogen ratios, and are most likely to house a healthy oocyte. An androgenic milieu antagonizes estrogen-induced granulosa proliferation and, if sustained, promotes degenerative change in the oocyte.

The steroids present in follicular fluid can be found in concentrations often several orders of magnitude higher than those in plasma and reflect the functional capacity of the surrounding granulosa and thecal cells. The synthesis of steroid hormones is functionally compartmentalized within the follicle—the two-cell mechanism. (9–13)

Though each compartment (theca and granulosa) retains the ability to produce progestins, androgens, and estrogens, the aromatase activity of the granulosa far exceeds that observed in the theca.

In the antral follicle, LH receptors are present only on the thecal cells and FSH receptors only on the granulosa cells. In response to LH, thecal tissue is stimulated to produce androgens which can then be converted, through FSH-induced aromatization, to estrogens in the granulosa cells.

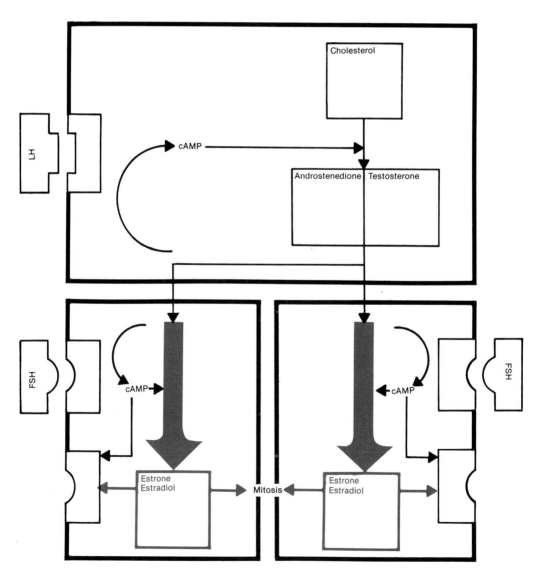

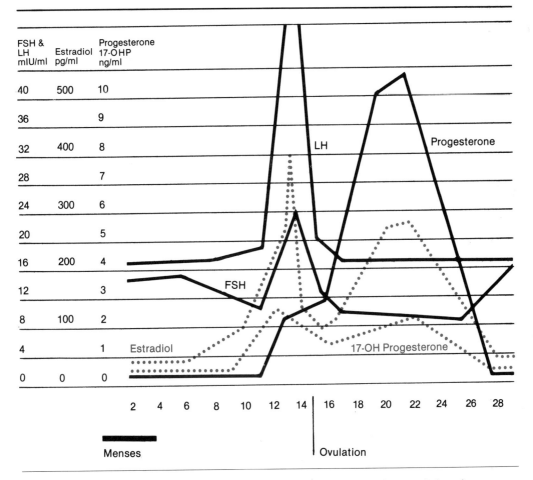

FSH & LH mIU/ml	Estradiol pg/ml	Progesterone 17-OHP ng/ml
40	500	10
36		9
32	400	8
28		7
24	300	6
20		5
16	200	4
12		3
8	100	2
4		1
0	0	0

LH

Progesterone

FSH

Estradiol

17-OH Progesterone

2   4   6   8   10   12   14   16   18   20   22   24   26   28

Menses

Ovulation

The interaction between the granulosa and thecal compartments, with resulting accelerated estrogen production, is not fully functional until later in antral development. Like preantral granulosa cells, the granulosa of small antral follicles exhibits an in vitro tendency to convert significant amounts of androgen to the more potent 5α-reduced form. In contrast, granulosa cells isolated from large antral follicles readily and preferentially metabolize androgens to estrogens. The conversion from an androgen microenvironment to an estrogen microenvironment (a conversion essential for further growth and development) is dependent upon a growing sensitivity to FSH because of the rapid accumulation of FSH receptors in the granulosa layer brought about by the combined action of FSH and estrogen.

The successful conversion to an estrogen dominant follicle marks the "selection" of a follicle destined to ovulate, a process whereby, with rare exception, only a single follicle succeeds. This selection process is the result of two estrogen actions: 1) a local interaction between estrogen and FSH within the follicle, and 2) the effect of estrogen on pituitary secretion of FSH. While estrogen exerts a positive influence on FSH action within the maturing follicle, its negative feedback relationship with FSH at the hypothalamic-pituitary level serves to withdraw gonadotropin support from the other less developed follicles. (14) The fall in FSH leads

81

to a decline in FSH-dependent aromatase activity, limiting estrogen production in the less mature follicles. Even if a lesser follicle succeeds in achieving an estrogen environment, decreasing FSH support would interrupt granulosa proliferation and function, promote a conversion to an androgenic microenvironment, and thereby induce irreversible atretic change. Indeed, the first event in the process of atresia is a reduction in FSH receptors in the granulosa layer.

An asymmetry in ovarian estrogen production, an expression of the emerging dominant follicle, can be detected in ovarian venous effluent as early as cycle day 5–7, corresponding with the gradual fall of FSH levels observed at midfollicular phase. (15) This is a crucial time in the cycle. Exogenous estrogen, administered even after selection of the dominant follicle, disrupts preovulatory development and induces atresia by reducing FSH levels below the sustaining level. (16) Because the lesser follicles have entered the process of atresia, loss of the dominant follicle during this period of time requires beginning over, with recruitment of another set of preantral follicles. (17)

The negative feedback of estrogen on FSH serves to inhibit the development of all but the dominant follicle, but the selected follicle remains dependent on FSH and must complete its preovulatory development in the face of declining plasma levels of FSH. The dominant follicle, therefore, must escape the consequences of FSH suppression induced by its own accelerating estrogen production. The dominant follicle has a significant advantage, a greater content of FSH receptors acquired because of a rate of granulosa proliferation that surpasses that of its cohorts. As a result, the stimulus for aromatization, FSH, can be maintained, while at the same time it is being withdrawn from among the less developed follicles. A wave of atresia among the lesser follicles is therefore seen to parallel the rise in estrogen.

In addition, the accumulation of a greater mass of granulosa cells is accompanied by advanced development of the thecal vasculature. By day 9, thecal vascularity in the dominant follicle is twice that of other antral follicles. (18) This may allow a preferential delivery of FSH to the follicle. These events allow the dominant follicle to retain FSH responsiveness and permit continued development and function despite waning gonadotropin levels.

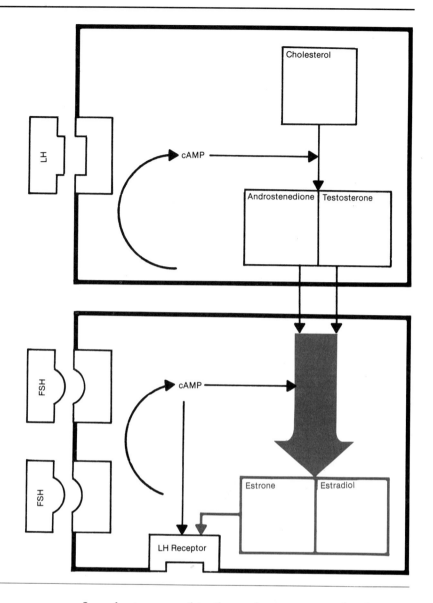

In order to respond to the ovulatory surge and to become a successful corpus luteum, the granulosa cells must acquire LH receptors. FSH induces LH receptor development on the granulosa cells of the large antral follicles. Here again estrogen serves as the chief coordinator. With increasing concentrations of estrogen within the follicle, FSH changes its focus of action, from its own receptor to the LH receptor. The capacity for continued response to declining levels of FSH and a high local estrogen environment in the dominant follicle provide optimal conditions for LH receptor development.

Although prolactin is always present in follicular fluid, there is no evidence to suggest that prolactin is important during normal ovulatory cycles in the primate.

The Feedback System. Through its own estrogen production, the dominant follicle assumes control of its own destiny. By altering gonadotropin secretion through feedback mechanisms it optimizes its own environment to the detriment of the lesser follicles.

As reviewed in Chapter 2, gonadotropin releasing hormone (GnRH) plays only a permissive, though obligatory, role in the control of gonadotropin secretion. The pattern of gonadotropin secretion observed in the menstrual cycle is the result of feedback modulation of steroids originating in the dominant follicle, acting directly on the anterior pituitary. Experimental evidence suggests that the estrogen positive feedback mechanism involves an increase in GnRH receptor concentration, while the negative feedback action operates through a different and uncertain system. (19) Estrogen exerts its inhibitory effects in both the hypothalamus and the anterior pituitary, decreasing both GnRH secretion and GnRH response. (20) Progesterone also operates in two sites. Its inhibitory action is at the hypothalamic level, and, like estrogen, its positive action is directly on the pituitary. (21)

The secretion of FSH is very sensitive to the negative inhibitory effects of estrogen even at low levels. At higher levels, suppression of FSH is profound and sustained. In contrast, the influence of estrogen on LH release varies with concentration and duration of exposure. At low levels, estrogen commands a negative feedback relationship with LH. At higher levels, however, estrogen is also capable of exerting a positive stimulatory feedback effect on LH release.

The transition from suppression to stimulation of LH release occurs as estradiol rises during the midfollicular phase. There are two critical features in this mechanism: 1) the concentration of estradiol and 2) the length of time during which the estradiol elevation is sustained. In women, the estradiol concentration necessary to achieve a positive feedback is over 200 pg/ml, and this concentration must be sustained for approximately 50 hours. (22) The estrogen stimulus must be applied until after the surge actually begins. Otherwise, the LH surge is abbreviated or fails to occur at all.

Further suppression of FSH is attributed to a nonsteroidal inhibitor present in follicular fluid. Folliculostatin is a peptide synthesized by granulosa cells and secreted into the follicular fluid and ovarian venous effluent. It is capable of exerting suppressive action on FSH and may participate in the changes observed in the menstrual cycle. (23) A loss of this peptide due to old follicles of low quality may explain the rise in FSH seen in the perimenopausal period despite the continued presence of menstrual bleeding. Furthermore, the inability to suppress gonadotropins to a normal range during estrogen replacement therapy may be due to the absence of folliculostatin.

84

Variation in the pattern of gonadotropin release is the result of the feedback modulation of gonadal steroids. Within the well-established monthly pattern, the gonadotropins are secreted in a pulsatile fashion with a frequency and magnitude that vary with the phase of the cycle. Pulsatile increments in gonadotropin release occur every 60–90 minutes throughout most of the cycle but decrease in frequency to every 3 or 4 hours during the mid and late luteal phase. Pulse amplitude is greatest during the midcycle surge and least in the late follicular phase. The pulsatile pattern is directly due to a similar pulsatile secretion of GnRH, but amplitude and frequency modulation is probably the consequence of steroid feedback.

There is another, newly appreciated action of estrogen. A disparity exists between the patterns of LH secretion during the gonadotropin surge as determined by radioimmunoassay and bioassay, suggesting that the LH released at midcycle is a more biologically active molecule than that secreted at other times in the cycle. (24) This behavior, bioactivity vs. immunoactivity, is determined by the molecular structure of the gonadotropin molecule, a concept referred to in Chapter 1 as heterogeneity of the tropic hormone. There is a well-established relationship between the activity and half-life of glycoprotein hormones and their sialic acid content. The feedback effects of estrogen include modulation of sialylation and the size and activity of the gonadotropins subsequently released. It certainly makes sense to intensify the gonadotropin effect at midcycle. The positive feedback action of estrogen therefore, both increases the quantity and the quality (the bioactivity) of LH.

Summary of events in the antral follicle.

1. Peripheral levels of estradiol begin to rise significantly by cycle day 7, shortly after the process of selection of the dominant follicle has occurred.

2. Derived primarily from the dominant follicle, estradiol levels increase steadily and, through negative feedback effects, exert progressively greater suppressive influence on FSH release.

3. While directing a decline in FSH levels, the midfollicular rise in estradiol exerts a positive feedback influence on LH.

4. LH levels rise steadily during the late follicular phase, stimulating androgen production in the theca.

5. A unique responsiveness to FSH allows the dominant follicle to utilize the androgen as substrate and further accelerate estrogen production.

6. Enhanced by increasing exposure to estrogen, FSH induces the appearance of LH receptors on granulosa cells.

7. The positive action of estrogen also includes a modulation of the gonadotropin molecule, increasing the quality (the bioactivity) as well as the quantity of LH at midcycle.

The Preovulatory Follicle

Granulosa cells in the preovulatory follicle enlarge and acquire lipid inclusions while the theca becomes vacuolated and richly vascular, giving the preovulatory follicle a hyperemic appearance. The oocyte resumes meiosis, approaching completion of its reduction division.

Approaching maturity, the preovulatory follicle produces increasing amounts of estrogen. During the late follicular phase, estrogens rise slowly at first, then rapidly, reaching a peak approximately 24–36 hours prior to ovulation. (25) Concomitant with the rise in estrogens there is a decline in FSH to its nadir. In contrast LH increases steadily, and then rapidly in a surge-like burst at midcycle, accompanied by a lesser but similar surge of FSH. In the absence of FSH or adequate estrogen, follicles respond to an LH bolus with atresia rather than luteinization. The premature administration of human chorionic gonadotropin (HCG) (as used for the induction of ovulation) may disrupt development and result in the failure of ovulation. (26) In providing the ovulatory stimulus to the selected follicle, the LH surge may serve to seal the fate of the remaining follicles with their lower estrogen and FSH content.

Acting through its own receptors, LH promotes luteinization of the granulosa, resulting in the production of progesterone. An increase in progesterone can be detected in the venous effluent of the ovary bearing the preovulatory follicle 24–48 hours before ovulation. (15) A significant rise in circulating levels of progesterone occurs on the day of the LH peak, 12–24 hours prior to ovulation. (27) This small but significant increase in the production of progesterone in the preovulatory period has immense physiologic importance.

Progesterone affects the positive feedback response to estrogen in both a time and dose dependent manner. When introduced after adequate estrogen priming, progesterone facilitates the positive feedback response, and in the presence of subthreshold levels of estradiol can induce a characteristic LH surge. (28–30) Hence, the surprising onset of ovulation occasionally observed in an anovulatory, amenorrheic patient administered a progestin challenge. When administered before the estrogen stimulus or in high doses, progesterone blocks the midcycle LH surge.

In addition to its facilitory action on LH, progesterone at midcycle is responsible for the FSH surge. (29, 30) This action of progesterone can be viewed as a further step in ensuring completion of FSH action on the follicle, specifically making sure that a full complement of LH receptors is in place in the granulosa layer.

When the lesser follicles fail to achieve full maturity and

undergo atresia, the thecal cells return to their origin as a component of stromal tissue, retaining, however, an ability to respond to LH with steroid production. Because the products of thecal tissue are androgens, the increase in stromal tissue in the late follicular phase is associated with a rise in androgen levels in the periphal plasma at midcycle, a 15% increase in androstenedione and a 20% increase in testosterone. (31, 32)

Androgen production at this stage in the cycle may serve two purposes: 1) a local role within the ovary to enhance the process of atresia, and 2) a systemic effect to stimulate libido.

Intraovarian androgens accelerate granulosa cell death and follicular atresia. The mechanism for this action is an interference with estrogen and its vital duties in enhancing FSH action. Therefore, androgens may play a regulatory role in ensuring that only a dominant follicle reaches the point of ovulation.

It is well known that libido can be stimulated by androgens. If the midcycle rise in androgens affects libido, then an increase in sexual activity should coincide with this rise. Previous studies failed to demonstrate a consistent pattern in coital frequency in women because of the effect of male partner initiation. If only sexual behavior initiated by women is studied, a peak in female-initiated sexual activity is seen during the ovulatory phase of the cycle, and no such peak is noted in users of birth control pills. (33) Therefore the midcycle rise in androgens may serve to increase sexual activity at the time most likely to achieve pregnancy.

Summary of events in the preovulatory follicle:

1. Estrogen production becomes sufficient to achieve and maintain peripheral threshold concentrations of estradiol in order to induce the LH surge.

2. Acting through its receptors, LH initiates luteinization and progesterone production in the granulosa layer.

3. The preovulatory rise in progesterone facilitates the positive feedback action of estrogen and is required to induce the midcycle FSH peak.

4. A midcycle increase in local and peripheral androgens occurs, derived from the thecal tissue of lesser, unsuccessful follicles.

Ovulation

The preovulatory follicle, through the elaboration of estradiol, provides its own ovulatory stimulus. Considerable variation in timing exists from cycle to cycle, even in the same woman. A reasonable and accurate estimate places ovulation approximately 10–12 hours after the LH peak and 24–36 hours after peak estradiol levels are attained. (25, 34, 35) The onset of the LH surge appears to be the

87

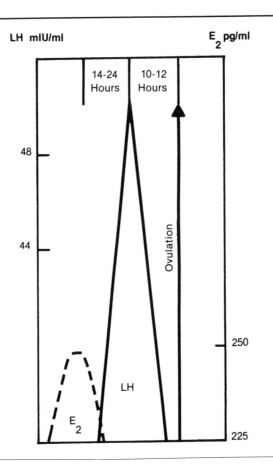

LH mIU/ml   E₂ pg/ml

most reliable indicator of impending ovulation, occurring 28–32 hours prior to follicle rupture.

The LH surge initiates the resumption of meiosis in the oocyte, luteinization of granulosa cells, and the synthesis of prostaglandins essential for follicle rupture. Premature oocyte maturation and luteinization are prevented by local factors. (23) LH-induced cyclic AMP activity overcomes the local inhibitory action of oocyte maturation inhibitor (OMI) and luteinization inhibitor (LI). These nonsteroidal substances are different from folliculostatin in that they act locally rather than through a central mechanism.

With the LH surge, levels of progesterone in the follicle continue to rise up to the time of ovulation. The progressive rise in progesterone may act to terminate the LH surge as a negative feedback effect is exerted at higher concentrations. (36) In addition to its central effects, progesterone may increase the distensibility of the follicle wall. (37) A change in the elastic properties of the follicular wall seems necessary to explain the rapid increase in follicular fluid volume which occurs just prior to ovulation, unaccompanied by any significant change in intrafollicular pressure. The escape of the ovum is associated with degenerative changes of the collagen in the follicular wall so that just prior to ovulation the follicular wall becomes thin and stretched. LH and/or progesterone may enhance the activity of proteolytic enzymes, resulting in digestion of collagen in the follicular wall and increasing its distensibility. Proteolytic enzymes such as collagenase and plasmin are present in follicular fluid and are capable of increasing follicle wall distensibility in vitro.

Prostaglandins of the E and F series increase markedly in the preovulatory follicular fluid, reaching a peak concentration at ovulation. Inhibition of prostaglandin synthesis blocks follicle rupture without affecting the other LH-induced processes of luteinization and oocyte maturation. (38) The mechanism by which prostaglandins induce follicle rupture is unknown. They may act to free lysosomal enzymes which digest the follicular wall. Smooth muscle cells have been identified in the ovary, and prostaglandins may serve to contract this tissue, thereby aiding the extrusion of the oocyte-cumulus cell mass. (39) This role of prostaglan-

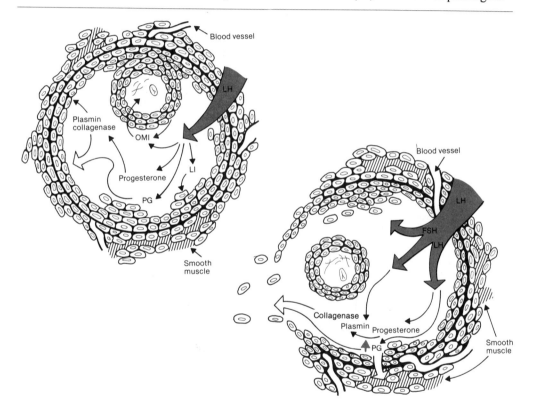

dins is so well demonstrated that infertility patients should be advised to avoid the use of drugs which inhibit prostaglandin synthesis.

Estradiol levels plunge as LH reaches its peak. This may be a consequence of LH down regulation of its own receptors on the follicle. Thecal tissue derived from healthy antral follicles exhibits marked suppression of steroidogenesis when exposed to high levels of LH whereas exposure over a low range stimulates steroid production. (10) The low midcycle level of progesterone exerts an inhibitory action on further granulosa cell multiplication, and the drop in estrogen may also reflect this local follicular role for progesterone.

The FSH peak, dependent on the preovulatory rise of progesterone, may have several functions. Plasminogen activator is required for conversion of plasminogen to the active proteolytic enzyme, plasmin, involved in the breakdown of the follicle wall. Its production is more sensitive to FSH than to LH. (40) Expansion of the cumulus allows the oocyte-cumulus cell mass to become free-floating in the antral fluid just before follicle rupture. The process involves the deposition of a hyaluronic acid matrix, the synthesis of which is stimulated by FSH in vitro. (41) Finally, an adequate FSH peak ensures an adequate complement of LH receptors on the granulosa layer. It should be noted that a shortened or inadequate luteal phase is observed in cycles when FSH levels are low or selectively suppressed at any point during the follicular phase. (42)

The ovulatory period is also associated with a rise in plasma levels of 17α-hydroxyprogesterone. This steroid does not appear to have a role in cyclic regulation, and its appearance in the blood may simply represent the secretion of an intermediate product.

The mechanism that shuts off the LH surge is unknown. Within hours after the rise in LH, there is a precipitous drop in the plasma estrogens. The decrease in LH may be due to a loss of the positive stimulating action of estradiol or to an increasing negative feedback of progesterone. The abrupt fall in LH levels may also reflect a depletion in pituitary LH content due to down regulation of GnRH receptors. Finally, LH may further be controlled by "short" negative feedback of LH upon the hypothalamus. Direct LH suppression of hypothalamic releasing hormone production has been demonstrated.

An adequate gonadotropin surge does not ensure ovulation. The follicle must be at the appropriate stage of maturity in order for it to respond to the ovulating stimulus. In the normal cycle, gonadotropin release and final maturation of the follicle coincide because the timing of the gonadotropin surge is controlled by the level of estradiol, which in turn is a function of follicular growth and maturation. Therefore, gonadotropin release and morphologic maturity are usually coordinated and coupled in time. In the majority of human cycles, the requisite feedback relationships in this system allow only one follicle to reach the point of ovulation.

Multiple births may, in part, reflect the random statistical chance of more than one follicle fulfilling all the requirements for ovulation.

Summary of the ovulatory events:

1. The LH surge stimulates completion of reduction division in the oocyte, luteinization of the granulosa, and synthesis of progesterone and prostaglandins within the follicle.

2. Progesterone enhances the activity of proteolytic enzymes responsible, together with prostaglandins, for digestion and rupture of the follicular wall.

3. The progesterone-dependent midcycle rise in FSH serves to free the oocyte from follicular attachments and to ensure that sufficient LH receptors are present to allow an adequate, normal luteal phase.

Luteal Phase

After rupture of the follicle and release of the ovum, the granulosa cells increase in size, and assume a characteristic vacuolated appearance associated with the accumulation of a yellow pigment, lutein, which lends its name to the process of luteinization and the new anatomical subunit, the corpus luteum. During the first 3 days after ovulation, the granulosa cells enlarge. In addition, theca-lutein cells may differentiate from the surrounding theca and stroma to become part of the corpus luteum. (43)

Capillaries penetrate into the granulosa layer, reaching the central cavity and often filling it with blood. By day 8 or 9 after ovulation, a peak of vascularization is reached, associated with peak levels of progesterone and estradiol in the blood. The primate corpus luteum is unique in that it synthesizes all three classes of sex steroids, androgens, estrogens, and progestins.

Normal luteal function requires optimal preovulatory follicular development. Suppression of FSH during the follicular phase is associated with lower preovulatory estradiol levels, depressed midluteal progesterone production, and a decrease in luteal cell mass. Experimental evidence supports the contention that the accumulation of LH receptors during the follicular phase predetermines the extent of luteinization and the subsequent functional capacity of the corpus luteum. (44) The successful conversion of the avascular granulosa of the follicular phase to the vascularized luteal tissue is also of importance. Because progesterone production is dependent upon low density lipoprotein (LDL) transport of cholesterol, the vascularization of the granulosa layer is essential to allow LDL-cholesterol to reach the luteal cells. (45)

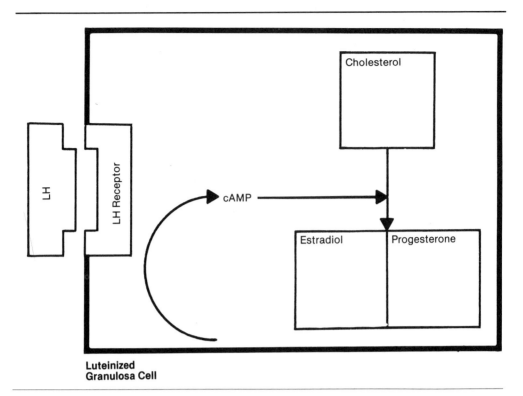

Luteinized
Granulosa Cell

The life span and steroidogenic capacity of the corpus luteum are dependent on continued tonic LH secretion. Studies in hypophysectomized women have clearly demonstrated that normal corpus luteum function requires the continuous presence of small amounts of LH. (46) There is no evidence that other luteotropic hormones, such as prolactin, play a role in the human menstrual cycle.

Progesterone levels normally rise sharply after ovulation reaching a peak approximately 8 days after the LH surge. Progesterone acts both locally and centrally to suppress new follicular growth. If progesterone concentrations are monitored in ovarian venous effluents following luteectomy in the monkey, ovulation in the subsequent cycle uniformly occurs on the side opposite the higher progesterone level and contralateral to the previous corpus luteum. (47) If circulating progesterone levels are maintained after luteectomy, the subsequent ovulation again occurs in the ovary having a lower progesterone concentration in its venous effluent. (48) Because progesterone antagonizes estrogen action (through depletion of estrogen receptors), it is not surprising that estrogen-dependent follicular mechanisms may be inhibited. Initiation of new follicular growth during the luteal phase is further inhibited by the low levels of gonadotropins due to the negative feedback actions of both estrogen and progesterone. Under normal circumstances, therefore, a woman probably ovulates from alternate sides. This mechanism obviously must be overwhelmed when only one ovary is present.

In the normal cycle the time period from the LH midcycle surge to menses is consistently close to 14 days. It is well known that the variability in cycle length among women is due to the varying number of days required for follicular growth and maturation in the follicular phase. The luteal phase cannot be extended indefinitely even with progressively increasing LH exposure, indicating that the demise of the corpus luteum is due to an active luteolytic mechanism.

The corpus luteum rapidly declines 9–11 days after ovulation, and the mechanism of the degeneration remains unknown. In certain nonprimate mammalian species, a luteolytic factor originating in the uterus (probably prostaglandin $F_{2\alpha}$) regulates the life span of the corpus luteum. No definite luteolytic factor has been identified in the primate menstrual cycle; however, the morphologic regression of luteal cells may be induced by the estradiol produced by the corpus luteum. There is considerable evidence to support a role for estrogen in the decline of the corpus luteum. The premature elevation of circulating estradiol levels in the early luteal phase results in a prompt fall in progesterone concentrations. (49) Direct injections of estradiol into the ovary bearing the corpus luteum induces luteolysis while

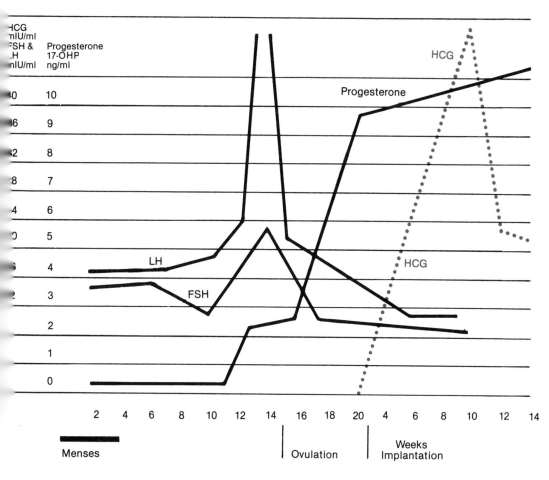

similar treatment of the contralateral ovary produces no effect. (50) Estrogen-induced luteolysis may be due to a prostaglandin-mediated effect on LH receptors, because it can be blocked by inhibiting prostaglandin synthesis. (51, 52)

There is another possible role for the estrogen produced by the corpus luteum. In view of the known estrogen requirement for the synthesis of progesterone receptors, luteal phase estrogen may be necessary to allow the progesterone-induced changes in the endometrium after ovulation. Inadequate progesterone receptor content due to inadequate estrogen priming of the endometrium is an additional possible mechanism for infertility or early abortion, another form of luteal phase deficiency. (53)

Degeneration of the corpus luteum is inevitable unless pregnancy intervenes. With pregnancy, survival of the corpus luteum is prolonged by the emergence of a new stimulus of rapidly increasing intensity, HCG. This new stimulus first appears at the peak of corpus luteum development (9–13 days after ovulation), just in time to prevent luteal regression. (54) HCG serves to maintain the vital steroidogenesis of the corpus luteum until approximately the 9th or 10th week of gestation, by which time placental steroidogenesis is well established. The mechanism appears to be a counter action of the estrogen-induced prostaglandin effect on the adenylate cyclase enzyme, specifically a coupling action as discussed in Chapter 1. (55, 56) In some pregnancies placental steroidogenesis will be sufficiently established as early as the 7th week of gestation.

Summary of events in the luteal phase:

1. Normal luteal function requires optimal preovulatory follicular development and continued tonic LH stimulation.

2. Progesterone acts both centrally and within the ovary to suppress new follicular growth.

3. Regression of the corpus luteum appears to involve the luteolytic action of its own estrogen production, mediated by an alteration in local prostaglandin concentrations.

4. In early pregnancy, HCG maintains luteal function until placental steroidogenesis is well established.

Key Events in the Human Menstrual Cycle

The human menstrual cycle is a recycling system dependent upon essential changes in estradiol levels at key moments in time. Estradiol plays a principal role in the following events:

1. The beginning of the cycle is initiated by a rise in FSH which occurs in response to the decline in estradiol in the preceding luteal phase.

2. Estradiol maintains follicular sensitivity to FSH by aiding FSH in increasing the follicle's content of FSH receptors.

3. At high local concentrations estradiol enhances follicular response to LH by working synergistically with FSH to induce LH receptors.

4. Ovulation is triggered by the rapid peripheral rise in estradiol at midcycle.

5. Regression of the corpus luteum may depend upon its own estradiol production and a local luteolytic effect.

The coordination of this complex system can be understood, therefore, by an appreciation for the essential role of estrogen. The interplay between the follicle and the brain depends upon estradiol functioning as a classic hormone, i.e. to transmit the messages of negative and positive feedback, and also upon the local effect of estradiol within the follicle to insure gonadotropin sensitivity. Events which prevent estrogen production, block estrogen action, or obtund the necessary fluctuations in circulating levels will interfere with the normal reproductive cycle.

References

1. **Peters H, Byskov AG, Himelstein-Graw R, Faber M,** Follicular growth: the basic event in the mouse and human ovary, J Reprod Fertil 45:559, 1975.

2. **McNatty KP, Makris A, DeGrazia C, Osathanondh R, Ryan KJ,** The production of progesterone, androgens, and estrogens by granulosa cells, thecal tissue, and stromal tissue from human ovaries in vitro, J Clin Endocrinol Metab 49:687, 1979.

3. **Richards JS,** Hormonal control of ovarian follicular development: a 1978 perspective, Recent Prog Horm Res 35:343, 1979.

4. **Daniel SAJ, Armstrong DT,** Enhancement of follicle-stimulating hormone-induced aromatase activity by androgens in cultured rat granulosa cells, Endocrinology 107:1027, 1980.

5. **Hillier SG, DeZwart FA,** Evidence that granulosa cell aromatase induction/activation by follicle stimulating hormone is an androgen receptor-regulated process in vitro, Endocrinology 109:1303, 1981.

6. **McNatty KP, Makris A, Reinhold VN, DeGrazia C, Osa-thanondh R, Ryan KJ,** Metabolism of androstenedione by human ovarian tissues in vitro with particular reference to reductase and aromatase activity, Steroids 34:429, 1979.

7. **Hillier SG, Van Den Boogaard AMJ, Reichert LE, Van Hall EV,** Intraovarian sex steroid hormone interactions and the regulation of follicular maturation: aromatization of androgens by human granulosa cells in vitro, J Clin Endocrinol Metab 50:640, 1980.

8. **McNatty KP, Smith DM, Makris A, Osathanondh R, Ryan KJ,** The microenvironment of the human antral follicle: inter-relationships among the steroid levels in antral fluid, the population of granulosa cells, and the status of the oocyte in vivo and in vitro, J Clin Endocrinol Metab 49:851, 1979.

9. **Hillier SG, Reichert LE, Van Hall EV,** Control of preovulatory follicular estrogen biosynthesis in the human ovary, J Clin Endocrinol Metab 52:847, 1981.

10. **McNatty KP, Makris A, Osathanondh R, Ryan KJ,** Thecal tissue from human ovarian follicles in vitro, Steroids 36:53, 1980.

11. **Tsang BK, Armstrong DT, Whitfield JF,** Steroid biosynthesis by isolated human ovarian follicular cells in vitro, J Clin Endocrinol Metab 51:1407, 1980.

12. **Dorrington JH, Armstrong DT,** Effects of FSH on gonadal functions, Recent Prog Horm Res 35:301, 1979.

13. **McNatty KP, Makris A, DeGrazia C, Osathanondh R, Ryan KJ,** Steroidogenesis by recombined follicular cells from the human ovary in vitro, J Clin Endocrinol Metab 51:1286, 1980.

14. **Zeleznik AJ,** Premature elevation of systemic estradiol reduces serum levels of follicle stimulating hormone and lengthens the follicular phase of the menstrual cycle in rhesus monkeys, Endocrinology 109:352, 1981.

15. **diZerega GS, Marut EL, Turner CK, Hodgen GD,** Asymmetrical ovarian function during recruitment and selection of the dominant follicle in the menstrual cycle of the rhesus monkey, J Clin Endocrinol Metab 51:698, 1980.

16. **Clark JR, Dierschke DJ, Wolf RC,** Hormonal regulation of ovarian folliculogenesis in rhesus monkeys: III. Atresia of the preovulatory follicle induced by exogenous steroids and subsequent follicular development, Biol Reprod 25:332, 1981.

17. **diZerega GS, Hodgen GD,** Folliculogenesis in the primate ovarian cycle, Endocr Rev 2:27, 1981.

18. **Zeleznik AJ, Schuler HM, Reichert LE,** Gonadotropin-binding sites in the rhesus monkey ovary: role of the vasculature in the selective distribution of human chronic gonadotropin to the preovulatory follicle, Endocrinology 109:356, 1981.

19. **Adams TE, Norman RL, Spies HG,** Gonadotropin-releasing hormone receptor binding and pituitary responsiveness in estradiol-primed monkeys, Science 213:1388, 1981.

20. **Chappel SC, Resko JA, Norman RL, Spies HG,** Studies in rhesus monkeys on the site where estrogen inhibits gonadotropins: delivery of 17-estradiol to the hypothalamus and pituitary gland, J Clin Endocrinol Metab 52:1, 1981.

21. **Wildt L, Hutchinson JS, Marshall G, Pohl CR, Knobil E,** On the site of action of progesterone in the blockade of the estradiol-induced gonadotropin discharge in the rhesus monkey, Endocrinology 109:1293, 1981.

22. **Young JR, Jaffe RB,** Strength-duration characteristics of estrogen effects on gonadotropin response to gonadotropin-releasing hormone in women: II. Effects of varying concentrations of estradiol, J Clin Endocrinol Metab 42:432, 1976.

23. **Channing CP, Schaerf FW, Anderson LD, Tsafriri A,** Ovarian follicular and luteal physiology, Int Rev Physiol 22:117, 1980.

24. **Marut EL, Williams RF, Cowan BD, Lynch A, Lerner SP, Hodgen GD,** Pulsatile pituitary gonadotropin secretion during maturation of the dominant follicle in monkeys: estrogen positive feedback enhances the biological activity of LH, Endocrinology 109:2270, 1981.

25. **Pauerstein CJ, Eddy CA, Croxatto HD, Hess R, Siler-Khodr TM, Croxatto HB,** Temporal relationships of estrogen, progesterone, and luteinizing hormone levels to ovulation in women and infrahuman primates, Am J Obstet Gynecol 130:876, 1978.

26. **Williams RF, Hodgen GD,** Disparate effects of human chorionic gonadotropin during the late follicular phase in monkeys: normal ovulation, follicular atresia, ovarian acyclicity, and hypersecretion of follicle-stimulating hormone. Fertil Steril 33:64, 1980.

27. **Moghissi KS, Syner FN, Evans TN,** A composite picture of the menstrual cycle, Am J Obstet Gynecol 114:405, 1972.

28. **Terasawa E, Rodriguez-Sierra JF, Dierschke DJ, Bridson WE, Goy RW,** Positive feedback effect of progesterone on luteinizing hormone (LH) release in cyclic female rhesus monkeys: LH response occurs in two phases, J Clin Endocrinol Metab 51:1245, 1980.

29. **March CM, Goebelsmann U, Nakamura RM, Mishell DR,** Roles of estradiol and progesterone in eliciting the midcycle luteinizing hormone and follicle-stimulating hormone surges, J Clin Endocrinol Metab 49:507, 1979.

30. **March CM, Marrs RP, Goebelsmann U, Mishell DR,** Feedback effects of estradiol and progesterone upon gonadotropin and prolactin release, Obstet Gynecol 58:10, 1981.

31. **Judd HL, Yen SSC,** Serum androstenedione and testosterone levels during the menstrual cycle, J Clin Endocrinol Metab 38:475, 1973.

32. **Abraham GE,** Ovarian and adrenal contribution to peripheral androgens during the menstrual cycle, J Clin Endocrinol Metab 39:340, 1974.

33. **Adams DB, Gold AR,** Rise in female-initiated sexual activity at ovulation and its suppression by oral contraceptives, N Engl J Med 229:1145, 1978.

34. **World Health Organization Task Force Investigators,** Temporal relationships between ovulation and defined changes in the concentration of plasma estradiol-17β, luteinizing hormone, follicle stimulating hormone, and progesterone, Am J Obstet Gynecol 138:383, 1980.

35. **Garcia JE, Jones GS, Wright GL,** Prediction of the time of ovulation, Fertil Steril 36:308, 1981.

36. **Helmond FA, Simons PA, Hein PR,** The effects of progesterone on estrogen-induced luteinizing hormone and follicle-stimulating hormone release in the female rhesus monkey, Endocrinology 107:478, 1980.

37. **Peters H, McNatty KP,** *The Ovary*, Ch 6, University of California Press, Los Angeles, 1980, pp 75–84.

38. **O'Grady JP, Caldwell BV, Auletta FJ, Speroff L,** The effects of an inhibitor of prostaglandin synthesis (indomethacin) on ovulation, pregnancy, and pseudopregnancy in the rabbit, Prostaglandins 1:97, 1972.

39. **Virutomosen P, Wright KH, Wallach EE,** Effects of prostaglandin E_2 and $F_{2\alpha}$ on ovarian contractility in the rabbit, Fertil Steril 26:678, 1972.

40. **Stickland S, Beers WH,** Studies on the role of plasminogen activator in ovulation, J Biol Chem 251:5694, 1976.

41. **Eppig JJ,** FSH stimulates hyaluronic acid synthesis by oocyte-cumulus cell complexes from mouse preovulatory follicles, Nature 281:483, 1979.

42. **diZerega GS, Turner CK, Stouffer RL, Anderson LD, Channing CP, Hodgen GD,** Suppression of follicle stimulating hormone-dependent folliculogenesis during the primate ovarian cycle, J Clin Endocrinol Metab 52:451, 1981.

43. **Peters H, McNatty KP,** *The Ovary*, University of California Press, Los Angeles, 1980, pp 12–35.

44. **Stouffer RL, Hodgen GD,** Induction of luteal phase defects in rhesus monkeys by follicular fluid administration at the onset of the menstrual cycle, J Clin Endocrinol Metab 51:669, 1980.

45. **Carr BR, McDonald PC, Simpson ER,** The role of lipoproteins in the regulation of progesterone secretion by the human corpus luteum, Fertil Steril 38:303, 1982.

46. **Vande Wiele RL, Bogumil J, Dyrenfurth I, Ferin M, Jewelewicz R, Warren M, Rizkallah R, Mikhail G,** Mechanisms regulating the menstrual cycle in women, Recent Prog Horm Res 26:63, 1970.

47. **diZerega GS, Lynch A, Hodgen GD,** Initiation of asymmetrical ovarian estradiol secretion in the primate ovarian cycle after luteectomy, Endocrinology 108:1233, 1981.

48. **diZerega GS, Hodgen GD,** The interovarian progesterone gradient: a spatial and temporal regulator of folliculogenesis in the primate ovarian cycle, J Clin Endocrinol Metab 54:495, 1982.

49. **Karsch JF, Krey LC, Weick RF, Dierschke DJ, Knobil E,** Functional luteolysis in the rhesus monkey: the role of estrogen, Endocrinology 92:1148, 1973.

50. **Karsch FJ, Sutton GP,** An intra-ovarian site for the luteolytic action of estrogen in the rhesus monkey, Endocrinology 98:553, 1976.

51. **Auletta FJ, Caldwell BV, Speroff L,** Estrogen-induced luteolysis in the rhesus monkey: reversal with indomethacin, Prostaglandins 11:745, 1976.

52. **Auletta FJ, Agins H, Scommegna A,** Prostaglandin F mediation of the inhibitory effect of estrogen on the corpus luteum of the rhesus monkey, Endocrinology 103:1183, 1978.

53. **Goldstein D, Zuckerman H, Harpaz S, Barkai J, Geva A, Gordon S, Shalev E, Schwartz M,** Correlation between estradiol and progesterone in cycles with luteal phase deficiency, Fertil Steril 37:348, 1982.

54. **Catt KJ, Dufau ML, Vaitukaitis JL,** Appearance of hCG in pregnancy plasma following the initiation of implantation of the blastocyst, J Clin Endocrinol Metab 40:537, 1975.

55. **Behrman HR, Hall AK, Preston SL, Gore SD,** Antagonistic interactions of adenosine and prostaglandin $F_{2\alpha}$ modulate acute responses of luteal cells to luteinizing hormone, Endocrinology 110:38, 1982.

56. **Balmaceda JP,** Effects of hCG on prostaglandin synthesis and function of corpus luteum, Obstet Gynecol 57:505, 1981.

4

The Ovary from Conception to Senescence

The physiologic responsibilities of the ovary are the periodic release of gametes (eggs) (oocytes) and the production of the steroid hormones, estradiol and progesterone. Both activities are integrated in the continuous repetitive process of follicle maturation, ovulation, and corpus luteum formation and regression. The ovary, therefore, cannot be viewed as a relatively static endocrine organ whose size and function expand and contract depending on the vigor of stimulating tropic hormones. Rather, the female gonad is an envelope containing subunits (follicle, corpus luteum, stroma) with different and variable biologic properties, a heterogenous ever-changing tissue whose cyclicity is measured in weeks, rather than hours. The activity of the human ovary at any given time is defined by a single subunit during the brief period of its dominance.

In this chapter, the development and differentiation of the ovary will be described with emphasis on that most critical functioning subunit of the gonad, the follicle. Events within the ovary will be traced from early embryonic formation to final senescent atrophy. Correlations of morphology with reproductive and steroidogenic functions will be emphasized. Finally, the menopause and the rationale for therapy of this physiologic state will be examined in the light of information on endogenous estrogen production and the impact of estrogen on nonreproductive functions of the female.

101

Embryology and Differentiation of the Ovary

During fetal life, the development of the human ovary can be traced through four stages. These are: 1) the indifferent gonadal stage, 2) the differentiation and cortical supremacy state, 3) the period of oogonal multiplication, and finally 4) the stage of follicle formation.

Indifferent Gonadal State

At approximately 5 weeks of intrauterine life, the paired gonads are structurally consolidated prominences overlying the mesonephros, forming the gonadal ridge. At this point, although sexual characterization of this tissue is possible by nuclear sex chromatin studies, the gonad is morphologically indistinguishable as a primordial testis or ovary. The gonad is composed of primitive germ cells intermingled with coelomic surface epithelial cells and an inner core of medullary mesenchymal tissue. Just below this ridge lies the mesonephric duct. The germ cells originate in the primitive endoderm of the yolk sac and hindgut, and are recognizable at this site before the mesonephros is formed. They migrate to the gonadal ridge, the one and only site where they survive, in a journey which is completed by the 5th week. The germ cells are the direct precursors of sperm and ova, and by the 6th week, on completion of the indifferent state, these germ cells have multipled by mitosis to a total of 100,000.

Differentiation and Cortical Supremacy Stage

If the indifferent gonad is destined to become a testis, differentiation along this line will take place at 4–6 weeks. The absence of testicular evolution (formation of medullary primary sex cords, primitive tubules, and incorporation of germ cells) gives implicit evidence of the existence of a primitive, albeit momentarily quiescent, ovary. Despite apparent morphologic inactivity, the cortical dominance over the medulla has been asserted, and estradiol synthesis begins. Although ovarian estrogen is minor compared to the overall production by the placenta, local estrogen may be important in later ovarian differentiation. In contrast to the male, female internal and external genitalia differentiation precedes ovarian maturation. These events are related to the genetic constitution of the germ cells and the territorial receptivity of the mesenchyme. If either factor is deficient or defective, improper development occurs. As has been noted, primitive germ cells appear unable to survive in locations other than the gonadal ridge. If partial or imperfect gonadal tissue is formed, the resulting abnormal nonsteroidal and steroidal events have wide ranging morphologic, reproductive, and behavioral effects. In the indifferent stage, the Müllerian duct system is preserved, and the Wolffian potential is unrealized.

Stage of Oogonal Multiplication and Maturation

At 6–8 weeks, the first signs of ovarian differentiation are expressed by the onset of rapid mitotic multiplication of oogonia, reaching 6–7 million germ cells by 20 weeks. This represents the maximum oogonal content of the gonad. From this point in time germ cell content will irretrievably decrease until, some 50 years later, the store of germ cells will be finally exhausted. The egg depletion process by

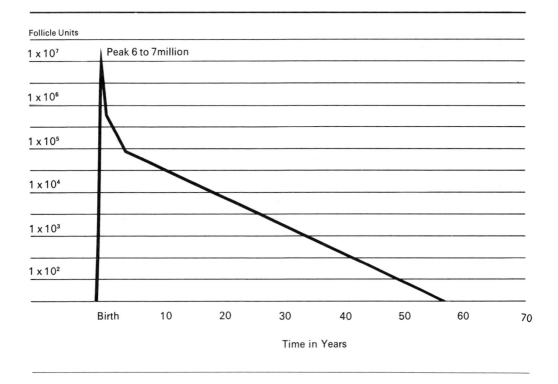

Follicle Units

1×10^7 Peak 6 to 7 million

1×10^6

1×10^5

1×10^4

1×10^3

1×10^2

Birth 10 20 30 40 50 60 70

Time in Years

atresia begins at about 15 weeks of gestation when evidence of nuclear maturation is first seen. The oogonia are transformed to oocytes as they enter the first meiotic division and arrest in prophase.

Stage of Follicle Formation

When nuclear maturation within germ cells becomes noticeable, the gonad is composed of an expanded dense sheet of oogonia and oocytes in huge numbers. At 20 weeks, this highly cellular cortex is gradually perforated by vascular channels originating in the deeper medullary areas. As the finger-like vascular projections enter the cortex, the cortex takes on the appearance of secondary sex cords. As the blood vessels invade and penetrate, they divide the previously solid cortical cell mass into smaller and smaller segments. Drawn in with the blood vessels are perivascular cells which are both mesenchymal and epithelial in origin. These cells surround the oocyte in layers. The resulting unit is the primordial follicle—an oocyte arrested in prophase of meiosis enveloped by a single layer of pregranulosa (primitive epithelial) and an outer less organized matrix of mesenchymal cells (the pretheca cells). Eventually all oocytes are covered in this fashion. Residual mesenchyme not utilized in primordial follicle formation is noted in the interstices between follicles, forming the primitive ovarian stroma. The granulosa cells differentiate from mesonephric precursors, and like the germ cells, they must migrate to the gonadal ridge.

As soon as the oocyte is surrounded by the rosette of pregranulosa cells it may resume meiosis and the entire follicle undergoes variable degrees of maturation before

103

arresting and becoming atretic. These events include in sequence: oocyte cytoplasmic enlargement, eccentric migration of the nucleus, and proliferation of several layers of granulosa cells by mitosis. As a result, a primary follicle is formed. Less frequently, but by no means rarely, further differentiation is expressed as more complete granulosa proliferation. Call-Exner body formation, coalescence to form the antrum, and occasionally a minor thecal layer system may be seen.

Even in fetal life the cycle of follicle formation, variable ripening, and atresia occurs. Although these steps are precisely those typical of adult reproductive life, full maturity, as expressed in ovulation, does not occur. However, the ovary at birth may contain several cystic follicles of varying size, undoubtedly stimulated by the reactive gonadotropin surge accompanying the withdrawal of the neonatal pituitary from negative feedback of massive fetoplacental steroids.

The initiation of follicle maturation and atresia has a profound effect on germ cell endowment. As a result of prenatal follicle differentiation, the total cortical content of germ cells has fallen to 1–2 million by birth. This huge depletion of germ cell mass (close to 4–5 million) has occurred over as short a time as 20 weeks. No similar rate of depletion will be seen again. Studies with the scanning electron microscope have indicated that the major mechanism for the loss of eggs during intrauterine life is elimination through the surface of the ovary into the peritoneal cavity. (1) Clusters of oogonia and oocytes make their way through the ovarian stroma and can be seen emerging from the ovarian surface. Due to the fixed initial endowment of germ cells the newborn female enters life, still far from reproductive potential, having lost 80% of her oocytes.

Neonatal Ovary

At birth, the ovary is approximately 1 cm in diameter, although sizable cystic follicles may enlarge the total dimensions. Compartmentalization of the gonad into cortex and a small residual medulla has been achieved. In the cortex almost all the oocytes are involved in primordial follicle units. Varying degrees of maturation in some units can be seen as in the prenatal state.

Adult Ovary

At the onset of puberty, the germ cell mass has been reduced to 300,000 units. During the next 35–40 years of reproductive life, these units will be depleted further to a point at menopause where only a few thousand units remain. In this period of time the typical cycle of follicle maturation, including ovulation and corpus luteum formation, will be realized. This results from the complex but well-defined sequence of hypothalamic-pituitary-gonadal interactions in which follicle and corpus luteum steroid and pituitary gonadotropin production are integrated to yield ovulation. These important events are described in detail in Chapter 3. For the moment, our attention will be exclusively directed to a description of the events as the gonad is driven inex-

104

orably to final and complete exhaustion of its germ cell supply. The major feature of this reproductive period of the ovary's existence is the full maturational expression of some follicle units in ovulation and corpus luteum formation, and the accompaniment of varying steroid output of estradiol and progesterone. For every follicle which ovulates, close to 1000 will pursue abortive growth periods of variable length.

Follicle Growth

In the adult ovary, the two stages of follicle development noted even in the prenatal period are repeated, but to a more complete degree. Initially the oocyte enlarges and the granulosa cells proliferate markedly. A solid sphere of cells encasing the oocyte is formed. At this point the theca interna is noted in initial stages of formation. The zona pellucida begins to form. In this stage of development gonadotropins must be available, but these events are not the result of an input of gonadotropin (follicle-stimulating hormone (FSH)) activity. If gonadotropin increments are available, as may be seen early in the cycle, a second, gonadotropin-dependent stage of follicle maturation is seen. The number of follicles that mature is dependent on the amount of FSH and luteinizing hormone (LH) available to the gonad and the sensitivity of the follicles to gonadotropins.

The sequence of maturation in this second phase of follicle growth proceeds in the following order. The antrum appears as a coalescence of numerous intragranulosa cavities (Call-Exner bodies). Whether this represents liquefaction or granulosa cell secretion is uncertain. At first the cavity is filled with a coagulum of cellular debris. Soon a liquor accumulates, which is essentially a transudation of blood filtered through the avascular granulosa from the thecal vessels. With antral formation, the theca interna develops more fully, expressed by increased cell mass, increased vascularity, and the formation of lipid-rich cytoplasmic vacuoles within the theca cells. As the follicle expands, the surrounding stroma is compressed and is called the theca externa.

At any point in this development, individual follicles become arrested and eventually regress in the process known as atresia. At first the granulosa component begins to disrupt. The antral cavity constituents are resorbed, and the cavity collapses and obliterates. The oocyte degenerates in situ. Finally, a ribbon-like scarred streak surrounded by theca is seen. Eventually this theca mass loses its lipid and becomes indistinguishable from the growing mass of stroma. Prior to regression, the cystic follicle may be retained in the cortex for variable periods of time.

The local concentrations of estradiol within the microenvironment of the differentiating follicle appear to exert a major influence on the possibility of its emergence as the dominant follicle destined to ovulate. Antral fluid estradiol concentrations increase as a result of interplay between theca and granulosa cells (the two-cell explanation), reviewed in detail elsewhere (Chapters 1 and 3). The relevant issue is that thecal androgen is aromatized to estrogen in granulosa cells. The capacity for aromatization reflects the number of granulosa cells and the biochemical differentiation of the aromatase enzyme system of these cells. These granulosa cell reactions are FSH-induced and catalyzed by local estradiol. The more local estrogen, the more "receptivity" (more cells, more FSH receptors, more aromatase, more estrogen) and the greater the likelihood of that follicle becoming dominant and avoiding atresia. Steroid and peptide concentrations found in human follicle fluid sustain this concept; as the follicle grows, androgens decrease, but FSH and estradiol increase. In anovulation, unruptured follicle cysts contain relatively high androgens and *low* estradiol and FSH.

Local concentrations of estrogen also have been implicated in the mechanism by which, in most cases, only a single unit is selected for the final burst of maturity expressed as ovulation. As FSH quantities diminish prior to ovulation, it appears that the most mature follicle, the most efficient estrogen producer, selectively binds available FSH better than its less successful sisters. As a result, the limited FSH supplies are directed to a single maturing follicle.

Ovulation

Of the several follicle units thrust to varying degrees of maturity, one unit will advance to ovulation if gonadotropin stimulation is adequate. Morphologically these events include distension of the antrum by increments of antral fluid, and compression of the granulosa against the limiting membrane separating the avascular granulosa and the luteinized, vascularized theca interna. In addition, the antral fluid increment gradually pinches off the tongue of granulosa enveloping the oocyte as the cumulus oophorus. The events associated with the thinning of the theca over the surface of the now protruding, distended follicle, the creation of an avascular area weakening the ovarian capsule, and the final acute distension of the antrum with rupture and extrusion of the oocyte in its cumulus, are unknown at this time. Repeated evaluation of intrafollicular pressures has failed to indict an explosive factor in this crucial event.

In a variety of animal experiments, the physical expulsion of the oocyte appears to be dependent upon a preovulatory surge in prostaglandin synthesis within the follicle. (2) Inhibition of this prostaglandin synthesis produces a corpus luteum with an entrapped oocyte. Both prostaglandins and the midcycle surge of gonadotropins are thought to increase the concentration of local proteases, such as plasminogen conversion to plasmin. As a result of generalized tissue weakening (loss of intercellular gap junction integrity and disruption of elastic fibers), there is swift accumulation of antral fluid and rupture of the tissue envelope surrounding the follicle.

Corpus Luteum	Shortly after ovulation profound alterations in cellular organization occur in the ruptured follicle that go well beyond simple repair. After tissue integrity and continuity are retrieved, the granulosa cells hypertrophy markedly, gradually filling in the cystic, sometimes hemorrhagic, cavity of the early corpus luteum. In addition, for the first time the granulosa becomes markedly luteinized by incorporation of lipid-rich vacuoles within its cytoplasm. Also, for the first time, vascularization occurs in the granulosa. Both these properties had been the exclusive features of the theca prior to ovulation. For its part, the theca of the corpus luteum becomes less prominent, vestiges being noted eventually only in the interstices of the typical scalloping of the mature corpus luteum. As a result, a new yellow body is formed now dominated by the enlarged, lipid-rich, fully vascularized granulosa. In the 14 days of its life, dependent on the low but important quantities of LH available in the luteal phase, this unit produces estrogen and progesterone. Failing a new enlarging source of LH-like human chorionic gonadotropin (HCG) from a successful implantation, the corpus luteum rapidly ages. Its vascularity and lipid content wane, and the sequence of scarification (albicantia) ensues.
Correlation of Follicle Maturation, Follicle Availability, and Estrogen Production	If one considers the effects of increments of endogenous estrogen production on the body, certain categorical effects can be seen as varying estrogen thresholds are reached. As biologic levels of estrogen increase, the sequence of formation and maintenance of secondary sexual characteristics, cervical mucus and vaginal cornification, endometrial proliferation and menses, and finally ovulation, is achieved. Each event requiring quantum increments in estrogen production is bound to the evolving, increased maturation of the follicle units.

As we trace estrogen effects over a life span, with increased follicle maturation, female phenotype is asserted early, growth spurt is stimulated, and appearance of secondary sex characteristics is also seen. As individual follicles undergo greater and greater maturity, menarche and the first ovulation are achieved in short order. For the next 30 years, estrogen production and follicle maturation work hand in hand to sustain adult reproductive efficiency via repeated (about 400) monthly ovulations. At this level of steroid production all other estrogen-dependent systems are more than sufficiently sustained.

At approximately age 38–42, ovulation is clinically known to reduce in frequency. It has been suggested that the residual follicle units, now only thousands in number, are the least sensitive to gonadotropin stimulation, and hence are less likely to achieve successful and complete maturation. As numbers of follicle units decrease and resistant factors increase, less and less estrogen is produced from the surviving stimulated units. Eventually the recession in estrogenicity no longer proliferates endometrium to yield menstruation, and menopause ensues. Further retreat in estrogen production threatens even the most basic tissues which are estrogen dependent. |

107

Relative Biological
Levels of Estrogen

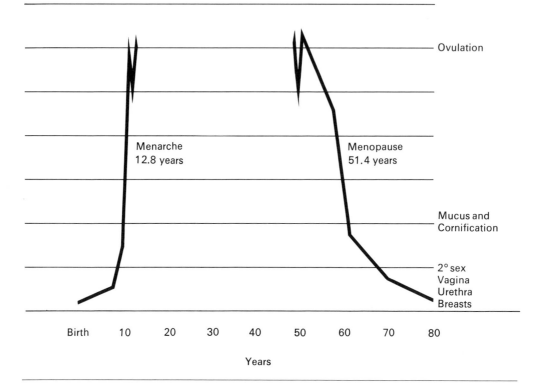

Birth 10 20 30 40 50 60 70 80

Years

At one point during pubescence, enough follicle maturation has yielded sufficient estrogen to cause the first period (menarche). In this respect, menarche is only one point on a curve of ascending estrogen production. Similarly, the climacteric defines a more prolonged period of estrogen withdrawal, starting with the first decrease in frequency of ovulation, and ending in atrophy of secondary sex characteristics. A single point in that curve, when insufficient follicle maturity results in inadequate estrogen and no menses, is the menopause.

Hormone Production after Follicle Exhaustion

Some residual follicles exist within the gonads even after the menopause is reached. Their performance in terms of both steroidogenesis and morphological change is a matter of degree. Even prior to menopause, the remaining follicles begin to perform less well. During the perimenopausal period, women who are having regular periods may have lower estradiol levels and higher levels of FSH, and the cycle begins to change, mainly because of a shortening of the follicular phase. (3) This is a time period during which postmenopausal levels of FSH (greater than 40 mIU/ml) may be seen despite continued menstrual bleeding, while LH levels usually remain in the normal range. It is likely that the elevated FSH levels are an indicator of a significant reduction in the number of follicles remaining, and those remaining have diminished ability to produce estrogen.

Relative Biological
Levels of Estrogen

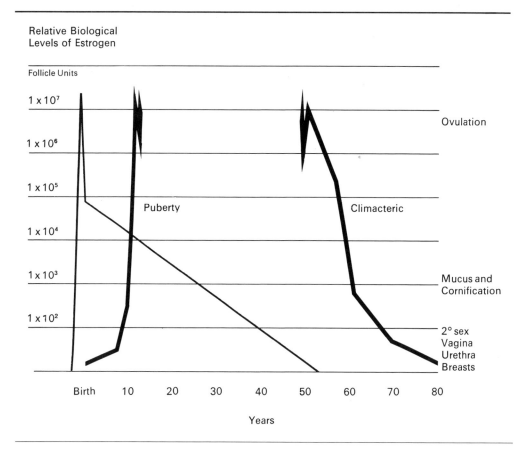

Follicle Units

1×10^7		Ovulation
1×10^6		
1×10^5		
1×10^4	Puberty	Climacteric
1×10^3		Mucus and Cornification
1×10^2		$2°$ sex Vagina Urethra Breasts

Birth   10   20   30   40   50   60   70   80

Years

However, FSH may also be regulated in part by the negative feedback action of a nonsteroid substance (folliculostatin) produced by granulosa cells, a situation which would be similar to the action in the male of inhibin, a peptide produced in the testicular Sertoli cells. Occasionally corpus luteum formation and function occur. As cycles become irregular, vaginal bleeding occurs at the end of an inadequate luteal phase or after a peak of estradiol without subsequent ovulation or corpus luteum formation. Eventually there is a 10–20-fold increase in FSH and approximately a 3-fold increase in LH, reaching a maximum level 1–3 years after menopause, after which there is a gradual and slight decline. Elevated levels of both FSH and LH at this time in life appear to be conclusive evidence of ovarian failure.

After menopause, the circulating level of androstenedione is about one half that seen prior to menopause. (4, 5) Most of this postmenopausal androstenedione is derived from the adrenal gland, with only a small amount secreted from the ovary. Testosterone levels do not fall appreciably, and, in fact, the postmenopausal ovary secretes more testosterone than the premenopausal ovary. (4, 5) With the disappearance of follicles and estrogen, the elevated gonadotropins probably drive the remaining stromal tissue in the ovary to a level of increased testosterone secretion.

The circulating estradiol level after menopause is approximately 10–20 pg/ml, most of which is derived from peripheral conversion of estrone. (6) The circulating level of estrone in the postmenopausal women is higher than that of estradiol, the mean level being approximately 30–70 pg/ml. (5, 6) The average production rate of estrogen is approximately 45 μg/24 hours; almost all, if not all, being estrone derived from the peripheral conversion of adrostenedione. (6, 7) With increasing age, a decrease can be measured in the circulating levels of dehydroepiandrosterone (DHA) and its sulfate (DHAS), whereas the circulating levels of androstenedione, testosterone, and estrogen remain relatively constant. (8).

The percent conversion of androstenedione to estrogen correlates with body weight. (7, 8) Increased production of estrogen from androstenedione with increasing body weight is probably due to the ability of fat to aromatize androgens. This fact may be the basis for the well-known association between obesity and the development of endometrial cancer. Evidence suggests that the actual site for aromatization in fat is not the adipose cell itself, but the surrounding stromal tissue. (9) Body weight, therefore, has a positive correlation with the circulating levels of estrone and estradiol. In addition, obesity, by an unknown mechanism, independently suppresses sex hormone binding globulin (SHBG) levels in both men and women, thus increasing free steroid levels. (10) The increased estrogen impact associated with obesity arises, therefore, from two sources: increased peripheral conversion of androstenedione to estrone, and increased free estrogen levels due to decreased SHBG.

Estrogen production by the ovaries does not continue beyond the menopause; however, estrogen levels in postmenopausal women continue to be significant, principally due to the extraglandular conversion of androstenedione to estrone. The clinical impact of this estrogen will vary from one postmenopausal individual to another, depending upon the degree of extraglandular production, probably modified by a variety of factors.

The two major influences are:

1. An increase in substrate (e.g. stress induced increases in adrenal production of androstenedione).

2. An increase in the percent conversion of androstenedione to estrone (e.g. with an accumulation of adipose tissue).

Estrogen derived from extraglandular production may be sufficient to sustain breasts and estrogen-stimulated surfaces such as urethra and vagina.

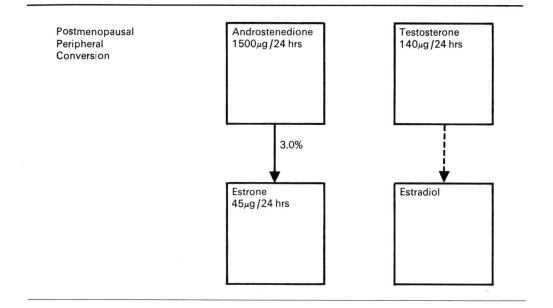

Postmenopausal Peripheral Conversion

Androstenedione 1500μg/24 hrs

Testosterone 140μg/24 hrs

3.0%

Estrone 45μg/24 hrs

Estradiol

Based on this review of the physiology of the perimenopause, particularly with respect to mechanisms of hormone production during this period, the physician gains appreciation for mechanisms involved in the clinical diversity of symptomatology seen in practice. Among these are the mechanisms whereby:

—Young castrates may have more serious risk of long-term estrogen deprivation.
—Postmenopausal women may not display signs of progressive genital atrophy.
—Thin women are more likely to have estrogen deprivation symptoms than are obese women.
—Obese women are more prone to dysfunctional uterine bleeding, endometrial hyperplasia, and neoplasia.
—Hot flushes and elevated gonadotropins may appear before true menopause (and yet be followed by episodes of ovulatory cycles).
—Stress (acute and/or chronic) may induce a menstrual flow in postmenopausal women.
—Hirsutism may recur or primarily appear after the menopause.
—Endometrial hyperplasia and carcinoma may occur in untreated, oophorectomized women.

Eventually, the ovarian stroma is exhausted and, despite huge reactive homeostatic increments in FSH and LH, no further steroidogenesis of importance results from gonadal activity. With increasing age, the adrenal contribution of precursors for estrogen production proves inadequate. In this final stage of estrogen availability, levels are insufficient to sustain secondary sex tissues.

The Premenstrual Syndrome. It is commonly recognized that behavioral changes may be associated with the menstrual cycle. The first description of this syndrome is attributed to Frank in 1931. The definition appears to be a common sense description: symptoms or behavior which interfere with one's ability to function in daily life and which appear in a cyclic fashion related to menstruation. The most frequently encountered symptoms include the following: abdominal bloating, anxiety, breast tenderness, crying spells, depression, fatigue, irritability, thirst and appetite changes, and weight gain. (11)

The prevalence is totally unknown, in that all estimates have been derived from selected populations of women, such as women attending special clinics or undergoing gynecological surgery. A further problem, and a major difficulty in evaluating studies and in dealing with individual cases, is that behavior is usually related to menstruation in a retrospective fashion, and this is prone to considerable subjective bias. For example, there are studies in the literature that point out that some women do not actually experience problems in relation to menstruation, but they believe that they do.

There has been significant publicity given to the use of progesterone treatment by injection (100 mg daily) or suppository (400 mg daily), long proposed and promoted by Dalton. (12) It is disappointing that this proponent of progesterone treatment has not offered us any scientific evidence to support her claims over 25 years.

Others have tried to substantiate her claims. One laboratory has reported a lower progesterone/estrogen ratio (13) whereas no impressive correlation has been reported between premenstrual symptoms and blood progesterone levels in two other properly controlled studies. (14, 15) There have been two double-blind controlled studies of progesterone therapy for premenstrual symptoms. Smith showed no difference in 14 cases of premenstrual depression when progesterone, spironolactone, or placebo were used. (16) Sampson administered progesterone suppositories to women attending a premenstrual syndrome clinic, and in this double-blind, controlled trial the placebo appeared to be more effective, although there was no statistically significant difference between the two groups. (17) Several investigators reported the effect of synthetic progestins, and only one claimed a high rate of success (but the study was not blinded). (18–20) A review of a variety of other treatment regimens (diuretics, oral contraceptives, spironolactone, pyridoxine, bromocriptine, monomine oxidase inhibitors) fails to reveal any clear cut benefits. (11, 21)

While depression and mood lability may be associated with oral contraceptive use, an opposite stabilizing effect may also be achieved. In extreme circumstances, complete elimination of sex steroid variability may be achieved with the daily use of an oral contraceptive, as in the treatment of endometriosis, or with the administration of Provera, 150 mg intramuscularly every 3 months or 10–30 mg daily and orally. Others have used pyridoxine (200 mg daily), inhibitors of prostaglandin synthesis, and spironolactone (50 mg daily). On occasion, we have experienced beneficial and gratifying results in patients with incapacitating emotional swings. But in view of the vague and subjective nature of this syndrome, any such empiric therapeutic treatment must be pursued in full consideration of the information noted above. If a patient is willing to undergo an empiric trial, we are willing. In doing so, however, neither partner in this contract should be deceived; we must remember that the placebo response may be the underlying basis for any positive response.

Dysmenorrhea. Primary dysmenorrhea is due to myometrial contractions induced by prostaglandins originating in the endometrium. (22) Other symptoms associated with menstrual flow, such as headache, nausea, and diarrhea, can be explained by entry of the prostaglandins into the systemic circulation. There is a 3-fold increase in prostaglandin levels in the endometrium from the follicular phase to the luteal phase, with a further increase during menstruation.

Prostaglandin $F_{2\alpha}$ ($PGF_{2\alpha}$) is the responsible agent for dysmenorrhea. It always stimulates uterine contractions, while the E prostaglandins inhibit contractions in the non-pregnant uterus. Uterine muscle from both normal and dysmenorrheic women is sensitive to $PGF_{2\alpha}$, and the amount of $PGF_{2\alpha}$ produced is the major factor. Dysmenorrheic women clearly have more prostaglandins in their menstrual fluid than nondysmenorrheic women.

The clinical benefit seen with the pharmacological use of inhibitors of prostaglandin synthesis depends upon a significant decrease in prostaglandin production in the endometrium. An additional role may be attributed to decreased prostaglandins from the platelets participating in the clotting of menstrual blood. The best explanation for the benefit seen with oral contraceptives is decreased prostaglandin synthesis associated with the atrophic decidualized endometrium.

While the fenamates offer a theoretical advantage in that they also have an antagonistic action, competing for prostaglandin binding sites, comparative studies have shown no significant advantage over other prostaglandin inhibitors. Indeed, there may be some disadvantage in that the fenamates have more side effects, usually blurred vision, headaches, dizzyness, and gastrointestinal discomfort. Gastrointestinal side effects can be reduced by taking the medication with milk or food. All of the new agents are more potent than aspirin, because the uterus is relatively insensitive to aspirin.

About 80% of dysmenorrheic women are relieved by prostaglandin inhibitors. Improvement is noted in a constellation of symptoms associated with menses, specifically cramping, backache, nausea, vomiting, dizziness, leg pain,

113

insomnia, and headache. (23) Initially it was felt that better relief was achieved if treatment was started 2–3 days before menses in order to lower the tissue level of prostaglandins before breakdown of the tissue which might prevent entry of the inhibitor into the tissue. Fortunately, studies have indicated that treatment is just as effective if begun at the sign of first bleeding, thus avoiding the possibility of taking one of these agents early in pregnancy. (24) Another benefit of prostaglandin inhibition is a reduction in the amount of blood lost with periods, and the agents may be used to treat menorrhagia, even that associated with an intrauterine device (IUD). (25) Most women do not need to take the medication more than 2–3 days.

Climacteric (Menopause and Postmenopause): Clinical Implications and Rationale for Estrogen Replacement Therapy

After 3 decades of ovulatory menstrual function, accompanied by full biologic estrogen maintenance of dependent tissues, at approximately 40 years of age, the frequency of ovulation decreases. This initiates a period of waning ovarian function called the climacteric, which will last as long as 30 years, and will carry the woman through decreased fertility, menopause, and manifestations of progressive tissue atrophy and aging. The major factor in this evolving picture is the decrease in estrogen production associated with this period of life. Menopause occurs in the United States between ages 48 and 55 with the median age being 51.4. In contrast to a decline in the age of menarche during modern times, a review of medieval sources has indicated that the age of menopause has not changed signficantly for hundreds of years. (26)

The population of postmenopausal women is increasing. Current census figures estimate that in the 1980s we are approaching a figure of 50 million women over 50 years of age. An American woman at the age of 50 can expect to live another 30 years; therefore, women in our country now live approximately one-third of their lives after ovarian failure. The problems of the postmenopausal period, by virtue of the older population size alone, have achieved the status of a major public health concern.

In this section, the clinical implications of estrogen withdrawal will be reviewed. A policy supporting replacement therapy, consistent with cautious medical practice and based on supporting data, will be offered.

Clinical Implications of Progressive Estrogen Withdrawal

Although estrogen does not wane in a straight line function, its progressive diminution over time leads to a sequential loss of estrogenic dependent functions: ovulation, menstrual function, vaginal and vulvar tissue strength, and finally generalized atrophy of all estrogen-dependent tissues.

This estrogen loss is due to the continued attrition in the numbers of residual follicle units in the 5th decade of life. Because fewer follicles are available, less and less estrogen production is possible. It must be remembered that these oldest follicle units have perhaps remained in the ovary unstimulated by gonadotropin not entirely by chance, but possibly due to their inherent refractoriness to otherwise appropriate gonadotropin stimulation. When these are finally activated, the degree of differentiation each is likely to experience is limited. Thus, each follicle growth period will be increasingly blunted, with less estrogen produced. Eventually even the older and sluggish follicles are exhausted, and estrogen production is now at a low level, resulting almost entirely from indirect resources, the peripheral conversion of ovarian stromal and adrenal precursors to active estrogen in nonendocrine tissue sites.

Finally the gonadal resource becomes defunct, the ovary shrivels to an atrophic mass of fibrous tissue. Estrogenicity, now at marginally sustaining levels, is the product of adrenal activity. As peripheral tissues age (now in the 7th, 8th and 9th decade) even these low levels wane still further.

The symptoms frequently seen and related to estrogen loss in this protracted climacteric are:

1. Disturbances in menstrual pattern, including anovulation and reduced fertility, decreased flow or hypermenorrhea, and irregular frequency of menses.

2. Vasomotor instability (hot flushes and sweats). Hot flushes are not well understood, but apparently are the result of instability between the hypothalamus and the autonomic nervous system, brought about by a decline in estrogen. They are especially disturbing at night, perhaps because the hypothalamus is relatively unoccupied.

3. Psychological symptoms, including anxiety, increased tension, mood depression, and irritability.

4. Atrophic conditions: atrophy of vaginal epithelium; urethral caruncles, dyspareunia and pruritus due to vulvar, introital, and vaginal atrophy; general skin atrophy; urinary difficulties such as urgency and cystitis.

5. A variety of complaints such as headaches, insomnia, myalgia, changes in libido, and palpitations. Lower back pain may be due to osteoporosis.

A precise understanding of the symptom complex the individual patient may display is often difficult to achieve. Some patients will show severe multiple reactions that may be disabling. Others will show no reactions, or minimal reactions, which go unnoticed until careful medical evaluation. The majority of patients (50–60%) require medical assistance and support for intermittent difficulties of moderate severity.

It appears that three factors are at work in all climacteric women. The symptomatic reaction is the sum of the impact of these three components:

1. The amount of estrogen depletion and the rate at which estrogen is withdrawn.

2. The collective inherited and acquired propensities to succumb or withstand the impositions of the overall aging process.

3. The psychologic impact of aging and the individual's reaction to the emotional implications of "a change of life."

Clearly good medical practice obligates the concerned physician to support patients in all aspects of the sometimes prolonged climacteric period. We have found it helpful to classify the hormonal problems in three categories:

1. Those associated with *estrogen deprivation* such as flushes, atrophic vaginitis, urethritis, and osteoporosis.

2. Those associated with relative *estrogen excess* such as dysfunctional uterine bleeding, endometrial hyperplasia, and endometrial carcinoma.

3. Those associated with *estrogen replacement* therapy.

The Problems of Estrogen Deprivation

Altered Menstrual Function. Oligomenorrhea followed by amenorrhea is usually the first clinical evidence of the female climacteric, although fertility has declined since age 30, and many premenopausal women note the transient presence of hot flushes prior to the cessation of menses. The diagnosis of permanent loss of menses requires sufficient follow-up time for retrospective confirmation. Usually 6–12 months of amenorrhea in a woman over 45 years of age is the commonly accepted rule of thumb for diagnosis of the menopause. Only rarely will vaginal bleeding reappear; when it does, organic pathology must be ruled out. Many patients will insist that pregnancy be ruled out and confirmation of postmenopausal status (hypergonadotropism) be obtained.

Vasomotor Symptoms. The vasomotor flush is viewed as the hallmark of the female climacteric, experienced to some degree by at least 85% of postmenopausal women. The term "hot flush" is descriptive of a sudden onset of reddening of the skin over the head, neck, and chest, accompanied by a feeling of intense body heat and concluded by sometimes profuse perspiration. Their duration varies from a few seconds to several minutes, and rarely for an hour. Their frequency may be rare to recurrent every 10–30 minutes. Finally, flushes appear to be more frequent and severe at night (when the woman may be awakened from sleep) or during times of stress. Although the flush may occur in the premenopause, it is a major feature of postmenopause, lasting in most women for 1–2 years but, in some (as many as 25–50%) for longer than 5 years.

The flush coincides with a surge of LH (not FSH) and is preceded by a subjective prodromal awareness that a flush is beginning. (27, 28) This aura is followed by measurable increased heat over the entire body surface. Core temperature falls. In short, the flush is not a release of accumulated body heat but is a sudden inappropriate excitation of heat release mechanisms. Its relationship to the LH surge and temperature change within the brain is not understood. The observation that flushes occur after hypophystectomy indicates that the mechanism is not dependent or due directly to LH release. In other words, the same hypothalamic event that causes flushes also elevates LH.

The correlation between the onset of flushes and estrogen reduction is clinically supported by the effectiveness of estrogen replacement therapy and the absence of flushes in hypoestrogen states, such as gonadal dysgenesis. Only after estrogen is administered and withdrawn do hypogonadal patients experience the hot flush. Curiously, control of this symptom may require estrogen doses in excess of premenopausal physiologic levels. Although the clinical impression that premenopausal castrates suffer more severe vasomotor reactions is widely held, this is not borne out in objective studies. (29)

Osteoporosis. Although the hot flush is the most common problem of the postmenopause, it presents no inherent health hazard. Osteoporosis, a change of bone structure characterized by a reduction in quantity rather than chemical composition, results in mechanical fragility with subsequent compression and fracture. Bones get their strength from a structure of protein fibers combined with hard calcium phosphate crystals. A reduction of both bone protein and calcium results in osteoporosis. The osteoporotic disabilities sustained by castrate or postmenopausal women include fractures of the vertebral body, humerus, upper femur, distal forearm, and ribs; back pain; and decreased height and mobility. Cross sectional studies (30–33) of white women reveal:

1. Spinal compression fracture: symptomatic spinal osteoporosis causing pain and loss of height. Approximately 25% of white women over 60 years of age display spinal compression fractures. The average nontreated postmenopausal white woman can expect to shrink 2½ inches.

2. Colles fracture: there is a 10-fold increase in distal forearm fractures in white women (not men) as they progress from age 35 to 60 years.

3. Head of femur fracture: the incidence of hip fractures also increases with age in white women, rising from 0.3/1000 to 20/1000 from 45 to 85 years. The incidence is about 10

times that of endometrial cancer in postmenopausal women. Eighty percent of all hip fractures are associated with osteoporosis. This fracture carries a heavy risk of morbidity and mortality. In most studies, between 15 and 20% of patients with hip fracture die due to the fracture or its complications (surgical, embolic, cardiopulmonary) within 3 months, but Beals found that only half of hip fracture victims in Portland, Oregon, survived for 1 year. (34) In addition the survivors are frequently severely disabled and may become permanent invalids.

Loss of mineral content of bone happens in all aging individuals. However, white and oriental women start losing bone earlier and at a more rapid rate than black women; thus, not only a sexual but also a racial difference is displayed. The problem is particularly severe in thin, cigarette smoking women castrated early in life, or those with gonadal dysgenesis.

Unquestionably, exercise and diet have a beneficial effect on bone integrity. Equally impressive is the accumulating evidence not only that postmenopausal osteoporosis is related to estrogen loss, but also that estrogen therapy has prophylactic value in retarding the process. The mechanism of this salutary action is thought to be an interference with the parathyroid hormone influence on bone resorption, requiring that calcium homeostasis be achieved in three ways: (35, 36)

1. Increased intestinal absorption of dietary calcium.

2. Reduced urinary loss due to increased renal tubular reabsorption of calcium, and

3. Inhibition of bone resorption.

Estrogen also increases calcitonin levels. This potent inhibitor of bone resorption restricts calcium loss from bone during estrogen treatment.

Long-term follow-up of postmenopausal and castrated women reveals a significantly lower rate of bone mineral loss in those women receiving estrogen therapy. (33) A pioneering double-blind prospective study showed that women receiving mestranol replacement also displayed marked reduction in the loss of mineral content of bone. (37) In response to the pivotal question of whether estrogen therapy has an effect on bone turnover dynamics and reduces fracture risk, the answer is "yes." (38–42) Users in every age group 50–75 can expect a 50–60% reduction in the risk of fracture of the hip or arm. (38) This decrease in fracture risk is identical with both 0.625- and 1.25-mg doses of conjugated estrogens. However, this protection is maintained only while women continue taking estrogens.

It is now clear that if estrogen therapy is discontinued, bone loss resumes and the reduced mineral content of previously treated women rapidly reaches the low levels of nontreated controls. (43) In other words, the same accelerated rate of bone loss occurs in the immediate years after stopping estrogen as seen in the first 3 postmenopausal years. (43, 44) Therefore, as a prophylaxis against osteoporosis, estrogen therapy must be started before the process has reached clinical significance, and it must be continued virtually indefinitely. Unfortunately, estrogen therapy does not reverse the inroads of advanced osteoporosis, although further bone loss can be reduced.

Although it has been estimated that, at the present time, 20% of castrate women and 30% of women experiencing natural menopause do not lose significant bone, (33) it is not possible (aside from racial factors) to designate which individual is not at risk for osteoporosis. Patients who already have osteoporosis should be screened for other conditions which lead to osteoporosis:

1. Serum calcium and phosphorus and alkaline phosphatase— for primary hyperparathyroidism.

2. Renal function tests—for secondary hyperparathyroidism with chronic renal failure.

3. Blood count and smear, and sedimentation rate—for multiple myeloma.

4. Thyroid function tests—for thyrotoxicosis.

The prevention of osteoporosis in the aging women now constitutes a major public health problem. By virtue of the large number of women living their postmenopausal years, a significant reduction in the clinical manifestations of osteoporosis will have a very large impact on our health care system and our patients in terms of quality of life, mortality, and money saved.

An aggressive approach is necessary for two reasons. First, therapy is more effective the closer it is initiated to menopause, and, second, once significant amounts of bone have been lost, complete retrieval can never be achieved. The prospective study, however, by Nachitigall et al. (42) merits special attention. The patients treated with both estrogen and progestin demonstrated an actual gain in bone mass, a gain which was greater in those women in whom treatment started within 3 years after menopause. These results are even more significant in that patients in both the placebo and treatment groups were receiving a supplement of 2 g of dietary calcium per day.

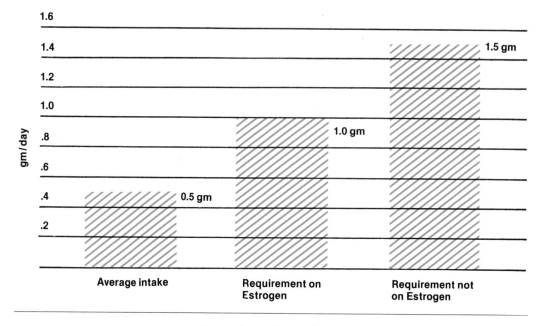

Calcium requirement
for zero balance (45)

An analysis of an aging women's calcium needs indicates a greater requirement than previously appreciated. (45) In order to remain in zero calcium balance, women on estrogen replacement require approximately 1.0 gm of calcium per day, while untreated women require 1.5 gm/day. In other words, estrogen therapy alone may not avoid a negative calcium balance.

In an excellent prospective study, the effect of supplementary calcium, with and without combinations of vitamin D, estrogen and sodium fluoride, on the rate of vertebral fractures was studied. (46) Whereas calcium supplementation significantly reduced the number of fractures, it was even more effective when combined with estrogen (80% reduction). The lowest fracture rate was achieved by combining calcium, estrogen and sodium fluoride (90% reduction). Because fluoride is a potent stimulator of bone formation and estrogen inhibits bone reabsorption, it is not surprising that an additive effect results. However, a high rate (40%) of side affects is encountered with fluoride supplementation, including joint and tendon inflammation, anemia, and gastrointestinal disturbances. The addition of vitamin D to the therapeutic regimens did not significantly affect the fracture rate, but was associated with problems of hypercalcemia or hypercalciuria. Therefore, the optimum regimen is a combination of estrogen and calcium.

Finally, we would be remiss if we did not promote the benefits of exercise. Physical activity, as little as 30 minutes a day for 3 days a week, will increase the bone mineral content in older women. (47) The exercise need not be extreme. Walking and ordinary calisthenics will suffice.

Menopausal Syndrome. As noted, the major extragenital problems of the menopause are the hot flush and osteoporosis. There are additional problems encountered in the early postmenopause that are seen frequently, but their causal relation with estrogen is uncertain. Called the menopausal syndrome, these problems include fatigue, nervousness, headaches, insomnia, depression, irritability, joint and muscle pain, dizziness, palpitations, and formication. Attempts to study the effects of estrogen on these problems have been hampered by the subjectivity of the complaints (high placebo reactions) and the "domino effect" of what reduction of hot flushes would do to frequency of insomnia or irritability. Using a double-blind crossover prospective study format, Campbell and Whitehead (48) have concluded that many symptomatic "improvements" ascribed to estrogen therapy result from relief of hot flushes—a domino effect. On the other hand, a tonic effect—improvement in memory and reduction of anxiety—was also noted in these observations. The unreliability of claims regarding skin dryness or wrinkles was underscored. Fatigue, irritability, headache, and depression are not thought to be estrogen-related phenomena.

Emotional stability during the perimenopausal period may be disrupted by poor sleep patterns. Estrogen therapy improves the quality of sleep, decreasing the time to onset of sleep and increasing the rapid eye movement (REM) sleep time. (49) Perhaps flushing may be insufficient to awaken a women, but sufficient to affect the quality of sleep, thereby diminishing the ability to handle the next day's problems and stresses.

Finally, there is a general clinical consensus that certain physical changes—redistribution of fat deposits, muscle tone loss, and loss of elastic tissue of the skin with wrinkling—are due to aging rather than to estrogen deprivation.

Cardiovascular Effects. The apparent sex difference between men and women with respect to coronary artery disease and stroke is a phenomenon characteristic only of affluent populations carrying a high burden of other risk factors, i.e. hyperlipidemia, diabetes, hypertension, and cigarette smoking. Inspection of the apparent sex difference in national mortality statistics shows that there is no abrupt change in the incidence of coronary mortality in women at the time of the menopause. The observed decrease in the ratio of male to female deaths is not due to an acceleration in female mortality but is due to a slowing in the rate in the male population with increasing age. Where the overall coronary mortality is low, sex differentials diminish. Nev-

121

ertheless, the question of whether cessation of ovarian function is associated with an increased incidence of heart disease persists with vexing uncertainty.

Several factors account for this inconclusive status. Most important are the results of the Framingham study, reporting data derived from biannual examination of 3000 women over a 24-year span. (50) These data reveal a marked increase in incidence of heart disease at the menopause regardless of age. The increase is substantial, abrupt, and continues, but only very slowly thereafter. Estrogen therapy did not reduce morbidity or mortality in this population. These data, however, are derived from a time when estrogen therapy was uncommon, and it is likely that dosage was relatively high. Studies have indicated that women who are castrated prior to the menopause have a higher incidence of coronary heart disease. (51) In addition, recent case-control studies have noted a general reduction in cardiovascular disease with estrogen replacement therapy. (40, 52) An excellent study, utilizing a very large retirement community, demonstrated significant protection against death by ischemic heart disease with estrogen therapy. (52) This protection was observed with both the 0.625 mg and 1.25 mg dose of conjugated estrogens, and it was effective even in cigarette smokers, changing a high risk to a risk less than that of controls. This protective relationship coincides with a decrease in mortality rates from ischemic heart disease among American white women during the time of increased estrogen use in recent years. This decrease in women is greater than the decrease in men over the same period of time, despite a greater decrease in cigarette smoking in men compared to women. (53) The mechanisms of this protection may be related to the decrease in levels of serum low density lipoprotein (LDL) cholesterol and the increase in high density lipoprotein (HDL) cholesterol seen with low doses of estrogen. (54) Particularly in older age groups, an inverse relationship exists between HDL cholesterol and coronary mortality. (55)

In the United States, the death rate from ischemic heart disease is over 4 times the combined death rates of breast cancer and endometrial cancer. The protective effect of replacement estrogen, if real, would be a significant benefit of therapy.

Finally, when estrogen replacement therapy is administered in the usual dosage to postmenopausal women, there is no increase observed in stroke, thromboembolism, or myocardial infarction. (56–59) These data reinforce the dose-response relationship between estrogen and thrombosis (also discussed in Chapter 15), and it is not surprising that relatively physiologic doses of estrogen are free of thrombotic side effects.

Atrophic Changes. With extremely low estrogen production in the late postmenopausal period, or many years after castration, atrophy of all mucosal surfaces takes place, accompanied by vaginitis, pruritus, dyspareunia, and stenosis. Genitourinary atrophy leads to a variety of symptoms which affect the ease and quality of living. Urethritis with dysuria, urgency incontinence, and urinary frequency are further results of mucosal thinning, in this instance, of the urethra. Vaginal relaxation with cystocele, rectocele, and uterine prolapse, and vulvar dystrophies are not a consequence of estrogen deprivation.

Unless dermatologic conditions exist masquerading as menopausal atrophy, estrogen replacement is invariably successful in reversing these atrophic problems. Relief from these problems often results in significant improvements in general well-being. Dyspareunia seldom brings older women to our offices. A basic reluctance to discuss sexual behavior still permeates our society, even among older patients and physicians. Gentle questioning may lead to estrogen treatment of atrophy and enhancement of sexual enjoyment. Objective measurements have demonstrated that vaginal factors which influence the enjoyment of sexual intercourse can be maintained by appropriate doses of estrogen. (60)

Problems of Excess Estrogen

Not all climacteric women experience symptoms or signs of estrogen deprivation. Most are asymptomatic; some actually manifest estrogen excess via the presence of uterine bleeding—dysfunctional uterine bleeding.

Throughout the usual period of life identified with perimenopause (40–60), there is a significant incidence of dysfunctional uterine bleeding. Although the greatest concern provoked by this symptom is endometrial neoplasia, the usual finding is nonneoplastic tissue displaying estrogen effects unopposed by progesterone. This results from anovulation in the premenopausal woman and from extragonadal endogenous estrogen production or estrogen administration in the postmenopausal woman. There are four mechanisms which could result in increased endogenous estrogen levels:

1. Increased precursor androgen (functional and nonfunctional endocrine tumors, liver disease, stress).

2. Increased aromatization (obesity, hyperthyroidism, liver disease).

3. Increased direct secretion of estrogen (ovarian tumors).

4. Decreased levels of SHBG (sex hormone binding globulin) leading to increased levels of free estrogen.

In all women, whether premenopausal or postmenopausal, whether on or off hormone therapy, specific organic causes

123

(intrauterine tumor, carcinoma, complications of unexpected pregnancy, or bleeding from extrauterine sites) must be ruled out. In addition to careful history and physical examination dysfunctional uterine bleeding occurring beyond the age of 35 is evaluated by multiple-specimen endometrial aspiration biopsy. In the absence of organic disease, appropriate management is dependent upon the age of the patient and endometrial tissue findings. In the perimenopausal woman with dysfunctional uterine bleeding associated with proliferative or hyperplastic endometrium, (uncomplicated by atypical or dysplastic constituents), periodic oral progestin therapy is mandatory. Provera, 10 mg, is given daily the first 10 days of each month. Follow-up aspiration biopsy is required, and if histologic regression is not observed, a formal curettage is essential.

When monthly progestin therapy reverses hyperplastic changes and controls irregular bleeding, treatment should be continued until withdrawal bleeding ceases. This is a reliable sign (in effect, a bioassay) indicating the onset of estrogen deprivation and the need for the addition of estrogen. If vasomotor disturbances begin before the cessation of menstrual bleeding, the combined estrogen-progestin program may be initiated to control the flushes.

Problems of Estrogen Therapy

General and Metabolic. In the foregoing paragraphs, it was apparent that substantial benefits may accrue if estrogen deprivation conditions are treated with estrogen replacement. But, as in all clinical situations, benefits of therapy must be balanced by evaluating the liabilities of adverse effects of the hormone. Considerable information of this type has accumulated in relation to the use of oral contraceptives. The increased incidence of thromboembolic disease, hypertension, and altered carbohydrate metabolism during oral contraceptive usage is well documented and considered attributable to the estrogen component of the pill. Probably as a result of the lower dosage of estrogen, these metabolic effects are not seen with postmenopausal replacement therapy. Postmenopausal women on estrogen therapy are not at risk for myocardial infarction, idiopathic thromboembolism, or breast tumors. (58, 59) As with contraception, however, estrogen replacement therapy does carry an increased incidence of gallbladder disease, and careful monitoring for the appearance of symptoms and signs of biliary tract disease is necessary.

Obviously, the general area of metabolic effects cannot be dismissed; patients with high-risk features need special attention when a decision is made in favor of estrogen treatment. Metabolic contraindications to estrogen replacement therapy include chronically impaired liver function, acute vascular thrombosis (with or without emboli), and neurophthalmologic vascular disease. Relative contraindications (estrogens may have adverse effects on some patients) include seizure disorders, hypertension, familial hyperlipidemias, migraine headaches, and thromboembolic problems.

Breast Cancer. The possibility that estrogen use increases the risk of breast cancer must be intensively scrutinized. The epidemiologic data on the scope of human female breast cancer are astonishing: 1 of every 11 women will develop breast cancer in her lifetime. It is the leading type of cancer in women (26%), and the leading cause of cancer death in women (20%), about 10 times the number of deaths from endometrial cancer. The mortality rate from breast cancer of 23:100,000 female population has not changed in 45 years.

Evidence for the involvement of endogenous estrogen in human breast cancer is persuasive (even if the mechanism is unknown):

1. The condition is 100 times more frequent in women than in men.

2. Breast cancer invariably occurs after puberty.

3. Gonadal dysgenesis and breast cancer are mutually exclusive.

4. Breast cancer frequently contains estrogen and progestin receptors, and these respond beneficially to endocrine ablative therapy.

5. Breast cancer risks decrease by 70% if castration occurs prior to the age of 35 years.

6. There is increased risk if first pregnancy is delayed beyond 30 years of age.

Although the relationship between endogenous estrogen and breast cancer does not require or imply a cause and effect carcinogenic action of the estrogen, it does suggest a permissive or supportive role of the hormone in the disease process. What of exogenous estrogen hormone and its effects on breast cancer incidence? There are several retrospective case control studies (61–66) which have shown no significant association between estrogen use and breast cancer risk. For a full critical analysis of all of these studies, the reader is referred to Horwitz and Feinstein (67) and Hertz. (68)

A practice-based follow-up study showed slightly increased rates (not statistically significant) in high dose estrogen users after approximately 10–15 years. (69) In two case control studies, a slightly increased risk for developing breast cancer was noted if there was a high dose or prolonged exposure to estrogen. (70, 71) At particular risk were patients who had pre-existing benign breast disease or who developed surgically proven benign breast disease during estrogen replacement therapy.

The incidence of breast cancer in general has not risen dramatically in the United States despite a massive increase in the use of estrogen during the 1960s and early 1970s in this country. However, the latency period before breast cancer is clinically manifested may be prolonged, and may be greater than 10–20 years. Some reassurance has come from the 1977–1979 Connecticut survey, showing no increased risk to estrogen users in a hospital based study. (72)

In a large long-term prospective study, there has been no evidence that estrogen therapy increases the risk of breast cancer. Even more impressive, as this study approached 15 years of follow-up, the incidence of breast cancer in women using an estrogen-progestin combination program was significantly lower than the incidence in women using estrogen alone. (73) It is logical to expect that the same mechanism of estrogen receptor depletion should operate in both the endometrium and the breast, and that protection against abnormal mitotic activity should exist in both target tissues. The unique progestin-induced breast neoplasia observed in the Beagle dog is discussed in Chapter 15.

Despite the acknowledged deficiencies and uncertainties in the accumulated epidemiologic data, prudent management of estrogen replacement therapy should include these elements with respect to the potential breast cancer problem:

1. Routine replacement dosage should not exceed 0.625 mg of conjugated estrogens (or its potency equivalent).

2. The development of surgically proven benign breast disease on therapy warrants consideration of avoidance of further estrogen.

3. In view of the significant potential offered by periodic exposure to progestin, a combined program of estrogen-progestin should be utilized for all patients, including those women who have undergone hysterectomy.

4. A family history of breast cancer does not preclude estrogen replacement, but periodic follow-up with mammography is warranted.

Endometrial Cancer. Within the last few years, the relationship between estrogen replacement therapy and the risk of recipients developing endometrial hyperplasia and carcinoma has been revealed, (74–76) emphasized, (77) evaluated, (78) and given clinical perspective. (79, 80) As a result of this scrutiny, extensive modifications of diagnostic and treatment regimens were proposed, and preliminary evidence for their beneficial impact demonstrated. (81–83) Clinicians have witnessed similar rapid swings of the informational pendulum before. They have learned to "hold" decisions on management until time has passed and all the facts are in. Nevertheless, the swiftness of the evolution and outcome of the medical dialectic operating in the estrogen therapy-endometrial carcinoma issue was impressive. The catalysts compelling the solution were the prevalence of estrogen use, the pressures for informed consent, and the need to rationalize the polarizing elements of high utility vs. presumed high risk and, fortunately, the ease of diagnostic access to the endometrial cavity. The outcome?—low dose, cyclic, sequential estrogen and progestin therapy and diagnostic biopsy when indicated.

Estrogen normally promotes mitotic growth of the endometrium. Abnormal progression of growth through cystic hyperplasia, adenomatous hyperplasia, atypia, and early carcinoma have been associated with unopposed estrogen activity. Some 10% of women with adenomatous hyperplasia progress to frank cancer, and adenomatous hyperplasia is observed to antedate adenocarcinoma in 25–30% of cases. (84) Although a majority of cancers are found associated with inactive or atrophic endometrium appropriate for the age and hormonal condition of the patient, the morphologic progression from hyperplasia to carcinoma in situ represents a disease continuum catalyzed by unopposed estrogen stimulation. The practicing gynecologist is impressed with this potential; hysterectomy is legitimate treatment for endometrial adenomatous hyperplasia in the perimenopausal woman.

Attention has focused on the relationships of this histologic progression to the use of estrogen replacement therapy. Retrospective studies have estimated that the risk of endometrial cancer in women on estrogen replacement therapy is increased by a factor of 4–8. In America, the actual incidence of endometrial cancer would therefore increase from 1 per 1000 postmenopausal women per year to 4–8 per 1000 per year. The risk appears to increase with duration of exposure and dose of estrogen, and decreases after estrogen is stopped. When adjusted for the recognized risk of obesity, hypertension, and diabetes, the increased risk with estrogen matched the risk associated with these conditions.

Estrogen replacement therapy based on the amount of sales of estrogen in the United States more than doubled from 1965 to 1974, and this has been reflected in a higher incidence of endometrial cancer in various parts of the country. The increase, however, is confined to early, highly localized disease. (85) While incidence is increasing, mortality from endometrial cancer is decreasing. Does estrogen increase early diagnosis of otherwise-silent disease (selection bias)? Are pathologists "overdiagnosing" adenomatous hyperplasia (observation bias or misclassification)? Are women at intrinsically higher risk being treated with estrogen (confounding factor bias)?

The data on this issue do not need to be definitive or conclusive. For the present time it is clear that estrogen is associated with an increased risk of endometrial cancer, even though several biases may have falsely increased the magnitude of the association, and that risk is related to dosage, duration, and continuous as opposed to cyclic therapy, and may be reduced by the addition of progestin therapy.

127

Whereas estrogen promotes the growth of endometrium, progestins inhibit that growth. This counter effect is accomplished by progestin reduction in cystoplasmic receptors for estrogens (by diminished replenishment) and by induction of a target cell enzyme (estradiol dehydrogenase) that converts estradiol to estrone. In addition, progestational agents stimulate estrogen sulfotransferase activity. (86) The actions of estradiol dehydrogenase and the sulfotransferase are closely coupled, producing an increase in estrone sulfate which is rapidly excreted from target cells. As a result, the number of estrogen receptor complexes that are translocated and retained in the endometrial nucleus is decreased, as is the overall intracellular availability of the powerful estradiol.

Reports of the clinical impact of adding progestin in sequence with estrogen replacement therapy include the reversal of hyperplasia and a diminished incidence of endometrial cancer. (87, 88) Not all studies support this salutary effect; clearly, the dose and duration of progestin are important. Recent information indicates that a 10-day course of progestin achieves a maximal antiestrogenic effect. (81, 89, 90)

Is there a "high-risk" group for endometrial cancer? Such a group surely would include obese individuals, those with high endogenous estrogen levels, and those with other constitutional features that predispose them for the endometrial disease. If there is any concern, a pretherapy biopsy to document endometrial activity should be performed. Treatment of all dysfunctional uterine bleeding of perimenopause with progestins only (after biopsy) is a necessary added precaution. Once on estrogen replacement therapy, the cost effectiveness of periodic endometrial biopsy must be considered. Many patients and physicians opt for biopsy every 1–3 years to ensure endometrial stability, regardless of the high overall cost and relatively low case identification rates. In the high risk patient, a combined estrogen-progestin program is safer than leaving the patient to prolonged and uninterrupted endogenous estrogen exposure.

Postmenopausal Estrogen Replacement Therapy

In view of the above considerations, our opinion is as follows: There is little question that women who suffer from hot flushes or atrophy of reproductive tract tissues can and should be relieved of their problems by use of estrogens. It also is now definite that the long-term disabilities of osteoporosis can be largely prevented by therapy with estrogen. The protective effects afforded by estrogen must be weighed against the increased incidence of cancer that may be associated with hormone use. We suggest treatment with estrogen for all women showing any stigmata of hormone deprivation, and advocate hormonal prophylaxis against osteoporosis. The lowest dose of estrogen that reverses the deficiency should be used and monthly addition of a progestin is mandatory. In practice, we exclude from therapy those patients in whom estrogen is specifically contraindicated (estrogen dependent tumors, impaired liver metabolism, and sometimes, in a diffi-

cult matter of clinical judgment, patients with thromboembolic problems or conditions predisposing to thromboembolism). The decision to use or not to use estrogen belongs to the patient, and it should be based on the information available in this chapter. The recommendation that replacement therapy be given for the shortest period of time appears short sighted in view of the impressive evidence that therapy has a profound impact on osteoporosis, and there are more beneficial than harmful effects.

Patients Under the Age of 40 (Castrates and Patients with Gonadal Dysgenesis)

In these women, the duration of estrogen deprivation is prolonged and the loss of estrogen may be acute. The cyclic use of estrogen is recommended for short-term reduction of vasomotor symptoms and for long-term prophylaxis against osteoporosis and target organ atrophy. In many young patients, 0.625 mg of conjugated estrogens is insufficient to allow menstrual bleeding. Because women of this age ordinarily are exposed to estrogen levels which stimulate endometrial growth and withdrawal bleeding, and for psychological reasons, a dose of 1.25 mg conjugated estrogens or its equivalent is utilized until the menopausal time of life. Progestin for the last 10 days is always added. In those patients castrated because of endometriosis, reoccurrence of endometriosis has not been a problem with this regimen.

Perimenopausal Dysfunctional Uterine Bleeding

After exclusion of other gynecologic causes, dysfunctional bleeding is treated by progestin therapy and biopsy surveillance. Vasomotor reactions appearing in women despite the presence of menstrual bleeding (presumably the flushes are due to a relative decrease in estrogen) can be treated by the usual estrogen-progestin regimen.

The Early Postmenopause

Progestin therapy is administered periodically (every month) until withdrawal bleeding does not occur. If vasomotor reactions begin, however, estrogen therapy is begun along with sequential progestin. Because there is no clinically useful diagnostic test to isolate those patients at risk for osteoporosis, the long-term postmenopausal use of hormone therapy depends heavily on the patient's own informed assessment of the special problems that this prospect represents. Should therapy be accepted, the sequential estrogen-progestin replacement program is initiated. At the low doses of estrogen recommended for replacement, increased growth of uterine fibroids, endometriosis, or breast reactions are rarely a concern.

As a result of immediate responses in early climacteric symptoms, the patient enters the climacteric more confident of herself emotionally, sexually, and physically. In our view, this establishes or cements good patient-physician interchange and relations. The follow-up of the patient on effective estrogen replacement is more secure and certain. The practitioner offering estrogen replacement has a better and more reliable opportunity to act as primary physician for these aging women. All monitoring of health systems will be improved as a result of this single involvement.

129

Bowel, breast, cardiac, and various metabolic functions are scrutinized periodically as consistent with good health practice.

The Late Postmenopause

The onset of atrophic conditions can be effectively treated with local or oral therapy in low maintenance doses. Is it beneficial to administer the replacement program to women who already have osteoporosis and who have not previously taken estrogen? If there is no apparent basis for the osteoporosis other than aging and ovarian failure, estrogen therapy and calcium supplementation are advisable. Further loss of bone mass may be prevented or slowed. In these older women, a higher dose of estrogen (1.25 mg) may be necessary. Assessment of impact or progress can be obtained by measuring bone density. Sensitive methods are now available, either photon absorptiometry measured at the lower radius, or limited computerized tomography (CT) scanning of the spine.

Method of Management

Which Drug Should Be Used? There currently is no evidence that one form of estrogen is superior to another. Any estrogen properly monitored and administered is acceptable. The specific estrogen does not appear to be as important as the duration, dose, and concomitant use of progestin. Which estrogen is administered is not as significant as the method with which it is used.

It is difficult to know the exact equivalent potency within the human body of the various estrogen preparations. Ethinyl estradiol in a dose of 5 μg is equivalent to 0.625 mg conjugated estrogens as measured by a variety of responses, including sex binding globulin, urinary calcium/creatinine ratios, gonadotropins, thyroxine binding globulin, corticoid steroid binding globulin, and renin substrate. (91)

How Do We Treat? Estrogens are administered on a cyclic basis, usually from the 1st through the 25th of each month, as a convenient aid to remembering the routine.

For the last 10 days of estrogen administration, a daily dose of 10 mg of medroxyprogesterone acetate (Provera) is added. Some patients develop unwanted reactions to this dose of progestin: weight gain, edema, or depression. Other progestins may be given and in lower doses, norethindrone 2.5 mg, norgestrel 150 μg. (89) The lower equivalent dose of medroxyprogesterone acetate has not been established by clinical studies, but 2.5 mg have been demonstrated to suppress endometrial estrogen receptor levels to baseline when used with 0.3 mg and 0.625 mg of conjugated estrogens (but not with 1.25 mg), while 5 mg and 10 mg were effective for all three doses of estrogen. (92) A possible disadvantage of the 19-nortestosterone progestins is an adverse effect on HDL cholesterol (a decrease) reversing the beneficial effect of the estrogen. (93) For this reason, medroxyprogesterone acetate is our drug of choice. Future studies may reveal that lower doses of 19-nortestosterone progestins do not decrease HDL cholesterol levels. Also in

130

the future, we may find that more than 10 days will be necessary for optimal prophylaxis.

In the absence of a uterus, some practitioners do not see the need to use cyclic administration of a progestin. However, in view of a possible impact on the breast, and for the reasons we have already noted, it seems best to adhere to a cyclic schedule including the terminal use of a progestin. There are no clinical studies to guide us in dealing with a woman who is symptomatic during the days off of medication. Our clinical judgment has led us to combine daily estrogen (every day through the month) with progestin daily for the first 14 days each month. The use of progestin for up to 10 days each month will not provide complete protection when estrogen is given continously. (89)

The dose of estrogen utilized is that which will provide sufficient estrogen to sustain physiologic functions, yet short of provoking a return of menstrual flow. An important principle of treatment is that relief of symptoms can usually be achieved by sub-bleeding doses of estrogen. For early climacteric, where there is still considerable endogenous estrogen present, the usual effective dose is 0.625 mg conjugated estrogens per day. In late climacteric where endogenous estrogen may be very low at best, a higher dose, 1.25 mg, may be necessary. Even at these doses there are inconsistent effects on various target tissues. There is a pharmacologic effect on the liver, and a subphysiologic effect on the vagina. (94) These doses do not cause significant elevation of blood pressure except for a rare idiosyncratic reaction. A dose of 0.625 mg is adequate for prophylaxis against osteoporosis. Because the average dietary intake of calcium is only 500 mg daily, for optimal protection against osteoporosis, the hormonal regimen is supplemented with another 500 mg calcium daily. If withdrawal bleeding occurs at the 0.625-mg dose, the estrogen dose is reduced to 0.3 mg, to be increased in later years as the requirement increases.

When estrogen is contraindicated, Depo-Provera (150 mg every 3 months) is effective in relieving vasomotor symptoms. Oral Provera (10–20 mg daily) also can be utilized. The effect on calcium excretion is less than that seen with estrogen, although progestins do exert some inhibition of bone loss. (95) When estrogen administration is not possible, calcium should be supplemented at the rate of 1.0 gm per day. Progestin will not improve vaginal atrophy and dyspareunia can be a problem.

Calcium supplementation can unmask asymptomatic hyperparathyroidism. Women receiving calcium supplementation should have their blood levels of calcium and phosphorus measured yearly for the first 2 years. If normal, no further surveillance is necessary.

Clonidine has been found to reduce the frequency of flushes, but it is less effective than either estrogen or a

131

progestin, and the dose required is associated with a high rate of side effects. (96) Propranolol is also ineffective. (97)

Estrogens are absorbed efficiently from the vagina and high blood levels are achieved with the usual recommended doses. Until dose response studies are available indicating the physiologic range for vaginal, parenteral, and other types of administration (e.g. transdermal) the oral program must be followed in the interests of patient safety.

A striking and consistent finding in most studies dealing with menopause and estrogen replacement, is a marked placebo response in a variety of symptoms including flushing. A significant clinical problem encountered in our referral practice is the following: Occasionally a woman will undergo an apparent beneficial response to estrogen, only to have the response wear off in several months. This leads to a sequence of periodic visits to the physician and ever-increasing doses of estrogen therapy. When a patient reaches a point of requiring large doses of estrogen (2.5 mg conjugated estrogens or more), a careful inquiry must be undertaken for a basic psychoneurotic problem.

Hormonal treatment for decreased libido should be discouraged in that psychosocial reasons are usually the blame. However, we have found that occasionally the addition of androgen (methyltestosterone, up to 5 mg daily), in addition to the estrogen, may provide an increased sense of well-being, along with an increase in libido. The patient should be cautioned that hirsutism may develop.

We find no need to monitor dosage by any means other than symptoms and bleeding; assessing vaginal cytology is not useful.

When to Biopsy? Aspiration endometrial biopsy is recommended prior to instituting therapy in the perimenopausal period. This aggressive approach will identify those cases in which hyperplasia is already present. If hyperplasia is encountered, therapy is initiated and re-biopsy is performed 4 months later. This approach will isolate those patients with severe atypical changes resistant to progestin, allowing a clear-cut decision in favor of surgical treatment. The appearance of unscheduled, irregular, breakthrough bleeding demands biopsy at any time or at any age during postmenopausal estrogen therapy. In the absence of abnormal bleeding, sampling of the endometrium every 2–3 years is recommended by many authorities, but individualization is certainly in order, and a certain amount of trust in the protective effects of the progestin is justified.

The cost effectiveness of routine perimenopausal biopsies can be argued. It has been estimated that over 3000 biopsies are necessary to detect an invasive lesion in an asymptomatic woman. A reasonable economic moderation would be to limit pretreatment biopsies to patients at higher risk for endometrial changes. This would include those patients with conditions associated with chronic estrogen exposure such as obesity, dysfunctional uterine bleeding, anovulatory infertility, hirsutism, high alcohol intake, hepatic disease, metabolic problems such as diabetes mellitus and hypothyroidism, family history of endometrial cancer and breast cancer.

Conclusion. No one can hope to stay young forever, and hormones certainly will not prevent aging. There should be no misconceptions here. Some of the difficulties of menopause, however, can be softened with estrogen therapy, and several potentially disabling problems avoided. Unanswered questions remain. Practical clinical means are needed to identify which patients require estrogen. Controlled clinical studies are necessary in order to determine which route of administration of estrogen is best, what schedule of estrogen should be used, how much progestational agent is necessary, and how long a progestational agent should be given. Until these questions are answered, close clinical surveillance of our patients is necessary.

References

1. **Bonilla-Musoles F, Renau J, Hernandez-Yago J, Torres YJ,** How do oocytes disappear, Arch Gynaekol 218:233, 1975.

2. **LeMaire WJ, Yang NST, Behrman HR, Marsh JM,** Preovulatory changes in the concentration of prostaglandins in rabbit Graafian follicles, Prostaglandins 3:367, 1973.

3. **Sherman BM, West JH, Korenman SG,** The menopausal transition: analysis of LH, FSH, estradiol, and progesterone concentrations during menstrual cycles of older women, J Clin Endocrinol Metab 42:629, 1976.

4. **Vermeulen A,** The hormonal activity of the postmenopausal ovary, J Clin Endocrinol Metab 42:247, 1976.

5. **Judd HL,** Hormonal dynamics associated with the menopause, Clin Obstet Gynecol 19:775, 1976.

6. **Judd HL, Shamonki IM, Frumar AM, Lagasse LD,** Origin of serum estradiol in postmenopausal women, Obstet Gynecol 59:680, 1982.

7. **Siiteri PK, MacDonald PC,** Role of extraglandular estrogen in human endocrinology, in *Handbook of Physiology, Section 7, Endocrinology,* Geiger SR, Astwood EB, Greep RO, eds, American Physiology Society, Washington, DC, 1973.

8. **Meldrum DR, Davidson BJ, Tataryn IV, Judd HL,** Changes in circulating steroids with aging in postmenopausal women, Obstet Gynecol 57:624, 1981.

9. **Ackerman GE, Smith ME, Mendelson CR, MacDonald PC, Simpson ER,** Aromatization of androstenedione by human adipose tissue stromal cells in monolayer culture, J Clin Endocrinol Metab 53:412, 1981.

10. **Plymate SR, Fariss BL, Bassett ML, Matej L,** Obesity and its role in polycystic ovary syndrome, J Clin Endocrinol Metab 52:1246, 1981.

11. **Hoffman PG,** Primary dysmenorrhea and the premenstrual syndrome, in *Office Gynecology*, Ed. 2, Glass RH, ed, Williams & Wilkins, Baltimore, 1981.

12. **Dalton K,** *The Premenstrual Syndrome and Progesterone Therapy*, Wm Heinemann, London, 1977.

13. **Backstrom T, Carstensen H,** Estrogen and progesterone in plasma in relation to premenstrual tension, J Steroid Biochem 5:257, 1974.

14. **Munday M,** Hormone levels in severe premenstrual tension, Curr Med Res Opin 4:16, 1977.

15. **Taylor JW,** The timing of menstruation-related symptoms assessed by a daily symptom rating scale, Acta Psychiatr Scand 60:87, 1979.

16. **Smith SL,** Mood and the menstrual cycle, in *Topics in Psychoendocrinology*, Sacher EJ, ed, Grune & Stratton, New York, 1975.

17. **Sampson GA,** Premenstrual syndrome: a double-blind controlled trial of progesterone and placebo, Br J Psychiatr 135:209, 1979.

18. **Swyer GIM,** Treatment of the premenstrual syndrome—value of ethisterone, mephenesin, and a placebo compared, Br Med J I:1410, 1955.

19. **Jordheim O,** The premenstrual syndrome—clinical trials of treatment with a progestogen combined with a diuretic compared with both a progestogen alone and with a placebo, Acta Obstet Gynaecol Scand 51:77, 1972.

20. **Taylor RW,** The treatment of premenstrual tension with dydrogesteron (Duphaston), Curr Med Res Opin 4:35, 1977.

21. **Clare AW,** The treatment of premenstrual symptoms, Br J Psychiatr 135:576, 1979.

22. **Ylikorkala O, Dawood MY,** New concepts in dysmenorrhea, Am J Obstet Gynecol 130:833, 1978.

23. **Budoff PW,** Zomepirac sodium in the treatment of primary dysmenorrhea syndrome, N Engl J Med 307:714, 1982.

24. **Chan WY, Dawood MY, Fuchs F,** Prostaglandins in primary dysmenorrhea, comparison of prophylactic and non-prophylactic treatment with ibuprofen and use of oral contraceptives, Am J Med 80:535, 1981.

25. **Fraser IS, Pearse C, Shearman RP, Elliott PM, McIlveen J, Markham R,** Efficacy of mefenamic acid in patients with a complaint of menorrhagia, Obstet Gynecol 58:543, 1981.

26. **Amundsen DW, Diers CJ,** The age of menopause in medieval Europe, Hum Biol 45:605, 1973.

27. **Sturdee DW, Wilson KA, Pipila E, Crocker AD,** Physiologic aspects of the menopausal hot flush, Br Med J 2:79, 1978.

28. **Meldrum DR, Tataryn IV, Frumar E, Erlik Y, Lu KH, Judd HL,** Gonadotropins, estrogens and adrenal steroids during the menopausal hot flush, J Clin Endocrinol Metab 50:685, 1980.

29. **Aksel S, Schomberg DW, Tyrey L, Hammond CB,** Vasomotor symptoms, serum estrogens and gonadotropin levels in surgical menopause, Am J Obstet Gynecol 126:165, 1976.

30. **Albright F,** Postmenopausal osteoporosis, Trans Assoc Am Physicians 55:298, 1940.

31. **Meema S, Meema HE,** Loss of compact bone due to menopause, Obstet Gynecol 26:333, 1965.

32. **Knowelden J, Buhra J, Dunbar O,** Incidence of fractures in persons over 35 years of age, Br J Prev Soc Med 18:130, 1964.

33. **Meema S, Bunker ML, Meema HE,** Preventive effect of estrogen on postmenopausal bone loss, Arch Intern Med 135:1436, 1975.

34. **Beals RK,** Survival following hip fracture: long term follow-up of 607 patients, J Chronic Dis 25:235, 1972.

35. **Nordin BEC, Horsman A, Crilly RG, Marshall RG, Simpson M,** Treatment of spinal osteoporosis in postmenopausal women, Br Med J 280:453, 1980.

36. **Gallagher JC, Riggs BL, DeLuca HF,** Effect of estrogen on calcium absorption and serum vitamin D metabolites in postmenopausal osteoporosis, J Clin Endocrinol Metab 51:1359, 1980.

37. **Lindsay R, Aitken JM, Anderson JB, Hart DM, MacDonald EB, Clarke AC,** Long-term prevention of postmenopausal osteoporosis by oestrogen, Lancet 1:1038, 1976.

38. **Weiss N, Ure L, Ballard JH, Williams AR, Daling JR,** Estimated incidence of fractures of lower forearm and hip in postmenopausal women, N Engl J Med 303:1195, 1980.

39. **Hutchinson TA, Polansky SM, Feinstein AR,** Postmenopausal estrogens protect against fractures of hip and distal radius, a case controlled study, Lancet 2:705, 1979.

40. **Hammond CB, Jelovsek FR, Lee KL, Creasman WT, Parker RT,** Effects of long-term estrogen replacement therapy: I. Metabolic effects, Am J Obstet Gynecol 133:525, 1979.

41. **Johansson BW, Kaij L, Kullander S, Lenner HC, Svanberg L, Astedt B,** On some late effects of bilateral oophorectomy in the age range 15–30 years, Acta Obstet Gynecol Scand 54:449, 1975.

42. **Nachtigall LE, Nachtigall RH, Nachtigall RD, Beckman EM,** Estrogen replacement therapy: I. A 10-year prospective study of the relationship to osteoporosis, Obstet Gynecol 53:277, 1979.

43. **Lindsay R, MacLean A, Kroszewski A, Clark AC, Garwood J,** Bone response to termination of oestrogen treatment, Lancet 1:1325, 1978.

44. **Horsman A, Nordin BEC, Crilly RG,** Effect on bone of withdrawal of oestrogen therapy, Lancet 2:33, 1979.

45. **Heaney RP, Recker RR, Saville PD,** Menopausal changes in calcium balance performance, Lab Clin Med 92:953, 1978.

46. **Riggs BL, Seeman E, Hodgson SF, Taves DR, O'Fallon WM,** Effect of the fluoride/calcium regimen on vertebral fracture occurrence in postmenopausal osteoporosis, N Engl J Med 306:446, 1982.

47. **Smith EL,** Exercise for prevention of osteoporosis: a review, Physician and Sportsmedicine 10:72 (Mar), 1982.

48. **Campbell S, Whitehead M,** Estrogen therapy and the menopausal syndrome, Clin Obstet Gynecol 4:31, 1977.

49. **Schiff I, Regestein Q, Tulchinsky D, Ryan KJ,** Effects of estrogens on sleep and psychological state of hypogonadal women, JAMA 242:2405, 1979.

50. **Gordon T, Kannel WB, Hjortland MC, McNamara PM,** Menopause and coronary heart disease, Ann Intern Med 89:157, 1978.

51. **Oliver MF,** The menopause and coronary heart disease, in *The Management of the Menopause and Postmenopausal Years*, Campbell S, ed, University Park Press, Baltimore, 1976, pp 175–184.

52. **Ross RK, Mack TM, Paganini-Hill A, Arthur M, Henderson BD,** Menopausal oestrogen therapy and protection from death from ischaemic heart disease, Lancet 1:858, 1981.

53. **Kannel WB,** Meaning of the downward trend in cardiovascular mortality, JAMA 247:877, 1982.

136

54. **Wallace RB, Hoover J, Barrett-Conner E, Rifkind BM, Hunninghake DB, Mackenthun A, Heiss G,** Altered plasma lipid and lipo-protein associated with oral contraceptive and oestrogen use, Lancet 2:112, 1979.

55. **Yaari S, Even-Zohar S, Goldbourt U, Neufeld HN,** Associations of serum high density lipoprotein and total cholesterol with total, cardiovascular, and cancer motality in a 7-year prospective study of 10,000 men, Lancet 1:1011, 1981.

56. **Pfeffer RI, Whipple GH, Kurosaki TT, Chapman JM,** Coronary risk and estrogen use in postmenopausal women, Am J Epidemiol 107:479, 1978.

57. **Pfeffer RI, Kurosaki TT, Charlton SK,** Estrogen use and blood pressure in later life, Am J Epidemiol 110:469, 1979.

58. **Rosenberg L, Armstrong B, Jick H,** Myocardial infarction and estrogen therapy in post-menopausal women, N Engl J Med 294:1256, 1976.

59. **Pfeffer RI, Van Den Noort S,** Estrogen use and stroke risk in postmenopausal women, Am J Epidemiol 103:445, 1976.

60. **Semmens JP, Wagner G,** Estrogen deprivation and vaginal function in postmenopausal women, JAMA 248:445, 1982.

61. **Hammond CB, JeLovsek FT, Lee KL, Creasman WI, Parker R,** Effects of long-term estrogen replacement therapy: II. Neoplasia, Am J Obstet Gynecol 133:537, 1979.

62. **Craig TJ, Comstock GW, Geiser PB,** Epidemiologic comparison of breast cancer patients with early and late onset of malignancy and general population control, JNCI 53:1577, 1974.

63. **Casagrande J, Gerkins V, Henderson BE, Mack T, Pike MC,** Brief communication: Exogenous estrogens and breast cancer in women with natural menopause, JNCI 56:839, 1976.

64. **Sartwell PE, Arthes FG, Tonascia JA,** Exogenous hormones, reproductive history, and breast cancer, JNCI 59:1589, 1977.

65. **Wynder EL, MacCornack FA, Stellman SD,** The epidemiology of breast cancer in 785 United States caucasian women, Cancer 41:2341, 1978.

66. **Brinton LA, Williams RR, Hoover RN, Stegens NL, Feinleib M, Fraumeni FJ Jr,** Breast cancer risk factors among screening program participants, JNCI 62:37, 1979.

67. **Horwitz R, Feinstein AR,** The clinical epidemiology of breast and uterine cancer, in *The Menopause and Postmenopause*, Pasello N, Paoli UR, Ambrus JL, eds, MTD Press, Ltd, Lancaster, England, 1980.

68. **Hertz R,** The steroid cancer hypothesis, J Steroid Biochem 11:435, 1979.

69. **Hoover R, Gray LA, Cole P, MacMahon B,** Menopausal estrogens and breast cancer, N Engl J Med 295:401, 1976.

70. **Ross RK, Paganini-Hill A, Gerkins V, Mack TM, Pfeffer R, Arthur M, Henderson BE,** A case-control study of menopausal estrogen therapy and breast cancer, JAMA 243:1635, 1980

71. **Jick H, Walker AM, Watkins RN, D'Ewart DC, Hunter JR, Danford A, Madsen S, Dinan BJ, Rothman KJ,** Replacement estrogens and breast cancer, Am J Epidemiol 112:586, 1980.

72. **Kelsey JL, LaVolsi V,** Estrogen replacement therapy and breast cancer incidence, JNCI 67:327, 1981.

73. **Gambrell RD Jr,** The menopause: benefits and risks of estrogen-progestogen replacement therapy, Fertil Steril 37:457, 1982.

74. **Smith DC, Prentice R, Thompson DJ, Hermann WL,** Association of exogenous estrogens and endometrial carcinoma, N Engl J Med 293:1164, 1975.

75. **Ziel AK, Finkle WD,** Increased risk of endometrial carcinoma among users of conjugated estrogens, N Engl J Med 293:1167, 1975.

76. **Mack TM, Pike MC, Henderson BE, Pfeffer RI, Gerkins VR, Arthur M, Brown SE,** Estrogens and endometrial cancer in a retirement community, N Engl J Med 294:1262, 1976.

77. **Antunes CMF, Stolley PD, Rosenshein NB, Davies JL, Tonascia JA, Brown C, Burnett L, Rutledge A, Pokempner M, Garcia R,** Endometrial cancer and estrogen use. Report of a large case-control study, N Engl J Med 300:9, 1979.

78. **Horwitz RI, Feinstein AR,** Alternative analytic methods for case control studies of estrogens and endometrial cancer, N Engl J Med 299:1089, 1978.

79. **Sturde DW, Wade-Evans T, Paterson MEL, Thom M, Studd JWW,** Relations between bleeding pattern, endometrial histology, and oestrogen treatment in menopausal women, Br Med J 1:1575, 1978.

80. **Cramer DW, Knapp RC,** Review of epidemiologic studies of endometrial cancer and exogenous estrogen, Obstet Gynecol 54:521, 1979.

81. **Gambrell RD Jr, Massey FM, Castaneda TA, Ugenas AJ, Ricci CA,** Reduced incidence of endometrial cancer among postmenopausal women treated with progestogens, J Am Geriatr Soc 27:389, 1979.

82. **Campbell S, McQueen J, Minardi J, Whitehead MI,** The modifying effect of progestogen and the response of the postmenopausal endometrium to exogenous estrogen, Postgrad Med J Sup(2), 54:59, 1978.

83. **Paterson MEL, Wade-Evans T, Sturdee DW, Thom MH, Studd JWW,** Endometrial disease after treatment with oestrogens and progestogens in the climacteric, Br Med J 1:822, 1980.

84. **Gusberg S,** The individual at high risk for endometrial carcinoma, Am J Obstet Gynecol 126:535, 1976.

85. **Hulka BS,** Effect of exogenous estrogen on postmenopausal women: the epidemiological evidence, Obstet Gynecol Surv 35:389, 1980.

86. **Clarke CL, Adams JB, Wren BG,** Induction of estrogen sulfotransferase in the human endometrium by progesterone in organ culture, J Clin Endocrinol Metab 55:70, 1982.

87. **Thom MH, White PJ, Williams RM, Sturdee DW, Paterson MEL, Wade-Evans T, Studd JWW,** Prevention and treatment of endometrial disease in climacteric women receiving estrogen, Lancet 2:455, 1979.

88. **The British Gynaecological Cancer Group,** Oestrogen replacement and endometrial cancer, Lancet 1:1359, 1981.

89. **Whitehead MI, Townsend PT, Pryse-Davies J, Ryder TA, King RJB,** Effects of estrogens and progestins on the biochemistry and morphology of the postmenopausal endometrium, N Engl J Med 305:1599, 1981.

90. **Gambrell RD Jr, Massey FM, Castenda TA, Ugenes AJ, Ricci CA, Wright JM,** Use of the progestogen challenge test to reduce the risk of endometrial cancer, Obstet Gynecol 55:732, 1980.

91. **Mandel FP, Geola FL, Lu JK, Eggena P, Sambhi MP, Hershman JM, Judd HL,** Biologic effects of various doses of ethinyl estradiol in postmenopausal women, Obstet Gynecol 59:673, 1982.

92. **Gibbons WE, Lobo RA, Roy S, Mishell DR,** Evaluation of estrogen receptor status in the endometria of postmenopausal women on sequential estrogen-progestin therapy, The Endocrine Society Program, Abstract 1079, 1982.

93. **Hirvonen E, Malkonen M, Manninen V,** Effects of different progestogens on lipoproteins during postmenopausal replacement therapy, N Engl J Med 304:560, 1981.

94. **Geola FL, Frumar AM, Tartaryn IV, Lu KH, Hershman JM, Eggena P, Samhli MP, Judd HL,** Biologic effects of various doses of conjugated equine estrogens in postmenopausal women, J Clin Endocrinol Metab 51:620, 1980.

95. **Lindsay R, Hart DM, Purdie D, Ferguson MM, Clark AS, Kraszeweki A,** Comparative effects of oestrogen and a progestogen on bone loss in postmenopausal women, Clin Sci Mol Med 54:193, 1978.

96. **Laufer LR, Erlik Y, Meldrum DR, Judd HL,** Effect of clonidine on hot flashes in postmenopausal women, Obstet Gynecol 60:583, 1982.

97. **Cooper J, Williams S, Patterson JS,** A study of the effectiveness of propranolol in menopausal hot flushes, Br J Obstet Gynaecol 85:472, 1978.

5 Amenorrhea

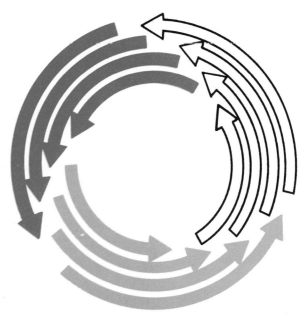

Few problems in gynecologic endocrinology are as challenging or taxing to the clinician as amenorrhea. The physician must be concerned with an array of potential diseases and disorders involving, in many instances, unfamiliar organ systems, some carrying morbid and even lethal consequences for the patient. Not infrequently, the otherwise confident and experienced gynecologist dismisses the problem as too complex for his busy practice and refers the patient to a "specialist" in the field. In doing so, the nonavailability of sophisticated endocrine laboratory techniques is often cited as necessitating the costly and frequently inconvenient transfer of the patient.

The intent of this chapter is to provide a simple mechanism for differential diagnosis of amenorrhea of all types and chronology, utilizing procedures available to all physicians. Strict adherence to this design will unerringly pinpoint the organ system locus of disorder leading to the presenting symptom of amenorrhea. Once this is accomplished, the detailed evidence confirming the diagnosis can be sought and the assistance of appropriate specialists (neurosurgeon, internist, endocrinologist, psychiatrist) confidently chosen. In the end, the patient receives the most reliable diagnosis and therapy at minimum cost and optimum convenience. The majority of patients with amenorrhea have relatively simple problems which can be easily managed by the patient's primary care physician.

The "workup" to be described is not new. With minor modifications, it has been continuously and successfully applied for several decades. Before presenting the diagnostic workup in detail, it is necessary to provide a definition of amenorrhea designating the appropriate selection of patients. In addition, a brief review of the physiologic mechanisms by which a menstrual flow is produced is presented to clarify the logic of the various steps in the diagnostic procedure.

Definition of Amenorrhea

Any patient fulfilling the following criteria should be evaluated as having the clinical problem of amenorrhea:

1. No period by age 14 in the absence of growth or development of secondary sexual characteristics.

2. No period by age 16 regardless of the presence of normal growth and development with the appearance of secondary sexual characteristics.

3. In a woman who has been menstruating, the absence of periods for a length of time equivalent to a total of at least 3 of the previous cycle intervals, or 6 months of amenorrhea.

Having affirmed the traditional criteria, let us now point out that strict adherence to these criteria may result in improper management of individual cases. There is no reason to defer the evaluation of a young girl who presents with the obvious stigmata of Turner's syndrome. Similarly, the 14-year-old girl with an absent vagina who is otherwise completely normal should not be told to return in 2 years. A patient deserves a considerate evaluation whenever her anxieties or those of her parents bring her to a physician. Finally, the possibility of pregnancy should always be considered.

Another tradition has been to categorize amenorrhea as primary or secondary in nature. While these stipulations are inherent in the classic definitions noted above, experience has shown that premature categorization of this sort leads to diagnostic omission in certain instances, and frequently, unnecessary and expensive diagnostic procedures. Because the prescribed workup to be detailed here applies comprehensively to all amenorrheas, the classic distinctions are not retained.

Basic Principles in Menstrual Function

The clinical presence of menstrual function depends on visible external evidence of the menstrual discharge. This requires an intact outflow tract which connects the internal genital source of flow with the outside. As such, the outflow tract requires patency and continuity of the vaginal orifice, the vaginal canal, and the endocervix with the uterine cavity. The presence of a menstrual flow depends on the existence and development of the endometrium lining the uterine cavity. This tissue is stimulated and regulated by the proper quantity and sequence of the steroid hormones, estrogen and progesterone. The secretion of these hormones originates in the ovary, but more specifically in the evolving spectrum of follicle development, ovulation, and corpus luteum function. This essential maturation of the follicular apparatus is guided by the stimuli provided by the sequence and magnitude of the gonadotropins, follicle-stimulating hormone (FSH) and luteinizing hormone (LH), originating in the anterior pituitary. The secretion of these hormones is in turn dependent upon gonadotropin releasing hormone (GnRH), the specific peptide releasing hormone produced in the median eminence area of the basal hypothalamus and blood borne via the portal vessels of the stalk to action points within the anterior pituitary. The entire system is regulated by a complex mechanism which integrates biophysical and biochemical information comprised of feedback levels of ovarian steroids and pituitary gonadotropins as well as neurohumors derived from higher hypothalamic and other CNS resources.

The basic principles underlying the physiology of menstrual function permit formulation of several discrete compartmental systems on which proper menstruation depends. It is useful to employ a diagnostic evaluation which segregates causes of amenorrhea into the following compartments:

Compartment I:
Disorders of outflow tract or uterine target organ.

Compartment II:
Disorders of the ovary.

Compartment III
Disorders of the anterior pituitary.

Compartment IV:
Disorders of CNS (hypothalamic) factors.

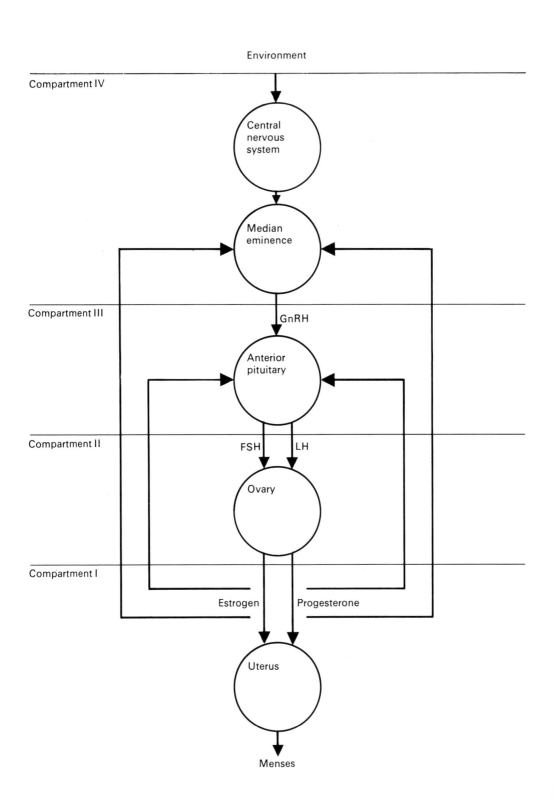

Evaluation of Amenorrhea

A careful history and physical examination should seek the following: evidence for psychological dysfunction or emotional stress, family history of apparent genetic anomalies, signs of a physical problem with a focus on nutritional status, abnormal growth and development, the presence of a normal reproductive tract, and evidence for CNS disease. A patient with amenorrhea is then exposed to a combined therapeutic and laboratory dissection according to the depicted flow diagrams. Because a significant number of patients with amenorrhea also have galactorrhea, and there are similarities in the evaluation of these two conditions, the workup as described is appropriate for patients who have amenorrhea or galactorrhea, or both. Galactorrhea is also considered in Chapter 9.

Amenorrhea and galactorrhea are the sole pertinent initial items of information. Although additional data are undoubtedly available at this time, achieved by history and physical examination and evaluation of other endocrine glands such as the thyroid and adrenal, these items should not be utilized for diagnostic purposes until the entire workup is completed. Experience has shown that premature diagnostic bias at this point, while frequently accurate, not uncommonly leads to erroneous judgments as well as inappropriate, costly, and useless testing.

Step 1

The initial step in the workup of the amenorrheic patient includes a measurement of thyroid stimulating hormone (TSH), a prolactin level, and a progestational challenge. The initial step in the patient presenting with galactorrhea, regardless of menstrual history, also includes TSH and prolactin measurement, but adds a coned down, lateral x-ray view of the sella turcica.

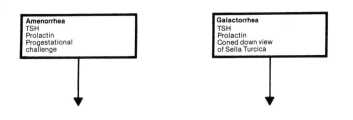

Only a few patients presenting with amenorrhea and/or galactorrhea will have hypothyroidism which is not clinically apparent. Although it seems rather extravagant to measure TSH in such a large number of patients for such a small return, treatment for hypothyroidism is so simple and is rewarded by such a prompt return of ovulatory cycles, and if galactorrhea is present, by a disappearance of the breast secretions, TSH measurement is warranted. It is not sufficient to measure the routine thyroid function tests. A patient may be in a compensated state with normal thyroxine (T_4) levels achieved by increased TSH secretion. With regard to the mechanism of the galactorrhea, the duration of the hypothyroidism is important; the longer the duration the higher the incidence of galactorrhea and the

145

higher the prolactin levels. (1) This is thought to be associated with declining hypothalamic content of dopamine with on-going hypothyroidism. This would lead to an unopposed TRH stimulatory effect on the pituitary cells which secrete prolactin. In our experience, prolactin levels associated with primary hypothyroidism have always been less than 100 ng/ml.

The constant stimulation of the pituitary by hypothalamic releasing hormones results in hypertrophy or hyperplasia. The x-ray picture of a tumor, therefore, may be seen with hypothyroidism, and in patients with elevated GnRH and gonadotropin secretion due to premature ovarian failure. (2, 3)

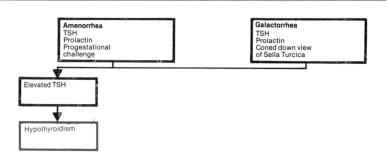

The purpose of the progestational challenge is to assess the level of endogenous estrogen and the competence of the outflow tract. A course of a progestational agent totally devoid of estrogenic activity is administered. There are two choices: parenteral progesterone in oil (200 mg) or orally active medroxyprogesterone acetate (Provera), 10 mg daily for 5 days. The use of an orally active agent avoids an unpleasant intramuscular injection (although this might be necessary when compliance is a concern). Other hormonal preparations, such as birth control pills, are not appropriate since they do not exert a purely progestational effect.

Within 2–7 days after the conclusion of progestational medication, the patient will either bleed or not bleed. If the patient bleeds, one has reliably and securely established a diagnosis of anovulation. The presence of a functional outflow tract and a uterus lined by reactive endometrium sufficiently prepared by endogenous estrogen are confirmed. With this demonstration of the presence of estrogen, minimal function of the ovary, pituitary, and CNS is established. In the absence of galactorrhea, with a normal prolactin level, and a normal TSH, further evaluation is unnecessary. Approximately 50–60% of patients with anovulation are amenorrheic. All anovulatory patients require therapeutic management and with this minimal evaluation, therapy can be planned immediately. The systematic analysis of this problem is the subject of Chapter 6. If, at any time, an anovulatory patient develops a failure to have withdrawal bleeding, this is a sign (providing the patient is not pregnant) that she has moved to the negative withdrawal bleed category, and the remainder of the workup must be pursued. The progestational challenge will occasionally trigger an ovulation in an anovulatory patient. The tip-off will be a later withdrawal bleed, 14 days after the progestational challenge!

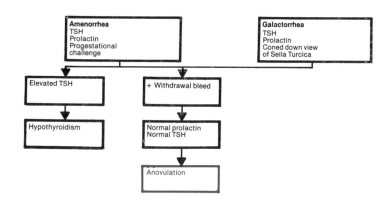

In the absence of galactorrhea, if the serum prolactin level is normal (less than 20 ng/ml in some laboratories, and 30 ng/ml in others), further evaluation for the presence of a pituitary tumor is unnecessary when the patient has undergone a withdrawal bleed. Random single samples for prolactin are sufficient as variations in the amplitude of the spikes of secretion and the sleep-related increase appear to be abolished in both functional and tumor hyperprolactinemic states. If the prolactin is elevated, x-ray evaluation of the sella turcica by a coned down view is essential (discussed below). Likewise, the presence of galactorrhea, regardless of the bleeding pattern or the prolactin level, requires a coned down view. At this point in the workup, the following statement is a useful clinical rule of thumb: *A positive withdrawal bleeding response to progestational medication, the absence of galactorrhea, and a normal prolactin level together effectively rule out the presence of a significant pituitary tumor.*

How much bleeding constitutes a positive withdrawal response? The appearance of only a few blood spots following progestational medication implies marginal levels of endogenous estrogen. Such patients should be followed closely and periodically re-evaluated, since the marginally positive response may progress to a clearly negative response, placing the patient in a new diagnostic category. Bleeding in any amount beyond a few spots is considered a positive withdrawal response.

147

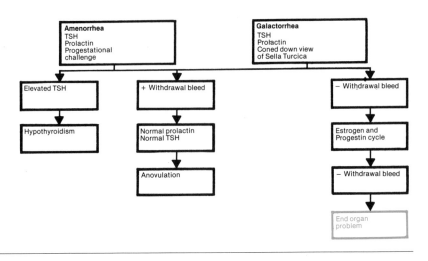

Amenorrhea TSH Prolactin Progestational challenge			**Galactorrhea** TSH Prolactin Coned down view of Sella Turcica	

Elevated TSH   + Withdrawal bleed   – Withdrawal bleed

Hypothyroidism   Normal prolactin / Normal TSH   Estrogen and Progestin cycle

Anovulation   – Withdrawal bleed

End organ problem

Step 2	If the course of progestational medication does not produce withdrawal flow, either the target organ outflow tract is inoperative or preliminary estrogen preparation of the endometrium has not occurred. Step 2 is designed to clarify this situation. Orally active estrogen is administered in quantity and duration certain to stimulate endometrial proliferation and withdrawal bleeding provided that a completely reactive uterus and patent outflow tract exist. An appropriate dose is 2.5 mg conjugated estrogens daily for 21 days. The terminal addition of an orally active progestational agent (Provera 10 mg daily for the last 5 days) is useful to achieve withdrawal. In this way the capacity of Compartment I is challenged by exogenous estrogen. In the absence of withdrawal flow, a validating second course of estrogen is a wise precaution.

As a result of the pharmacologic test of Step 2, the patient with amenorrhea will either bleed or not bleed. If there is no withdrawal flow, the diagnosis of a defect in the Compartment I systems (endometrium, outflow tract) can be made with confidence. If withdrawal bleeding does occur, one can assume that Compartment I systems have normal functional abilities if properly stimulated by estrogen.

In a patient with normal external and internal genitalia by pelvic examination, and in the absence of a history of infection or trauma (such as curettage), Step 2 can be safely omitted. Abnormalities in the systems of Compartment I are not commonly encountered.

Step 3	With the elucidation of the amenorrheic patient's inability to provide adequate stimulatory amounts of estrogen, the physiologic mechanisms responsible for the elaboration of this steroid must be tested. In order to produce estrogen, gonads containing a normal follicular apparatus and sufficient pituitary gonadotropins to stimulate that apparatus are required. Step 3 is designed to determine which of these two crucial components (gonadotropins or follicular activity) is functioning improperly.

Clinical State	Serum FSH	Serum LH
Normal adult female	5–30 mIU/ml, with the ovulatory midcycle peak about 2 times the base level	5–20 mIU/ml with the ovulatory midcycle peak about 3 times the base level
Hypogonadotropic state: Prepubertal, Hypothalamic and Pituitary Dysfunction	Less than 5 mIU/ml	Less than 5 mIU/ml
Hypergonadotropic state: Postmenopausal, Castrate and Ovarian Failure	Greater than 40 mIU/ml	Greater than 25 mIU/ml

This step involves an assay of the level of gonadotropins in the patient. Two important points must be made at this point in the workup. Since Step 2 involved administration of exogenous estrogen, endogenous gonadotropin levels may be artificially and temporarily altered from their true baseline concentrations. Hence, a delay of 2 weeks following Step 2 must ensue before doing Step 3, the gonadotropin assay. The second point relates to the type of assay to be done. The total urinary gonadotropin assay performed on a 24-hour urine specimen should be abandoned. Even in a normal patient the urinary assay may return with a zero level or a postmenopausal level. In recent years physicians have turned to the more precise radioimmunoassay of gonadotropins in serum. The convenience of a single blood specimen is matched by the reliability of the method. One should keep in mind that the midcycle surge of LH is approximately 3 times the baseline level. Therefore, if the patient does not bleed 2 weeks after the blood sample was obtained, the high level can be safely interpreted as abnormal.

Step 3 is designed to determine whether the lack of estrogen is due to a fault in the follicle (Compartment II) or in the CNS-pituitary axis (Compartments III and IV). The result of the gonadotropin assay in the amenorrheic woman who does not bleed following a progestional agent will be abnormally high, abnormally low, or in the normal range.

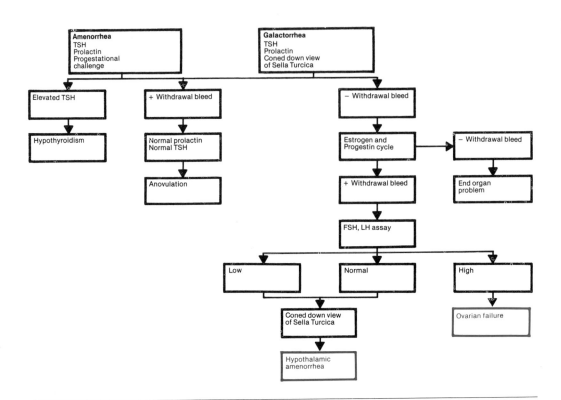

High Gonadotropins

The association between castrate or postmenopausal levels of gonadotropins and ovarian failure is very reliable. However, there are several rare situations in which high gonadotropins may be accompanied by ovaries that contain follicles.

1. On rare occasions, tumors can produce gonadotropins. This situation is usually associated with lung cancer and is so infrequent, that with a normal history and physical examination, routine chest x-ray is not warranted in amenorrheic patients.

2. There are conditions in which there is a single gonadotropin deficiency. In such a case, primary amenorrhea is associated with a high LH level and undetectable FSH, or vice-versa.

3. During the perimenopausal period, it is normal for FSH levels to begin to rise even before bleeding has ceased. (4) This can be true whether the perimenopausal period is premature at age 25–35 or at the usual time. It is believed that FSH is under the negative feedback control of a peptide (folliculostatin) produced by granulosa cells. This situation is analogous to the peptide called inhibin produced by the Sertoli cells in the testicle. During the perimenopausal period the remaining follicles may be viewed as the least sensitive of all follicles because they have remained in place and failed to respond to gonadotropins for many years. As these remaining follicles begin to respond to the rising gonadotropin levels during the perimenopause, the produc-

150

tion of the peptide responsible for the negative feedback may be inadequate, and the patient may have elevated levels of FSH despite continued bleeding or a recent onset of amenorrhea. Attention must be paid to this situation because a period of postmenopausal levels of FSH may be followed by a pregnancy. The value of measuring both FSH and LH is emphasized in that this special perimenopausal condition is usually associated with a high FSH, but a normal LH.

4. The resistant or insensitive ovary syndrome is a condition in which a patient with amenorrhea has elevated gonadotropins despite the presence of ovarian follicles. It is believed that this condition represents an absence of gonadotropin receptors on the follicles. In these cases laparotomy is the only way to evaluate the ovaries adequately, because follicles are contained deep within the ovary, yielding only to a full thickness biopsy. (5–7) Because this condition is vary rare, and the chance of achieving pregnancy is probably impossible even with added exogenous gonadotropins, laparotomy is NOT recommended.

5. The final rare clinical situation associated with high gonadotropins, but normal ovarian follicles is an enzymatic deficiency in both the ovaries and the adrenal glands, the 17-hydroxylase deficiency. Such a patient would present with absent secondary sexual development because sex steroids could not be produced. Because of the enzyme block in the adrenal glands, this patient would also be hypertensive and have high blood levels of progesterone.

All patients under the age of 30 who have been assigned the diagnosis of ovarian failure on the basis of elevated gonadotropins must have a karyotype determination. The presence of mosaicism with a Y chromosome requires laparotomy and excision of the gonadal areas because the presence of any testicular component within the gonad carries with it a 25% chance of malignant tumor formation. Approximately 30% of patients with a Y chromosome will not develop signs of virilization. Therefore, even the normal appearing adult with elevated gonadotropin levels must be karyotyped. Even if the karyotype is normal, as an added precaution, all patients with ovarian failure should have an annual pelvic examination. Such preventive care is also indicated because these patients will be on hormone replacement therapy. Over the age of 30, amenorrhea with high gonadotropins is best labeled premature menopause. Genetic evaluation is unnecessary because it is essentially unheard of to have a gonadal tumor appear in these patients after the age of 30.

Premature Ovarian Failure: A Clinical Dilemma

In the past, patients with elevated gonadotropin levels were considered sterile, a judgment made with great confidence. In recent years, however, rare spontaneous pregnancies have been reported in patients with hypergonadotropic hypogonadism when placed on estrogen therapy. (6) In some patients, return of normal ovarian function with

151

pregnancy has occurred spontaneously. (7) The return of function with estrogen replacement therapy may reflect estrogen enhancement of receptor formation in the follicles, or it may be coincidental. Regardless, these cases are rare compared to the number of patients who develop hypergonadotropic amenorrhea. Is it worthwhile or justified to perform laparotomy and ovarian biopsy on all of these patients?

A number of cases of ovarian failure have been reported with autoimmune disorders, including hypoparathyroidism, thyroiditis, rheumatoid arthritis, myasthenia gravis, Addison's disease, pernicious anemia, and diabetes mellitus. Some of these patients, but not all, have detectable ovarian antibodies. Circulating immunoglobulins can inhibit FSH binding to ovarian follicular receptors. (8) The result is hypergonadotropic amenorrhea in the presence of primordial follicles in the ovaries.

In view of this recent experience, a reasonable approach would be the following: In young patients who desire pregnancy, a few selected blood tests for autoimmune disease are in order:

Calcium
Phosphorus
A.M. cortisol
Free T_4
TSH and thyroid antibodies
Complete blood count and sedimentation rate
Total protein, albumin/globulin ratio
Rheumatoid factor
Antinuclear antibody

Testing for ACTH reserve (with metyrapone, see Chapter 21) seems debatable if clinical appearance and other laboratory tests are normal. Blood gonadotropins and estradiol should be measured weekly on 4 occasions. If FSH is not higher than LH, and if estradiol is not in the postmenopausal range (less than 50 pg/ml), induction of ovulation can be considered. Prior to induction of ovulation, it seems legitimate to offer the patient a choice between a full thickness ovarian biopsy and empirical treatment. Empirical treatment, however, appears to outweigh the cost and risk of laparotomy, because only a rare woman with hypergonadotropic amenorrhea can be expected to conceive.

Normal Gonadotropins

Why is it that hypoestrogenic (negative progestational withdrawal) patients will frequently have normal circulating levels of FSH and LH as measured by the radioimmunoassay? If normal gonadotropins were truly present in the circulation, follicular growth should be maintained and estrogen levels would be adequate to provide a positive withdrawal bleed. The answer to this paradox lies in the heterogeneity of the glycoprotein hormones.

152

Experimental evidence indicates that the molecules of gonadotropins produced by these amenorrheic patients have increased amounts of sialic acid in the carbohydrate portion. (9) Therefore, the molecules are qualitatively altered and biologically inactive. The antibodies in the radioimmunoassay, however, are able to recognize a sufficient portion of the molecule to return a normal answer. A low estrogen environment is associated with higher levels of immunoreactive LH then bioactive LH. (10) Another very rare possibility is an inherited disorder of gonadotropin synthesis leading to the production of immunologically active, but biologically inactive hormones. (11)

The significant clinical point is the following: FSH and LH levels in the normal range in a patient with a negative progestational withdrawal test are consistent with pituitary-CNS failure. Indeed this is the more commonly encountered clinical situation in that extremely low or nondetectable gonadotropins are seldom found, usually only with large pituitary tumors or in patients with anorexia nervosa. Further evaluation, therefore, is in order, and follows the recommendations for low gonadotropins.

Low Gonadotropins

If the gonadotropin assay is abnormally low, or in the normal range, one final localization is required to distinguish between a pituitary (Compartment III) or CNS-hypothalmic (Compartment IV) cause for the amenorrhea. Skull films should be obtained to examine the sella turcica for signs of abnormal change.

X-ray Evaluation of the Sella Turcica. In recent years the radiologic evaluation of the pituitary area has undergone rapid change. At one time polytomography was the x-ray study of choice. Polytomography consists of tomographic sections (at approximately 1 mm increments) of the sella turcica in the lateral and anteroposterior projections, with movement which blurs structures not in the plane of the section, giving excellent focal resolution. Experience has indicated, however, that the accuracy of tomography is only 60% with both false positive and false negative readings. (12, 13) While it is true that most patients (as high as 90%) with the combination of abnormal polytomography and a prolactin over 100 ng/ml will have an adenoma, it is also true that patients with hypothyroidism or hypogonadism may have sellar changes similar to tumors (2) and patients with normal x-rays may have tumors. (12) Finally the continued development of computerized axial tomography (the CAT or CT scan) has led to the abandonment of the polytomogram. (14) The most modern CT scan (capable of high resolution 1 mm cuts) is able to evaluate the contents of the sella turcica as well as the suprasellar area.

The purpose of this workup is to isolate those few patients who require the sophisticated and expensive CT scan. There has been a growing conservatism with the management of small pituitary tumors, because the majority of these tumors never change. We have adopted a conservative approach of

153

close surveillance, recommending surgery only for those tumors that display rapid growth or those tumors that are already large. The initial x-ray evaluation of hypoestrogenic, hypogonadotropic, amenorrheic patients, with or without galactorrhea, is the coned down view of the sella turcia, in the lateral projection. *A double floor of the sella is often seen on the coned down view and, in the absence of enlargement and/or demineralization, is interpreted as a normal variation rather than asymmetrical depression of the sellar floor by a tumor.*

Combining this screening technique with the prolactin assay, we are able to select those few patients who require the modern CT scan. If the prolactin level is greater than 100 ng/ml, or if the coned down view of the sella turcia is abnormal, we recommend CT scan evaluation. If the CT scan rules out an empty sella syndrome, or a suprasellar problem, surgical intervention is then dictated by the patient's desires, the size of the tumor, and rapidity of growth of the tumor.

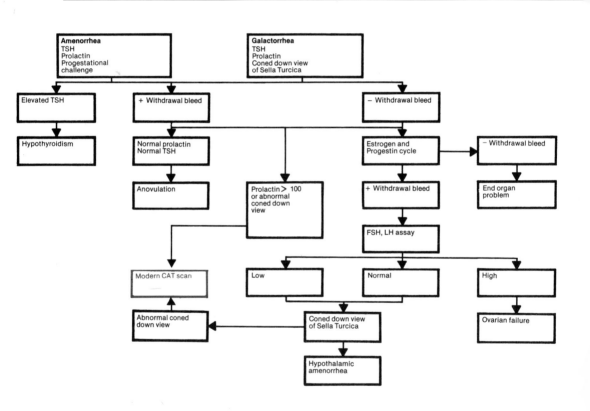

The above approach to the problem of pituitary tumors implies that patients with prolactin levels less than 100 ng/ml and with normal coned down views of the sella turcica are offered a choice between bromocriptine therapy and surveillance. An annual prolactin level and an annual coned down view are indicated for continued observation to detect an emerging and slow-growing tumor. Bromocriptine therapy is recommended for patients wishing to achieve pregnancy, and for those patients who have galactorrhea to the point of discomfort. The prolactin level of 100 ng/ml for determining a more aggressive approach has been empirically chosen. Both in our own experience, and that of others, large tumors are most frequently associated with prolactin levels greater than 100. (15)

Patients with amenorrhea and without galactorrhea who have reached this point in the workup and have normal x-rays are classified as hypothalamic amenorrhea. The mechanism of the amenorrhea is suppression of pulsatile GnRH secretion below its critical range. This is a diagnosis by exclusion because we can identify probable causes (e.g. anorexia and weight loss) but we cannot test, manipulate, or measure the hypothalamus to prove our diagnosis.

Evaluation of the Abnormal Sella Turcica and/or High Prolactin. The high incidence of pituitary tumors in patients with amenorrhea has prompted a search for a reliable method of diagnosing the condition. Expectations for the utilization of endocrine testing to discriminate between disorders of the hypothalamus and the anterior pituitary have not been realized. Tremendous variability in response is the rule, even to the degree that the patient with a pituitary tumor may or may not respond. These maneuvers include GnRH stimulation, thyroid releasing hormone (TRH) stimulation, and other steps to alter prolactin, growth hormone, and ACTH secretion. TRH stimulation of the prolactin response is the most consistently abnormal response (a blunter release of prolactin), but some patients with tumors respond normally. (12, 16, 17) A combined approach can be utilized, simultaneously testing the response of prolactin, TSH, gonadotropins, growth hormone, and ACTH. (16) The method is as follows: Bolus administration includes 200 μg TRH, 100 μg GnRH, and 0.15 unit/kg of insulin. Normal responses include:

Prolactin increment greater than 20 ng and double the baseline

TSH increment greater than 6 microunits/ml

LH increment greater than 4 mIU/ml

FSH increment double the baseline

Growth hormone increment greater than 8 ng/ml

Cortisol increment greater than 6 μg/dl

Frankly, the above endocrine maneuvers yield no more useful information than the two major screening procedures, the blood prolactin and the coned down view of the sella turcica. Visual field examination is not useful in screening for pituitary tumors because abnormalities are seen only with large tumors which are evident by prolactin and/or x-ray evaluation. If the coned down view is abnormal and/or the prolactin level is over 100, further evaluation and treatment require consultation with expert endocrine resources. These patients are rare, and accumulated experience which can provide the necessary clinical judgment can be found only with the referral resource. On the other hand, our workup easily deals with the vast majority of patients, and the few who require a multidisciplinary team approach are readily identified.

Specific Disorders within Compartments

With only modest effort, expense, and time the problem of amenorrhea has been dissected into compartments of dysfunction which positively correlate with specific organ systems. At this point, with the specific anatomic locus of the defect defined, the clinician can now undertake steps to elucidate the specific disorder leading to amenorrhea. Within each anatomic compartment certain diagnostic frequencies are observed.

Compartment I

Asherman's Syndrome. Secondary amenorrhea follows destruction of the endometrium (Asherman's syndrome). (18) This condition generally is the result of an overzealous postpartum curettage resulting in intrauterine scarification. A typical pattern of multiple synechiae is seen on a hysterogram. In the presence of normal ovarian function, the basal body temperature will be biphasic. The adhesions may partially or completely obliterate the endometrial cavity, the internal cervical os, or the cervical canal, or combinations of these areas. Surprisingly, despite stenosis or atresia of the internal os, hematometra does not inevitably occur. (19) The endometrium, perhaps in response to a buildup of pressure, becomes refractory and simple cervical dilatation cures the problem. Asherman's syndrome can also occur following uterine surgery, including cesarean section, myomectomy, or metroplasty. Very severe adhesions have been noted following postpartum curettage and postpartum hypogonadism, e.g. in Sheehan's syndrome.

Patients with Asherman's syndrome may present with other problems besides amenorrhea, including abortions, dysmenorrhea, or hypomenorrhea. They may even have normal menses. Infertility may be present with mild adhesions, an association not readily explainable. Patients with repeated abortions, infertility, or pregnancy wastage should have investigation of the endometrial cavity by hysterogram or hysteroscopy.

Impairment of the endometrium resulting in amenorrhea can be caused by tuberculosis, a rare but still present condition in the United States. Diagnosis is made by culture of the menstrual discharge or tissue obtained by endometrial biopsy. Uterine schistosomiasis is another rare cause of end organ failure, and eggs may be found in urine, feces, rectal scrapings, menstrual discharge, or endometrium. In recent years, we have seen the syndrome following intra-uterine device (IUD)-related infections, and severe pelvic infections.

Asherman's syndrome can be treated with a dilatation and curettage to break up the synechiae, and if necessary an on-the-table hysterogram to ensure a free uterine cavity. Advocates of the hysteroscope claim that direct lysis of adhesions yields better results than the "blind" dilatation and curettage. (20) At operation, a method should be utilized to prevent the sides of the uterine cavity from adhering. Previously an IUD was used for this purpose; however, a pediatric Foley catheter appears to be a better method. The bag is filled with 3 ml of fluid, and the catheter is removed after 7 days. A broad-spectrum antibiotic is started preoperatively and maintained for 10 days. The patient is treated for 2 months with high stimulatory doses of estrogen (e.g. conjugated estrogens 10 mg daily 3 weeks out of 4 with Provera 10 mg daily added during the 3rd week). When the initial attempt fails to reestablish menstrual flow, repeated attempts are worthwhile. Persistent treatment with repeated procedures may be necessary to regain reproductive potential. In recent reports approximately 70–80% of patients with this condition have achieved a successful pregnancy. Pregnancy is frequently complicated by premature labor, placenta accreta, placenta previa, and postpartum hemorrhage.

Müllerian Anomalies. In primary amenorrheas, discontinuity by segmental disruptions of the Müllerian tube should be ruled out. Good clinical practice demands a survey which begins distally and works proximally. Thus, imperforate hymen, obliteration of the vaginal orifice, and lapses in continuity of the vaginal canal must be ruled out by direct observation. The cervix or the entire uterus may be absent. Far less common, the uterus may be present, but the cavity absent, or, in the presence of a cavity, the endometrium may be congenitally lacking. With the exception of the latter abnormalities, the clinical problem of amenorrhea due to obstruction is compounded by the painful distension of hematocolpos, hematometra, or hematoperitoneum. In all instances an effort must be made to incise and drain from below at the points of closure of the Müllerian tube. Even in complicated circumstances re-establishment of Müllerian duct continuity can usually be achieved surgically. The unfortunate consequences of operative extirpation of painful masses from above with danger to bladder, ureter, and rectum, as well as irretrievable loss of distended but otherwise healthy, reproductive organs are rare but well remembered.

Müllerian Agenesis. Lack of Müllerian development (Mayer-Rokitansky-Kuster-Hauser syndrome) is the diagnosis for the individual with primary amenorrhea and no apparent vagina. (21) This is a relatively common cause of primary amenorrhea, more frequent than testicular femin-

157

ization, and second only to gonadal dysgenesis. These patients have an absence or hypoplasia of the vagina. The uterus may be normal, but lacking a conduit to the introitus, or there may only be rudimentary, bicornuate cords present. If a partial endometrial cavity is present, cyclic abdominal pain may be a complaint. Because of the similarity to some types of male pseudohermaphroditism, it is worthwhile to demonstrate the normal female karyotype. Ovarian function is normal, and can be documented with basal body temperatures or peripheral levels of progesterone. Growth and development are normal. Although usually sporadic, occasional occurrence may be noted within a family.

Further evaluation should include radiologic studies. Approximately one third have urinary tract abnormalities and 12% or more have skeletal anomalies, most involving the spine. (21) Renal tract abnormalities include ectopic kidney, renal agenesis, horseshoe kidney, and abnormal collecting tracts. When the presence of a uterine structure is suspected on examination, ultrasound can be utilized to depict the size and symmetry of the structure. Laparoscopic visualization of the pelvis is not necessary and extirpation of the Müllerian remnants is certainly not necessary unless they are causing a problem such as uterine fibroid growth, hematometra, endometriosis, or symptomatic herniation into the inguinal canal.

Because of the difficulties and complications experienced in surgical series, we favor, when possible, abandonment of the surgical construction of an artificial vagina. Instead, we encourage the use of progressive dilatation as first described by Frank (22) and later by Wabrek et al. (23). Beginning first in a downward posterior direction, and then after 2 weeks changing upward to the usual line of the vaginal axis, pressure with commercially available glass vaginal dilators is carried out for 20 min daily to the point of modest discomfort. Utilizing increasingly larger dilators, a functional vagina can be created in approximately 6–12 weeks. Plastic syringe covers can be used instead of the expensive commercial glass dilators. Operative treatment should be reserved for those women in whom a well-formed uterus is present and fertility might be preserved. The symptoms of retained menstruation should identify these patients. Unless it is the relatively simple problem of an imperforate hymen or a transverse vaginal septum, some have recommended against trying to preserve fertility in the presence of complete vaginal agenesis. (24) The morbidity subsequent to surgery argues for removal of the Müllerian structures at the time of construction of a neovagina. Patients with a transverse vaginal septum, which is a failure of canalization of the distal third of the vagina, usually present with symptoms of obstruction and urinary frequency. A transverse septum can be differentiated from an imperforate hymen by a lack of distension at the introitus with Valsalva's maneuver.

Distal obstruction of the genital tract is the only condition in this category which can be considered an emergency. Delay in surgical treatment can lead to infertility due to inflammatory changes and endometriosis. Definitive surgery should be accomplished as soon as possible. Diagnostic needling should be avoided because a hematocolpos can be converted into a pyocolpos.

Reassurance and support are necessary to carry a patient through these procedures. Problems with body image and sexual enjoyment can be avoided and, although infertile, a full and normal life as a woman can be achieved.

Testicular Feminization. Testicular feminization is the likely diagnosis when a blind vaginal canal is encountered and the uterus is absent. The patient with testicular feminization is a male pseudohermaphrodite. The adjective male refers to the gonadal sex; thus, the individual has testes and an XY karyotype. Pseudohermaphrodite means that the genitalia are opposite of the gonads; thus, the individual is phenotypically female, but with absent or meager pubic and axillary hair.

The male pseudohermaphrodite is a genetic and gonadal male with failure of virilization. Failures in male development can be considered as a spectrum with incomplete forms of testicular feminization being represented by some androgen response. Transmission of this disorder is by means of an X-linked recessive gene that is responsible for the androgen intracellular receptor. Clinically the diagnosis should be considered in: 1) a female child with inguinal hernias, since the testes are frequently partially descended; 2) a patient with primary amenorrhea and an absent uterus; and 3) a patient with absent body hair.

These patients appear normal at birth, except for the possible presence of an inguinal hernia, and most patients are not seen by a physician until puberty. Growth and development are normal, although overall height is usually greater than average and there may be a eunuchoidal tendency (long arms, big hands and feet). The breasts, although large, are abnormal; actual glandular tissue is not abundant and the nipples are small and the areolae are pale. More than 50% have an inguinal hernia; the labia minora are usually underdeveloped, and the blind vagina is less deep than normal. Rudimentary Fallopian tubes are composed of fibromuscular tissue with only occasional epithelial lining.

Perhaps urological evaluation in these patients has been inadequately pursued. Horseshoe kidneys in two phenotypic females with XY karyotypes have been reported. (25)

The testes may be intra-abdominal, but often are in a hernia. They are similar to any cryptorchid testis except that they may be nodular. After puberty, the testis has immature tubular development, and tubules are lined by immature germ cells and Sertoli cells. There is no spermatogenesis. The incidence of neoplasia in these gonads is high. In 50 reported cases, there were 11 malignancies, 15 adenomas, and 10 benign cysts, a 22% incidence of malignancy and a 52% incidence of neoplasia. (26) Therefore, once full development is attained after puberty, the gonads should be removed and the patient placed on hormonal replacement therapy. This is the only exception to the rule that gonads with a Y chromosome should be removed prior to puberty. The reason is the development achieved with hormonal replacement does not seem to match the smooth pubertal changes due to endogenous hormones. When testicular feminization was first studied, it was found the the urinary 17-ketosteroids were normal, and it was suggested that there might be a resistance to androgen action rather than an absence of androgens—a congenital androgen insensitivity. Indeed, the plasma levels of testosterone are in the normal to high male range, and the plasma clearance and metabolism of testosterone are normal. Thus, these patients produce testosterone, but they do not respond to androgens, either their own or those given locally or systemically. Therefore, the critical steps in sexual differentiation which require androgens fail to take place and development is totally female.

Appropriately this condition is now referred to as the congenital androgen insensitivity syndrome. It is marked by a unique combination:

1. Normal female phenotype.

2. Normal male karyotype, 46,XY.

3. Normal or slightly elevated male blood testosterone levels.

Cases of incomplete testicular feminization represent individuals with some androgen effect. These individuals may have clitoral enlargement, or a phallus may even be present. Axillary and pubic hair develop along with breast growth. Gonadectomy should not be deferred in such cases, because it will obviate unwanted further virilization. Patients with a deficit in testicular 17-dehydrogenase activity will have impaired testosterone production, and present clinically as incomplete testicular feminization. Since treatment is the same, precise diagnosis is not essential.

Conventional wisdom warns against unthinking and needless disclosure of the gonadal and chromosomal sex to a patient with testicular feminization. Although infertile, these patients are certainly completely female in their gender identity, and this should be reinforced rather than challenged. There are exceptions to every rule, however, and certain situations may call for a more straightforward, accurate discussion. One example in our own practice was a student nurse who pointed out that she would much rather have learned the facts from her parents and physician than from the textbooks she was reading in school.

160

**Differences between
Müllerian Agenesis and
Testicular Feminization**

	Müllerian Agenesis	**Testicular Feminization**
Karyotype	46,XX	46,XY
Heredity	Not known	Maternal X-linked recessive; 25% risk of affected child, 25% risk of carrier
Sexual hair	Normal female	Absent to sparse
Testosterone level	Normal female	Normal to slightly elevated male
Other anomalies	Frequent	Rare
Gonadal neoplasia	Normal incidence	Over 25% incidence of malignant tumors

Compartment II

Turner's Syndrome. Turner's syndrome is a well-known and thoroughly discussed entity. The characteristics of short stature, webbed neck, shield chest, and increased carrying angle at the elbow, combined with hypergonadotropic hypoestrogenic amenorrhea, make a correct diagnosis usually possible on the most superficial evaluation. However, special attention must be given to the less common variations of this syndrome. Coarctation of the aorta and various renal collecting system anomalies must be ruled out. A karyotype should be performed on all patients with elevated gonadotropins, despite the appearance of a typical case of Turner's syndrome. The presence of a pure syndrome, 45,X chromosome single cell line, should be confirmed. This expensive test cannot be viewed just as a step toward academic perfection.

Mosaicism. The presence of mosaicism (multiple cell lines of varying sex chromosome composition) must be ruled out for a very important reason. The presence of a Y chromosome in the karyotype requires laparotomy and excision of the gonadal areas, on the basis that the presence of any medullary (testicular) component within the gonad is a predisposing factor to tumor formation and to heterosexual development (virilization). Only in the patient with the complete form of testicular feminization can laparotomy be deferred until after puberty, since the individual is resistant to androgens. In all other patients with a Y chromosome, gonadectomy should be performed before puberty to avoid virilization. One should be aware that approximately 30% of patients with a Y chromosome will not develop any signs of virilization. Therefore, even the normal appearing adult patient with elevated serum levels of gonadotropins must be karyotyped to detect a silent Y chromosome, so that prophylactic gonadectomy can be performed before neoplastic changes occur. Assays for the H-Y antigen are neither generally available nor totally reliable. The fully stained and banded karyotype continues to be the best method to detect the presence of testicular tissue or other mosaic combinations.

161

The impact of mosaicism, even in the absence of a Y-containing line, is significant. With an XX component (e.g. XX/XO), functional cortical (ovarian) tissue can be found within the gonad, leading to a variety of responses, including some degree of female development, and, on occasion, even menses and reproduction. These individuals may appear normal, attaining normal stature before premature menopause is experienced. The menopause is early, presumably because the number of functioning follicles undergoes an accelerated rate of atresia because of the abnormal chromosomal constitution. More commonly, these patients are short, as most patients with missing sex chromosome material are less than 63 inches in height.

This complex array of gonadal dysgenesis variations, from the typical pure form to an otherwise normal appearing and functioning woman with premature menopause, is the result of a variety of mosaicism which produces a complex mixture of cortical and medullary gonadal tissue. The clinical importance of this information justifies obtaining karyotypes in all cases of elevated gonadotropins in women under age 30. All patients with absent ovarian function and quantitative alterations in the sex chromosomes are categorized as having *gonadal dysgenesis*.

XY Gonadal Dysgenesis. A patient with an XY karyotype who has a palpable Müllerian system, normal female testosterone levels, and lack of sexual development has Swyer's syndrome. Tumor transformation in the gonadal ridge can occur at any age, and extirpation of the gonadal streaks should be performed as soon as the diagnosis is made.

Gonadal Agenesis. No complicated clinical problems accompany the gonadal failure due to agenesis. Without precise information, only conjecture as to the causes of absent development can be made. Thus, viral and metabolic influences in early gestation are suspected events. Nevertheless, the final result is irretrievable—hypergonadotropic hypogonadism.

The Resistant Ovary Syndrome. There is a rare patient with amenorrhea who has elevated gonadotropins despite the presence of ovarian follicles. To arrive at a correct diagnosis, laparotomy is necessary to achieve adequate histological evaluation of the ovaries (since laparoscopic biopsy is not representative). (5–7) Because of the rarity of this condition, and the very low chance of achieving pregnancy even with high doses of exogenous gonadotropins, we do not feel it is worthwhile to perform a laparotomy for the purpose of ovarian biopsy on every patient with amenorrhea, high gonadotropins, and a normal karyotype.

Premature Ovarian Failure. The etiology of premature ovarian failure is unknown. It is useful to explain to the patient that it is probably a genetic disorder with either a reduced number of primordial follicles or an increased rate of disappearance. The latter is most likely as even 45,X

(Turner's syndrome) patients begin with a full complement of germ cells, but undergo an acceleration of the atretic process. The only other possibility is destruction of follicles, perhaps by infections such as mumps oophoritis, or a physical insult such as irradiation or chemotherapy. A high incidence of hypergonadotropic hypogonadism has been reported in women with abnormal galactose metabolism. (27) In addition to the above explanations, there may be an autoimmune basis (as previously discussed).

The problems can present at varying ages, as well as in many forms depending upon the number of follicles left. It is a useful concept to view the various presentations as representing a stage in the process of the perimenopausal change. If loss of follicles has been rapid, then primary amenorrhea and lack of sexual development will be present. If loss of follicles takes place during puberty, or later, the onset of secondary amenorrhea will vary accordingly.

Those cases, in whom ovarian failure is not permanent, most likely represent individuals who have a limited number of follicles present which respond after exposure to a period of time to estrogen or elevated gonadotropins or both. Accelerated atresia may be due to a genetic problem within the germ cells, or, because primordial follicle number correlates with fetal levels of gonadotropins, there may have been a deficiency of gonadotropin secretion during fetal life. The patients reported to have temporary failure may be the victims of viral infections of the ovary, with a slow but eventual recovery.

In view of the increasing case reports documenting resumption of normal function, (6, 7) we cannot guarantee that these patients will be sterile forever. On the other hand, laparotomy and full thickness ovarian biopsy surely is not necessary for all of these patients. We believe that a minimal approach, with a survey for autoimmune disease and an assessment of ovarian-pituitary activity, can serve as a guide for an attempt at induction of ovulation (see p. 152).

Compartment III

Disorders of the hypothalamic-pituitary axis must first focus on the problem of the pituitary tumor. Through the appearance of amenorrhea, the patient with a slowly growing pituitary tumor may present years before the tumor becomes evident by radiologic techniques. Fortunately, malignant tumors are almost never encountered, but growth of a benign tumor can cause problems because it is in a confined space. As the tumor grows, it grows upward, compressing the optic chiasm and producing the classic findings of bitemporal hemianopsia. With small tumors, however, abnormal visual fields are rarely encountered. In contrast, other tumors of this region (e.g. craniopharyngioma, usually calcified on x-ray) may be associated with the early development of blurring of vision and visual field defects because of their close proximity to the optic chiasm.

Sometimes the suspicion of a pituitary tumor is increased because of clinical signs of acromegaly due to excessive secretion of growth hormone, or Cushing's disease due to excessive secretion of ACTH. Amenorrhea and/or galactorrhea may precede the eventual full clinical expression of a tumor which secretes ACTH or growth hormone. If clinical criteria suggest Cushing's disease, ACTH levels and the 24-hour urinary levels of free cortisol should be measured, and the rapid suppression test (Chapter 7) should be utilized. If acromegaly is suspected, growth hormone should be measured in the fasting state and during an oral glucose tolerance test. Though usually a problem in adult life, prolactin secreting tumors may be seen in preadolescent and adolescent children, and thus be a cause of failure of growth and development or primary amenorrhea.

Not all intrasellar masses are neoplastic. Gummas, tuberculomas, and fat deposits have been reported as causes of pituitary compression leading to hypogonadotropic amenorrhea. Nearby lesions such as internal carotid artery aneurysms and obstruction of the aqueduct of Sylvius may also cause amenorrhea. Pituitary insufficiency may be secondary to ischemia and infarction, and appear as a late sequela to obstetrical hemorrhage—the well-known Sheehan's syndrome. These problems as well as genetic disorders, such as Laurence-Moon-Biedl and Prader-Willi syndromes, are so rarely encountered that consultation with textbooks and colleagues is necessary.

Pituitary Prolactin-secreting Adenomas

Prolactin-secreting adenomas are the most common pituitary tumors. Tumors less than 1 cm in diameter are referred to as microadenomas, those greater than 1 cm, macroadenomas. Classically pituitary adenomas have been grouped according to their staining ability as eosinophilic, basophilic, or chromophobic. This classification is misleading and of no clinical usefulness. Pituitary adenomas should be classified according to their function, e.g. prolactin-secreting adenoma.

With the utilization of the serum prolactin assay and the increased sensitivity of the new x-ray techniques, the association of amenorrhea and small pituitary tumors has become recognized as a relatively common problem. This does not appear to be a new phenomenon, rather it reflects more sensitive diagnostic techniques. Attempts to link the problem to other factors, such as oral contraceptive use, have proved negative. (28)

The exact incidence of this clinical problem is unknown. In autopsy series the number of pituitary glands found to contain adenomas ranges from 9 to 27%. (13, 29–32) The age distribution ranged from 2 to 86, with the greatest incidence in the 6th decade of life. The sex distribution was equal. However, clinical manifestations, mainly a disruption of the reproductive cycle, are almost exclusively a problem of women, probably due to estrogen-induced activity of the pituitary lactotrophs.

A high prolactin level may be encountered in about one third of women with no obvious cause of amenorrhea. (12) Only one third of patients with high prolactin levels will have galactorrhea, probably because the low estrogen environment associated with the amenorrhea prevents a normal response to prolactin. Such patients may present with primary amenorrhea and no galactorrhea. About one third of women with galactorrhea have normal menses. (15) As the prolactin increases, a patient may progress sequentially from normal ovulation to an inadequate luteal phase to intermittent anovulation to total anovulation to complete amenorrhea.

Possibly as many as one third of patients with secondary amenorrhea will have a pituitary adenoma, and if galactorrhea is also present, half will have an abnormal sella turcica. (15) The clinical symptoms do not always correlate with the prolactin level, and patients with normal prolactins may have pituitary tumors. (33) The highest prolactin levels, however, are associated with amenorrhea, with or without galactorrhea.

The amenorrhea associated with elevated prolactin levels appears to be due to prolactin inhibition of the pulsatile secretion of GnRH. The pituitary glands in these patients respond normally to GnRH, or in augmented fashion (perhaps due to increased stores of gonadotropins), thus, indicating that the mechanism of the amenorrhea is a decrease in GnRH. (34) This is supported by experiments in monkeys, in which animals with destroyed hypothalami and very high prolactin levels were able to respond with normal ovulatory cycles to pulsatile GnRH administration. (35) Regardless of the mechanism, treatment which lowers the circulating levels of prolactin restores ovarian responsiveness and menstrual function. This is true whether the treatment consists of removal of a prolactin-secreting tumor or suppression of prolactin secretion.

The increased ability to detect pituitary tumors has been accompanied by the development of a surgical technique which very effectively removes the small tumors with a high margin of safety. This technique is the transsphenoidal approach to the sella turcica utilizing the operating microscope. (36) The transsphenoidal approach is via a sublabial incision (under the upper lip), with dissection under the nasal mucosa, removal of the nasal septum to expose the sphenoidal sinus, and resection of the floor of the sphenoid sinus to expose the sella turcica. Tumor tissue is usually distinguishable from the yellow-orange, firm tissue of the normal anterior pituitary. However, because pituitary adenomas do not have a capsule, the borderline between tumor and normal tissue is often vague. The ideal time for excision is when the adenoma is a small nodule. When enlarged it becomes more difficult to distinguish normal from pathological tissue. Once the adenoma grows beyond the sella, total removal is essentially impossible.

The development of transsphenoidal surgery was paralleled by the availability and clinical application of the drug, bromocriptine, which specifically suppresses prolactin secretion. For a while, appropriate decisions between the surgical approach and medical treatment were difficult to make. With increasing experience, some perspective has been achieved, and reasonable clinical judgments are now possible. Let us first consider results with surgery, then examine bromocriptine.

Results with Surgery

Transsphenoidal neurosurgery achieves complete resolution of hyperprolactinemia with resumption of cyclic menses in about 40% of patients with macroadenomas and 80–90% of patients with microadenomas. (17, 36–38) Besides an inability to achieve a complete cure, surgery may be followed by recurrence of tumor and a still unknown but significant percentage (perhaps as high as 10–30% after surgery for macroadenomas) of development of panhypopituitarism. Other complications of surgery include, cerebrospinal fluid leaks, an occasional case of meningitis, and the frequent postoperative problem of diabetes insipidus. The diabetes insipidus is a transient problem, rarely lasting as long as 6 months.

There are three possible explanations for the recurrence or persistence of hyperprolactinemia after surgery.

1. The prolactin producing tumor looks like the surrounding normal pituitary, and it is difficult to resect completely.

2. The tumor may be multifocal in origin.

3. There may be a continuing abnormality of the hypothalamus giving rise to chronic stimulation of the lactotrophs.

The following is our recommendation for patients who have had surgery.

1. If cyclic menses return: periodic evaluation for the problem of anovulation.

2. If amenorrhea or oligomenorrhea and hyperprolactinemia persist or recur: prolactin levels every 6 months and a limited (2 selected views) modern CT scan or coned down view yearly for 5 years, then every few years. If tumor growth becomes evident, treatment for an indefinite time with bromocriptine. Bromocriptine can be used to induce ovulation if pregnancy is desired.

Results with radiation therapy are less satisfactory than with surgery. In addition, response is very slow; prolactin concentration may take several years to fall. After radiation (including proton beam treatment) panhypopituitarism may occur as long as 10 years after treatment. Patients who have been treated with radiation therapy should be followed for a long time, and any symptoms suggestive of pituitary failure require investigation.

166

| Bromocriptine (Parlodel) | Bromocriptine is a lysergic acid derivative with a bromine substitute at position 2. (39) It is available as the methanesulfonate (mesylate) in 2.5-mg tablets. It is a dopamine agonist, binding to dopamine receptors, and, therefore, directly mimicking dopamine inhibition of pituitary prolactin secretion. Absorption from the gastrointestinal tract is rapid and complete; therefore, the side effect of vomiting is due to a central rather than a local effect. Bromocriptine is metabolized into at least 30 excretory products. Excretion is mainly biliary, and more than 90% appears in the feces over 5 days after a single dose of 2.5 mg. A small part, 6–7%, is excreted unchanged or as metabolites in the urine. |

Side effects can be minimized by slowly building tolerance toward the usual dose, 2.5 mg b.i.d. Treatment should be started with an initial dose of 2.5 mg, given at bedtime. The peak level is achieved 2 hours after ingestion, and the biological half-life is about 3 hours. If intolerance occurs with this initial dose, then the tablet should be cut in half, and an even slower program should be followed. Usually a week after the initial dose, the second 2.5-mg dose can be added at breakfast or lunch. About 1% of subjects are very sensitive to the first dose, but tolerate subsequent treatment without problems.

Nausea, headache, and faintness are the usual initial problems. The faintness is due to orthostatic hypotension which can be attributed to relaxation of smooth muscle in the splanchnic and renal beds, as well as inhibition of transmitter release at noradrenergic nerve endings and central inhibition of sympathetic activity. Neuropsychiatric symptoms, occasionally with hallucinations, occur in less than 1% of patients. This may be due to hydrolysis of the lysergic acid part of the molecule. Other side effects include dizziness, fatigue, vomiting, and abdominal cramps.

The dose that suppresses prolactin is 10 times lower than that which improves the symptoms of Parkinson's disease. Even higher doses are necessary for the treatment of acromegaly, and only a minority of patients with acromegaly show significant remission.

Results of Treatment. In 22 clinical trials, 80% of patients with amenorrhea/galactorrhea, associated with hyperprolactinemia but no demonstrable tumors, had menses restored. (40) The average treatment time to the initiation of menses was 5.7 weeks. Complete cessation of galactorrhea occurred in 50–60% of patients, in an average time of 12.7 weeks, and a 75% reduction of breast secretions was achieved in 6.4 weeks. Amenorrhea recurred in 41% of the patients within an average of 4.4 weeks of discontinuing treatment; galactorrhea recurred in 69% at an average of 6.0 weeks. About 5% of patients terminate treatment because of adverse reactions.

There are two bromocriptine treatment methods to follow in those patients seeking pregnancy. The first is simply daily administration of 2.5 mg b.i.d. until the patient is pregnant as judged by the basal body temperature chart. In the second method, bromocriptine is administered during the follicular phase, and the drug is stopped when a basal body temperature rise indicates that ovulation has occurred, thus avoiding high drug levels early in pregnancy. The drug is resumed at menses when it is apparent the patient is not pregnant. No comparative study has been performed to tell us whether the follicular phase only method is as effective as the daily method.

Regression of Tumors with Bromocriptine

There is no question that macroadenomas will regress with bromocriptine treatment. (40–45) In some there is prompt shrinkage with low dose treatment 5–7.5 mg daily; in others, prolonged treatment is required with higher doses. Visual improvement may be noted within several days. Very high prolactin levels, greater than 2000–3000 ng/ml, are probably the result of invasion of cavernous sinuses with release directly into the bloodstream. (46) Even these cases show remarkable resolution with bromocriptine treatment. (45)

A failure of bromocriptine to shrink a tumor may be due to the extrasellar escape of the tumor. Apparently the tumor tissue must be in contact with the hypothalamic-pituitary portal system for bromocriptine to work, suggesting that bromocriptine not only acts directly on the pituitary but on the hypothalamic tracts as well. (47)

The response of macroadenomas to bromocriptine is impressive, and a most compelling reason in favor of its use is that it has been successful when previous surgery or radiation has failed. The problem, however, is that it probably must be taken indefinitely, as there is yet to be a convincing report of complete disappearance and resolution of a tumor. Indeed recent evidence indicates that bromocriptine reduces cell size but does not bring about necrosis and loss of cells. (48) Long-term treatment will be easier with newer analogs which will require less frequent administration.

Long-term treatment of microadenomas with bromocriptine has not corrected the underlying cause or achieved an impressive record of resolution. (49) Generally prolactin levels return to an elevated state after discontinuation of the drug. There are cases of improvement in sellar x-rays. (49) However, the unreliability of polytomography (13) and the occasional spontaneous regression of prolactin-secreting tumors (50) make it impossible to attribute "cures" to bromocriptine. Recurrence of hyperprolactinemia has been observed after as many as 4–8 years of treatment.

Summary: Therapy of Pituitary Tumors

Macroadenomas. Currently bromocriptine treatment for as long as 1 year is advocated to precede surgery. It is expected that the tumor will be smaller, more circumscribed, and easier to remove after drug treatment. Whether such treatment will improve surgical results remains to be seen. Indefinite treatment with bromocriptine is a legitimate alternative to surgery.

Microadenomas. The treatment of microadenomas should be directed to alleviating one of two problems: infertility or breast discomfort. Bromocriptine is the method of choice. Some patients, deliberately and understandably, choose the surgical approach in hopes of achieving a cure and avoiding the worry and annoyance of continuing surveillance. The major therapeutic dilemma can be expressed by the following question: Should chronic bromocriptine treatment be utilized to retrieve ovarian function in those patients with hypoestrogenic amenorrhea, or should estrogen replacement be offered? Until a clear-cut benefit is demonstrated in the on-going clinical studies, we cannot advocate widespread bromocriptine therapy for those patients not interested in becoming pregnant. This conservative approach is supported by documentation of a benign clinical course in these patients. (51) Patients with hypoestrogenic amenorrhea are encouraged to be on an estrogen replacement program to maintain the health of the bones and vascular system. Estrogen-induced tumor expansion or growth has not been a problem.

Pregnancy and Pituitary Adenomas

Approximately 80% of hyperprolactinemic women achieve pregnancy with bromocriptine treatment. (52) Breast feeding, if desired, can be carried out normally without fear of stimulating tumor growth. (52–54) Interestingly, some women resume cyclic menses after pregnancy. This spontaneous improvement may be due to tumor infarction brought about by the expansion and shrinkage during and after pregnancy, or there may be a correction of a hypothalamic dysfunction followed by a disappearance of the associated pituitary hyperplasia.

Only 5–10% of women with hyperprolactinemia and presumed microadenomas will develop signs or symptoms suggestive of tumor growth during the pregnancy. (52–56) The risk is higher with macroadenomas, approximately 30–40%. (55, 56) Headaches usually precede visual disturbance, and both may occur in any trimester. There is no characteristic headache, as they are variable in intensity, location, and character. Bitemporal hemianopsia is the classic visual field finding, but other defects may occur. It has been argued in the past that a desire for pregnancy was a significant reason for the surgical approach. This argument hinged on the risk of tumor enlargement during pregnancy due to the well-known stimulatory effects of estrogen on the pituitary lactotrophs. As noted above, evaluation of this risk has indicated that only a minority of patients develop problems.

It is impossible to identify which patient is at risk for symptomatic expansion during pregnancy. Other than a very large tumor, the size is not critical in that both microadenomas and small macroadenomas may undergo uneventful pregnancies. There is no increase in abortions, or perinatal mortality and morbidity. It is virtually unheard of to develop a problem that results in perinatal damage or serious maternal sequelae.

Surveillance during pregnancy has traditionally consisted of monthly visual field and prolactin measurements. In our experience, this is unnecessary. The patient and the clinician can be guided by the development of symptoms. Assessment of visual fields, prolactin, and the sella turcica by limited CT scanning can await the onset of headaches or visual disturbances. Definite evidence of tumor expansion, as well as the symptoms of headaches and visual changes, promptly regress with bromocriptine treatment. Termination of pregnancy or neurosurgery, therefore, should rarely, if ever, be necessary. Although bromocriptine treatment profoundly lowers both maternal and fetal blood levels of prolactin, no adverse effects on the pregnancy or the newborn have been noted. (57)

The Empty Sella Syndrome

A patient may have an abnormal sella turcica, but rather than a tumor, she may have the empty sella syndrome. This is a condition in which there is a congenital incompleteness of the sellar diaphragm, allowing an extension of the subarachnoid space into the pituitary fossa. The pituitary gland is separated from the hypothalamus and is flattened. The sella floor may be demineralized due to pressure from the cerebrospinal fluid. The empty sella syndrome may also occur secondary to surgery or radiotherapy.

An empty sella is found in approximately 5% of autopsies, and approximately 85% are in women, previously thought to be concentrated in middle aged and obese women. (58) A closer look at the sella turcica, brought about by our pursuit of elevated prolactin levels, has revealed an incidence of empty sellas in 4–16% of patients who present with amenorrhea/galactorrhea. (3, 12, 33) Galactorrhea and elevated prolactins can be seen with an empty sella, and there may be a coexisting prolactin-secreting adenoma. (59) This suggests that the empty sella in these patients may have arisen because of tumor infarction.

This condition is benign; it does not progress to pituitary failure. The chief hazard to the patient is inadvertent treatment for a pituitary tumor. Even though enlargement of the sella turcica with a normal shape is more likely associated with an empty sella than a tumor, all patients should have examination by a modern CT scan prior to surgical intervention.

Because of the possibility of a coexisting adenoma, patients with elevated prolactins or galactorrhea and an empty sella should undergo annual surveillance (prolactin assay and coned down view) to detect tumor growth. Otherwise it is appropriate to offer hormone replacement or induction of ovulation.

Compartment IV

Hypothalamic Amenorrhea

Hypothalamic problems are usually diagnosed by exclusion of pituitary lesions and are the most common category of hypogonadotropic amenorrhea. Frequently there is an association with a stressful situation, such as in business or in school. There is also a higher proportion of underweight women and a higher occurrence of previous menstrual irregularity. Nevertheless, the physician is obliged to go through the process of exclusion prior to prescribing hormone replacement therapy, or attempting induction of ovulation to achieve pregnancy.

These patients are categorized by low or normal gonadotropins and a failure to demonstrate withdrawal bleeding. A good practice is to evaluate such patients annually. This annual surveillance should include a prolactin assay and the coned down view of the sella turcica. Even though a patient may not be currently interested in pursuing pregnancy, it is important to assure these patients that at the appropriate time treatment for the induction of ovulation will be available, and that fertility can be achieved. Concern with potential fertility is often an unspoken fear, especially in the younger patients, even teenagers. On the other hand, induction of ovulation should be carried out only for the purpose of producing a pregnancy. There is no evidence that cyclic hormone administration or induction of ovulation will stimulate the return of normal function.

Anorexia

A special example of hypothalamic amenorrhea is that associated with weight loss. It is true that obesity may be associated with amenorrhea, but amenorrhea in an obese patient is usually due to anovulation, and a hypogonadotropic state is not encountered unless the patient also has a severe emotional disorder. Acute weight loss, on the other hand, in some unknown way, can lead to the hypogonadotropic state. Again the physician must pursue the presence of a tumor, and the diagnosis is made by exclusion.

Clinically a spectrum is encountered which ranges from a limited period of amenorrhea associated with a crash diet, to the severely ill patient with the life-threatening attrition of anorexia nervosa. It is a common experience for the gynecologist to be the first to recognize anorexia nervosa in a patient presenting with the complaint of amenorrhea. It is also not infrequent that a gynecologist will evaluate and manage an infertility problem due to hypogonadotropism and not be aware of a developing case of anorexia. It is important that attention be directed to this syndrome which is associated with a mortality rate of 5–15%. In England, the prevalence is estimated to be 1 in 200 high school girls. (60)

Diagnosis of Anorexia Nervosa.

1. Onset between ages 10 and 30.

2. Weight loss of 25%, or weight 15% below normal for age and height.

3. Special attitudes:
—Denial,
—Distorted body image,
—Unusual hoarding or handling of food.

4. At least one of the following:
—Lanugo,
—Bradycardia,
—Overactivity,
—Episodes of overeating (bulimia),
—Vomiting, which may be self-induced.

5. Amenorrhea.

6. No known medical illness.

7. No other psychiatric disorder.

8. Other characteristics:
—Constipation,
—Low blood pressure,
—Hypercarotenemia,
—Diabetes insipidus.

Anorexia nervosa occurs almost exclusively in young white middle to upper class girls under age 25. The families of anorexics are success-achievement-appearance oriented. Serious problems may be present within the family, but the parents make every effort to maintain an apparent marital harmony, glossing over or denying conflicts. In one psychiatric interpretation, each parent, in secret dissatisfaction with the other, expects affection from their "perfect" child. Anorexia begins when the role of the perfect child becomes too difficult. The pattern usually starts with a voluntary diet to control weight. This brings a sense of power and accomplishment, soon followed by a fear that weight cannot be controlled if discipline is allowed to relax.

At puberty, the normal weight gain may be interpreted as excessive, and this can trip the teenager over into true anorexia nervosa. The children are characteristically over-achievers and strivers. They seldom give any trouble, but are judgmental and demand that others live up to their rigid value system, often resulting in social isolation.

Besides amenorrhea, constipation is a common symptom, often severe and accompanied by abdominal pain. The preoccupation with food may manifest itself by large intakes of lettuce, raw vegatables, and low calorie foods. Hypotension, hypothermia, rough, dry skin, soft lanugo-type hair on the back and buttocks, bradycardia, and edema are the most commonly encountered signs. Long-term diuretic and laxative abuse may produce significant hypokalemia. An elevation of the serum carotene is not always associated with a large intake of yellow vegetables, suggesting that a defect in vitamin A utilization is present. (61) The yellowish coloration of the skin is usually seen on the palms.

The serious case of anorexia nervosa is seen more often by an internist than by a gynecologist. However, the borderline anorexic frequently presents to the gynecologist as a teenager who has low body weight, amenorrhea, and hyperactivity (excellent grades and many extracurricular activities). The amenorrhea can precede, follow, or appear coincidentally with the weight loss.

The various problems associated with anorexia represent dysfunction of the body mechanisms regulated by the hypothalamus: appetite, thirst and water conservation, temperature, sleep, autonomic balance, and endocrine secretion. (62, 63) Endocrine studies can be summarized as follows: FSH and LH levels are low, cortisol levels are elevated due to decreased clearance in the face of a normal production rate, prolactin levels are normal, TSH and thyroxine (T_4) levels are normal, but the 3,5,3'-triiodothyronine (T_3) level is low and reverse T_3 is high. Indeed many of the symptoms can be explained by relative hypothyroidism (constipation, cold intolerance, bradycardia, hypotension, dry skin, low metabolic rates, hypercarotenemia). There appears to be a compensation to the state of undernourishment, with diversion from formation of the active T_3 to the inactive metabolite, reverse T_3. With weight gain, all of the metabolic changes revert to normal. Even though normal gonadotropin secretion may be restored with weight gain, 30% of patients remain amenorrheic. (62)

This is one of the rare conditions in which gonadotropins may be undetectable (large pituitary tumors and genetic deficiencies being the others). If necessary, a high plasma cortisol can differentiate this condition from pituitary insufficiency.

The central origin for the amenorrhea is suggested by the demonstration that the response to GnRH is regained at approximately 15% below the ideal weight, and this return to normal responsiveness occurs before the resumption of menses. (64). Patients with anorexia nervosa have persistent low levels of gonadotropins similar to prepubertal children. With weight gain, sleep-associated episodic secretion of LH appears, similar to the early pubertal child. With full recovery the 24-hour pattern is similar to that of an adult, with fluctuating peaks. This is a pattern expected of increasing and decreasing pulsatile secretion of GnRH.

173

Extensive laboratory testing in these patients is not necessary. Adherence to our scheme for the evaluation of amenorrhea is indicated to rule out other pathological processes. Further endocrine assessment, however, is not essential for patient management. A careful and gentle revelation to the patient of the relationship between the amenorrhea and the low body weight is often all that is necessary to stimulate the patient to return to normal weight and normal menstrual function. Occasionally it is necessary to see the patient frequently and become involved in a program of daily calorie counting (a minimum intake of 2600 calories) in order to break the patient's established eating habits. If progress is slow, hormone replacement therapy should be initiated. In an adult weighing less than 100 pounds, continued weight loss requires psychiatric consultation.

Going away to school or the development of a relationship with a male friend often are turning points for young women with mild to moderate anorexia. This is also true of pregnancy, and once pregnancy is achieved, its course is not influenced by the past history of anorexia. A failure to respond to these life changes is relatively ominous, predicting a severe problem with a protracted course.

Several characteristics have been described which are associated with a poor prognosis: (65)

1. Long duration of illness.

2. Older age at the onset.

3. Very low weight during the illness.

4. Presence of bulimia, vomiting, and anxiety when eating with others.

5. Poor childhood social adjustment.

6. Low socioeconomic status.

7. Poor parental relationship.

It is disappointing that despite the impressive studies on anorexia there is no specific or new therapy available. This only serves to emphasize the need for early recognition to allow psychologic intervention before the syndrome is entrenched in its full severity. Physicians (and parents) should pay particular attention to weight and diet in young women with amenorrhea.

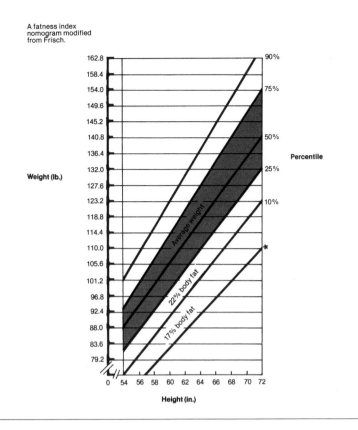

A fatness index nomogram modified from Frisch.

Weight (lb.)

162.8 158.4 154.0 149.6 145.2 140.8 136.4 132.0 127.6 123.2 118.8 114.4 110.0 105.6 101.2 96.8 92.4 88.0 83.6 79.2

90% 75% 50% 25% 10%

Percentile

Average weight

22% body fat

17% body fat

Height (in.)

Exercise and Amenorrhea

The magnitude of the problem of exercise and amenorrhea has changed considerably in the last decade. In the early 1970s, a woman jogger was a curiosity. Today millions of women are running, over a million girls play soccer, and more than one third of high school athletes are female. In addition to competitive female athletes, women engaged in strenuous recreational exercise and women engaged in other forms of demanding activity such as ballet and modern dancing have a high incidence of menstrual irregularity and amenorrhea, in the pattern called hypothalamic suppression.

There appear to be two critical influences: a critical level of body fat and the effect of stress itself. Young women who weigh less than 115 pounds and lose more than 10 pounds while exercising are the women most likely to develop the problem, (66) an association which supports the critical weight concept of Frisch. (67) The critical weight hypothesis states that onset and regularity of menstrual function necessitate maintaining weight above a critical level, and therefore above a critical amount of body fat. In dealing with patients, it is helpful to use the nomogram derived from Frisch (67), which is based on the calculation of the amount of total body water as a percentage of body weight. This relates to the percentage of body fat and, therefore, is an index of fatness. The 10th percentile at age 16 is equivalent to about 22% body fat, the minimal weight for height

175

necessary for sustaining menstruation, and the 10th percentile at age 13 is equivalent to 17% body fat, the minimum for initiating menarche. A loss of body weight in the range of 10–15% of normal weight for height represents a loss of about one third of the body fat, which will result in a drop below the 22% line and may result in amenorrhea. Of course there is significant individual variation, and the nomogram cannot be used to give definitive predictions.

The competitive female athlete has about 50% less body fat than the noncompetitor. Indeed, the mean is very much under the 10th percentile for secondary amenorrhea (the 22% body fat line). This change in body fat can occur with no discernable change in total body weight, as fat is converted to lean muscle mass.

In addition to the role of body fat, stress and energy expenditure appear to play an independent role. Warren (68) has pointed out that dancers will have a return of menses during intervals of rest, despite no change in body weight or percent body fat. High energy output and stress, therefore, may act independently, as well as additively to low body fat, in suppressing reproductive function. It is not surprising that a woman with low body weight who is engaged in competitive activity (athletic or aesthetic) is highly susceptible for amenorrhea.

Recent studies have indicated that this amenorrhea is due to hypothalamic dysfunction similar to that which is more marked in the classic cases of anorexia nervosa. It is tempting to relate the endocrine changes to the newly described central neuroendocrine mechanisms. In running circles, there is frequent talk about the runner's "high," the feeling of euphoria and exhilaration after competition or an extensive workout. A convincing explanation for this emotional reaction is the involvement of endogenous opiates. Exercise is associated with increases in prolactin, ACTH, growth hormone, and various sex steroids, while gonadotropins are decreased. (69) With a progressive training program of vigorous exercise, the circulating levels of β-endorphin, β-lipotropin, and ACTH become greater with each exercise session. (70) The increased prolactin and decreased gonadotropins found after exercise may be mediated, therefore, by endogenous opiate release. Suppression of GnRH pulsatile secretion is the central feature, and this is the general effect on the arcuate nucleus exerted by endorphins. By suppressing the arcuate nucleus, endorphins not only suppress GnRH but also increase prolactin levels by suppressing hypothalamic dopamine secretion. How this suppression is further intensified or activated by a state of low body fat is unknown.

In the subculture of exercise and amenorrhea, the characteristics strikingly remind one of anorexia nervosa: significant physical exercise, a necessity for control of the body, striving for artistic and technical proficiency, and the consequent preoccupation with the body—together with the stressful pressures of performing and competition. (71)

Individuals in this life-style are prone to develop what can be called the anorectic reaction. Fries (72) has described four stages of dieting behavior which can form a continuum:

1. Dieting for cosmetic reasons.

2. Dieting due to neurotic fixation on food intake and weight.

3. The anorectic reaction.

4. True anorexia nervosa.

There are several important distinctions between the anorectic reaction and true anorexia nervosa. Psychologically the patient with true anorexia nervosa has a misperception of reality and a lack of insight into the disease and her problem. She does not consider herself underweight and displays an impressive lack of concern over her dreadful physical condition and appearance. The doctor-patient relationship is difficult with no visible emotional involvement and a great deal of mistrust. Patients with the anorectic reaction have the capability for self-criticism. They can see the problem and describe it with insight and an absence of denial. The exercising woman and the competing athlete or dancer can develop an anorectic reaction. The anorectic reaction develops consciously and voluntarily just as in anorexia nervosa, as the exercising woman deliberately makes an effort to decrease body weight. A physician may be the first to be aware of the problem having encountered the patient because of the presenting complaint of either amenorrhea or weight loss. Early recognition, concentrated counseling, and confidential support may intercept and prevent a progressive problem.

Prognosis is excellent with early recognition, and simple weight gain may reverse the state of amenorrhea. However, these patients often are unwilling to give up their routines of exercise. Hormone replacement therapy is therefore encouraged for these amenorrheic patients, because it appears that the exercise is not sufficient to balance the loss of estrogen protection against osteoporosis. When pregnancy is desired, a reduction in the amount of exercise and a gain in weight should be recommended, or induction of ovulation must be pursued.

Amenorrhea and Anosmia. A rare condition in females is the syndrome of hypogonadotropic hypogonadism associated with anosmia. A similar syndrome in the male is hereditary and known as Kallmann's syndrome. In the female, this problem is characterized by primary amenorrhea, infantile sexual development, low gonadotropins, a normal female karyotype, and the inability to perceive odors, e.g. coffee grounds or perfume. (73) The gonads can respond to gonadotropins, therefore induction of ovulation with exogenous gonadotropins has been successful. However, clomiphene is ineffective.

Postpill Amenorrhea. It has been assumed that amenorrhea may reflect persistent suppressive effects of oral contraceptive medication or the use of the intramuscular depot form of medroxyprogesterone acetate (Depo-Provera). It is now recognized that the fertility rate is normal following discontinuance of either of these forms of contraception (Chapter 15), and attempts to identify a cause-effect relationship in case-control studies have failed. (74, 75) Therefore, amenorrhea following the use of steroids for contraception requires investigation as described in order to avoid missing a significant problem. This investigation should be pursued if a patient is still amenorrheic 6 months after discontinuing oral contraception or 12 months after the last injection of Depo-Provera.

Hormone Replacement Therapy

The patient who is hypoestrogenic and who is not a candidate for induction of ovulation deserves hormone replacement therapy. This includes patients appropriately evaluated and diagnosed as having gonadal failure, patients with hypothalamic amenorrhea, and postgonadectomy patients. Measurements of bone density in young women with secondary amenorrhea associated with hyperprolactinemia reveal that these young women lose bone density at a rate equivalent to that of postmenopausal women. (76) A decrease in bone mass with an even greater decrement in spinal trabecular bone compared to peripheral bone has been observed in young women with amenorrhea from a variety of causes. (77) The same arguments that apply to hormone replacement in older women (Chapter 4) can be convincingly used to encourage these younger women to replace the estrogen they are lacking.

A good schedule is the following: on days 1 through 25 of each month, take 1.25 mg of conjugated estrogens; on days 16 through 25, add 10 mg of medroxyprogesterone acetate. Beginning medication on the first of every month establishes an easily remembered routine. Menstruation generally occurs 3 days after the last medication, the 28th of each month. In a few individuals, the estrogen dosage must be reduced because of bothersome estrogenic effects such as fluid retention. If the progestational agent is responsible for side effects the daily dose can be decreased to 5 mg. Bleeding which occurs at any time other than the usual expected time, the 28th of the month, may be a sign that endogenous function has returned. The hormone replacement program should be discontinued and the patient monitored for the resumption of ovulation.

The importance of monthly menstruation to a young woman cannot be overemphasized. Regular and visible menstrual bleeding is often a gratifying experience in the young patient with gonadal dysgenesis and serves to reinforce her identification with the feminine gender role. The estrogen dose in the replacement regimen must be sufficient to achieve menstruation in a young woman; therefore a 1.25 mg dose is used compared to the usual dose of 0.625 mg in the postmenopausal woman.

Patients with hypothalamic amenorrhea must be cautioned that replacement therapy will not protect against pregnancy in the event that normal function unknowingly returns. In the occasional patient who must have the most effective contraception possible, it is reasonable to utilize a low dose oral contraceptive to provide the missing estrogen.

References

1. **Contreras P, Generini G, Michelson H, Pumarino H, Campino C,** Hyperprolactinemia and galactorrhea: spontaneous versus iatrogenic hypothyroidism, J Clin Endocrinol Metab 53:1036, 1981.

2. **Danziger J, Wallace S, Handel S, Samaan NG,** The sella turcica in primary end organ failure, Radiology 131:111, 1979.

3. **Nachtigall RD, Monroe SE, Wilson CB, Jaffe RB,** Prolactin-secreting pituitary adenomas in women: VI. Absence of demonstrable adenomas in patients with altered menstrual function and abnormal sellar polytomography. Am J Obstet Gynecol 140:303, 1981.

4. **Sherman BM, Korenman SG,** Hormonal characteristics of the human menstrual cycle throughout reproductive life, J Clin Invest 55:699, 1975.

5. **Sutton C,** The limitations of laparoscopic ovarian biopsy, J Obstet Gynecol Br Commonwlth 81:317, 1974.

6. **Tulandi T, Kinch RA,** Premature ovarian failure, Obstet Gynecol Surv 36:521, 1981.

7. **Rebar RW, Erickson GF, Yen SSC,** Idiopathic premature ovarian failure: clinical and endocrine characteristics, Fertil Steril 37:35, 1982.

8. **Chiauzzi V, Cigorraga S, Escobar ME, Rivarola MA, Charreau EH,** Inhibition of follicle-stimulating hormone receptor binding by circulating immunoglobins. J Clin Endocrinol Metab 54:1221, 1982.

9. **Peckham WD, Knobil ED,** The effects of ovariectomy, estrogen replacement, and neuraminidase treatment on the properties of the adenohypophysial glycoprotein hormones of the rhesus monkey, Endocrinology 98:1054, 1976.

10. **Lucky AQ, Rebar RW, Rosenfield RL, Roche-Bender N, Helke J,** Reduction of the potency of luteinizing hormone by estrogen, N Engl J Med 300:1034, 1979.

11. **Axelrod L, Neer RM, Kliman B,** Hypogonadism in a male with immunologically active, biologically inactive luteinizing hormone: an exception to a venerable rule. J Clin Endocrinol Metab 48:279, 1979.

12. **Schlechte J, Sherman B, Halmi N, Van Gilder J, Chapler FK, Dolan K, Granner D, Duello T, Harris C,** Prolactin-secreting pituitary tumors, Endocr Rev 1:295, 1980.

13. **Burrow GN, Wortzman G, Rewcastle NB, Holgate RC, Kovacs K.** Microadenomas of the pituitary and abnormal sellar tomograms in an unselected autopsy series, N Engl J Med 304:156, 1981.

14. **Syvertsen A, Haughton VM, Williams AL, Cusick JF,** The computed tomographic appearance of the normal pituitary gland and pituitary microadenomas, Radiology 133:385, 1979.

15. **Kleinberg, DL, Noel GL, Frantz AG,** Galactorrhea: a study of 235 cases, including 48 with pituitary tumors, N Engl J Med 296:589, 1977.

16. **Shewchuk AB, Adamson GD, Lessard P, Ezrin C,** The effect of pregnancy on suspected pituitary adenomas after conservative management of ovulation defects associated with galactorrhea, Am J Obstet Gynecol 136:659, 1980.

17. **Woosley RE, King JS, Talbert L,** Prolactin-secreting pituitary adenomas: neurosurgical management of 37 patients, Fertil Steril 37:54, 1982.

18. **Schenker JG, Margalioth EJ,** Intrauterine adhesions: an updated appraisal, Fertil Steril 37:593, 1982.

19. **Toaff R, Ballas S,** Traumatic hypomenorrhea-amenorrhea (Asherman's syndrome), Fertil Steril 30:379, 1978.

20. **March CM, Israel R, March AD,** Hysteroscopic management of intrauterine adhesions, Am J Obstet Gynecol 130:653:1978.

21. **Griffin JE, Edwards C, Ladden JD, Harrod MJ, Wilson JD,** Congenital absence of the vagina, Ann Intern Med 85:224, 1976.

22. **Frank RT,** Formation of artificial vagina without operation, Am J Obstet Gynecol 35:1053, 1938.

23. **Wabrek AJ, Millard PR, Wilson WB Jr, Pion RJ,** Creation of a neovagina by the Frank nonoperative method, Obstet Gynecol 37:408, 1971.

24. **Maciulla GJ, Heine MW, Christian CD,** Functional endometrial tissue with vaginal agenesis, J Reprod Med 21:373, 1978.

25. **Swanson JA, Chapler FK,** Renal anomalies in the XY female, Obstet Gynecol 51:237, 1978.

26. **Morris JM, Mahesh VB,** Further observations on the syndrome "testicular feminization," Am J Obstet Gynecol 87:731, 1963.

27. **Kaufman F, Kogut MD, Donnell GN, Koch R, Goebelsmann U,** Ovarian failure in galactosaemia, Lancet 2:737, 1979.

28. **Coulam CB, Annegers JF, Abboud CF, Laws ER Jr, Kurland LT,** Pituitary adenoma and oral contraceptives: a case-control study, Fertil Steril 31:25, 1979.

29. **McCormick WF, Halmi NS,** Absence of chromophobe adenomas from a large series of pituitary tumors, Arch Pathol 92:231, 1971.

30. **Kraus HE,** Neoplastic diseases of the human hypophysis, Arch Pathol 39:343, 1945.

31. **Sheline GE,** Untreated and recurrent chromophobe adenomas of the pituitary, Radiology 112:768, 1971.

32. **Costello RT,** Subclinical adenoma of the pituitary gland, Am J Pathol 12:191, 1936.

33. **Speroff L, Levin RM, Haning RV Jr, Kase NG,** A practical approach for the evaluation of women with abnormal polytomography or elevated prolactin levels, Am J Obstet Gynecol 135:896, 1979.

34. **Monroe SE, Levine L, Chang RJ, Keye WR Jr, Yamamoto M, Jaffe RB,** Prolactin-secreting pituitary adenomas: V. Increased gonadotropin responsivity in hyperprolactinemic women with pituitary adenomas, J Clin Endocrinol Metab 52:1171, 1981.

35. **Knobil E,** The neuroendocrine control of the menstrual cycle, Recent Prog Horm Res 36:53, 1980.

36. **Hardy J, Beauregard H, Robert F,** Prolactin-secreting pituitary adenomas: transsphenoidal microsurgical treatment, in *Progress in Prolactin Physiology and Pathology*, Robyn C, Harter M, eds, Elsevier-North Holland, Amsterdam, 1978, pp 361–369.

37. **Post KD, Biller BJ, Adelman LS, Molitch ME, Wolpert SM, Reichlin S,** Selective transsphenoidal adenomectomy in women with galactorrhea-amenorrhea, JAMA 242:158, 1979.

38. **Tucker HS, Grubb SR, Wigand JP, Taylon A, Lankford HV, Blackard WG, Becker DP,** Galactorrhea-amenorrhea syndrome: follow-up of 45 patients after pituitary tumor removal, Ann Intern Med 94:302, 1981.

39. **Parkes D,** Bromocriptine, N Engl J Med 301:873, 1979.

40. **Cuellar FG,** Bromocriptine mesylate (Parlodel) in the management of amenorrhea/galactorrhea associated with hyperprolactinemia, Obstet Gynecol 55:278, 1980.

41. **Wass JAH, Mout PJA, Thorner MO, Dacie JE, Charlesworth M, Jones AE, Besser GM,** Reduction of pituitary-tumor size in patients with prolactinomas and acromegaly treated with bromocriptine with or without radiotherapy, Lancet 2:66, 1979.

181

42. **Thorner MO, Martin WH, Rogol AD, Morris JL, Perryman RL, Conway BP, Howards SS, Wolfman MG, MacLeod RM,** Rapid regression of pituitary prolactinomas during bromocriptine treatment, J Clin Endocrinol Metab 51:438, 1980.

43. **Corenblum B, Hanley DA,** Bromocriptine reduction of prolactinoma size, Fertil Steril 36:716, 1981.

44. **Choidini P, Luizzi A, Cozzi R, Verge G, Oppizzi G, Dallabonzana D, Spelta B, Silvestrini F, Borghi G, Luccarelli G, Rainer E, Horowski R,** Size reduction of macroprolactinomas by bromocriptine or lisuride treatment, J Clin Endocrinol Metab 53:737, 1981.

45. **Velentzas C, Carras D, Vassilouthis J,** Regression of pituitary prolactinoma with bromocriptine administration, JAMA 245:1149, 1981.

46. **Shucart WA,** Implications of very high serum prolactin levels associated with pituitary tumors, J Neurosurg 52:226, 1980.

47. **Spark RF, Baker R, Beinfang DC, Berland R,** Bromocriptine reduces pituitary tumor size and hypersecretion: requiem for pituitary surgery? JAMA 247:311, 1982.

48. **Thorner MO, Tindall GT, Kovacs K, Horvath E,** Human prolactinomas and bromocriptine: a histologic immunocytochemical, ultrastructure and morphometric study, The Endocrine Society Program, Abstract 227, 1982.

49. **Archer DF, Lattanzi DR, Moore EE, Harger JH, Herbert DL,** Bromocriptine treatment of women with suspected pituitary prolactin-secreting microadenomas, Am J Obstet Gynecol 143:620, 1982.

50. **Vaughn TC, Haney AF, Wiebe RH, Kramer RS, Hammond CB,** Spontaneous regression of prolactin-producing pituitary adenomas, Am J Obstet Gynecol 136:980, 1980.

51. **Koppelman MCS, Jaffe MJ, Rieth KG, Caruso RC, Loriaux DL,** Natural history of hyperprolactinemia, galactorrhea and amenorrhea, The Endocrine Society Program, Abstract 22, 1982.

52. **Crosignani PG, Ferrari C, Scarduelli C, Picciotti MC, Caldara R, Malinverni A,** Spontaneous and induced pregnancies in hyperprolactinemic women, Obstet Gynecol 58:708, 1981.

53. **Bergh T, Nillius SJ, Wide L,** Clinical course and outcome of pregnancies in amenorrheic women with hyperprolactinaemia and pituitary tumors, Br Med J 1:875, 1978.

54. **Jewelewicz R, Vande Wiele RL,** Clinical course and outcome of pregnancy in twenty-five patients with pituitary microadenomas, Am J Obstet Gynecol 136:339, 1980.

55. **Magyar DM, Marshall JR,** Pituitary tumors and pregnancy, Am J Obstet Gynecol 132:739, 1978.

56. **Gemzell C, Wang CF,** Outcome of pregnancy in women with pituitary adenoma, Fertil Steril 31:363, 1979.

57. **Turkalj I, Braun P, Krupp P,** Surveillance of bromocriptine in pregnancy, JAMA 247:1589, 1982.

58. **Hodgson SF, Randall RV, Holman CB, MacCarty CS,** Empty sella syndrome, Med Clin North Am 56:897, 1972.

59. **Swanson JA, Sherman BM, Van Gilder JC, Chapler FK,** Coexistent empty sella and prolactin-secreting microadenoma, Obstet Gynecol 53:258, 1979.

60. **Crisp AH, Palmer RL, Kalucy RS,** How common is anorexia nervosa: a prevalence study, Br J Psychiatr 128:549:1976.

61. **Robboy MS, Sato AS, Schwabe AD,** The hypercarotenemia in anorexia nervosa: a comparison of vitamin A and carotene levels in various forms of menstrual dysfunction and cachexia, Am J Clin Nutr 27:362, 1974.

62. **Warren MP, Vande Wiele RL,** Clinical and metabolic features of anorexia nervosa, Am J Obstet Gynecol 117:435, 1973.

63. **Vigersky RA, Andersen AE, Thompson RH, Loriaux DL,** Hypothalamic dysfunction in secondary amenorrhea, associated with simple weight loss, N Engl J Med 297:1141, 1977.

64. **Warren MP, Jewelewicz R, Dyrenfurth I, Ans R, Khalaf S, Vande Wiele RL,** The significance of weight loss in the evaluation of pituitary response to LH-RH in women with secondary amenorrhea, J Clin Endocrinol Metab 40:601, 1975.

65. **Hsu LKG, Crisp AH, Harding B,** Outcome of anorexia nervosa, Lancet 1:61, 1979.

66. **Speroff L, Redwine DB,** Exercise and menstrual function, Physician Sportsmed 8:42, 1980.

67. **Frisch RE,** Food intake, fatness, and reproductive ability, in *Anorexia Nervosa*, Vigersky RA, ed, Raven Press, New York, 1977, pp 149–160.

68. **Warren MP,** The effects of exercise on pubertal progression and reproductive function in girls, J Clin Endocrinol Metab 51:1150, 1980.

69. **Shangold MM, Gatz ML, Thysen B,** Acute effects of exercise on plasma concentrations of prolactin and testosterone in recreational women runners, Fertil Steril 35:699, 1981.

70. **Carr DB, Bullen BA, Skrinar GS, Arnold MA, Beitins IZ, Martin JB, McArthur JW,** Physical conditioning facilitates the exercise-induced secretion of beta-endorphin and beta-lipotropin in women, N Engl J Med 305:560, 1981.

71. **Smith NJ,** Excessive weight loss and food aversion in athletes simulating anorexia nervosa, Pediatrics 66:139, 1980.

72. **Fries H,** Secondary amenorrhea, self-induced weight reduction and anorexia nervosa, Acta Psychiatr Scand, Suppl 248, 1974.

73. **Tagatz G, Fialkow PJ, Smith D, Spadoni L,** Hypogonadotropic hypogonadism associated with anosmia in the female, N Engl J Med 282:1326, 1970.

74. **Jacobs HS, Knuth UA, Hull MGR, Franks S,** Postpill amenorrhea—cause or coincidence? Br Med J 2:940, 1977.

75. **Tolis G, Ruggere D, Popkin DR, Chow J, Boyd ME, De Leon A, Lalonde AB, Asswad A, Hendelman M, Scali V, Koby R, Arronet G, Yufe B, Tweedie FJ, Fournier PR, Naftolin F,** Prolonged amenorrhea and oral contraceptives, Fertil Steril 32:265, 1979.

76. **Kilbanski A, Neer RM, Beitins IZ, Ridgway EC, Zervas NT, McArthur JW,** Decreased bone density in hyperprolactinemic women, N Engl J Med 303:1511, 1980.

77. **Cann CE, Martin MC, Genant KH,** Detection of premenopausal amenorrheic women at risk for the development of osteoporosis, The Endocrine Society Program, Abstract 747, 1982.

6   Anovulation

Anovulation is a very common problem which presents itself in a variety of clinical manifestations, including amenorrhea, irregular menses, and hirsutism. Serious consequences of chronic anovulation are infertility and a greater risk for developing carcinoma of the endometrium and the breast. The physician must appreciate the clinical impact of anovulation and undertake therapeutic management of all anovulatory patients to avoid these unwanted consequences.

Normal ovulation requires coordination of the menstrual system at all levels, the central hypothalamic-pituitary axis, the feedback signals, and local responses within the ovary. The loss of ovulation may be due to any one of a variety of factors operating at each of these levels. The end result is a dysfunctional state: anovulation. *In this chapter, we will discuss the variety of mechanisms by which dysfunction of the ovulatory cycle can occur and how the clinical expressions of the resulting abnormal menstrual function are produced.*

Pathogenesis of Anovulation

During menses, escape from the negative feedback of estrogen results in increased follicle-stimulating hormone (FSH) secretion by the anterior pituitary. This initial increase in FSH is essential for follicular growth and steroidogenesis. With continued growth of the follicle, estradiol production within the follicle maintains follicular sensitivity to FSH allowing conversion from a microenvironment dominated by androgens to one dominated by estrogen, a change necessary for a complete and successful follicular life span. Continuing and combined action of FSH and estradiol leads to the appearance of luteinizing hormone (LH) receptors on the granulosa cells, a prerequisite for luteinization and ovulation. Ovulation is triggered by the rapid rise in circulating levels of estradiol. A positive feedback response at the level of the anterior pituitary results in the midcycle surge of LH necessary for expulsion of the egg and formation of the corpus luteum. A rise in progesterone follows ovulation along with a second rise in estradiol, producing the well-known 14-day luteal phase characterized by low FSH and LH levels. The demise of the corpus luteum, concomitant with a fall in hormone levels, allows FSH to increase again, thus initiating a new cycle.

This recycling mechanism is regulated largely by estradiol. The negative feedback relationship between estradiol and FSH results in the critical initial rise in that gonadotropin during menses, and the positive feedback relationship between estradiol and LH is the ovulatory stimulus. Within the ovary, estradiol induces follicular receptor responses necessary for growth and function. Estradiol is, therefore, properly viewed as the critical agent for appropriate hypothalamic-pituitary-ovarian responses. Dysfunction in the cycle may be due to an abnormality in one of the various roles for estradiol, or an inability to respond to estradiol signals. Problems in normal function may be conveniently organized into central defects, abnormalities in the feedback signals, and abnormal function within the ovary itself.

Central Defects

The hypothalamic-pituitary axis may be unable to respond, even if given adequate and appropriately timed feedback signals. A pituitary tumor represents an obvious example of a central defect in menstrual function, and is discussed in Chapter 5, "Amenorrhea."

Although difficult to demonstrate definitively, malfunction within the hypothalamus is both a likely, as well as a favorite, explanation for ovulatory failure. Normal pituitary ovulatory response to the follicle's steroid signals requires the presence of gonadotropin releasing hormone (GnRH) pulsatile secretion within a critical range. The teenager between menarche and the onset of ovulation cannot generate a normal cycle until full GnRH pulsatile secretion is achieved. Increasing intensity of GnRH suppression is associated with increasing dysfunction and a changing clinical presentation. A variety of problems, such as stress and anxiety, borderline anorexia nervosa, and acute weight loss after a crash diet are thought to inhibit normal GnRH pulsatile secretion so that the gonadotropin surge is not possible and only homeostatic pituitary-ovarian function is maintained.

At least one specific clinical syndrome has been recognized: hyperprolactinemia. Increasing levels of prolactin can cause a woman to progress through a spectrum, beginning with an inadequate luteal phase to anovulation to the amenorrhea associated with complete GnRH suppression. A search for galactorrhea and measurement of the prolactin level are important screening procedures for all women who are not ovulating normally.

Abnormal Signals

Abnormal cycles can be due to failures within the system, or due to the introduction of confounding factors. It is instructive to focus on the blood estradiol concentration as the critical signal for the machinery of the ovulatory cycle. In order to achieve the appropriate changes within the cycle, estradiol levels must rise and fall in synchrony with morphologic events. Therefore, two possible signal failures may occur: 1) estradiol levels may not fall low enough to allow sufficient FSH response for the initial growth stimulus, and 2) levels of estradiol may be inadequate to produce the positive stimulatory effects necessary to induce the ovulatory surge of LH.

1. **Loss of FSH Stimulation.** In order to achieve recycling, a nadir in blood sex steroid levels must occur so that the initial event in the cycle, the rise in FSH, may take place. Sustained estrogen at such a key moment would not permit FSH stimulation of follicular growth and maturation, and recycling would be thwarted. The necessary decline in blood estrogen requires reduction of secretion, appropriate clearance and metabolism, and the absence of a significant contribution of estrogen to the circulation by extragonadal sources.

   Persistent Estrogen Secretion. The most common clinical example of anovulation associated with continued secretion of estrogen is pregnancy. Persistent and elevated secretion of estrogen can be encountered rarely with an ovarian or adrenal tumor. In such a case, anovulation or amenorrhea may bring the patient to a physician's attention.

   Abnormal Estrogen Clearance and Metabolism. The clearance and metabolism of estrogen can be impaired by other pathologic conditions, such as thyroid or hepatic disease. It is for this reason that a careful history and physical examination are important elements in the differential diagnosis of anovulation. Both hyperthyroidism and hypothyroidism can cause persistent anovulation by altering not only metabolic clearance, but also the peripheral conversion rates among the various steroids. The subtle presence of hypothyroidism, which may be associated with elevated prolactin levels, demands screening of anovulatory and amenorrheic women with a thyroid stimulating hormone (TSH) level.

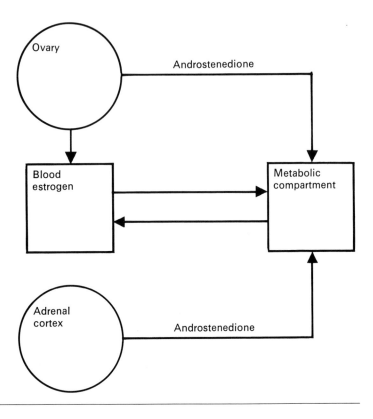

Extraglandular Estrogen Production. Extragonadal contribution to the blood estrogen level can reach significant proportions. While the adrenal gland does not secrete appreciable amounts of estrogen into the circulation, it indirectly contributes to the total estrogen level. This is accomplished by the extragonadal peripheral conversion of C-19 androgenic precursors, mainly androstenedione, to estrogen. In this manner psychologic or physical stress may increase the adrenal contribution of estrogenic precursor, and subsequent conversion to estrogen may sustain the blood level of estrogen at a time when a decline is necessary for successful recycling of the menstrual cycle. Adipose tissue is capable of converting androstenedione to estrogen, hence the percent conversion increases with increasing body weight. (1) This is at least one mechanism for the well-known association between obesity and anovulation.

2. **Loss of LH Stimulation.** A failure in gonadal production of estrogen need not be absolute. Obviously the patient with gonadal dysgenesis and ovarian failure will present with amenorrhea and infertility because of a total lack of estrogen secretion. More commonly, the clinician is concerned with the patient who has gonadotropin and estrogen production, but does not ovulate. The failure to achieve a critical midcycle level of estradiol necessary to trigger the gonadotropin surge may be due to a relative deficiency in steroid production. The perimenopausal woman undergoes a terminal period of anovulation which may represent a

steroidogenic refractoriness within the remaining elderly follicles. This inadequacy may be due to intrinsic follicular weaknesses or an impairment in the follicular-gonadotropin interaction. In any case, the end result is the same—a failure to achieve critical signal levels of estradiol at the appropriate time in midcycle.

Local
Ovarian
Conditions

An understanding of the critical role for estradiol within the follicle indicates possible points of failure which may lead to anovulation. Estradiol prevents atresia despite declining FSH levels by enhancing the action of FSH in increasing the number of FSH receptors within the follicle, thus increasing follicular sensitivity to FSH. In addition, estradiol enhances the induction of LH receptors by FSH, making it possible for the follicle to respond to the LH surge at midcycle. A follicle can fail to grow and ovulate either because of inadequate estradiol production within the follicle, or because of interference with the action of estradiol.

The factors which control follicular production of estradiol are now understood in terms of the two-cell explanation described in Chapter 3. Surely a very precise coordination is necessary between morphologic development and hormonal stimulation. Pertubations may arise from an infectious process, from the presence of endometriosis, by abnormal qualitative or quantitative changes in tropic hormone receptors (ovarian insensitivity), or the necessary biologic effects may be blocked by an improper molecular constitution of the gonadotropins (heterogeneity of the glycopeptide hormones).

Local ovarian androgens induce follicular atresia. Whereas this action in the normal cycle may be important in ensuring that only one follicle reaches the point of ovulation, an excessive concentration of androgens can prevent normal cycling. This effect of androgens can be mediated by interference with the key actions of estradiol. Thus, the important effects of estradiol on gonadotropin receptors will be impeded, leading to chronic anovulation. This may be another mechanism by which obesity leads to persistent anovulation. Obese women depress their sex hormone binding globulin (SHBG) levels out of proportion to changes in estrogen or testosterone when compared to normal weight patients. (2) This change also has been noted in men, but the mechanism is unknown. Thus, obesity itself would increase free sex steroid levels, and the resulting increase in free testosterone could serve as the factor which acts locally within the ovary to prevent normal follicular growth and ovulation.

Precise Etiology

The normal ovulatory function of the menstrual system relies on a dynamic coordination of complex actions. Abnormal function may represent discordance at all of the levels reviewed in the above paragraphs. Thus, a minor deficiency in the estradiol signal will be associated with a subnormal central response, and an impaired or inappropriate degree of follicular growth and function. Dysfunction is sustained by the internal feedback mechanisms within the system, and anovulation may become a persistent problem.

It is usually impossible to reduce the issue of etiology to a single factor of abnormal menstrual function, except in severe disease states such as pituitary tumors, anorexia nervosa, gonadal dysgenesis, and perhaps hyperprolactinemia and obesity. Regardless of the nature of the initial cause of the problem, the final clinical statement of the dysfunction is predictable, and easily diagnosed and managed. Not only is it often impossible, but it is also often unnecessary, to define the precise etiology. In patients who have abnormal or absent menstrual function, but are otherwise medically well, the diagnosis will fall into one of three categories:

1. **Ovarian Failure.** Hypergonadotropic hypogonadism, the inability of the ovary to respond to any gonadotropic stimulation, usually due to the absence of follicular tissue on a genetic basis (discussed in Chapter 5).

2. **Central Failure.** Hypogonadotropic hypogonadism, hypothalamic or pituitary suppression as expressed in abnormally low or normal serum gonadotropins (discussed in Chapter 5).

3. **Anovulatory Dysfunction.** The patient who has asynchronous gonadotropin and estrogen production and does not ovulate presents with a variety of clinical manifestations. The associated clinical signs and symptoms depend upon the level of gonadal function preserved, and are represented by the following principal problems:

    Endometrial hyperplasia and cancer (Chapter 4)

    Amenorrhea (Chapter 5)

    Hirsutism (Chapter 7)

    Dysfunctional uterine bleeding (Chapter 8)

    Breast disease (Chapter 9)

    Infertility and induction of ovulation (Chapter 20)

    The polycystic ovary (this chapter).

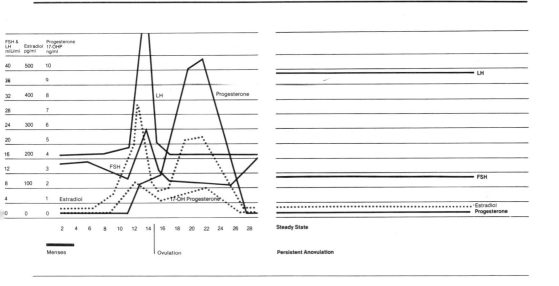

FSH & LH mIU/ml	Estradiol pg/ml	Progesterone 17-OHP ng/ml		
40	500	10		
36		9		
32	400	8		
28		7		
24	300	6		
20		5		
16	200	4		
12		3		
8	100	2		
4	1			
0	0	0		

Menses   Ovulation   Steady State   Persistent Anovulation

The Polycystic Ovary

In 1935 Stein and Leventhal first described a symptom complex due to anovulation. Acceptance of this syndrome as a singular clinical entity led to a rather rigid approach to this problem for many years. Only those women qualified who had a history of oligomenorrhea, hirsutism, and obesity, together with a demonstration of enlarged, polycystic ovaries. It is far more useful clinically to avoid the use of eponyms and even the term polycystic ovary syndrome. It is better to consider this problem as one of persistent anovulation with a spectrum of etiologies and clinical manifestations.

A question which has puzzled gynecologists and endocrinologists for many years is what causes polycystic ovaries. The answer is now apparent. The characteristic polycystic ovary emerges when a state of anovulation persists for any length of time. Because there are many causes of anovulation, there are many causes of polycystic ovaries. A similar clinical picture and ovarian condition may reflect any of the dysfunctional states discussed above. In other words, the polycystic ovary is the result of a functional derangement, not a specific central or local defect.

In contrast to the characteristic picture of fluctuating hormone levels in the normal cycle, a "steady state" of gonadotropins and sex steroids can be depicted in association with persistent anovulation. This steady state is only relative, and is being exaggerated here to present a concept of this clinical problem.

In patients with persistent anovulation, the average daily production of estrogen and androgens is both increased and dependent upon LH stimulation. This is reflected in higher circulating levels of testosterone, androstenedione, dehydroepiandrosterone (DHA), dehydroepiandrosterone sulfate (DHAS), 17-hydroxyprogesterone, and estrone. (3, 4) The testosterone, androstenedione, and DHA are secreted directly by the ovary while the DHAS is almost exclusively an adrenal contribution. (4) The ovary does not secrete increased amounts of estrogen, and estradiol levels are equivalent to early follicular phase concentrations. The increased estrogen is due to peripheral conversion of the increased amounts of androstenedione to estrone.

The levels of SHBG are controlled by a balance of hormonal influences on its synthesis in the liver; testosterone is inhibitory, estrogen and thyroxine are stimulatory. Due to the increased levels of testosterone in anovulatory patients, there is an approximate 50% reduction in SHBG. Indeed, in hirsute females the mean SHBG concentration is similar to that of males. (5)

When compared to levels found in normal women, patients with this condition have higher mean concentrations of LH, but low or low-normal levels of FSH. (3, 6, 7) The elevated levels of LH can be in the range of the midcycle surge or equivalent to postmenopausal values. Evidence (an augmented response to GnRH) indicates that the elevated LH levels are due to an increased sensitivity of the pituitary to releasing hormone stimulation. (7) This is consistent with the concepts discussed in Chapter 2, linking a high estrogen environment with anterior pituitary secretion of LH and suppression of FSH.

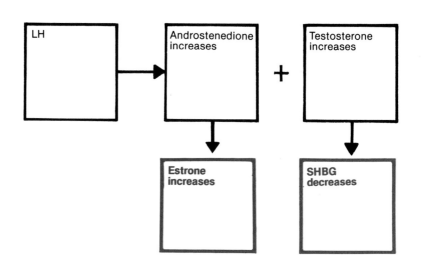

This increased sensitivity can be attributed to the increased estrone levels, (8) but a newly appreciated factor is the impact of the decreased SHBG concentration. Despite no increase in estradiol secretion, free estradiol levels are increased because of the significant decrease in SHBG. The increased LH secretion as expressed by the LH:FSH ratio is positively correlated with the increased free estradiol. (9) The lower FSH levels represent the sensitivity of the FSH negative feedback system to the elevated estrogen, both free estradiol and the estrone formed from peripheral conversion of androstenedione. The clinical consequences of uninterrupted estrogen stimulation (endometrial and breast cancer) as well as the increased LH are the result of the two estrogenic influences, increased estrone levels from peripheral conversion of androstenedione and increased free estradiol levels.

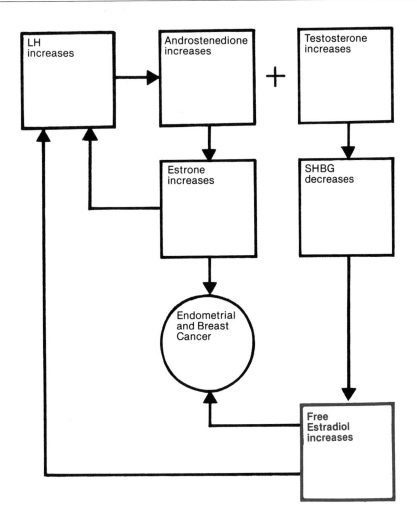

Because the FSH levels are not totally depressed, new follicular growth is continuously stimulated, but not to the point of full maturation and ovulation. Despite the fact that full growth potential is not realized, follicular life span may extend several months in the form of multiple follicular cysts, 2–6 mm in diameter. These follicles are surrounded by hyperplastic theca cells, often luteinized in response to the high LH levels. The accumulation of follicular tissue in various stages of development allows an increased and relatively constant production of steroids in response to the gonadotropin stimulation. This condition is self-sustaining. As various follicles undergo atresia, they are immediately replaced by new follicles of similar limited growth potential.

The tissue derived from follicular atresia is also sustained by the steady state, and now contributes to the stromal compartment of the ovary. In terms of the two-cell explanation of follicular steroidogenesis, atresia is associated with a degenerating granulosa, leaving the theca cells to contribute to the stromal compartment of the ovary. It is not surprising, therefore, that this functioning stromal tissue secretes significant amounts of androstenedione and testosterone, the usual products of theca cells. In response to the elevated LH levels, the androgen production rate is increased. In turn, in a vicious cycle, the elevated androgen levels, through the process of extraglandular conversion and by suppressing synthesis of SHBG, result in elevated estrogen levels. In addition, the decrease in SHBG is associated with a twofold increase in free testosterone.

The elevated androgens contribute to the morphologic effect within the ovary by blocking the actions of estradiol on the granulosa cells, preventing normal follicular development and inducing premature atresia. Indeed, in another vicious cycle, the local androgen block appears to be the major obstacle which maintains this steady state of persistent anovulation. The ovulatory response to wedge resection of the ovaries follows a sustained reduction in testosterone levels, indicating that the intraovarian androgen effect is the principal factor in preventing normal cycling. (10–12)

In this manner the classic picture of the polycystic ovary is attained, displaying numerous follicles in the early stages of development and atresia, and dense stromal tissue. The loss of recycling has resulted in a hormonal steady state causing persistent anovulation which may be associated with the increased production of androgens.

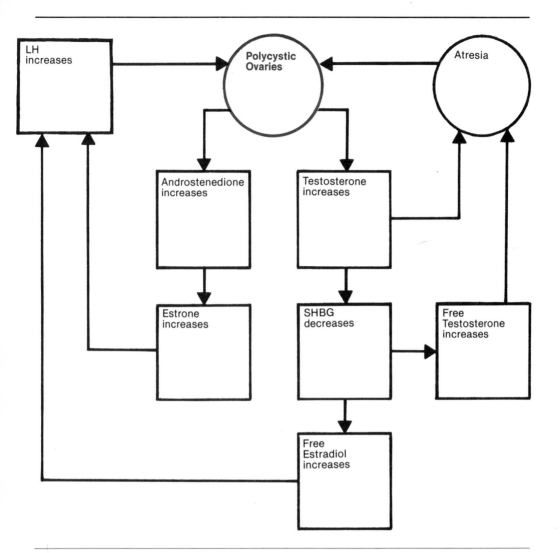

The polycystic ovary is usually enlarged and is characterized by a smooth pearly white capsule. For years, it was erroneously believed that the thick sclerotic capsule acted as a mechanical barrier to ovulation. A more accurate concept is that the polycystic ovary is a consequence of the loss of ovulation and the achievement of the steady state of persistent anovulation. The characteristics of the ovary reflect this dysfunctional state (13):

1.   The surface area is doubled, giving an average volume increase of 2.8 times.

2.   The same number of primordial follicles are present, but the number of growing and atretic follicles (up to the secondary follicle stage), is doubled. Each ovary may contain 20–100 cystic follicles.

3. There is a 50% increase in the thickness of the tunica.

4. There is a one third increase in cortical stromal thickness and a 5-fold increase in subcortical stroma. The increased stroma is due both to hyperplasia and to increased formation subsequent to the excessive follicular maturation and atresia.

5. There are 4 times more ovarian hilus cell nests (hyperplasia).

Hyperthecosis refers to patches of luteinized theca-like cells scattered throughout the ovarian stroma. It is characterized by the same histologic findings as seen with polycystic ovaries. (13) The clinical picture of more intense androgenization is a result of greater androgen production. This condition is associated with lower LH levels, which is a likely consequence of the higher testosterone levels blocking estrogen action at the pituitary level. (14, 15) It seems appropriate to view hyperthecosis as a manifestation of the same process, persistent anovulation, but with greater intensity.

The typical histologic changes of the polycystic ovary can be encountered with any size ovary. There is a spectrum of time involved in the development of this condition, and it is useful to view the attainment of high LH levels and large ovaries as a stage of maximal effect of persistent anovulation. Increased size of the ovaries is not a critical feature, nor is it necessary for diagnosis. The key to understanding this clinical problem is an appreciation for the disruption in ovulatory recycling function.

There is no specific defect. The hypothalamic-pituitary response is entirely appropriate, a response to chronically elevated estrogen feedback. The changes are a functional derangement brought about by accumulated and increased androgen due to a failure of ovulation, whatever the reason. Hence, the polycystic ovary may be associated with extragonadal sources of androgens (16) or with ovarian androgen-producing tumors. (17)

The functional problem can be understood in terms of the two-cell explanation of steroidogenesis (Chapter 3). The follicles are unable to successfully change their microenvironment from androgen dominance to estrogen dominance, the change that is essential for continued follicular growth and development. (18) The functional picture that emerges, incompetent granulosa cells and very active theca cells, corresponds to the morphologic histology of underdeveloped granulosa and hyperplastic and luteinized theca. Granulosa cells obtained from the small follicles of polycystic ovaries produce negligible amounts of estradiol, but show a dramatic increase in estrogen production when FSH is added. (19) In terms of the two-cell explanation, this behavior is consistent with deficient FSH receptors and granulosa function, not an intrinsic enzyme defect. Successful treatment depends, therefore, on altering the ratio of FSH to androgens; either increasing FSH (with clomiphene) or decreasing androgens (wedge resection) to overcome the androgen block at the granulosa level. This permits development of aromatization to bring about conversion of the microenvironment to estrogen dominance. Because anovulation with polycystic ovaries is a functional derangment, it is not surprising that these patients occasionally may ovulate spontaneously. Indeed, ovulation is unpredictable and contraception may be necessary.

At least one group of patients with this condition inherits the disorder, possibly by means of an X-linked dominant transmission. There is a 2-fold higher incidence of hirsutism and oligomenorrhea with paternal transmission, but with marked variability of phenotypic expression. (20)

The adrenal gland is involved in this problem. Higher circulating levels of DHAS, almost exclusively an adrenal product, testify to adrenal participation. The mechanism and the clinical importance of this involvement will be discussed in Chapter 7, "Hirsutism."

Clinical Consequences

Anovulation is the key feature of this condition and presents as amenorrhea in approximately 55% of cases, and with irregular, heavy bleeding in 28%. (21) True virilization is rare, but 70% of anovulatory patients complain of cosmetically disturbing hirsutism. The development of hirsutism depends not only on the concentration of androgens in the blood, but on the genetic sensitivity of hair follicles to androgens. Obesity has been classically regarded as an important feature, but in view of the concept of persistent anovulation arising from many causes, its presence is extremely variable and has no diagnostic value.

While an elevated LH value in the presence of a low or low-normal FSH may be diagnostic, the diagnosis is easily made by the clinical presentation alone. Indeed, the androgen impact may be such that the estrogen-induced LH secretion is suppressed. About 10–20% of patients with this condition do not have elevated LH levels with reversal of the LH:FSH ratio. We do not routinely measure FSH and LH levels in anovulatory patients.

The symptoms are a consequence of the loss of ovulation: dysfunctional bleeding, amenorrhea, hirsutism, and infertility. They each require a specific diagnostic and therapeutic approach, as discussed in separate chapters in this book.

There are potentially severe clinical consequences of the steady state of hormone secretion. Besides the problems of bleeding, amenorrhea, hirsutism, and infertility, the effect of the unopposed and uninterrupted estrogen is to place the patient in considerable risk for cancer of the endometrium and cancer of the breast. (22) If left unattended, patients with persistent anovulation develop clinical problems, and therefore, appropriate therapeutic management is essential for all anovulatory patients.

The typical patient presents with anovulation and irregular menses, or amenorrhea with withdrawal bleeding after a progestational challenge. If there is no hirsutism or virilism, evaluation of androgen production is not necessary. There is no need for urinary 17-ketosteroids, blood testosterone, blood DHAS, or any other laboratory procedures. In the patient whose only problem is long-standing anovulation, and especially if the patient is over 35, an endometrial biopsy (with extensive sampling) is a wise precaution. The well-known association between this syndrome and abnormal endometrial changes must be kept in mind. Documentation of anovulation is usually unnecessary, especially in view of menstrual irregularity with periods of amenorrhea.

Therapy of most anovulatory patients can be planned at the first visit. If the patient desires pregnancy, she is a candidate for the medical induction of ovulation (Chapter 20). If the patient presents with amenorrhea, an investigation must be pursued as outlined in Chapter 5. The management of significant dysfunctional uterine bleeding is discussed in Chapter 8, and hirsutism in Chapter 7.

For the patient who does not wish to become pregnant and does not complain of hirsutism, but is anovulatory and has irregular bleeding, therapy is directed toward interruption of the steady state effect on the endometrium and breast. The use of Provera (10 mg daily for the first 10 days of every month) is favored to ensure complete withdrawal bleeding, and to prevent endometrial hyperplasia and atypia. The monthly 10-day duration has been shown to be essential to protect the endometrium from cancer in women on estrogen replacement therapy. Until specific clinical data are available, it seems logical that young, anovulatory women also require 10 days of progestational exposure every month. The patient will be aware of the onset of ovulatory cycles because bleeding will occur at a time besides the expected withdrawal bleed. The use of oral contraception medication for therapy in these patients requires individual patient judgment. In our opinion, when reliable contraception is essential, the use of low dose combination oral contraception in the usual cyclic fashion is appropriate.

References

1. **Siiteri PK, MacDonald PC,** Role of extraglandular estrogen in human endocrinology, in *Handbook of Physiology, Section 7, Endocrinology,* Geyer SR, Astwood EB, Greep RO, eds, American Physiology Society, Washington DC, 1973, pp 615–629.

2. **Plymate SR, Fariss BL, Bassett ML, Matej L,** Obesity and its role in polycystic ovary syndrome, J Clin Endocrinol Metab 52:1246, 1981.

3. **DeVane GW, Czekala NM, Judd HL, Yen SSC,** Circulating gonadotropins, estrogen and androgens in polycystic ovarian disease, Am J Obstet Gynecol 121:496, 1975.

4. **Laatikainen TJ, Apter DL, Paavonen JA, Wahlstrom TR,** Steroids in ovarian and peripheral venous blood in polycystic ovarian disease, Clin Endocrinol 13:125, 1980.

5. **Moll GW Jr, Rosenfield RL, Helke JH,** Estradiol-testosterone binding interactions and free plasma estradiol under physiological conditions, J Clin Endocrinol Metab 52:868, 1981.

6. **Kletzky OA, Davajan V, Nakamura RM, Thorneycroft IH, Mishell DR Jr,** Clinical categorization of patients with secondary amenorrhea using progesterone induced uterine bleeding and measurement of serum gonadotropin levels, Am J Obstet Gynecol 121:695, 1975.

7. **Rebar R, Judd HL, Yen SSC, Rakoff J, Vandenberg G, Naftolin F,** Characterization of the inappropriate gonadotropin secretion in polycystic ovary syndrome, J Clin Invest 57:1320, 1976.

8. **Chang RJ, Mandel FP, Lu JK, Judd HL,** Enhanced disparity of gonadotropin secretion by estrone in women with polycystic ovarian disease, J Clin Endocrinol Metab 54:490, 1982.

9. **Lobo RA, Granger L, Goebelsmann U, Mishell DR Jr,** Elevations in unbound serum estradiol as a possible mechanism for inappropriate gonadotropin secretion in women with PCO, J Clin Endocrinol Metab 52:156, 1981.

10. **Judd HL, Rigg LA, Anderson DC, Yen SSC,** The effects of ovarian wedge resection on circulating gonadotropin and ovarian steroid levels in patients with polycystic ovary syndrome, J Clin Endocrinol Metab 43:347, 1976.

11. **Mahesh VB, Bratlid D, Lindabeck T,** Hormone levels following wedge resection in polycystic ovary syndrome, Obstet Gynecol 51:64, 1978.

12. **Katz M, Carr PJ, Cohen BM, Milhin RP,** Hormonal effects of wedge resection of polycystic ovaries, Obstet Gynecol 51:437, 1978.

13. **Hughesdon PE,** Morphology and morphogenesis of the Stein-Leventhal ovary and of so-called "hyperthecosis," Obstet Gynecol Surv 37:59, 1982.

14. **Judd HL, Scully RE, Herbst AL, Yen SSC, Ingersol FM, Kliman B,** Familial hyperthecosis: comparison of endocrinologic and histologic findings with polycystic ovarian disease, Am J Obstet Gynecol 117:979, 1973.

15. **Nagamani M, Lingold JC, Gomez LG, Barza JR,** Clinical and hormonal studies in hyperthecosis of the ovaries, Fertil Steril 36:326, 1981.

16. **Kase N, Kowal J, Perloff W, Soffer LJ,** In vitro production of androgens by a virilizing adenoma and associated polycystic ovaries, Acta Endocrinol 44:15, 1963.

17. **Zourlas PA, Jones HW Jr,** Stein-Leventhal syndrome with masculinizing ovarian tumors, Obstet Gynecol 34:861, 1969.

18. **McNatty KP, Smith DM, Makris A, DeGrazia C, Tulchinsky D, Osathanondh R, Schiff I, Ryan KJ,** The intraovarian sites of androgen and estrogen formation in women with normal and hyperandrogenic ovaries as judged by in vitro experiments, J Clin Endocrinol Metab 50:755, 1980.

19. **Erickson GF, Hsueh AJN, Quigley ME, Rebar R, Yen SSC,** Functional studies of aromatase activity in human granulosa cells from normal and polycystic ovaries, J Clin Endocrinol Metab 49:514, 1979.

20. **Givens JR,** Hirsutism and hyperandrogenism, Adv Intern Med 21:221, 1976.

21. **Prunty FTG,** Hirsutism, virilism, and apparent virilism, and their gonadal relationships, J Endocrinol 38:203, 1967.

22. **Cowan LD, Gordis L, Tonascia JA, Jones GES,** Breast cancer incidence in women with a history of progesterone deficiency, Am J Epidemiol 114:209, 1981.

7 Hirsutism

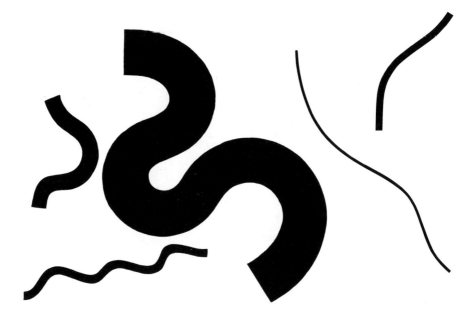

Excessive facial and body hair usually is associated with loss of cyclic menstrual function due to excess androgen production by anovulatory ovaries. The more severe states of virilism (clitoromegaly, deepening of the voice, balding, and changes in body habitus) are rarely seen and usually are secondary to adrenal hyperplasia or androgen-producing tumors of adrenal or ovarian origin. Although these are rare, diagnostic evaluation is required. Furthermore, a concerned and sympathetic approach must be offered to the patient. The responsible physician must view hirsutism both as an endocrine problem and as a cosmetic problem. To the affected woman, hair growth over the face, abdomen, or breasts is disturbing on several levels: Is there disease? Is sexuality changing? Is social acceptance altered? Is fertility impaired?

This chapter will review the biology of hair growth and the endocrine possibilities which may yield hirsutism. An uncomplicated, effective program for diagnostic evaluation and therapeutic management will be offered.

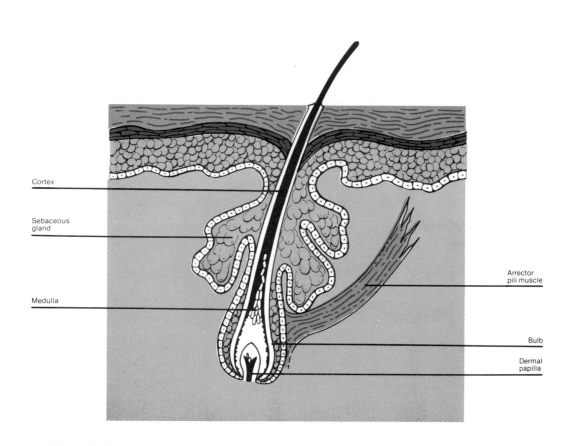

Cortex

Sebaceous
gland

Medulla

Arrector
pili muscle

Bulb

Dermal
papilla

**Biology of Hair
Growth**
Embryology

Each hair follicle develops at about 8 weeks of gestation as a derivative of the epidermis. It is composed initially of a solid column of cells which proliferates from the basal layers of the epidermis and protrudes downward into the dermis. As the column elongates it encounters a cluster of mesodermal cells (the dermal papilla) which it envelops at its bulbous tip (bulb). The solid epithelial column then hollows out to form a hair canal, and the pilosebaceous apparatus is laid down.

Hair growth begins with proliferation of the epithelial cells at the base of the column in contact with the dermal papilla. The lanugo hair present at this stage is lightly pigmented, thin in diameter, short in length, and fragile in attachment. Important to note here is the fact that the total endowment of hair follicles is made at an early gestational stage, and that no new hair follicles will be produced de novo. The concentration of hair follicles laid down per unit area of facial skin does not differ materially between sexes but does differ between races and ethnic groups (Caucasian > Oriental; Mediterranean > Nordic).

| Structure and Growth | Hair does not grow continuously, but rather in a cyclic fashion with alternating phases of activity and inactivity. The cycles are referred to by the following terms: |

Anagen—the growing phase.
Catagen—rapid involution phase.
Telogen—quiescent phase.

In the resting phase (telogen), the hair is short and loosely attached to the base of the epithelial canal. The bulb is formed around the dermal papilla. As growth begins (anagen), epithelial matrix cells at the base begin to proliferate and extend downward into the dermis. The bulb is reformed and the epithelial column elongates some 4–6 times from the resting state. Once downward extension is completed, continued rapid growth of the matrix cells pushes upward to the skin surface. The tenuous contact of the previous hair is broken, and that hair is shed. The superficial matrix cells differentiate forming a keratinized column. Growth continues as long as active mitoses persist in the basal matrix cells. When finished (categen), the column shrinks, the bulb shrivels, and the resting state is reachieved (telogen).

The length of hair is primarily determined by duration of the growth phase (anagen). Scalp hair remains in anagen for 2–6 years and has only a relatively short resting phase. Elsewhere (forearm) a short anagen and long telogen will lead to short hair of stable nongrowing length. The appearance of continuous growth (or periodic shedding) is determined by the degree to which individual hair follicles act asynchronously with their neighbors. Scalp hair is asynchronous and therefore always seems to be growing. The resting phase that some hairs are in is not apparent. If marked synchrony is achieved, then all hairs may undergo telogen at the same time leading to the appearance of shedding. Occasionally, women will complain of marked hair loss from the scalp, but this time period of shedding is usually limited, and normal growth resumes.

Factors which Influence Hair Growth

The dermal papilla is the director of the events which control hair growth. Despite major injury to the epithelial component of the follicle (such as freezing, x-rays, or a skin graft), if the dermal papilla survives, the hair follicle will regenerate and regrow hair. Injury to, or degeneration of, the dermal papilla are the crucial factors in permanent hair loss.

Sexual hair can be defined as that hair which responds to the sex steroids. Sexual hair grows on the face, lower abdomen, anterior thighs, the chest, the breasts, and in the axillae and pubic area. From animal studies and human disease patterns, the following list of hormonal effects can be compiled:

1. Androgens, particularly testosterone, initiate growth, increase the diameter and pigmentation of the keratin column, and probably increase the rate of matrix cell mitoses, in all but scalp hair.

203

2. Estrogens act essentially opposite from androgens, retarding the rate and initiation of growth, and leading to finer, less pigmented and slower growing hair.

3. Progestins have minimal direct effect on hair.

4. Pregnancy (high estrogen and progesterone) may increase the synchrony of hair growth, leading to periods of growth or shedding.

An important clinical characteristic of hair growth can be understood from studies of the effects of castration. If castration occurs before puberty, the male will not grow a beard. If castration occurs after puberty with beard and sexual hair distribution fully developed, then these hairs continue to grow albeit more slowly and with finer caliber. Clearly androgen stimulates sexual hair follicle conversion from lanugo to adult hair growth patterns, but *once established, these patterns persist despite withdrawal of androgen.* Hypertrichosis is a generalized increase in hair of the fetal vellus or lanugo type, associated with the use of drugs or malignancy. Hirsutism implies a vellus to terminal hair transformation.

Sexual and nonsexual hair growth can be affected by endocrine problems. In hypopituitarism, there is marked reduction of hair growth. Acromegaly will be associated with hirsutism in 10–15% of patients. While the impact of thyroid hormone is not clear, hypothyroid individuals sometimes display less axillary, pubic, and, curiously, lateral eyebrow hair.

Hair growth may be influenced by nonhormonal factors, such as local skin temperature, blood flow, edema, and stasis. Hair growth may be seen with CNS problems such as encephalitis, cranial trauma, multiple sclerosis, and with drugs.

Androgen Production

The production rate of testosterone in the normal female is 0.2 to 0.3 mg/day. Approximately 50% of testosterone arises from peripheral conversion of androstendione, while the adrenal gland and ovary contribute approximately equal amounts (25%) to the circulating levels of testosterone, except at midcycle when the ovarian contribution increases by 10–15%. Dehydroepiandrosterone sulfate (DHAS) arises almost exclusively from the adrenal gland, while 90% of dehydroepiandrosterone (DHA) is from the adrenal.

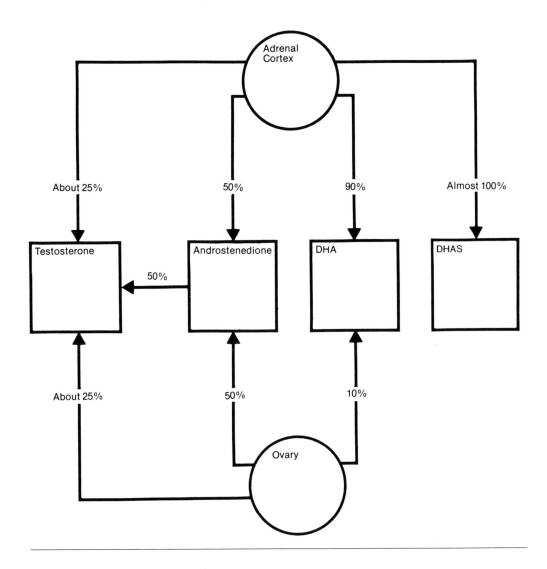

About 80% of circulating testosterone is bound to a β-globulin known as sex steroid hormone binding globulin (SHBG). Approximately 19% is loosely bound to albumin, leaving about 1% unbound. Androgenicity is dependent upon the unbound fraction which can move freely from the vascular compartment into the target cells. DHA, DHAS, and androstenedione are not significantly protein bound, and routine radioimmunoassay reflects their biologically available hormone activity. This is not the case with testosterone, for routine assays measure the total testosterone concentration, bound and unbound.

SHBG production in the liver is decreased by androgens. Hence, the binding capacity in men is lower than in normal women, and 2–3% of testosterone circulates in the free, active form in a man. SHBG is increased by estrogens and thyroid hormone. Therefore, binding capacity is increased in women, in hyperthyroidism, in pregnancy, and by estrogen-containing medication. In a hirsute woman, the SHBG level is depressed by the excess androgen, and the percent free and active testosterone is elevated as is the metabolic clearance rate of testosterone. The total testosterone concentration, therefore, may be in the normal range in a woman who is hirsute. There is no clinical need for a specific assay for the free portion of testosterone. The very presence of hirsutism or masculinization indicates increased androgen effects. One can reliably interpret a normal testosterone level in these circumstances as compatible with decreased binding capacity and increased free testosterone.

In hirsute women, only 25% of the circulating testosterone arises from peripheral conversion, and most is due to direct tissue secretion. Indeed, data overwhelmingly indicate that the ovary is the major source of increased testosterone in hirsute women. (1) The most common cause of hirsutism in women is anovulation and excessive androgen production by the ovaries. Adrenal causes are most uncommon.

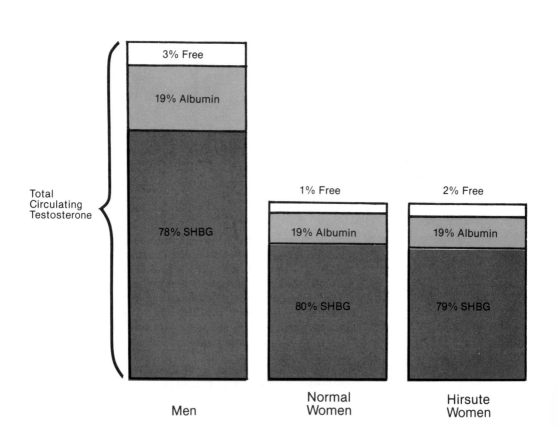

Evaluation of Hirsutism

Cosmetically disfiguring hirsutism is the end result of a number of factors:

1. The number of hair follicles present (Japanese women bearing androgen-producing tumors rarely are hirsute because of the low concentration of hair follicles per unit skin area).

2. The degree to which androgen has converted resting lanugo hair to adult hair.

3. The ratio of the growth to resting phases in the affected hair follicles.

4. The asynchrony of growth cycles in aggregates of hair follicles.

5. The thickness and degree of pigmentation of individual hairs.

The primary factor is an increase in androgen levels (primarily testosterone) which produces an initial growth stimulus and then acts to sustain continued growth. Essentially every woman with hirsutism will be found to have an increased production rate of testosterone and androstenedione if studied with sophisticated techniques. (2)

The most sensitive marker for increased androgen production is hirsutism. This is followed in order, according to the degree of androgen production, by acne and increased oiliness of the skin, menstrual irregularity, increased libido, clitoromegaly, and finally, masculinization. Masculinization and virilization are terms reserved for extreme androgen effects (usually, but not always, associated with a tumor) leading to the development of a male hair pattern, clitoromegaly, deepening of the voice, increased muscle mass, and general male body habitus.

The most common problem encountered is the hirsute woman with irregular menses, with the onset of hirsutism during puberty or in the early 20s, and a long, gradual worsening of the condition. About 70% of anovulatory women develop hirsutism. The picture is so characteristic that a careful history may be sufficient for the diagnosis.

A good history may reveal some of the rare causes of hirsutism: environmental factors producing chronic irritation or reactive hyperemia of the skin, the use of drugs, changes associated with Cushing's syndrome or acromegaly, or even the presence of pregnancy (indicating the possibility of a luteoma). Hair-stimulating drugs include methyltestosterone, anabolic agents such as Nilevar or Anavar, Dilantin, and danazol. The 19-nortestosterones in the current low dosage birth control pills rarely (if ever) cause acne or hirsutism. Especially important in the history is the rapidity of development. A woman who develops hirsutism after the age of 25 and demonstrates very rapid progression of masculinization over several months usually has an androgen-producing tumor.

207

Adrenal hyperplasia due to an enzymatic deficiency presenting in adult life is also very rare. Congenital adrenal hyperplasia which may lead to hirsutism is usually diagnosed and treated prior to puberty. Hirsutism in childhood is usually caused by congenital adrenal hyperplasia or androgen-producing tumors. Genetic problems, such as Y-containing mosaics or incomplete testicular feminization, will produce signs of androgen stimulation at puberty.

Virilization during pregnancy raises the suspicion of a luteoma, not a true tumor, but an exaggerated reaction of the ovarian stroma to chorionic gonadotropin. (3) The solid luteoma is usually unilateral and associated with a normal pregnancy, in contrast to the bilateral theca-lutein cysts seen with trophoblastic disease. Virilization due to theca-lutein cysts can also be seen with the high human chorionic gonadotropin (HCG) titers associated with multiple gestation. Since a luteoma regresses postpartum, the only risk is masculinization of a female fetus, which occurs in about 65% of cases. Subsequent pregnancies are normal.

Hirsutism, however, is rarely associated with anything but persistent anovulation. Although anovulatory ovaries are usually the source for excess androgens, a minimal workup is necessary, dedicated to ruling out the adrenal sources and tumors. It should be emphasized that hospitalization for extensive evaluation of hirsutism is required only rarely.

The Diagnostic Workup

For years, the mainstay of the diagnostic workup was a 24-hour urine collection for measurement of 17-ketosteroids and 17-hydroxysteroids. With the general availability of radioimmunoassays for blood steroids, the time has come to retire these old faithful urine measurements. Currently, the initial laboratory evaluation of hirsutism consists of the radioimmunoassay for the blood levels of testosterone and DHAS. In addition, as part of the evaluation for anovulation, prolactin levels and thyroid function should be measured, and a suction endometrial biopsy should be considered. Patients with intense androgen action may be amenorrheic due to endometrial suppression and may not demonstrate withdrawal bleeding after a progestational challenge.

Cushing's syndrome may present with hirsutism, and later masculinization. Remember that one of the most common referral diagnoses is Cushing's syndrome, but this is one of the least common final diagnoses. When clinical suspicion is high, a screen for Cushing's syndrome is indicated.

208

The Screen for Cushing's Syndrome

Cushing's syndrome, the persistent oversecretion of cortisol, can develop in three different ways: ACTH overproduction (Cushing's disease), ectopic ACTH overproduction by tumors, or autonomous cortisol-secreting adrenal tumors. A clinician must first make the diagnosis of Cushing's syndrome before determining the etiology.

The most useful measurements in the basal state to detect Cushing's syndrome are the 24-hour urinary free cortisol excretion (20–90 μg) and the late evening plasma cortisol level (<15 μg/dl). The urinary excretion of 17-ketosteroids and 17-hydroxysteroids and measurement of morning and afternoon plasma cortisol levels are less reliable because of a significant overlap between normal and abnormal patients.

The single dose overnight dexamethasone test is excellent because of the very low incidence of false results. Dexamethasone (1 mg) is given orally at bedtime, and blood is drawn at 8:00 the next morning for a plasma cortisol. A value less than 6 μg/dl rules out Cushing's syndrome. Cushing's syndrome is unlikely with intermediate values between 6 and 10 μg/dl, while a value higher than 10 μg/dl is diagnostic of adrenal hyperfunction. The number of patients with Cushing's syndrome who show a normal suppression in the single dose overnight test is negligible (less than 2%) and normal patients have a very low incidence of false positive results (less than 1%). (4) Obese patients, however, have a false positive rate up to 13%.

If the single dose overnight test is abnormal, go to the 2-mg low dose suppression test. Dexamethasone (0.5 mg every 6 hours) is administered for 2 consecutive days after 2 days of baseline urinary 17-hydroxysteroid measurements. Patients with Cushing's syndrome will not suppress their urine 17-hydroxysteroids below 4.0 mg/day. Combining the low dose test with the 24-hour urinary free cortisol and the 10 P.M. plasma cortisol should definitively provide the diagnosis of Cushing's syndrome.

The etiology of Cushing's syndrome can be established by combining an 8-mg high dose dexamethasone suppression test with measurement of the basal state blood ACTH level. Dexamethasone (2 mg every 6 hours) is administered for 2 days, and the urinary 17-hydroxysteroids on the 2nd day are compared with basal levels. If basal ACTH is undetectable, and the urinary steroids do not decrease by at least 40%, an adrenal tumor is likely. When ACTH is measurable in the blood, an ectopic ACTH producing tumor is unlikely if the 17-hydroxysteroids decrease by at least 40%. Cushing's disease is present when the blood ACTH level is in the normal range, a chest x-ray is normal, and CT scanning detects an abnormal sella turcica.

CT scanning is very accurate and reliable in detecting adrenal tumors (as small as 1.5 by 2.5 cm). (5) In addition, it reliably predicts which patients have an ectopic ACTH-producing tumor by detecting bilateral adrenal enlargement in such patients. The CT scan can differentiate between an adenoma (well rounded and circumscribed) and a carcinoma (irregular or lobulated with signs of infiltration into adjacent structures).

The DHAS Level

DHAS is the only blood assay which can be substituted for urinary 17-ketosteroids in the evaluation of hirsutism. A random sample is sufficient, needing no corrections for body weight, creatinine excretion, or random variation. Variations are minimized because of its high circulating concentration and its long half-life. A slow turnover rate results in a large and stable pool in the blood with insignificant variation.

DHAS circulates in higher concentration than any other steroid, and is derived almost exclusively from the adrenal gland. It is, therefore, a direct measure of adrenal androgen activity, correlating clinically with the urinary 17-ketosteroids. (6) The upper limit of normal in most laboratories is 250 μg/dl. As with urinary 17-ketosteroids, aging is associated with a decrease in the blood concentration of DHAS; the decrease accelerates after menopause and DHAS is almost undetectable after age 70. (7) This decline is 4 times greater than the age-related decline in cortisol, which suggests that there is an agent besides ACTH which controls DHAS secretion. Although there is a rapid decline associated with the menopause, the same decline has been observed in women over 65 and on estrogen replacement. Either a lack of estrogen is not responsible for the decline, or replacement estrogen does not mimic the estrogen milieu of the reproductive years.

Both 17-ketosteroids and circulating levels of DHAS are elevated in association with hyperprolactinemia. (8, 9) The mechanism is unknown, but both return to normal with prolactin suppression by bromocriptine. In addition, increased free testosterone levels associated with decreased SHBG are found in hyperprolactinemic women. (10, 11) This underscores the need to search for galactorrhea and to obtain a prolactin in all anovulatory women. The androgen changes are probably secondary to the persistant anovulatory state induced by the elevated prolactin, although direct prolactin effects on the adrenal, ovary, or SHBG are possible. Bromocriptine is a therapeutic option despite uncertainty over the cause of the hirsutism in this special circumstance.

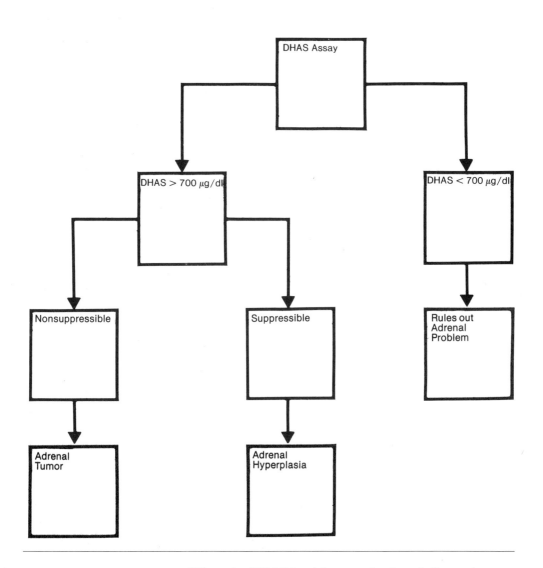

When the DHAS level is normal, adrenal disease is most unlikely, and the diagnosis of excess androgen production by the ovaries is established. There are only rare cases of adrenal tumors with normal 17-ketosteroids, and presumably normal DHAS levels, (12–14) and further evaluation of such cases would be indicated by the presence of markedly elevated blood levels of testosterone. These rare tumors are responsive to luteinzing hormone (LH), suggesting that they are derived from embryonic rest cells.

The clinical problem with DHAS measurement in the evaluation of hirsutism is the common finding of a moderately elevated DHAS level in anovulatory patients with polycystic ovaries. This is similar to the moderate elevations of 17-ketosteroids encountered in these patients. We believe that it is not worthwhile to subject these patients to a search for an adrenal enzyme defect, a search which requires an adrenal suppression and stimulation protocol. Clinical experience has established that a DHAS level of 700 µg/dl or below does not require further evaluation.

When the rare patient with a DHAS over 700 μg/dl is encountered, adrenal function must be suppressed with dexamethasone to reveal the nature and extent of the adrenal androgen contribution. Adequate adrenal androgen suppression requires a minimum of 4 days, and suppression can be carried out on an outpatient basis with 2.0 mg dexamethasone q.i.d. for 5 days. (15) On the last day of suppression a repeat DHAS determination is obtained. A lack of adrenal suppression is consistent with an autonomously functioning adrenal tumor. CT scan evaluation of the adrenal gland should be obtained.

If the DHAS suppresses to basal level (less than 50 μg/dl), adrenal hyperplasia is the diagnosis. A 21-hydroxylase or 11β-hydroxylase deficiency can be confirmed by elevated blood levels of 17-hydroxyprogesterone. This very infrequently encountered problem is the only one in which the patients should be treated with glucocorticoid compounds. For monitoring a patient with an enzyme deficiency adrenal hyperplasia, the blood 17-hydroxyprogesterone and urinary 17-ketosteroids are necessary, as the blood DHAS is not sensitive enough to provide good control.

Very few adults have a 3β-ol-dehydrogenase deficiency, which would be associated with normal 17-hydroxyprogesterone levels and only moderately elevated DHAS. The rarity of this subtle condition dictates an empirical approach discussed below.

Adrenal Gland Participation

Adrenal involvement in this syndrome of anovulation and hirsutism has long been recognized. Adrenal suppression, for example, will induce regular menses and ovulation in some patients, and empiric treatment with a glucocorticoid has been advocated in the past.

The important clinical questions are the following: Is excessive androgen secretion by the adrenal gland a primary disorder in these patients, or is it a secondary reaction to the hormonal milieu associated with anovulation? If the problem is primarily an adrenal enzyme deficiency, how common is it, and how necessary is it to pursue the diagnosis with endocrine testing?

One possibility is that the adrenal hyperactivity (as indicated by elevated DHAS levels) is due to an estrogen-induced 3β-ol-dehydrogenase insufficiency. Considerable effort has been devoted to demonstrating an estrogen influence on adrenal androgen secretion. Unfortunately there is no clear-cut conclusion, with both positive (16–19) and negative (20–22) results associated with the administration of estrogen.

Several recent studies have demonstrated a correlation between estrogen and serum levels of adrenal androgens. (19, 23) On the other hand, these same investigators have concluded that a small percentage of patients with high DHAS levels (and normal testosterone) have subtle 3β-ol-dehydrogenase deficiencies, identified only by abnormal $\Delta 5$ steroid to $\Delta 4$ steroid ratios in the blood after dexamethasone suppression and ACTH stimulation. (24) Others have compared adrenal function in normal women and women with polycystic ovaries and concluded that there is no overt enzyme defect. (25, 26)

It is attractive to explain adrenal hyperactivity (elevated DHAS) seen in anovulatory hirsute women as a secondary reaction induced and maintained by the constant estrogen state associated with persistent anovulation. This picture is similar to that of the fetal adrenal gland. Recent studies have demonstrated that the low level of 3β-ol-dehydrogenase activity and high secretion of DHA by the fetal adrenal cortex are due to estrogen. (27) The hyperplasia of the fetal adrenal cortex is the result of the high ACTH due to the relatively low cortisol levels, a consequence of the 3β-ol-dehydrogenase inhibition. Unfortunately, the adult anovulatory counterpart is not exactly similar, in that ACTH levels in women with polycystic ovaries are not elevated. (28) This can be explained, however, by evidence indicating the presence of a separate controlling agent for DHAS secretion, independent of ACTH, (7, 28), or very frequent sampling is necessary to detect a change in pulsatile secretion of ACTH.

The inconclusiveness of this situation and the rarity of a true adrenal enzyme deficiency in the adult make a cost-effective argument against endocrine testing (suppression and stimulation) in the pursuit of a definitive diagnosis. Accordingly we have adopted a blood DHAS level of 700 μg/dl, below which we do not pursue the possibility of a primary adrenal enzyme problem. An empirical approach should suffice. If the blood DHAS remains elevated after 6 months of progestational treatment, further diagnostic effort or treatment with a glucorticoid should be considered.

The use of cortisol and its derivatives to achieve adrenal suppression is not indicated in the vast majority of patients presenting with irregular menses and hirsutism. Not only is the long-term use of these drugs hazardous, it is also an indirect attack on the basic problem, the anovulatory ovary. In the absence of specific adrenal disease, the more reasonable approach is direct treatment of the menstrual dysfunction, either by medical induction of ovulation or progestin suppression of ovarian steroidogensis.

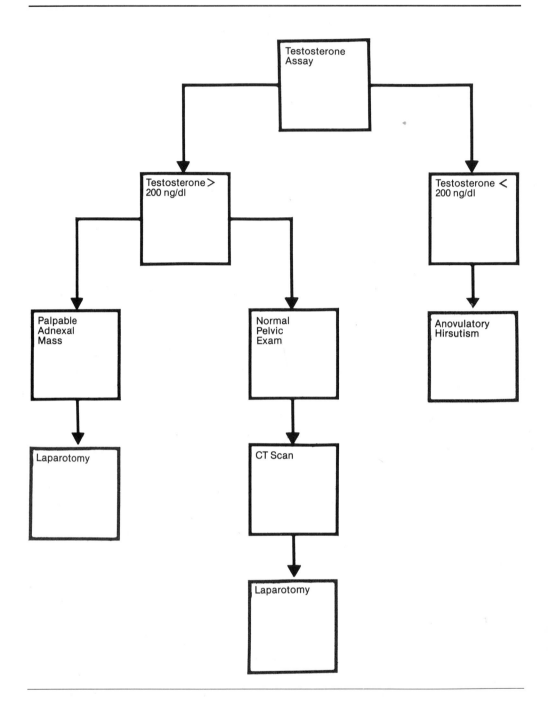

The Testosterone Level

Plasma testosterone levels (normal 20–80 ng/dl) are elevated in the majority of women (70%) with anovulation and hirsutism. Individual variation is great, however, largely due to the changes in the testosterone binding capacity of the sex binding globulin in the blood. Because the binding globulin levels are depressed by androgens, the total testosterone concentration can be in the normal range in a woman who is hirsute even though the percent unbound and active testosterone is elevated. Indeed, the unbound or free testosterone is approximately twice normal (an increase from 1% to 2%) in women with anovulation and polycystic ovaries. (29) Therefore a normal testosterone level in a hirsute woman is still consistent with elevated androgen production rates.

It is not necessary to measure the free testosterone (a technically difficult and expensive assay) because routine total testosterone assay adequately serves the purpose of screening for testosterone-secreting tumors and a single random blood sample is sufficient. Such tumors are associated with testosterone levels in the male range, (30, 31) and therefore the fine discrimination of the free testosterone level is unnecessary. *If the testosterone level exceeds 200 ng/ dl, an androgen-producing tumor must be suspected.*

Androgen-producing Tumors

There are two findings which should stimulate the clinician to suspect the presence of an androgen-producing tumor. One is a history of rapidly progressive masculinization. Hirsutism associated with anovulation is generally slow to develop, usually covering a time period of at least several years. Tumors are associated with a short time course, measured in months. Occasionally, virilization is encountered with a nonfunctional tumor due to tumor stimulation of androgen secretion in the surrounding stromal tissue. The second finding which should arouse suspicion is a testosterone level greater than 200 ng/dl.

In our view, androgen-producing tumors are one of medicine's vastly overrated problems. First, they are incredibly rare, and yet they attract an inordinate amount of attention at our meetings, and a disproportionate number of printed pages in texts and journals. Second, there is an endocrine mystique surrounding the functioning tumor. Actually it is a straightforward problem.

Functioning ovarian tumors are almost all palpable, and like any ovarian mass, rapid laparotomy and surgical removal are in order. The only diagnostic dilemma is when to explore a patient when a mass is not palpable. Suppression and stimulation tests, popular for many years, have been known to falsely lead to oophorectomy in the presence of a virilizing adrenocortical adenoma. (31) Selective angiography is not without problems. It is technically difficult to achieve bilateral catheterization of the ovaries, steroid secretion is episodic (especially by the adrenal gland), and the technique is not without risk.

When an androgen-producing tumor is suspected, an adnexal mass is not palpable, and the DHAS level is normal, CT scanning of the adrenal glands and the ovaries should be obtained. CT scanning of the adrenal has proven to be a sensitive diagnostic technique for small tumors producing Cushing's syndrome (5) as well as for virilizing adrenal adenomas. (31) Because ovarian functioning tumors are so rare, there is little experience thus far with CT scanning.

215

Selective angiography should be reserved for those patients with negative CT scans. We believe that angiography should be limited to the adrenal gland, relying upon surgical exploration and bivalving of the ovaries if adrenal angiography is negative.

Treatment of Hirsutism

Almost all patients presenting with hirsutism represent excess androgen production in association with the steady state of persistent anovulation. Treatment is directed toward interruption of the steady state. In those patients who wish to become pregnant, ovulation can be induced as discussed in Chapter 20. In patients in whom pregnancy is not desired, the steady state can be interrupted by suppression of ovarian steroidogenesis, by utilizing the potent negative feedback action on LH of progestational agents.

Androgen production in hirsute women is usually an LH-dependent process. (32) Suppression of ovarian steroidogenesis depends upon adequate LH suppression. We and others have found that plasma testosterone levels can be effectively decreased with any combination type birth control pill, including the new low dose pills. (33) In addition to the inhibitory action of the progestational component, further benefit is achieved by an increase in SHBG levels induced by the estrogen component. The increase in SHBG results in a greater testosterone binding capacity with a decrease in free testosterone levels. The testosterone value in hirsute patients decreases by 6 months of treatment. This reduction is associated with a gratifying clinical improvement in the progression of hirsutism.

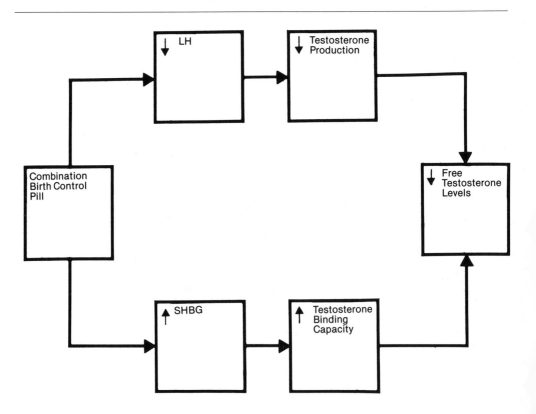

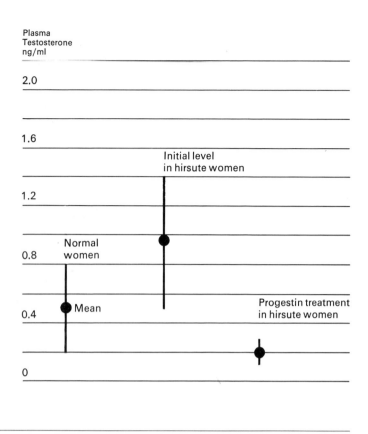

Plasma
Testosterone
ng/ml

2.0

1.6

Initial level
in hirsute women

1.2

Normal
0.8 women

Progestin treatment
0.4 ● Mean in hirsute women

0

In the patient in whom oral contraceptive pills are contraindicated or unwanted, good results can be achieved with the use of Depo-Provera, 150 mg intramuscularly every 3 months, or the use of oral Provera, 30 mg daily. The mechanism of action of Provera is slightly different from that of the birth control pill. Suppression of gonadotropins is less intense, hence ovarian follicular activity continues. Even though LH suppression is not as great, some reduction in LH results in a decreased testosterone production rate. In addition, testosterone clearance from the circulation is increased. (34) This latter effect is due to an induction of liver enzyme activity. The overall effect (decreased production and increased clearance) yields a clinical result comparable to that achieved with the birth control pill.

A noteworthy feature of this clinical problem is the slow response to treatment. The patient should be cautioned that treatment with a combination oral contraceptive will be necessary for 6 months to 1 year before an observable diminution in hair growth occurs. Combined treatment with electrolysis is not recommended, therefore, until hormone suppression has been used at least 6 months (except with extreme hirsutism).

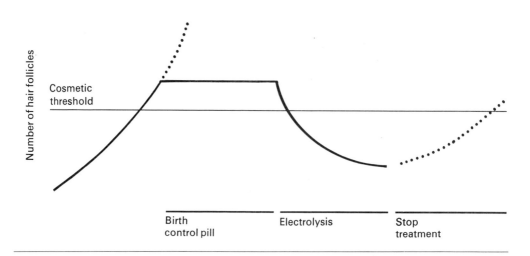

Number of hair follicles

Cosmetic threshold

Birth control pill | Electrolysis | Stop treatment

New hair follicles will no longer be stimulated to grow but hair growth which has been previously established will not disappear with hormone treatment alone. This may be affected temporarily by shaving, tweezing, waxing, or the use of depilatories. None of these tactics alters the inherent growth of the hair; therefore, they must be reapplied at frequent intervals. Permanent removal of hair can be accomplished only by electrocoagulation of dermal papillae. Some patients return after a period of treatment expressing disappointment because hair is still present. The effect of the treatment (prevention of new hair growth) may not be apparent unless the previously established hair is removed. The combination of ovarian suppression preventing new hair growth, and electrolysis removing the old hair, yields the most complete and effective treatment of hirsutism.

How long should treatment be continued? After 1–2 years it is worthwhile to stop the medication and observe the patient for a return of ovulatory cycles. Even in those patients who continue to be anovulatory, testosterone suppression may continue for 6 months to 2 years after discontinuing treatment.

The really resistent patient deserves further consideration. After 6 months of treatment, remeasurement of the blood DHAS is in order. If it is still elevated, one can either pursue the diagnosis of an adrenal enzyme deficiency (ACTH stimulation after an overnight dexamethasone suppression to identify an elevated $\Delta 5$ to $\Delta 4$ circulating steroid ratio) or offer empiric treatment with dexamethasone. Dexamethasone is given daily 0.5 mg at bedtime, to achieve maximum suppression of the CNS-adrenal axis which peaks during sleep. If this treatment suppresses the morning blood cortisol level below 2.0 μg/dl, the dose should be reduced to avoid an inability to react to stress.

218

In most patients DHAS levels are suppressed by progestational treatment. (35–37) The mechanism is not definitively known, but there are several possible explanations. If the original stimulus for the increased DHAS secretion is the steady estrogen state of anovulation, then the change in the endocrine milieu of the adrenal gland brought about by the suppression of ovarian sterodogenesis will restore a normal adrenal secretory pattern. With the combination pill, an effect on the adrenal by the estrogen may be blocked by the progestin component. A combination birth control pill may decrease ACTH stimulation of the adrenal gland by increasing serum binding of cortisol, thus lowering cortisol metabolic clearance.

The effectiveness of adrenal suppression in inducing ovulatory cycles in some anovulatory patients can be attributed to a lowering of circulating androgen levels due to a decrease in the adrenal contribution. The intraovarian androgen level is decreased, therefore lowering the inhibitory action of androgens on follicular growth and development. In terms of ovulation, the frequency of successful response with this type of treatment does not match that of the first drug of choice, clomiphene. In terms of treatment of hirsutism, progestin suppression of ovarian steroidogenesis is more effective and should remain the first therapeutic approach.

In an older woman who has no further desire for fertility, and in the woman in whom continued use of steroid medication is disturbing because of increasing risks with increasing age, serious consideration should be given to a surgical solution. A persistent problem of hirsutism, especially if it is progressive in severity, is a very reasonable indication for hysterectomy and bilateral salpingo-oophorectomy. Of course, the patient should accept an estrogen replacement program.

New Therapeutic Approaches

Several new approaches for the treatment of hirsutism are available. The most promising is the use of spironolactone, an aldosterone antagonist. (38, 39) Spironolactone has a 2-fold action, inhibiting the ovarian biosynthesis of androgens as well as competing for the androgen receptor in the hair follicle. Fortunately it has no effect on adrenal secretion, and the only side effect reported is diuresis in the first few days of use. There have been no dose response studies. The doses used range from 50 to 200 mg/day. As with progestational agents, the response is relatively slow and a maximal effect can be demonstrated only after 6 months of treatment. It is unknown whether results are superior to those obtained with progestational agents. We use spironolactone when patients find birth control pills or Provera unacceptable. One word of caution: with inhibition of androgen secretion, ovulation can occur. In view of the unknown impact of spironolactone on a fetus, effective contraception is important.

Cimetidine has been used to treat hirsutism in a dose of 300 mg, 5 times daily. (40) No change is detected in blood or urine androgens, therefore, it must function as a peripheral blocker at the receptor level.

Cyproterone acetate is an antiandrogen with progestational behavior used extensively in Europe to treat hirsutism. This agent is unavailable in the United States. While impressive results have been reported, its use is associated with the significant side effects of decreased libido and mental depression. (41, 42)

End Organ Hypersensitivity (Idiopathic Hirsutism)

There are some patients who present with hirsutism, but ovulate regularly. This category of patients has in the past been labeled idiopathic or familial hirsutism, and is more pronounced in certain geographic areas and among certain ethnic groups. The only satisfactory explanation for this distressing problem is hypersensitivity of the skin's hair apparatus to normal levels of androgens, perhaps due to altered androgen metabolism and receptor activity in the hair follicles. Because of this excessive sensitivity, normal levels of androgen stimulate hair growth. Even in these cases, hirsutism responds to ovarian suppression with a combination birth control pill. Suppression of normal female androgen levels to subnormal concentrations diminishes the stimulus to the hair follicles, yielding the same stabilizing results seen in other hirsute women. Spironolactone should also be effective for this group of patients. While hirsutism due to an endocrine disorder requires control, end organ hypersensitivity is treated only for the purpose of cosmetic improvement. Electrolysis is a useful adjunct in this group of patients.

Limitations and Pitfalls

1. Occasionally testosterone levels may be extremely elevated with anovulation, leading to very heavy hair growth and even masculinization. A level over 200 ng/dl does not absolutely indicate the presence of a tumor, but in the presence of a thorough, negative evaluation, surgical exploration of the ovaries is still warranted.

2. Enlarged ovaries are not necessary for the clinical syndrome of anovulation and excessive androgen production. On the other hand the presence of enlarged, polycystic ovaries does not assure the diagnosis of anovulation and excess ovarian production of androgens. Polycystic ovaries are the result of excess androgen, and may be associated with adrenal disease or exogenous androgen ingestion. Laparoscopy and ovarian biopsy are not indicated procedures.

3. The association of elevated testosterone production and hirsutism with normal ovulatory cycles is suspicious of an adrenal problem.

4. Suppression of elevated androgens by progestin treatment does not rule out the presence of an ovarian tumor, since functional ovarian tumors are usually gonadotropin-dependent and responsive.

5. Failure of progestin treatment to suppress hair growth and testosterone levels after 6–12 months indicates the need to further consider the presence of adrenal disease or a very small ovarian tumor.

References

1. **Kirschner MA, Zucker IR, Jespersen D,** Idiopathic hirsutism—an ovarian abnormality, N Engl J Med 294:637, 1976.

2. **Bardin CW, Lipsett M,** Testosterone and androstenedione blood production rates in normal women and women with idiopathic hirsutism and polycystic ovaries, J Clin Invest 46:891, 1967.

3. **Barcia-Bunuel R, Berek JS, Woodruff JD,** Luteomas of pregnancy, Obstet Gynecol 45:407, 1975.

4. **Crapo L,** Cushing's syndrome: a review of diagnostic tests, Metabolism 28:955, 1979.

5. **White FE, White MC, Drury PL, Fry IK, Besser GM,** Value of computed tomography of the abdomen and chest in investigation of Cushing's syndrome, Br Med J 284:771, 1982.

6. **Lobo RA, Paul WL, Goebelsmann U,** Dehydroepiandrosterone sulfate as an indicator of adrenal androgen function, Obstet Gynecol 57:69, 1981.

7. **Cumming DC, Rebar RW, Hopper BR, Yen SSC,** Evidence for an influence of the ovary on circulating dehydroepiandrosterone sulfate levels, J Clin Endocrinol Metab 54:1069, 1982.

8. **Carter JN, Tyson JE, Warne GL, McNeilly AS, Faiman C, Friesen HG,** Adrenocortical function in hyperprolactinemic women, J Clin Endocrinol Metab 45:973, 1977.

9. **Lobo RA, Kletsky OA, Kaptein EM, Goebelsmann U,** Prolactin modulation of dehydroepiandrosterone sulfate secretion, Am J Obstet Gynecol 138:632, 1980.

10. **Vermeulen A, Ando S, Verdonck L,** Prolactinomas, testosterone-binding globulin and androgen metabolism, J Clin Endocrinol Metab 54:409, 1982.

11. **Glickman SP, Rosenfield RL, Bergenstal RM, Helke J,** Multiple androgenic abnormalities, including elevated free testosterone, in hyperprolactinemic women, J Clin Endocrinol Metab 55:251, 1982.

12. **Larson BA, Vanderlaan WP, Judd HL, McCullough DL,** A testosterone-producing adrenal cortical adenoma in an elderly woman, J Clin Endocrinol Metab 42:882, 1976.

13. **Werk EE Jr, Sholiton LH, Kalejs L,** Testosterone-secreting adrenal adenoma under gonadotropin control, N Engl J Med 289:767, 1973.

14. **Givens JR, Andersen RN, Wiser WL, Coleman SA, Fish SA,** A gonadotropin-responsive adrenocortical adenoma, J Clin Endocrinol Metab 38:126, 1974.

15. **Abraham GE,** Ovarian and adrenal contribution to peripheral androgens during the menstrual cycle, J Clin Endocrinol Metab 39:340, 1974.

16. **Sabrino L, Kase N, Grunt J,** Changes in adrenocortical function in patients with gonadal dysgenesis after treatment with estrogen, J Clin Endocrinol Metab 33:110, 1971.

17. **Abraham G, Maroulis G,** Effect of exogenous estrogen on serum pregnenolone, cortisol and androgens in postmenopausal women, Obstet Gynecol 45:271, 1975.

18. **Lucky AW, Marynick SP, Rebar RW, Cutler GB, Glen M, Johnsonbaugh E, Loriaux DL,** Replacement oral ethinyloestradiol therapy for gonadal dysgenesis: growth and adrenal androgen studies, Acta Endocrinol 91:519, 1979.

19. **Lobo RA, March CM, Goebelsmann U, Mishell DR Jr,** The modulating role of obesity and of 17β-estradiol (E_2) on bound and unbound E_2 and adrenal androgens in oophorectomized women, J Clin Endocrinol Metab 54:320, 1982.

20. **Rosenfield RL, Fang IS,** The effects of prolonged physiologic estradiol therapy on the maturation of hypogonadal teenagers, J Pediatr 85:830, 1974.

21. **Anderson DC, Yen SSC,** Effects of estrogens on adrenal 3β-hydroxysteroid dehydrogenase in ovariectomized women, J Clin Endocrinol Metab 43:561, 1976.

22. **Rose DP, Fern M, Liskowski L, Milbrath JR,** Effect of treatment with estrogen conjugates on endogenous plasma steroids, Obst Gynecol 49:80, 1977.

23. **Lobo RA, Goebelsmann U, Brenner PF, Mishell DR Jr,** The effects of estrogen on adrenal androgens in oophorectomized women, Am J Obstet Gynecol 142:471, 1982.

24. **Lobo RA, Goebelsmann U,** Evidence of reduced 3β-ol-hydroxysteroid dehydrogenase activity in some hirsute women thought to have polycystic ovary syndrome, J Clin Endocrinol Metab 53:394, 1981.

25. **Lachelin GCL, Barnett M, Hopper BR, Brink G, Yen SSC,** Adrenal function in normal women and women with the polycystic ovary syndrome, J Clin Endocrinol Metab 49:892, 1979.

26. **Ayers JWT,** Differential response to adrenocorticotropin hormone stimulation in polycystic ovarian disease with high and low dehydroepiandrosterone sulfate levels, Fertil Steril 37:645, 1982.

27. **Fujieda K, Faiman C, Reyes FI, Winter JSD,** The control of steroidogenesis by human fetal adrenal cells in tissue culture: IV. The effects of exposure to placental steroids, J Clin Endocrinol Metab 54:89, 1982.

28. **Chang RJ, Mandel FP, Wolfren AR, Judd HL,** Circulating levels of plasma adrenocorticotropin in polycystic ovary disease, J Clin Endocrinol Metab 54:1265, 1982.

29. **Easterling WE Jr, Talbert LM, Potter HD,** Serum testosterone levels in the polycystic ovary syndrome, Am J Obstet Gynecol 120:385, 1974.

30. **Meldrum DR, Abraham GE,** Peripheral and ovarian venous concentrations of various steroid hormones in virilizing ovarian tumors, Obstet Gynecol 53:36, 1979.

31. **Gabrilove JL, Seman AT, Sabet R, Mitty HA, Nicolis GL,** Virilizing adrenal adenoma with studies on the steroid content of the adrenal venous effluent and a review of the literature, Endocr Rev 2:462, 1981.

32. **Givens JR, Andersen RN, Wiser WL, Umstot ES, Fish SA,** The effectiveness of two oral contraceptives in suppressing plasma androstenedione, testosterone, LH, and FSH, and in stimulating plasma testosterone-binding capacity in hirsute women, Am J Obstet Gynecol 124:333, 1976.

33. **Raj SG, Raj MH, Talbert LM, Sloan CS, Hicks B,** Normalization of testosterone levels using a low estrogen-containing oral contraceptive in women with polycystic ovary syndrome, Obstet Gynecol 60:15, 1982.

34. **Gordon GG, Southren AL, Tochimoto S, Olivo J, Altman K, Rand J, Lemberger L,** Effect of medroxyprogesterone acetate (Provera) on the metabolism and biological activity of testosterone. J Clin Endocrinol Metab 30:449, 1970.

35. **Madden JD, Milewich L, Parker CR Jr, Carr BR, Boyar RM, MacDonald PC,** The effect of an oral contraceptive treatment on the serum concentration of dehydroisoandrosterone sulfate, Am J Obstet Gynecol 132:380, 1978.

36. **Carr BR, Parker CR Jr, Madden JD, MacDonald PC, Porter JC,** Plasma levels of adrenocorticotropin and cortisol in women receiving oral contraceptive steroid treatment, J Clin Endocrinol Metab 49:346, 1979.

37. **Wild RA, Umstot ES, Andersen RN, Givens JR,** Adrenal function in hirsutism: II. Effect of an oral contraceptive, J Clin Endocrinol Metab 54:676, 1982.

38. **Boisselle A, Tremblay RR,** New therapeutic approach to the hirsute patient, Fertil Steril 32:276, 1979.

39. **Cumming DC, Yang JC, Rebar RW, Yen SSC,** Treatment of hirsutism with spironolactone, JAMA 247:1295, 1982.

40. **Vigersky RA, Mehlman I, Glass AR, Smith CE,** Treatment of hirsute women with cimetidine, N Engl J Med 303:1042, 1980.

41. **Kuttenn F, Rigaud C, Wright F, Maufais-Jarvis P,** Treatment of hirsutism by oral cyproterone acetate and percutaneous estradiol, J Clin Endocrinol Metab 51:1107, 1980.

42. **Frey H, Aakvaag A,** The treatment of essential hirsutism in women with cyproterone acetate and ethinyl estradiol, Acta Obstet Gynecol Scand 60:295, 1981.

8   Dysfunctional Uterine Bleeding

The thesis advanced in this chapter is that dysfunctional uterine bleeding, defined as a variety of bleeding manifestations of anovulatory cycles, can be confidently managed, without surgical intervention, by therapeutic regimens founded on sound physiologic principles. This formulation is based on knowledge of how the postovulatory menstrual function is naturally controlled, and utilizes pharmacologic application of sex steroids to reverse the abnormal tissue factors which lead to the excessive and prolonged flow typical of anovulatory cycles.

Three major categories of dysfunctional endometrial bleeding are dealt with:

1.   Estrogen breakthrough bleeding,

2.   Estrogen withdrawal bleeding, and

3.   Progestin breakthrough bleeding.

In each instance, the manner in which the endometrium deviates from the norm is depicted and specific steroid therapy is recommended to counter the difficulties each situation presents.

225

This mode of clinical management has been in regular use for many years, and failure to control vaginal bleeding with this therapy, despite appropriate application and utilization, excludes the diagnosis of dysfunctional uterine bleeding. If this occurs, attention is directed to a pathologic entity within the reproductive tract as the cause of abnormal bleeding.

In the following pages we will substantiate our thesis in a more detailed fashion. First, a review of the endometrial changes associated with an ovulatory cycle will be offered. Second, endometrial-sex steroid interactions will be listed. Finally, typical clinical situations will be presented, and specific acute and long-term management programs will be described.

Histologic Changes in Endometrium during an Ovulatory Cycle

The sequence of endometrial changes associated with an ovulatory cycle has been carefully studied by Noyes in the human and Bartelmez and Markee in the subhuman primate. (1–3) From these data a theory of menstrual physiology has developed based upon specific anatomic and functional changes within glandular, vascular, and stromal components of the endometrium. These changes will be discussed in five phases: 1) menstrual endometrium, 2) the proliferative phase, 3) the secretory phase, 4) preparation for implantation, and finally 5) the phase of endometrial breakdown. While these distinctions are not entirely arbitrary, it must be recalled that the entire process is an integrated evolutionary cycle of endometrial growth and regression, which is repeated some 300–400 times during the adult life of the human female.

Menstrual Endometrium

The menstrual endometrium is a relatively thin but dense tissue. It is composed of the stable, nonfunctioning basalis component and a variable amount of residual stratum spongiosum. At menstruation, this latter tissue displays a variety of functional states including disarray and breakage of glands, fragmentation of vessels and stroma with persisting evidence of necrosis, white cell infiltration, and red cell interstitial diapedesis. Even as the remnants of menstrual shedding dominate the overall appearance of this tissue, evidence of repair in all tissue components can be detected. The menstrual endometrium is a transitional state bridging the more dramatic exfoliative and proliferative phases of the cycle. Its density implies that the shortness of height is not entirely due to desquamation. Collapse of the supporting matrix also contributes significantly to the shallowness. Reticular stains in rhesus endometrium confirm this "deflated" state. Nevertheless, as much as two thirds of the functioning endometrium may be lost during menstruation. The more rapid the tissue loss, the shorter the duration of flow. Delayed or incomplete shedding is associated with heavier flow and greater blood loss.

226

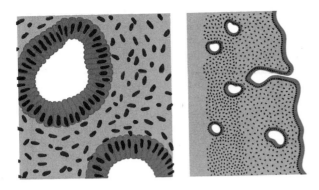

| Proliferative Phase | The proliferative phase is associated with ovarian follicle growth and increased estrogen secretion. Undoubtedly as a result of this steroidal action, reconstruction and growth of the endometrium are achieved. The glands are most notable in this response. At first they are narrow and tubular, lined by low columnar epithelium cells. Mitoses become prominent and pseudostratification is observed. As a result, the glandular epithelium extends peripherally and links one gland segment with its immediate neighbor. A continuous epithelial lining is formed facing the endometrial cavity. The stromal component evolves from its dense cellular menstrual condition through a brief period of edema to a final loose syncytial-like status. Coursing through the stroma, spiral vessels extend unbranched to a point immediately below the epithelial binding membrane. Here they form a loose capillary network. |

During proliferation, the endometrium has grown from approximately 0.5 mm to 3.5–5.0 mm in height. Restoration of tissue constituents has been achieved by estrogen-induced new growth as well as incorporation of ions, water, and amino acids. The stromal ground substance has reexpanded from its menstrual collapse. While true tissue growth has occurred, a major element in achievement of endometrial height is "reinflation" of the stroma.

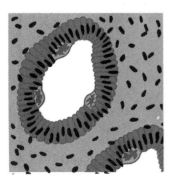
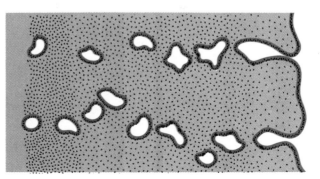

227

Secretory Phase

The endometrium now demonstrates a combined reaction to estrogen and progesterone activity. More impressive is that total endometrial height is fixed at roughly its preovulatory extent despite continued availability of estrogen. This restraint or inhibition is believed to be induced by progesterone. Individual components of the tissue continue to display growth, but confinement in a fixed structure leads to progressive tortuosity of glands and intensified coiling of the spiral vessels. The secretory events within the glandular cells, with progression of vacuoles from intracellular to intraluminal appearance, are well-known and take place approximately over a 7-day postovulatory interval. At the conclusion of these events the glands appear exhausted, the tortuous lumina variably distended, and individual cell surfaces fragmented and lost (sawtooth appearance). Stroma is increasingly edematous and spiral vessels are prominent and densely coiled.

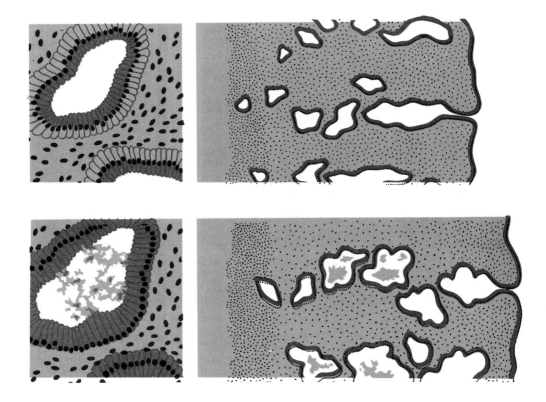

Implantation Phase	Significant changes occur within the endometrium from the 8th to 13th day postovulation. At the onset of this period, the distended tortuous secretory glands have been most prominent with little intervening stroma. By 13 days postovulation, the endometrium has differentiated into three distinct zones. Something less than one fourth of the tissue is the unchanged basalis fed by its straight vessels and surrounded by indifferent spindle-shaped stroma. The midportion of the endometrium (approximately 50% of the total) is the lace-like stratum spongiosum, composed of loose edematous stroma with tightly coiled but ubiquitous spiral vessels and exhausted dilated glandular ribbons. Overlying the spongiosum is the superficial layer of the endometrium (about 25% of the height) called the stratum compactum. Here the prominent histologic feature is the stromal cell which has become large and polyhedral. In its cytoplasmic expansion one cell abuts the other forming a compact, structurally sturdy layer. The necks of the glands traversing this segment are compressed and less prominent. The subepithelial capillaries and spiral vessels are engorged.
Phase of Endometrial Breakdown	In the absence of fertilization, implantation, and the consequent lack of sustaining quantities of human chorionic gonadotropin from the trophoblast, the otherwise fixed life span of the corpus luteum is completed and estrogen and progesterone levels wane. The withdrawal of estrogen and progesterone initiates three endometrial events: vasomotor reactions, tissue loss, and menstruation. The most prominent immediate effect of this hormone withdrawal is a modest shrinking of the tissue height and remarkable spiral arteriole vasomotor responses. The following vascular sequence has been constructed from direct observations of rhesus endometrium. With shrinkage of height, blood flow within the spiral vessels diminishes, venous drainage is decreased, and vasodilatation ensues. Thereafter, the spiral arterioles undergo rhythmic vasoconstriction and relaxation. Each successive spasm is more prolonged and profound, leading eventually to endometrial blanching. Within the 24 hours immediately preceding menstruation, these reactions lead to endometrial ischemia and stasis. White cells migrate through capillary walls, at first remaining adjacent to vessels, but then extending throughout the stroma. During arteriolar vasomotor changes, red blood cells escape into the interstitial space. Thrombin-platelet plugs also appear in superficial vessels.

Eventually considerable leakage occurs as a result of diapedesis, and finally, interstitial hemorrhage occurs due to breaks in superficial arterioles and capillaries. As ischemia and weakening progress, the continuous binding membrane is fragmented and intercellular blood is extruded into the endometrial cavity. New thrombin-platelet plugs form upstream at the shedding surface, limiting blood loss. With further tissue disorganization, the endometrium shrinks further and coiled anterioles are buckled. Additional ischemic breakdown ensues with necrosis of cells and defects in vessels adding to the menstrual effluvium. A natural cleavage point exists between basalis and spongiosum and, once breached, the loose, vascular, edematous stroma of the spongiosum desquamates and collapses. In the end, the typical deflated shallow dense menstrual endometrium results. Menstrual flow stops as a result of the combined effects of prolonged vasoconstriction, tissue collapse, vascular stasis and estrogen-induced "healing." Resumption of estrogen secretion with its healing effects leads to clot formation over the decapitated stumps of endometrial vessels. Within 13 hours, the endometrial height shrinks from 4 mm to 1.25 mm. (4)

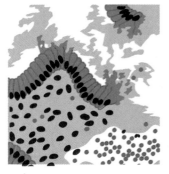
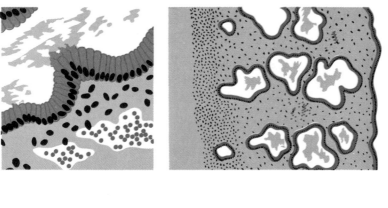
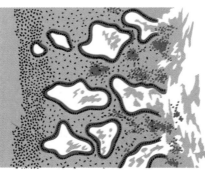

Teleologic Theory of Endometrial-Menstrual Events

An unabashedly teleologic view of the events just described has been offered by Rock et al. (5). The basic premise of this thesis is that every endometrial cycle has, as its only goal, support of an early embryo. Failure to accomplish this objective is followed by orderly elimination of unutilized tissue and prompt renewal to achieve a more successful cycle.

The ovum must be fertilized within 12–24 hours of ovulation. Over the next 2 days, it remains unattached within the tubal lumen utilizing tubal fluids and residual cumulus cells to sustain nutrition and energy for early cellular cleavage. After this stay, the solid ball of cells (morula) which is the embryo leaves the tube and enters the uterine cavity. Here the embryo undergoes another 2–3 days of unattached, but active existence. Fortunately, by this time endometrial

230

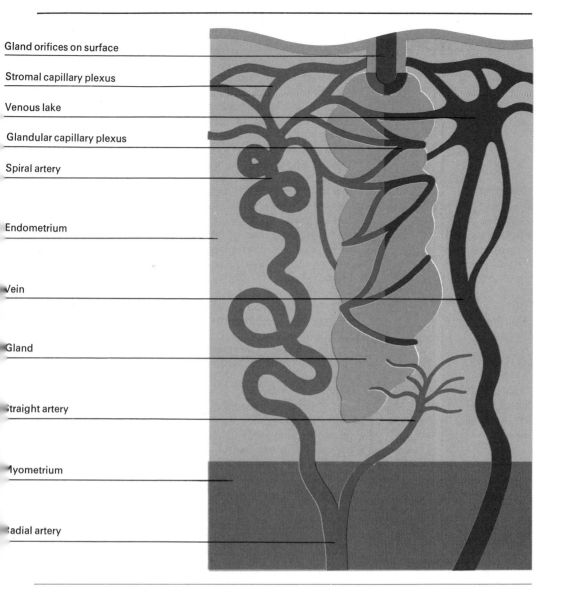

Gland orifices on surface

Stromal capillary plexus

Venous lake

Glandular capillary plexus

Spiral artery

Endometrium

Vein

Gland

Straight artery

Myometrium

Radial artery

gland secretions have filled the cavity and they bathe the embryo in nutrients. This is the first of many neatly synchronized events that mark the egg-endometrial relationship. By 6 days after ovulation the embryo (now a blastocyst) is ready to attach and implant. At this time it finds an endometrial lining of sufficient depth, vascularity, and nutritional richness to sustain the important events of early placentation to follow. Just below the epithelial lining, a rich capillary plexus has been formed and is available for creation of the trophoblast-maternal blood interface. Later, the surrounding zona compactum, occupying more and more of the endometrium, will provide a sturdy splint to retain endometrial architecture despite the invasive inroads of the burgeoning trophoblast.

231

Failure of the appearance of human chorionic gonadotropin (HCG), despite otherwise appropriate tissue reactions, leads to the vasomotor changes associated with estrogen-progesterone withdrawal and menstrual desquamation. However, not all the tissue is lost, and, in any event, a residual basalis is always available, making resumption of growth with estrogen a relatively rapid process. Indeed, even as menses persists, early regeneration can be seen. As soon as follicle maturation occurs (in as short a time as 10 days), the endometrium is ready to perform its reproductive function.

Endometrial Responses to Steroid Hormones: Physiologic and Pharmacologic

Obviously estrogen and progesterone withdrawal is not the only type of endometrial bleeding provoked by the presence of sex steroids and their effects on the endometrium. There are clinical examples for estrogen withdrawal bleeding and estrogen breakthrough bleeding, as well as for progesterone withdrawal and breakthrough bleeding. These events can be summarized.

Estrogen Withdrawal Bleeding

This category of uterine bleeding can occur after bilateral oophorectomy, radiation of mature follicles, or administration of estrogen to a castrate and then discontinuation of therapy. Similarly, the bleeding that occurs postcastration can be delayed by concomitant estrogen therapy. Flow will occur on discontinuation of exogenous estrogen.

Estrogen Breakthrough Bleeding

Here a semiquantitative relationship exists between the amount of estrogen stimulating the endometrium and the type of bleeding that can ensue. Relatively low doses of estrogen yield intermittent spotting which may be prolonged, but is generally light in quantity of flow. On the other hand, high levels of estrogen and sustained availability lead to prolonged periods of amenorrhea followed by acute, often profuse bleeds with excessive loss of blood.

Progesterone Withdrawal Bleeding

Removal of the corpus luteum will lead to endometrial desquamation. Pharmacologically, a similar event can be achieved by administration and discontinuation of progesterone or a nonestrogenic progestin derivative. Progesterone withdrawal bleeding occurs only if the endometrium is initially proliferated by endogenous or exogenous estrogen. If estrogen therapy is continued as progesterone is withdrawn, the progesterone withdrawal bleeding still occurs. Only if estrogen levels are increased 10–20-fold will progesterone withdrawal bleeding be delayed.

Progesterone Breakthrough Bleeding

Progesterone breakthrough bleeding occurs only in the presence of an unfavorably high ratio of progesterone to estrogen. In the absence of sufficient estrogen, continuous progesterone therapy will yield intermittent bleeding of variable duration, similar to low dose estrogen breakthrough bleeding noted above.

Of all the types of hormonal-endometrial relationships, the most stable endometrium and the most reproducible menstrual function in terms of quantity and duration occurs with postovulatory estrogen-progesterone withdrawal bleeding. It is so controlling that many women over the years come to expect a certain characteristic flow pattern. Any slight deviations, such as plus or minus 1 day in duration or minor deviation from expected napkin or tampon utilization, are causes for major concern in the patient. So ingrained is the expected flow that considerable physician reassurance may be required in some instances of minor variability. The usual duration of flow is 4–6 days, but many women flow as little as 2 days, and as much as 8 days. While the postovulatory phase averages 14 days, greater variability in the proliferative phase produces a distribution in the duration of a menstrual cycle. The normal volume of menstrual blood loss is 30 ml. (6). Greater than 80 ml is abnormal. Most of the blood loss occurs during the first 3 days of a period, so that excessive flow may exist without prolongation of flow. (7, 8).

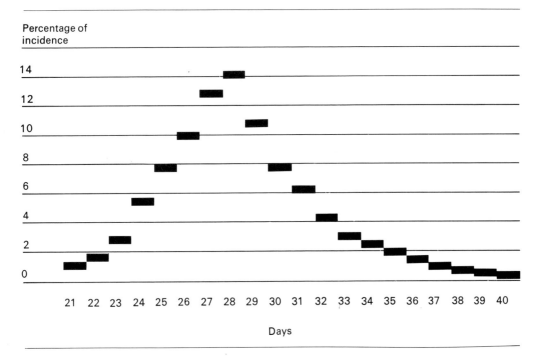

There are three reasons for the self-limited character of estrogen-progesterone withdrawal bleeding:

1. It is a universal endometrial event. Because the onset and conclusion of menses are related to a precise sequence of hormonal events, menstrual changes occur almost simultaneously in all segments of the endometrium.

233

2. The endometrial tissue which has responded to an appropriate sequence of estrogen and progesterone is structurally stable, and random breakdown of tissue due to fragility is avoided. Furthermore, the events leading to ischemic disintegration of the endometrium are orderly and progressive, being related to rhythmic waves of vasoconstriction of increasing duration.

3. Inherent in the events that start menstrual function following estrogen-progesterone are the factors involved in stopping menstrual flow. Just as waves of vasoconstriction initiate the ischemic events provoking menses, so will prolonged vasoconstriction abetted by the stasis associated with endometrial collapse enable clotting factors to seal off the exposed bleeding sites. Additional and significant effects are obtained by resumed estrogen activity.

Platelets and fibrin play a direct part in the hemostasis achieved in a bleeding menstrual endometrium. Deficiencies in these constituents cause the increased blood loss seen in von Willebrand's disease and in thrombocytopenia. The blood loss at menses in afibrinogenemia indicates the importance of fibrin generating and fibrinolytic factors in the menstrual process. Intravascular thrombi are observed in the functional layers and are localized to the shedding surface of the tissue. These are known as impeding "plugs" in that blood may flow past these only partially occlusive barriers. Therefore, thrombi continue to develop within the menstrual blood accounting for the empty vesicular platelets and large amounts of fibrin found in this effluent. Fibrinolysis occurs in the endometrial tissue, limiting fibrin deposition in the proximal, still unshed layer. Despite large holes in vessel walls, with blood exposed to collagen surfaces, no occlusive surface binding thrombus is formed. After early dependence on thrombin plugs to restrain blood loss, later generalized vasoconstrictive hemostasis without thrombin plugs occurs. The healing endometrium is pale, collapsed, and disorderly, but no thrombi and no fibrin deposits are seen.

The mechanisms of tissue breakdown, as well as clearance of debris and restructuring of the endometrium, are thought to proceed via sex steroid effects on the endometrial cell lysosomes. (9) With reduced steroids, lysosomal membrane destabilization and leakage of lysosomal prostaglandin synthetase enzymes, proteases, and collagenases occur. These cause breakdown of endometrial structures, dissolution of ground substance and cell walls, and vasoconstriction. Further "liquefaction" permits efficient absorption and possible recycling of protein components.

Most instances of anovulatory bleeding are examples of estrogen withdrawal or estrogen breakthrough bleeding. Furthermore, the heaviest bleeding is secondary to high sustained levels of estrogen associated with the polycystic ovary syndrome, obesity, immaturity of the hypothalamic-pituitary-ovarian axis as in postpubertal teenagers, and late anovulation, usually involving women in their late 30s and early 40s. Unopposed estrogen induces a progression of endometrial responses in the following pattern: proliferative hyperplasia, adenomatous hyperplasia, and in some, over the course of many years, atypia and carcinoma. In the absence of growth limiting progesterone and periodic desquamation, the endometrium attains an abnormal height without concomitant structural support. The tissue increasingly displays intense vascularity, back to back glandularity, but without an intervening stromal support matrix. This tissue is fragile, and will suffer spontaneous superficial breakage and bleeding. As one site heals, another, and yet another new site of breakdown will appear. The typical clinical picture is that of a pale frightened teenager who has bled for weeks. Also frequently encountered is the older woman with prolonged bleeding who is deeply concerned over this experience as a manifestation of cancer.

In these instances the usual endometrial control mechanisms are missing. This bleeding is not a universal event, but rather it involves random portions of the endometrium at variable times and in asynchronous sequences. The fragility of the vascular adenomatous hyperplastic tissue is responsible for this experience, in part because of excessive growth, but mostly because of irregular stimulation in which the structural rigidity of a well-developed stroma or stratum compactum does not occur. Finally, the flow is prolonged and excessive not only because there is a large quantity of tissue available for bleeding, but more importantly because there is a disorderly, abrupt, random, accidental breakdown of tissue with consequent opening of multiple vascular channels. There is no vasoconstrictive rhythmicity, no tight coiling of spiral vessels, no orderly collapse to induce stasis. The anovulatory tissue can only rely on the "healing" effects of endogenous estrogen to stop local bleeds. However, this is a vicious cycle in that this healing is only temporary. As quickly as it rebuilds, tissue fragility and breakdown recur at other endometrial sites.

Alternate Hypothesis

Another explanation for the control of postovulatory endometrial bleeding and regeneration has been presented. (10) Based on light and scanning electron microscopy of hysterectomy specimens, this thesis favors nonhormone-related regeneration of surface epithelium from basal glands and cornual area residual tissue with restoration of the continuous binding membrane as the critical events in cessation of blood flow. By this account, estrogen withdrawal or breakthrough bleeding is uncontrolled because there is insufficient stimulus (loss of tissue) for binding surface restoration to occur. Furthermore, curettage is effective in this condition by reachieving sufficient basal glandular denudation (as is seen also in combined estrogen and progestin withdrawal) which stimulates regeneration of surface integrity, and thus controls blood flow.

Additional studies are needed to clarify the difference of opinion concerning the pathophysiology of dysfunctional uterine bleeding. The therapeutic approach favored in this book utilizes hormonal control of endometrial events and rarely finds it necessary to resort to surgery.

Treatment Program for Anovulatory Bleeding

The immediate objective of medical therapy in anovulatory bleeding is to retrieve the natural controlling influences missing in this tissue: universal, synchronous endometrial events, structural stability, and vasomotor rhythmicity.

Progestin Therapy

Most women will, at sometime, either fail to ovulate or not sustain adequate corpus luteum function or duration. This occurs with increased frequency in the decade prior to menopause. The usual clinical presentation is oligomenorrhea with terminal bouts of menorrhagia or polymenorrhea. Women correctly seek medical advice promptly because these menstrual aberrations suggest unplanned pregnancy or uterine pathology. Therefore, it is uncommon to find significant blood loss or excessive tissue proliferation in these women. Under most circumstances, progestin therapy will suffice to control the abnormality once uterine pathology is ruled out.

Progesterone and progestins are powerful antiestrogens when given in pharmacologic doses. Gurpide has shown that progestin induces an enzyme, 17-hydroxysteroid dehydrogenase, in endometrial cells which converts estradiol to the less active estrone. (11) Progestins also diminish estrogen effects on target cells by inhibiting the augmentation of estrogen cytosol receptors which ordinarily accompanies estrogen action (receptor replenishment inhibition). (12) These influences account for the antimitotic, antigrowth impact of progestins on the endometrium (prevention and reversal of hyperplasia, limitation of growth postovulation, and the marked atrophy during pregnancy or in response to combined birth control pills).

In the treatment of oligomenorrhea, orderly limited withdrawal bleeding can be accomplished by administration of a progestin such as Provera 10 mg daily for 10 days every month. Absence of induced bleeding requires workup. In the treatment of dysfunctional menometrorrhagia or polymenorrhea, progestins are prescribed for 10 days to 2 weeks (to induce stabilizing predecidual stromal changes) followed by a withdrawal flow—the so-called "medical currettage." Thereafter, repeat progestin is offered cyclically the first 10 days of each month to ensure therapeutic effect. Failure of progestin to correct irregular bleeding requires diagnostic reevaluation.

Combined Birth Control Therapy	In young women, anovulatory bleeding may be associated with prolonged endometrial buildup, delayed diagnosis, and heavy blood loss. In these cases, combined progestin-estrogen therapy is used in the form of birth control pills. Any of the oral combination tablets are useful. Whatever dose is available or chosen, therapy is administered as one pill 4 times a day for 5–7 days. This therapy is maintained despite cessation of flow within 12–24 hours. If flow does not abate, other diagnostic possibilities (polyps, incomplete abortion, and neoplasia) should be reevaluated by examination under anesthesia, and dilatation and curettage (D and C).

If flow does diminish rapidly, the remainder of the week of treatment can be given over to the evaluation of causes of anovulation, investigation of hemorrhagic tendencies, and blood replacement or initiation of iron therapy. In addition, the week provides time to prepare the patient for the progestin-estrogen withdrawal flow that will soon be induced. For the moment, therapy has produced the structural rigidity intrinsic to the compact pseudodecidual reaction. Continued random breakdown of formerly fragile tissue is avoided and blood loss stopped. However, a large amount of tissue remains to react to progestin-estrogen withdrawal. The patient must be warned to anticipate a heavy and severely cramping flow 2–4 days after stopping therapy. If not prepared in this way, it is certain that the patient will view the problem as recurrent disease or failure of hormonal therapy.

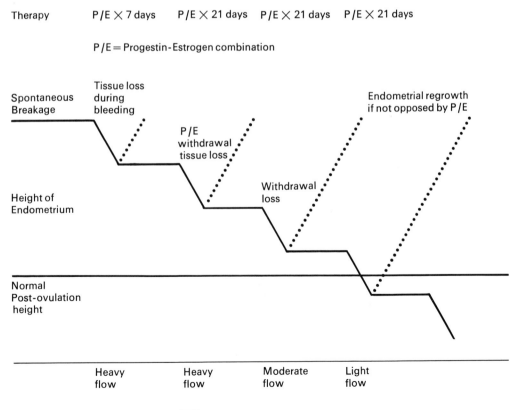

Therapy P/E × 7 days   P/E × 21 days   P/E × 21 days   P/E × 21 days

P/E = Progestin-Estrogen combination

Spontaneous Breakage

Tissue loss during bleeding

Endometrial regrowth if not opposed by P/E

P/E withdrawal tissue loss

Withdrawal loss

Height of Endometrium

Normal Post-ovulation height

Heavy flow   Heavy flow   Moderate flow   Light flow

237

In successful therapy, on the 5th day of flow, a low dose cyclic combination birth control medication (one pill a day) is started. This will be repeated for several (usually three) 3-week treatments, punctuated by 1-week withdrawal flow intervals. A decrease in volume and pain with each successive cycle is reassuring. Birth control pills reduce menstrual flow by at least 60% in normal uteri. (13) Early application of the progestin-estrogen combination limits growth and allows orderly regression of excessive endometrial height to normal controllable levels. If the progestin-estrogen combination is not applied, abnormal endometrial height and persistent excessive flow will recur.

In the patient not exposed to potential pregnancy, in whom cyclic progestin-estrogen for 3 months has reduced endometrial tissue to normal height, the pill may be discontinued and unopposed endogenous estrogen permitted to reactivate the endometrium. In the absence of spontaneous menses, the recurrence of the anovulatory state is suspected, and a brief preemptive course of an orally active progestin is administered to counter endometrial proliferation. Once pregnancy is ruled out, Provera 10 mg orally daily for 10 days is given monthly. Reasonable flow (progestin withdrawal flow) will occur 2–7 days after the last pill. With this therapy, excessive endometrial buildup is avoided, and an increased risk of endometrial and breast cancer is avoided. If contraception is desired, routine use of birth control pills is warranted and will also be of prophylactic value.

Estrogen Therapy

Intermittent vaginal spotting is frequently associated with minimal (low) estrogen stimulation (estrogen breakthrough bleeding). In this circumstance, where minimal endometrium exists, the beneficial effect of progestin treatment is not achieved, because there is insufficient tissue on which the progestin can exert action. A similar circumstance also exists in the younger anovulatory patient in whom prolonged hemorrhagic desquamation leaves little residual tissue.

In these circumstances, high dose estrogen therapy is applied using as much as Premarin 25 mg intravenously every 4 hours until bleeding abates (up to three doses can be given). (14) This is the sign that the "healing" events are initiated to a sufficient degree. Progestin treatment must be started at that time. Where bleeding is less, lower oral doses of estrogen (1.25 mg of conjugated estrogens daily for 7–10 days) can be prescribed initially. All estrogen therapy must be followed by progestin coverage.

Estrogen therapy is also useful in two examples of problems associated with progestin breakthrough bleeding. These are the breakthrough bleeding episodes occurring with use of birth control pills or with depot forms of progestational derivatives. In the absence of sufficient endogenous and exogenous estrogen, the endometrium shrinks by pharmacologically induced pseudoatrophy. Furthermore, it is composed almost exclusively of pseudodecidual stroma and blood vessels with minimal glands. Peculiarly, experience has shown that this type of endometrium also leads to the fragility bleeding more typical of pure estrogen stimulation. The usual clinical story is a patient on long-standing oral contraception who, after experiencing marked diminution or absence of withdrawal flow in the pill free interval, begins to see breakthrough bleeding while on medication.

Another frequently encountered problem is the progestin breakthrough bleeding experienced with chronic depot administration of progestin. This therapy is used not only for contraception, but also in the treatment of endometriosis and the prevention of menses during chemotherapy. In 75% of recipients, continuous therapy is not associated with abnormal menstrual bleeding. In the remainder, breakthrough progestin bleeding occurs. Judicious use of estrogen is the appropriate and effective therapy in these instances.

Estrogen therapy (ethinyl estradiol 20 μg or conjugated estrogens 2.5 mg daily for 7 days) during, and in addition to, the usual birth control pill administration is useful. This rejuvenates the endometrium and intermenstrual flow stops.

The Use of Antiprostaglandins

There seems little doubt that prostaglandins (PG) have important actions on the endometrial vasculature and presumably on endometrial hemostasis. The concentrations of PGE_2 and $PGF_{2\alpha}$ increase progressively in human endometrium during the menstrual cycle, and PG synthetase inhibitors decrease menstrual blood loss (15) perhaps by altering the balance between the platelet proaggregating vasoconstrictor thromboxane A_2 (TXA_2) and the antiaggregating vasodilator prostacyclin (PGI_2).

Whatever the exact mechanism, PG synthetase inhibitors diminish menstrual bleeding in normal women as well as in the bleeding of chronic endometritis secondary to intrauterine device (IUD) use.

Summary of Key Points in Therapy of Anovulatory (Dysfunctional) Bleeding

Teenager	Adult
Preliminary: Pelvic or rectal examination	*Preliminary:* Pelvic examination PAP smear Endometrial biopsy

1.   Intense progestin-estrogen therapy for 7 days

2.   Cyclic low dose oral contraceptive for 3 months

3.   If exposed to pregnancy, continue oral contraception

4.   If not exposed to pregnancy, Provera, 10 mg daily for 10 days every month.

If bleeding has been prolonged:
If biopsy yields minimal tissue:
If patient is on progestin medication:
If follow-up is uncertain:
Premarin, 25 mg intravenously every 4 hours until bleeding stops, or significantly slows, then proceed to Step 1 above. If no response in 12–24 hours, proceed to D and C.

The clinical problem of dysfunctional bleeding is associated with either anovulation and estrogen withdrawal or breakthrough bleeding, or with anovulation due to exogenous progestin medication and bleeding due to progestational endometrial breakthrough. Both categories of bleeding lack the three important characteristics of normal estrogen-progesterone withdrawal bleeding:

1.   Universal, simultaneous change in all segments of the endometrium;

2.   An orderly progression of events involving a rigid, compact structure; and

3.   Vasomotor rhythmicity with vasoconstriction, structural collapse, and clotting.

After evaluation and examination, including biopsies where appropriate, therapy involves an initial choice between intensive progestin-estrogen combination medication or high doses of estrogen. The progestin-estrogen combination will be ineffective unless endometrium of sufficient quantity and responsiveness to allow the formation of pseudodecidual tissue is present. Therefore, the intial choice of therapy should be high doses of estrogen (Premarin, 25 mg intravenously every 4 hours until bleeding stops or for 24 hours) in the following situations:

1. When bleeding has been heavy for many days and it is likely that the uterine cavity is now lined only by a raw basalis layer;

2. When the endometrial curet yields minimal tissue;

3. When the patient has been on progestin medication (oral contraceptives, intramuscular progestins) and the endometrium is shallow and atrophic; and

4. When follow-up is uncertain, because estrogen therapy will temporarily stop all categories of dysfunctional bleeding.

If high dose estrogen therapy does not significantly abate flow within 12–24 hours, reevaluation is mandatory, and the need for curettage is likely.

Once the acute bleeding episode in an anovulatory patient is under control, the patient should not be forgotten. With persistent anovulation, recurrent hemorrhage is a common pattern and, more importantly, chronic unopposed estrogen stimulation to the endometrium can eventually lead to atypical tissue changes. It is absolutely necessary that the patient undergo periodic progestational withdrawal, either with a routine oral contraceptive regimen, or if exposure to pregnancy is not a consideration, a progestational agent (Provera, 10 mg daily for 10 days) should be administered every month.

Curettage is *not* the first line of defense, but rather the last. The utilization of appropriate steroids for the clinical management of dysfunctional bleeding is based upon a physiologic understanding of the endometrium and its responses to hormones. Adherence to this program will avoid D and C except in a rare case of dysfunctional bleeding, and except in those cases where bleeding is due to a pathologic entity within the reproductive tract where D and C is truly indicated and necessary.

If a patient has recurrent bleeding despite repeated medical therapy, submucous myomas or endometrial polyps must be suspected. Thorough currettage can miss such pathology and further diagnostic study can be helpful. Either hysterosalpingography with slow instillation of dye and careful fluoroscopic examination or hysteroscopy may reveal a myoma or polyp. A pathologic problem such as this should especially be suspected in the puzzling case of the patient who has abnormal bleeding and ovulatory cycles.

References

1. **Noyes RW, Hertig AW, Rock J,** Dating the endometrial biopsy, Fertil Steril 1:3, 1950.

2. **Bartlemez GW,** The phases of the menstrual cycle and their interpretation in terms of the pregnancy cycle, Am J Obstet Gynecol 74:931, 1957.

3. **Markee JE,** Morphological basis for menstrual bleeding, Bull NY Acad Med 24:253, 1948.

4. **Sixma JJ, Cristiens GCML, Haspels AS,** The sequence of hemostatic events in the endometrium during normal menstruation, in *WHO Symposium on Steroid Contraception and Endometrial Bleeding,* Diczfalusy E, Fraser IS, Webb FTG, eds, 1980, p 86.

5. **Rock J, Garcia CR, Menkin M,** A theory of menstruation, Ann NY Acad Sci 75:830, 1959.

6. **Hallberg L, Hogdahl A, Nilsson L, Rybo G,** Menstrual blood loss—a population study, Acta Obstet Gynecol Scand 45:320, 1966.

7. **Rybo G,** Menstrual blood loss in relation to parity and menstrual pattern, Acta Obstet Gynecol Scand 7:119, 1966.

8. **Haynes PJ, Hodgson H, Anderson ABM, Turnbull AC,** Measurement of menstrual blood loss in patients complaining of menorrhagia. Br J Obstet Gynecol 84:763, 1977.

9. **Wilson EW,** Lysosome function in normal endometrium and endometrium exposed to contraceptive steroids, in *WHO Symposium on Steroid Contraception and Endometrial Bleeding,* Diczfalusy E, Fraser IS, Webb FTG, eds, 1980, p 201.

10. **Ferenczy A,** Studies on the cytodynamics of human endometrial regeneration: I. Scanning electron microscopy. Am J Obstet Gynecol 124:64, 1976.

11. **Gurpide E, Gusberg S, Tseng L,** Estradiol binding and metabolism in human endometrial hyperplasia and adenocarcinoma, J Steroid Biochem 7:891, 1976.

12. **Hsueh AJW, Peck EJ, Clark JH,** Progesterone antagonism of the estrogen receptor and estrogen-induced uterine growth. Nature 254:337, 1975.

13. **Nelson L, Rybo G,** Treatment of menorrhagia. Am J Obstet Gynecol 110:713, 1971.

14. **DeVore GR, Owens O, Kase N,** Use of intravenous premarin in the treatment of dysfunctional uterine bleeding—a double-blind randomized control study, Obstet Gynecol 59:285, 1982.

15. **Anderson ABM, Haynes PJ, Guilleband J, Turnbull AC,** Reduction of menstrual blood loss by prostaglandin synthetase inhibitors, Lancet 1:774, 1976.

9   The Breast

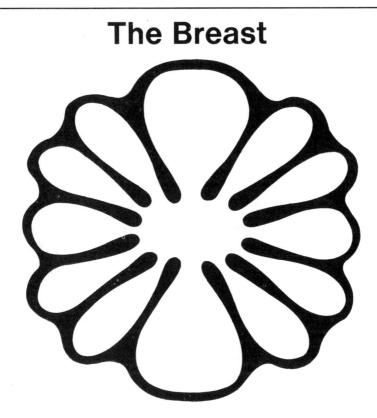

The form, function, and pathology of the human female breast are major concerns of medicine and society. As mammals, we define our biologic class by the function of the breast in nourishing our young. Breast contours occupy our attention. As obstetricians, we seek to enhance or diminish function, and as gynecologists, the appearance of inappropriate lactation (galactorrhea) is of grave concern. Cancer of the breast is a leading cause of death in women.

In this chapter, the factors involved in normal growth and development of the breast will be reviewed, including the physiology of normal lactation. A description of the numerous factors leading to inappropriate lactation will follow, and finally, the endocrine aspects of breast cancer will be considered.

Growth and Development

The basic component of the breast lobule is the hollow alveolus or milk gland lined by a single layer of milk-secreting epithelial cells, derived from an ingrowth of epidermis into the underlying mesenchyme at 10–12 weeks of gestation. Each alveolus is encased in a criss-crossing mantle of contractile myoepithelial strands. Also surrounding the milk gland is a rich capillary network.

The lumen of the alveolus connects to a collecting intralobar duct by means of a thin nonmuscular duct. Contractile muscle cells encase the intralobular ducts that eventually reach the exterior via 15–25 apertures in the areola.

Growth of this milk-producing system is dependent on numerous hormonal factors which occur in two sequences, first at puberty and then in pregnancy. Although there is considerable overlapping of hormonal influences, the differences in quantities of the stimuli in each circumstance and the availability of entirely unique inciting factors (human placental lactogen (HPL) and prolactin) during pregnancy permit this chronologic distinction.

Overall the major influence to breast growth at puberty is estrogen. In most girls, the first response to the increasing levels of estrogen is an increase in size and pigmentation of the areola and the formation of a mass of breast tissue just underneath the areola. Breast tissue binds estrogen in a manner similar to the uterus and vagina. The development of estrogen receptors in the breast does not occur in the absence of prolactin. The primary effect of estrogen in subprimate mammals is to stimulate growth of the ductal portion of the gland system. Progesterone in these animals appears to influence growth of the alveolar components of the lobule. However, neither hormone alone, or in combination, is capable of yielding optimum breast growth and development. Full differentiation of the gland requires insulin, cortisol, thyroxine, prolactin, and growth hormone. Changes occur routinely in response to the estrogen-progesterone sequence of a normal menstrual cycle. Consequently, breast examination is most effective during the follicular phase of the cycle.

The estrogen-induced impetus to mammary epithelial stem cell division requires the presence of insulin. Final differentiation of the alveolar epithelial cell into a mature milk cell is accomplished in the presence of prolactin, but only after prior exposure to cortisol and insulin. The complete reaction depends on the availability of minimal quantities of thyroid hormone. Thus, the endocrinologically intact individual in whom estrogen, progesterone, thyroxine, cortisol, insulin, prolactin, and growth hormone are available can have appropriate breast growth. Mild deficiencies in any of the hormones, short of severe restrictions or total absence, can be compensated for by excess prolactin. Furthermore, the growth of the breast and breast function can be incited by an excess of prolactin.

244

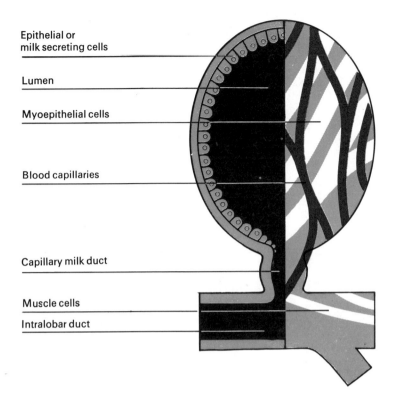

Epithelial or
milk secreting cells

Lumen

Myoepithelial cells

Blood capillaries

Capillary milk duct

Muscle cells

Intralobar duct

Abnormal Shapes
and Sizes

Early differentiation of the mammary gland anlage is under fetal hormonal control. Abnormalities in adult size or shape may reflect the impact of hormones (especially the presence or absence of testosterone) during this early period of development. Occasionally, the breast bud will begin to develop on one side first. Similarly, one breast may grow faster than the other. These inequalities usually disappear by the time development is complete. However, exact equalness in size usually is never attained. Significant asymmetry is correctable only by the plastic surgeon. Likewise hypoplasia and hypertrophy can be treated only by corrective surgery. A temporary decrease in breast hypertrophy can be achieved with danazol, however, and extended postoperative therapy may avoid recurrence. Hormone therapy is totally ineffective in producing a permanent change in breast shape or size. Of course in patients with primary amenorrhea secondary to deficient ovarian function, estrogen replacement will induce significant and gratifying breast growth.

Accessory nipples can be found anywhere from the knees to the neck. They occur in approximately 1% of the population and require no therapy.

The differentiation of terminal alveolar cells into active milk-secreting units requires the availability of insulin, prolactin, and cortisol, as well as estrogen and progesterone. (1) During pregnancy, prolactin levels rise to high concentrations, beginning about 8 weeks and reaching a peak of 200–400 ng/ml at term. (2) Made by the placenta and actively secreted into the maternal circulation from the 6th week of pregnancy, HPL rises progressively reaching a level of approximately 6000 ng/ml at term. Though displaying less activity than prolactin, HPL is produced in such large amounts that, although not conclusively demonstrated, it may exert a lactogenic effect.

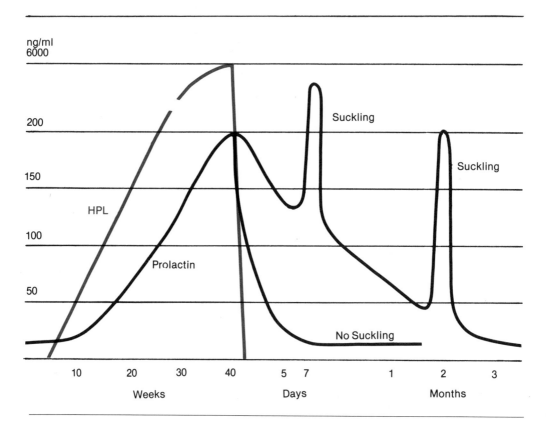

Although prolactin stimulates significant breast growth, and is available for lactation, only colostrum (composed of desquamated epithelial cells and transudate) is produced during gestation. Full lactation is inhibited by estrogen and progesterone which interfere with prolactin action at the alveolar cell prolactin receptor level. (3).

Amniotic fluid concentrations of prolactin parallel maternal serum concentration until the 10th week of pregnancy, rise markedly until the 20th week, and then decrease. Maternal prolactin does not pass to the fetus in significant amounts. Indeed the source of amniotic fluid prolactin is neither the maternal pituitary nor the fetal pituitary. The failure of bromocriptine to suppress amniotic fluid prolactin levels, and studies with in vitro culture systems, indicate a primary decidual source with transfer via amnion receptors to the amniotic fluid. This decidual synthesis of prolactin is under the control of the sex steroids, especially progesterone, rather than dopamine or thyroid releasing hormone (TRH). (4) There has been speculation that amniotic fluid prolactin plays a role similar to its regulation of sodium transport and water movement across the gills in fish (allowing the ocean dwelling salmon and steelhead to return to fresh water streams for reproduction). The protection of the fetus from dehydration by control of salt and water transport across the amnion is an attractive, but unproven, thesis.

There is marked variability in maternal prolactin levels in pregnancy, with a diurnal variation similar to that found in nonpregnant persons. The peak level occurs 4–5 hours after the onset of sleep. (5) The initial rise at 7–8 weeks of gestation correlates with the rising levels of estradiol, (6) which appear to act at the hypothalamic level to increase prolactin secretion. (7)

The principal hormone involved in milk biosynthesis is prolactin. Without prolactin, synthesis of the primary protein, casein, will not occur, and true milk secretion will be impossible. The hormonal trigger for initiation of milk production within the alveolar cell and its secretion into the lumen of the gland is the rapid disappearance of estrogen and progesterone from the circulation after delivery. The clearance of prolactin is much slower, requiring 7 days to reach nonpregnant levels in a nonbreastfeeding woman. These discordant hormonal events result in removal of the progesterone and estrogen inhibition of prolactin action on the breast. Breast engorgement and milk secretion begin 3–4 days postpartum when steroids have been sufficiently cleared. Maintenance of steroidal inhibition (estrogen, androgen, progestin) or rapid reduction of prolactin secretion (bromocriptine, 2.5 mg b.i.d. for 2 weeks) are effective in preventing postpartum milk synthesis and secretion. Augmentation of prolactin (by TRH or sulpiride, a dopamine receptor blocker) results in increased milk yield.

In the first postpartum week, prolactin levels in breastfeeding women decline approximately 50% (to about 100 ng/ml). Suckling elicits transient increases in prolactin, which are probably important in initiating milk production. Until 2–3 months postpartum, basal levels are approximately 40–50 ng/ml, and there are large (about 10–20-fold) increases after suckling. After 3–4 months, the basal levels are normal, but suckling still produces an increase that is essential for continuing milk production. The failure to lactate within the first 7 days postpartum may be the first sign of Sheehan's syndrome (hypopituitarism following intrapartum infarction of the pituitary gland).

Maintenance of milk production at high levels is dependent on the joint action of both anterior and posterior pituitary factors. By mechanisms to be described in detail shortly, suckling causes continued release of both prolactin and oxytocin, and in addition, thyroid stimulating hormone (TSH). (8) Prolactin sustains casein, fatty acids, lactose, and volume of secretion, while oxytocin contracts myoepithelial cells and empties the alveolar lumen, thus enhancing further milk secretion and alveolar refilling. The increase in TSH with suckling response suggests that TRH may play a role in the prolactin response to suckling (see below, "Prolactin Releasing Factor"). Again the optimum quantity and quality of milk are dependent upon the availability of thyroid, insulin, cortisol, and the dietary intake of nutrients and fluids.

Vitamin A, vitamin B_{12}, and folic acid are significantly reduced in the breast milk of women with poor dietary intake. As a general rule approximately 1% of any drug ingested by the mother appears in breast milk.

Frequent emptying of the lumen is an important feature in maintaining an adequate level of secretion. Indeed, after the 4th postpartum month, suckling appears to be the only stimulant required, but environmental and emotional states also are important for continued alveolar activity.

The ejection of milk from the breast does not occur as the result of a mechanically induced negative pressure produced by suckling. Tactile sensors concentrated in the areola activate, via thoracic sensory nerve roots 4, 5, and 6, an afferent sensory neural arc which stimulates the paraventricular and supraoptic nuclei of the hypothalamus to synthesize and transport oxytocin to the posterior pituitary, and to release oxytocin from the posterior pituitary. The efferent arc (oxytocin) is blood-borne to the breast alveolus-ductal systems to contract myoepithelial cells and empty the alveolar lumen. Milk contained in major ductal repositories is ejected from openings in the nipple. This rapid release of milk is called "letdown." In many instances, the activation of oxytocin release leading to letdown does not require initiation by tactile stimuli. The central nervous system can be conditioned to respond to the presence of the infant, or to the sound of the infant's cry, by inducing activation of the efferent arc.

The oxytocin effect is a release phenomenon acting on secreted and stored milk. For continued secretory replacement of ejected milk, at least in the first months of breast-feeding, prolactin must be available in sufficient quantities. As previously noted, suckling ensures adequate prolactin availability until the 4th postpartum month, after which elevated basal levels of prolactin are no longer necessary. Continued milk production, however, does require the transient prolactin increase associated with suckling. The amount of milk produced correlates with the amount removed by suckling. The breast can store milk for a maximum of 48 hours before production diminishes.

Adopting mothers occasionally request assistance in initiating lactation. Successful breastfeeding can be achieved approximately half the time by ingesting 25 mg chlorpromazine t.i.d. together with vigorous nipple stimulation every 1–3 hours. Milk production will not appear for several weeks.

Prolactin
Inhibiting
Factor (PIF)

Suckling suppresses the formation of a hypothalamic substance, prolactin inhibiting factor (PIF). This intrahypothalamic effect is either mediated by dopamine, or, in contrast to the peptide nature of other hypothalamic hormones, PIF is dopamine itself. (9) Dopamine is secreted by the basal hypothalamus into the portal system and conducted to the anterior pituitary. Dopamine suppresses secretion of prolactin into the general circulation; in its absence, prolactin is secreted. Suckling, therefore, acts to refill the breast by activating both portions of the pituitary (anterior and posterior) causing the breast to eject milk and to produce new milk.

Prolactin
Releasing
Factor (PRF)

Prolactin may also be influenced by a positive hypothalamic factor (prolactin releasing factor, PRF). PRF does exist in various fowl (e.g. pigeon, chicken, duck, turkey, and the tricolored blackbird). While the identity of this material has not been elucidated, or its function substantiated in normal human physiology, it is possible that TRH can be active as a PRF. Synthetic TRH is a potent stimulant of prolactin secretion in man. The smallest doses of TRH which are capable of producing an increase in TSH, also increase prolactin levels, a finding which supports a physiologic role for TRH in the control of prolactin secretion. (10) However, except in hypothyroidism, normal physiologic changes as well as abnormal prolactin secretion are best explained and understood in terms of variations in the inhibiting factor, PIF.

Cessation of
Lactation

Lactation can be terminated by discontinuing suckling. The primary effect of this cessation is loss of milk letdown via the neural evocation of oxytocin. With passage of a few days, the swollen alveoli depress milk formation, probably via a local pressure effect. With resorption of fluid and solute, the swollen engorged breast diminishes in size in a few days. In addition to the loss of milk letdown the absence of suckling reactivates dopamine (PIF) production so that there is less prolactin stimulation of milk secretion. However, after approximately 4 months of breastfeeding, prolactin probably serves only a permissive role, as levels gradually decline and response to suckling diminishes.

Contraceptive Effect
of Lactation

A moderate contraceptive effect accompanies lactation. (11) It is well known that this is temporary and at best an effect of low reliability. The contraceptive effectiveness of lactation, i.e. the length of the interval between births, depends on the level of nutrition of the mother (if low, the longer the contraceptive interval), the intensity of suckling, and the extent to which supplemental food is added to the infant diet. If suckling intensity and/or frequency is diminished, contraceptive effect is reduced. Approximately 40–75% of breastfeeding women resume menstrual function while still nursing and most will ovulate shortly therafter. The mechanism of the contraceptive effect is of interest because a similar interference with normal pituitary-gonadal function is seen with elevated prolactin levels in nonpregnant women, the syndrome of galactorrhea and amenorrhea.

Prolactin concentrations are increased in response to the repeated suckling stimulus of breastfeeding. Given sufficient intensity and frequency, prolactin levels will remain elevated; under these conditions, follicle-stimulating hormone (FSH) concentrations are in normal range (having risen from extremely low concentrations at delivery to follicular range in the 3 weeks postpartum). Luteinizing hormone (LH) values are low normal range but without pulsatile secretion. Despite the presence of gonadotropin, the ovary during lactational hyperprolactinemia does not display follicular development and does not secrete estrogen.

Earlier experimental evidence suggested that the ovaries might be refractory to gonadotropin stimulation during lactation, and in addition, the anterior pituitary might be less responsive to gonadotropin releasing hormone (GnRH) stimulation. Other studies, done later in the course of lactation, indicated, however, that the ovaries as well as the pituitary were responsive to adequate tropic hormone stimulation. (12)

These observations suggest that high concentrations of prolactin work at both central and ovarian sites to produce lactational amenorrhea and anovulation. Prolactin appears to affect granulosa cell function in vitro by inhibiting synthesis of progesterone. It also may change the testosterone:dihydrotestosterone ratio, thereby reducing aromatizable substrate and increasing local antiestrogen concentrations. Nevertheless, a direct effect of prolactin on ovarian follicular development does not appear to be a major factor. The central action seems to predominate. Prolactin excess has short loop positive feedback effects on dopamine. Increased dopamine could reduce GnRH by suppressing arcuate nucleus function. (13) While not totally settled, the bulk of evidence indicates that prolactin induces amenorrhea by suppressing pusatile GnRH secretion.

At weaning, when prolactin concentrations fall to normal, LH concentrations increase and estradiol secretion rises. This prompt resumption of ovarian function is also indicated by the occurrence of ovulation within 14–30 days of weaning. In nonlactating women, LH levels remain low during the early puerperium and return to normal concentrations during the 3rd to 5th week when prolactin levels have returned to normal. *In women treated with bromocriptine to suppress postpartum lactation, ovulation may occur by the 2nd postpartum week.*

Inappropriate Lactation-Galactorrheic Syndromes

Galactorrhea refers to the mammary secretion of a milky fluid which is nonphysiologic in that it is inappropriate (not immediately related to pregnancy or the needs of a child), persistent, and sometimes excessive. Although usually white or clear, the color may be yellow or even green. In the latter circumstance, local breast disease also should be considered. To elicit breast secretion, pressure should be applied to all sections of the breast beginning at the base of the breast and working up toward the nipple. The quantity of secretion is not an important criterion. Any galactorrhea demands evaluation in a nulliparous woman, and, if at least 12 months have ensued since the last pregnancy in a parous woman. Galactorrhea can involve both breasts, or just one breast. Amenorrhea does not necessarily accompany galacotrrhea, even in the most serious provocative disorders.

Differential Diagnosis

The differential diagnosis of galactorrhea syndromes is a difficult and complex clinical challenge. The difficulty arises from the multiple factors involved in the control of prolactin release. Before proceeding, it would be useful to reemphasize the mechanisms controlling prolactin secretion. In most pathophysiologic systems the final common pathway leading to galactorrhea is an inappropriate augmentation of prolactin release. Prolactin is under a chronic tonic inhibition due to the hypothalamic secretion into the pituitary portal system of PIF. The following considerations are important:

1. Excessive estrogen (e.g. birth control pills) can lead to milk secretion via hypothalamic suppression, causing reduction of PIF and release of pituitary prolactin. Galactorrhea developing during birth control pill administration may be most noticeable during the days free of medication (when the steroids are cleared from the body and the prolactin interfering action of estrogen wanes). Galactorrhea caused by excessive estrogen disappears within 3–6 months after discontinuing medication.

2. Prolonged intensive suckling can also release prolactin, via hypothalamic reduction of PIF. Similarly, thoracotomy scars, cervical spinal lesions, and herpes zoster can induce prolactin release by activating the afferent sensory neural arc, thereby simulating suckling.

251

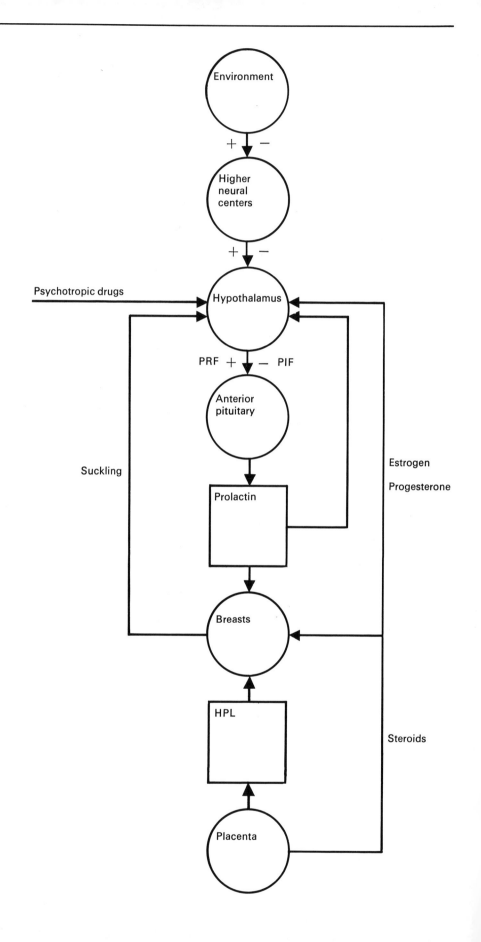

3. A variety of drugs can also inhibit hypothalamic PIF. (14) There are nearly 100 phenothiazine derivatives with indirect mammotropic activity of this type. In addition, there are many phenothiazine-like compounds, reserpine derivatives, amphetamines, and an unknown variety of other drugs (opiates, diazepams, butyrophenones, α-methyldopa, and tricyclic antidepressants such as Elavil and Tofranil) which can initiate galactorrhea via hypothalamic suppression. The final action of these compounds is either to deplete dopamine levels or to block dopamine receptors. Chemical features common to many of these drugs are an aromatic ring with a polar substituent as in estrogen and at least two additional rings or structural attributes making spatial arrangements similar to estrogen. Thus these compounds may act in a manner similar to estrogens to decrease PIF. In support of this conclusion, it has been demonstrated that estrogen and phenothiazine derivatives compete for the same receptors in the median eminence. Prolactin is uniformly elevated in patients on therapeutic amounts of phenothiazines. Approximately 30–50% will exhibit galactorrhea which should not persist beyond 3–6 months after drug treatment is discontinued.

4. Stresses can inhibit hypothalamic PIF, thereby inducing prolactin secretion and galactorrhea. Trauma, surgical procedures, and anesthesia can be seen in temporal relation to the onset of galactorrhea.

5. Hypothalamic lesions, stalk lesions, or stalk compression (events that physically reduce production or delivery of PIF to the pituitary) allow release of excess prolactin leading to galactorrhea.

6. Hypothyroidism (juvenile or adult) can be associated with galactorrhea. With diminished circulating levels of thyroid hormone, hypothalamic TRH is produced in excess and acts as a PRF to release prolactin from the pituitary. Juvenile hypothyroidism in association with breast development and galactorrhea can be seen. Reversal with thyroid is strong circumstantial evidence to support the conclusion that TRH stimulates prolactin.

7. Increased prolactin release may be a consequence of prolactin elaboration and secretion from pituitary tumors which function independently of the otherwise appropriate restraints exerted by PIF from a normally functioning hypothalamus. This infrequent, but potentially dangerous tumor, which has endocrine, neurologic, and ophthalmologic liabilities that can be disabling, makes the differential diagnosis of persistent galactorrhea a major clinical challenge. Beyond producing prolactin, the tumor may also suppress pituitary parenchyma by expansion and compression, interfering with the secretion of other tropic hormones.

253

8. Increased prolactin concentrations may result from nonpituitary sources such as lung and renal tumors. Severe renal disease requiring hemodialysis is associated with elevated prolactin levels.

Clinical Problem of
Galactorrhea

A variety of eponymic designations have been applied to variants of the lactation syndromes. These are based on the association of galactorrhea with intrasellar tumor (Forbes, Henneman, Griswold, and Albright, 1951), antecedent pregnancy with inappropriate persistence of galactorrhea (independently reported by Chiari and Frommel in 1852), and in the absence of previous pregnancy (Argonz and del Castillo, 1953). In all, the association of galactorrhea with eventual amenorrhea was noted.

On the basis of currently available information, categorization of individual cases according to these eponymic guidelines is neither helpful nor does it permit discrimination of patients who have serious intrasellar or suprasellar pathology.

Hyperprolactinemia may be associated with a variety of menstrual cycle disturbances, oligo-ovulation, corpus luteum insufficiency, as well as amenorrhea. (15) About one third of women with secondary amenorrhea will have elevated prolactin concentrations. Pathologic hyperprolactinemia inhibits the pulsatile secretion of GnRH. Baseline gonadotropin levels are normal or decreased, with LH reduction more common and occurring earlier than a lowering of FSH. Reduction of circulating prolactin levels restores menstrual function.

Mild hirsutism may accompany ovulatory dysfunction due to hyperprolactinemia. Whether excess androgen is stimulated by a proposed prolactin effect on adrenal cortex synthesis of DHA (dehydroepiandrosterone) and its sulfate (DHAS) or is primarily related to the chronic anovulation of these patients (and hence ovarian androgen secretion) is not settled.

Not all patients with hyperprolactinemia display galactorrhea. The reported incidence is about 33%. (15) The disparity may not be due entirely to the variable zeal with which the presence of nipple milk secretion is sought for during physical examination. The absence of galactorrhea may be due to the usual accompanying hypoestrogenic state. A more attractive explanation focuses on the concept of heterogeneity of tropic hormones (Chapter 1). The radioimmunoassay for prolactin may not discriminate between heterogenous molecules of prolactin. (16) A high circulating level of prolactin may not represent material capable of interacting with breast prolactin receptors. On the other hand, galactorrhea can be seen in women with normal prolactin serum concentrations. Episodic fluctuation and sleep increments may account for this clinical discordance, or, in this case, bioactive prolactin may be present which is immunoactively not detectable. In the pathophysiology of male hypogonadism, hyperprolactinemia is much less common and the incidence of actual galactorrhea quite rare. Hyperprolactinemia in men usually presents as decreased libido and potency.

Regardless of the clinical circumstances, if galactorrhea has been present for 6 months to 1 year, or hyperprolactinemia is noted in the process of working up menstrual disturbances, infertility, or hirsutism, the probability of a pituitary tumor must be recognized. The workup of hyperprolactinemia is presented in detail in Chapter 5, "Amenorrhea." Nevertheless, it is worth reemphasizing the salient clinical issues here.

With the current diagnostic techniques there is no difficulty in discovering and monitoring the size and function of a pituitary prolactin secreting "tumor." With few exceptions (such as false positive multidirectional polytomographic studies), the combination of elevation in basal levels of prolactin and radiographic imaging offers complete confidence in diagnosing sellar pathology. The major concern remains in determining management—medical, surgical, or expectant? The factors that influence management include:

1. Microadenomas, if exclusively prolactin producing, rarely progress to macroadenoma size. Most are exceedingly slow growing or stable.

2. The histology of many so-called tumors is clearly not one of neoplasia. Most contain normal pituitary tissue, others display nodular or diffuse hyperplasia of basically normal lactotropes.

3. It is possible that a primary hypothalamic dysfunction which drives the lactotrope to hyperfunction and hyperplasia is the fundamental factor in the genesis of these "tumors." Thus, uncertain long-term cures, recurrence, and new tumor formation remain possibilities.

4. Some tumors regress spontaneously. Medical therapy (the dopamine agonist, bromocriptine) shrinks tumors and can prevent growth, although complete elimination of a tumor by bromocriptine does not occur and rapid regrowth can follow discontinuation of bromocriptine treatment.

5. Transsphenoidal microsurgery is a very safe procedure with a high cure rate in microadenomas, but is less effective in larger tumors.

As a result of these considerations, many patients can be observed, others treated medically, and still others treated with surgery, with or without prior medically induced tumor size reduction (see Chapter 5).

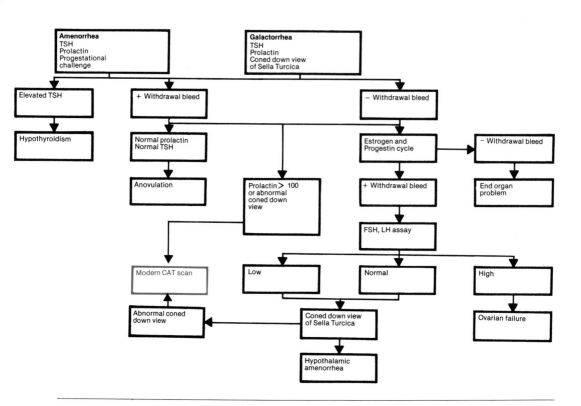

Amenorrhea		Galactorrhea
TSH Prolactin Progestational challenge		TSH Prolactin Coned down view of Sella Turcica

Boxes in flowchart:
- Elevated TSH → Hypothyroidism
- + Withdrawal bleed → Normal prolactin / Normal TSH → Anovulation
- Prolactin > 100 or abnormal coned down view → Modern CAT scan → Abnormal coned down view
- − Withdrawal bleed → Estrogen and Progestin cycle → − Withdrawal bleed → End organ problem
- Estrogen and Progestin cycle → + Withdrawal bleed → FSH, LH assay → Low / Normal / High
- High → Ovarian failure
- Normal → Coned down view of Sella Turcica → Hypothalamic amenorrhea

Treatment of Galactorrhea

Galactorrhea as an isolated symptom of hypothalamic dysfunction existing in an otherwise healthy woman does not require treatment. Periodic prolactin levels will, if within normal range, confirm the stability of the underlying process. However, some patients find the presence or amount of galactorrhea sexually, cosmetically, and emotionally burdensome. Treatment with combined birth control pills, androgens, danazol and progestins has met with variable success. Bromocriptine, therefore, is clearly the drug of choice. Even with normal prolactin concentrations and a normal skull x-ray, treatment with bromocriptine can eliminate galactorrhea.

We have adopted a conservative approach of close surveillance for pituitary prolactin-secreting adenomas, recommending surgery only for those tumors that display rapid growth or those tumors that are already large. If the prolactin level is greater than 100 ng/ml, or if the coned down view of the sella turcia is abnormal, we recommend CT scan evaluation, utilizing the most recently developed machine capable of 1 mm tomography. If the CT scan rules out an empty sella syndrome or a suprasellar problem, surgical intervention after preoperative bromocriptine treatment is then dictated by the patient's desires, the size of the tumor, and rapidity of growth of the tumor. Patients with prolactin levels less than 100 ng/ml and with normal coned down views of the sella turcia are offered a choice between bromocriptine therapy and surveillance. An annual prolactin level and annual coned down view are indicated for continued observation to detect a growing tumor. Bromocriptine therapy is recommended for patients wishing to achieve pregnancy, and for those patients who have galactorrhea to the point of discomfort.

The Management of Mastalgia

The cyclic occurrence of breast discomfort is a common problem and is usually associated with dysplastic, benign histologic changes in the breast. Medical treatment of mastalgia has historically included a bewildering array of options. Several clearly are of limited value. Diuretics have little impact, and thyroid hormone replacement is indicated only when hypothyroidism is documented. Steroid hormone treatment has been tried in many combinations, mostly unsupported by controlled studies. An old favorite, with many years of clinical experience testifying to its effectiveness, is testosterone. One must be careful, however, to avoid virilizing doses. A good practice is to start with small doses, such as 5 mg methyltestosterone every other day during the time of discomfort. In recent years, however, these methods have been supplanted by several new approaches. (17)

Danazol in a dose of 100–400 mg/day is effective in relieving discomfort as well as decreasing nodularity of the breast. A daily dose is recommended for a period of 6 months. This treatment may achieve long-term resolution of the histologic changes in addition to the clinical improvement. Doses below 400 mg daily do not assure inhibition of ovulation and a method of effective contraception is necessary. Significant improvement has been noted with vitamin E, 600 units/day of the synthetic tocopheral acetate. No side effects have been noted, and the mechanism of action is unknown. Bromocriptine and antiestrogens such as tamoxifen are also effective for treating mammary discomfort and benign disease.

Clinical observations have suggested that abstinence from methylxanthines leads to resolution of symptoms. Methylxanthines are present in coffee, tea, chocolate, and cola drinks.

Cancer of the Breast

Scope of the problem

One of every 11 women will develop breast cancer during her lifetime. The incidence has been increasing over the past 2 decades and mortality rates have remained constant. The breast is the leading site of cancer in women (28% of all cancers), and the leading cause of death from cancer in women is breast cancer (20% of cancer deaths). Breast cancer has an increasing frequency with age—a woman at age 70 has almost 10 times the risk as a 40-year-old woman. Over the years breast cancer has continued this deadly impact despite advances in surgical and diagnostic techniques. No more than 25% of breast cancer patients are "cured." Recently a growing appreciation for the hormonal influences on breast cancer has kindled a new hope for better therapeutic management.

Risk Factors

A constellation of factors influences the risk for breast cancer. (18) These include: reproductive experience, ovarian activity, benign breast disease, familial tendency, genetic differences, and specific endocrine factors.

Reproductive Experience. The risk of breast cancer increases with the increase in age at which a woman bears her first full-term child. A woman pregnant before the age of 18 has about one third the risk of one who first delivers after the age of 35. To be protective, pregnancy must occur before the age of 30. In fact, women over the age of 30 years at the time of their first birth have a greater risk than women who never become pregnant. Births after the first convey little or no additional protection.

The fact that pregnancy early in life is associated with reduced breast cancer implies that etiology factors are operating during that period of life. The protection afforded only by the first pregnancy and not substantially modified by subsequent births suggests that the first full-term pregnancy has a trigger effect which either produces a permanent change in the factors responsible for breast cancer, or changes the breast tissue and makes it less susceptible to malignant transformation. Lactation is not significant in this mechanism. Whether a patient breastfeeds or not has little if any effect on risk.

Ovarian Activity. Women who have an oophorectomy have a lower risk and the lowered risk is greater the younger a woman is ovariectomized. There is a 70% risk reduction in women who have surgery before age 35. This implies that ovarian activity plays a role in at least two thirds of breast cancer patients. There is a small increase in risk with early menarche and with late natural menopause, indicating that ovarian activity plays a continuing role throughout reproductive life. Obese women have earlier menarche and late menopause, higher estrone production rates and free estradiol levels (lower sex hormone binding globulin (SHBG)), and greater risk for breast cancer. (19)

Benign Breast Disease. Women with cystic mastitis have about 4 times the breast cancer rate of comparable normal women. Despite their risk, women with prior benign breast disease form only a small proportion of breast cancer patients—approximately 5%.

Familial Tendency. Female relatives of women with breast cancer have 2–3 times the rate of the general population. There is an excess of bilateral disease among patients with a family history of breast cancer. Relatives of women with bilateral disease have about a 45% lifetime chance of developing breast cancer.

Specific Endocrine Factors.

1. *Adrenal Steroids.* Subnormal levels of etiocholanolone (a urinary excretion product of androstenedione) have been found from 5 months to 9 years before the diagnosis of breast cancer in women living on the island of Guernsey, off the English coast. (20) A subnormal excretion of this 17-ketosteroid was also found in sisters of patients with breast cancer. A 6-fold increase in the incidence of breast cancer was found between women excreting less than 0.4 mg of etiocholanolone and those excreting over 1 mg/24 hours. Because approximately 25% of the population excretes less than 1 mg/24 hours, measurement of this 17-ketosteroid might be a useful screening procedure to detect a high risk group of patients, if these results are confirmed in additional studies.

2. *Endogenous Estrogen.* Estriol generally has failed to produce breast cancer in rodents, and in fact, estriol protects the rat against breast tumors induced by various chemical carcinogens. The hypothesis is that a higher estriol level protects against the more potent effects of estrone and estradiol. This might explain the protective effect of early pregnancies. Women having had an early pregnancy continue to excrete more estriol than nulliparous women. (21) Premenopausal healthy Asiatic women have a lower breast cancer risk than Caucasians, and also have a higher rate of urinary estriol excretion. (22) When Asiatic women migrate to the United States, however, their rate of breast cancer increases, and their urinary excretion of estriol decreases.

The notion that normal estrogen stimulation unopposed by adequate progesterone secretion was a factor in the pathogenesis of breast cancer was first stated by Sherman and Korenman. (23) Although theoretically appealing on the basis of presumed correlation with epidemiologic risks (infertility, late menopause) clinical research has not always confirmed the thesis. (24) Young women at high genetic risk for breast cancer had normal luteal phases, and a group of premenopausal women with breast cancer had normal luteal phases. On the other hand, a long-term follow-up study of infertile women with a history of progesterone deficiency indicated a 5.4 times increase in risk of premenopausal breast cancer. (25) The logic and epidemiologic

259

support for an estrogen link are impressive arguments. Whether the important factor is the total amount of estrogen, the estriol to estradiol ratio, the amount of estrogen unopposed by progesterone, or some other combination is not known.

3.   *Exogenous Estrogen.* Despite the failure to uncover an abnormal endogenous estrogen factor relating to increased breast cancer risk, epidemiologic and other information continues to suggest some estrogen-related promotor function. These include: a) the condition is 100 times more common in women than in men, b) breast cancer invariably occurs after puberty, c) untreated gonadal dysgenesis and breast cancer are mutually exclusive, d) a 65% excess rate of breast cancer has been observed among women who have had an endometrial cancer, (26) and e) breast tumors contain estrogen receptors which are biologically active as indicated by the presence of progesterone receptors in tumor tissue. Taken together, these data suggest an element of estrogen dependence, if not provocation, in many breast cancers. What is the evidence that exogenous estrogen therapy can provide the same stimulus in vulnerable recipients?

Early epidemiologic studies of the retrospective case control type did not reveal a significant relationship between estrogen therapy and breast cancer. (27, 28) Retrospective studies are unfortunately flawed by the difficulties of selection bias, i.e. comparing groups of patients followed by a single physician to an expected epidemiologic incidence rate in the general population as expressed in national surveys; nevertheless, the data are useful.

At least one study suggested that the relative risk increased with time, reaching 2.0 after 15 years of estrogen therapy. (29) The risk appeared to be greater with 1.25 mg conjugated estrogen than with 0.625 mg. Most impressively, the appearance of benign breast lesions during the period of treatment (surgically confirmed) was associated with an even higher risk. The presence of a benign breast lesion before therapy was likewise associated with an elevated relative risk.

In additional studies, the increased risk of prolonged dosage (1.25 mg greater than 5 years) has been reemphasized, and the presence of benign breast disease has been singled out as a major risk factor when combined with estrogen therapy. (30, 31) Some reassurance, however, has come from a hospital-based study using the respected Connecticut Registry, showing no increased risk for estrogen users. (32) As detailed elsewhere (Chapter 4), prudent practice dictates avoidance of excessive estrogen, and the addition of the protective 10 days of a progestational agent.

4.   *Thyroid, Prolactin, Various Nonestrogen Drugs.* Despite isolated suggestions of increased risk, hypothyroidism, reserpine, or prolactin excess, whether spontaneous or drug induced, are not related to an enhanced risk of breast cancer. (18)

5.   *Birth Control Pills and Breast Cancer.* The large number of women taking or having taken oral contraceptive steroids combined with the belief that steroids provoke or promote abnormal breast growth and possibly cancer has provided a source of major concern for years. Because the likelihood of a prolonged lag time between the induction and the clinical appearance of cancer, some reports have suggested that oral contraceptives might interact unfavorably with established risk factors for the disease. (33) Two recent and larger studies have provided results which are reassuring in at least two important respects: 1) breast cancer incidence was not altered by previous use of birth control pills (either positively or negatively) regardless of duration of use, age at initial use, or parity at initial use; and 2) women with breast cancer who had taken birth control pills survived significantly longer, had lower grade tumors, had smaller size primary tumors, and had fewer axillary metastases than nonuser breast cancer control patients. (34, 35) Over 800 user and control breast cancer subjects were involved in these studies beginning in 1968.

6.   *Breast Cancer in Diethylstilbestrol (DES)-exposed Women.* Exposure to DES occurred in association with 2 million live births; therefore, the risk for induction of breast cancer during a period of breast differentiation could be significant if DES were a true breast carcinogen. The major study on this subject reported on the follow-up of women who participated in a controlled trial of DES in pregnancy between 1950 and 1952 at the University of Chicago. In this study, no significant association between breast cancer and DES exposure was found. (36) The study involved information on 693 (90% of exposed group) and 668 (89% of the controls) of the original study patients. Reinterpretation post hoc in the public press led to a review of the original data and additional information from the national DESAD (DES plus adenosis) Project at the Mayo Clinic. (37) In this new study, among 408 women given DES, there were 8 confirmed cases of breast cancer, in comparison with an expected number of 8.1 based upon breast cancer incidence rates among parous women in the local population. The original Chicago report of no association was confirmed.

Stanley G. Korenman has promulgated a most interesting thesis concerning the endocrinology of breast cancer. (38, 39) Recognizing that the endocrine changes thought to be related to the promotion or provocation of breast cancer were small, inconsistent, did not persist in crossculture or single culture studies, and could hardly account for the 5-fold differential risk of breast cancer among populations, Korenman concluded that *endocrine status is related to breast cancer by influencing the patient's susceptibility to environmental carcinogens.* Recalling the dimethylbenzanthracene inducer-promoter model of rodents in which a favorable endocrine environment both increased susceptibility to a single exposure to a known carcinogen and thereafter provided favorable conditions for maintenance and growth of the tumor, the estrogen window hypothesis in humans has the following components:

1. Human breast cancer is induced by environmental carcinogens in a susceptible mammary gland.

2. Unopposed estrogen stimulation is the most favorable state for tumor induction (the "open" window).

3. The duration of exposure to estrogens determines risk (how long the window is "open").

4. There is a long latent period between tumor induction and clinical expression.

5. Susceptibility to induction ("inducibility") declines with the establishment of normal luteal phase progesterone secretion and becomes very low during pregnancy. (The "open" window is closed, but if tumor has been induced during a previous "open" window period, the hormones which reduce susceptibility nevertheless may promote maintenance and growth.)

The two main induction "open window" periods are the pubertal years prior to the establishment of regular ovulatory menstrual cycles and the perimenopausal period of waning ovulation and follicle maturation. The prolongation of these open windows by obesity, infertility, delayed pregnancy, earlier menarche, and later menopause would be associated with increased susceptibility to an environmental carcinogen. Opposed estrogen (as in birth control pill users and DES exposure during pregnancy) would not increase susceptibilty, but would not decrease breast cancer incidence.

If estrogens were given postmenopausally, extending the second window, the hypothesis would predict that after a latent period a greater incidence of breast cancer would appear. The breast cancer incidence peaks lend credence to both the open window incidence concept as well as the latent period. To be sure, the risk of breast cancer increases with age. However, the incidence rises between the ages of

25 and 45, then levels off between 45 and 55 and thereafter rises again to peak between ages 65–70. (40)

Korenman has cited independent support for the estrogen window hypothesis—breast cancer incidence studies of populations exposed to a single carcinogen superimposed on the normal environmental risks. Such data are reported in the extended life span study of atomic bomb survivors from Hiroshima and Nagasaki, and women with tuberculosis receiving repeated fluoroscopies. (41) Inducibility, the presence of windows, and a latency period between induction and clinical expression were demonstrated in each. In the A-bomb survivors, no breast cancer was seen in children irradiated under the age of 10; increased differences in risk occurred if exposure occurred between age 10 and 29 with an especially marked risk exposure period between 10 and 14 years—the period just before menarche. Excess risk due to irradiation decreased rapidly so that, if exposure occurred between 30 and 49 years of age, there was no significant breast cancer increase over nonradiated controls. After age 50, increased inducibility seemed to reappear.

In the repeatedly fluoroscoped women with tuberculosis, the greatest incremental risk of breast cancer over un-x-rayed controls occurred in those exposed in the 15–20-year age group with no increase after age 30. (42) The greatest risk appeared 15 years after exposure and persisted at least 40 years.

While the estrogen window hypothesis is not proven it has appealing clarity as well as partial supportive data. It explains many, but not all the elements of risk in breast cancer. It reminds us of duration as well as the intensity of inducer and promoter substances. It explains the lack of consistent hormonal findings in patients with established breast cancer even though a hormonal factor appears obvious in the pathogenesis of the disorder. It demands study of the relative benefit risk ratio of progestin therapy in estrogen replacement therapy with respect to breast cancer as well as endometrial disease.

Steroid Receptor Assays in Human Breast Cancer

Elsewhere (Chapter 1), the biochemical process by which steroid hormones produce effects on target cells has been reviewed in detail. Estrogen binds initially to specific cytoplasmic receptor protein; the steroid-protein complex is then translocated into the nucleus and binds specifically to receptor sites on the chromatin, thereby promoting biochemical processes involved in target tissue growth and function. This biochemical mechanism suggested that analysis of the estrogen receptor content of tumor tissue from breast cancers might provide a basis on which to predict response to endocrine therapy (steroid administration or glandular ablation). In the past decade, evidence has accumulated which supports the value of receptor assays in assessing the degree of differentiation, prognosis, response to endocrine therapy—in short, the management of patients with advanced breast cancer. (43, 44)

263

| Tissue Sampling and Assay Analysis | Tissue for receptor assay, taken from the periphery of the tumor, is frozen immediately in liquid nitrogen or solid carbon dioxide and sent to an established quality controlled receptor assay laboratory. The analysis should be done within 4 weeks. Prolonged storage beyond that time is discouraged. |

The assay can be performed on as little as 100–200 mg of fresh or frozen tissue. Tissue cytosol is prepared by homogenization and centrifugation and incubated with tritium-labeled estradiol. The levels of cytoplasmic estrogen-receptor protein are measured and reported as femtomoles of estradiol bound per milligram of total protein. A tumor with less than 3 femtomoles (fmol) is usually called estrogen receptor negative. One large study suggested improved clinical response to endocrine therapy correlated with the concentration of estrogen receptor; the rate of response (50% reduction in size of tumor) was 46% when the level exceeded 100 fmol. (45)

It has been suggested that some receptor positive patients fail to respond to endocrine manipulation because the presence of a receptor is a necessary but insufficient condition for response. The receptor may not be functional in certain tumors and hence endocrine therapy not useful. One reflection of the activity of the estrogen-receptor complex is the induction of progesterone receptors. Seventy-four percent of patients with both an estrogen and progesterone receptor have responded to endocrine therapy in collected series, whereas only 28% who were estrogen receptor positive and progesterone receptor negative reacted favorably. (46)

Estrogen Receptors and Clinical Prognosis

There is an excellent correlation between the presence of estrogen receptors and certain clinical characteristics of breast cancer. (45) Premenopausal and younger patients are more frequently receptor negative. Women within 4 years of menopause have the lowest receptor levels; receptors increase the more years the patient is postmenopausal. Patients with receptor positive tumors survive longer and have longer disease-free intervals after mastectomy than those with receptor negative tumors. The presence of an estrogen receptor correlates with increased disease-free interval regardless of the presence of axillary nodes, or the size and location of the tumors. Similarly, patients without axillary lymph node mestatases, but with an estradiol receptor negative tumor, have the same high rate of recurrence as do patients with axillary lymph node metastases.

It appears that patients with estrogen receptors are those with the more slowly growing tumors. Several reports indicate that estrogen receptor status correlates with the degree of differentiation of the primary tumor. A large proportion of highly differentiated Grade I carcinomas are receptor positive while the reverse is true of Grade III tumors.

| Treatment Selection | The estrogen receptor assay is a valuable prognostic indicator which combined with lymph node status and tumor histologic grade, can be used in management of patients with breast cancer. |

The correlation between the presence of an estrogen receptor and the clinical response to all types of endocrine therapy has been established. (45) Between 50 and 60% of receptor positive patients responded to ablation of hormones which is almost double the response rate in unselected patients with breast cancer. Less than 10% of receptor negative tumors showed a response (scored as tumor size regression of 50% for a period exceeding a month). Receptor negative patients can be spared unnecessary surgery and months of fruitless trials of hormone therapy by the prompt initiation of chemotherapy.

Mammography

Mammography is a means of detecting the nonpalpable cancer. In the past few years technical advancements have significantly improved the mammographic image. The major disadvantage of this screening procedure relates to radiation hazard, a possible increase in cancer induction through radiation. Cumulative dosage to the breast should be kept below 20 rad. The new techniques use approximately 1 rad per skin exposure, allowing at least 20 screening procedures. Further refinements are making it possible to lower doses to less than 0.5 rad per exposure. Thermography, while avoiding radiation exposure, can be considered as only an adjunctive procedure because its accuracy does not approach that of mammography. Ultrasound evaluation of the breast is still undergoing development.

Mammography cannot and should not replace examination by patient and physician. Cancer commonly presents as a solitary, solid, painless, hard, unilateral, irregular nonmobile mass. A cancer may be palpable yet not apparent on the mammogram. Mammography is an important component of preventive health care, however, as it can identify potential cancers at a preinvasive stage, 1–2 years before they reach a clinically palpable size. Between the ages of 35 and 50, every women should have baseline mammography. With a mammographic image consistent with a high risk of cancer, or with historical factors consistent with high risk, annual mammography should be obtained for a few years until no change is clearly apparent. Periodic mammography will then depend upon continuing evolution of technique with reduced radiation exposure, historical and endocrine factors of risk, patient concern and anxiety, and the degree of difficulty in accomplishing a reliable clinical examination of the breasts. The optimum screening approach will not be apparent until results are available from several large scale population studies now underway. Until then, in the absence of high risk factors, annual mammography is recommended only for women over the age of 50 years.

265

References

1. **Topper YL,** Multiple hormone interactions in the development of mammary gland in vitro, Recent Prog Horm Res 26:287, 1970.

2. **Tyson JE, Hwang P, Guyda H, Friesen HG,** Studies of prolactin secretion in human pregnancy, Am J Obstet Gynecol 113:14, 1972.

3. **Bruce JO, Ramirez VD,** Site of action of the inhibitory effects of estrogen upon lactation, Neuroendocrinology 6:19, 1970.

4. **Luciano AA, Maslar IA, Kusmik WF, Riddick DH,** Stimulatory activity of serum on prolactin production by human decidua, Am J Obstet Gynecol 138:665, 1980.

5. **Tyson JE, Friesen HG,** Factors influencing the secretion of human prolactin and growth hormone in menstrual and gestational women, Am J Obstet Gynecol 116:377, 1973.

6. **Barberia JM, Abu-Fadil S, Kletzky OA, Nakamura RM, Mishell DR Jr,** Serum prolactin patterns in early human gestation, Am J Obstet Gynecol 121:1107, 1975.

7. **Ehara Y, Siler TM, Yen SSC,** Effects of large doses of estrogen on prolactin and growth hormone release, Am J Obstet Gynecol 125:455, 1976.

8. **Dawood MY, Khan-Dawood FS, Wahl RS, Fuchs F,** Oxytocin release and plasma anterior pituitary and gonadal hormones in women during lactation, J Clin Endocrinol Metab 52:678, 1981.

9. **Macleod RM, Lehmeyer JE,** Studies on the mechanism of the dopamine-mediated inhibition of prolactin secretion, Endocrinology 94:1077, 1974.

10. **Noel GL, Dimond RC, Wartofsky L, Earll JM, Frantz AG,** Studies of prolactin and TSH secretion by continuous infusion of small amounts of thyrotropin-releasing hormone (TRH), J Clin Endocrinol Metab 39:6, 1974.

11. **McNeilly AS,** Effects of lactation on fertility, Br Med Bull 35:151, 1979.

12. **Tyson JE, Carter JN, Andreassen B, Huth J, Smith B,** Nursing mediated prolactin and luteinizing hormone secretion during puerperal lactation, Fertil Steril 30:154, 1978.

13. **Judd SJ, Rigg LA, Yen SSC,** The effects of ovariectomy and estrogen treatment on the dopamine inhibition of gonadotropin and prolactin release, J Clin Endocrinol Metab 49:182, 1979.

14. **Dickey RP, Stone SC,** Drugs that affect the breast and lactation, Clin Obstet Gynecol 18:95, 1975.

15. **Schlechte J, Sherman B, Halmi N, Van Gilder J, Chapler F, Dolan K, Granner D, Duello T, Harris C,** Prolactin-secreting pituitary tumors, Endocr Rev 1:295, 1980.

16. **Aubert ML, Grumbach MM, Kaplan SL,** The ontogenesis of human fetal hormones: III. Prolactin, J Clin Invest 56:155, 1975.

17. **London RS, Sundaram GS, Goldstein PJ,** Medical management of mammary dysplasia, Obstet Gynecol 59:519, 1982.

18. **Kelsey JL,** A review of the epidemiology of human breast cancer, Epidemol Rev 1:74, 1979.

19. **Sherman B, Wallace R, Bean J, Schlabaugh L,** Relationship of body weight to menarchael and menopausal age: implication for breast cancer risk, J Clin Endocrinol Metab 52:488, 1981.

20. **Bulbrook RD,** Urinary androgen excretion and the etiology of breast cancer, JNCI 48:1039, 1972.

21. **Cole P, Brown JB, MacMahon B,** Oestrogen profiles of parous and nulliparous women, Lancet 2:596, 1976.

22. **Dickinson LE, MacMahon B, Cole P, Brown JB,** Estrogen profiles of oriental and Caucasian women in Hawaii, N Engl J Med 291:1211, 1974.

23. **Sherman BM, Korenman SG,** Inadequate corpus luteum function: a pathophysiologic interpretation of human breast cancer epidemiology, Cancer 33:1306, 1974.

24. **McFayden IJ, Forrest APM, Prescott RJ, Golder MP, Groom GV, Fahmy DR,** Circulating hormone concentrations in women with breast cancer, Lancet 1:1100, 1976.

25. **Cowan LD, Gordis L, Tonascia JA, Jones GS,** Breast cancer incidence in women with a history of progesterone deficiency, Am J Epidemiol, 114:209, 1981.

26. **MacMahon B, Austin JH,** Association of carcinomas of the breast and corpus uteri, Cancer 23:275, 1969.

27. **Horwitz RE, Feinstein AR,** The clinical epidemiology of breast and uterine cancer, in *The Menopause and Postmenopause*, Passetto N, Paoletti R, Ambrus JL, eds. MTP Press, Lancaster, England, 1980.

28. **Hertz R,** The steroid-cancer hypothesis, J Steroid Biochem 11:435, 1979.

29. **Hoover R, Gray LA, Cole P, MacMahon B,** Menopausal estrogen and breast cancer, N Engl J Med 295:401, 1976.

30. **Ross RK, Paganini-Hill A, Gerkins V, Mack TM, Pfeffer R, Arthur M, Henderson BE,** A case-control study of menopausal estrogen therapy and breast cancer, JAMA 243:1635, 1980.

31. **Jick H, Walker AM, Watkins RN, D'Ewart DC, Hunter JR, Danford A, Madsen S, Dinan BJ, Rothman KJ,** Replacement estrogens and breast cancer, Am J Epidemiol 112:586, 1980.

32. **Kelsey JL, LaVolsi V,** Estrogen replacement therapy and breast cancer incidence, JNCI 67:327, 1981.

33. **Paffenbarger RS, Fasal E, Simmons ME, Kampert JM,** Cancer risk as related to use of oral contraceptives during fertile years, Cancer 39:1887, 1977.

34. **Vessey MP, McPherson K, Doll R,** Breast cancer and oral contraceptives: findings in Oxford-Family Planning Association contraceptive study, Br Med J 282:2093, 1981.

35. **Matthews PN, Millis RR, Haywood JL,** Breast cancer in women who have taken contraceptive steroids, Br Med J 282:774, 1981.

36. **Bibbo M, Haenszel W, Wied GL, Hubby M, Herbst AL,** A twenty-five year follow-up study of women exposed to DES during pregnancy, N Engl J Med 298:763, 1978.

37. **Brian OD, Tilley BC, LaBarthe DR, O'Fallon WM, Noller KL, Kurland LT,** Breast cancer in DES exposed mothers: absence of association, Mayo Clin Proc 55:89, 1980.

38. **Korenman SG,** The endocrinology of breast cancer, Cancer 46:874, 1980.

39. **Korenman SG,** Estrogen window hypothesis of the etiology of breast cancer, Lancet 1:700, 1980.

40. **DeWaard F, Baander-Van Halewijn EA, Huizinga J,** The bimodal age distribution of patients with mammary carcinoma, Cancer 17:141, 1964.

41. **Tokunaga M, Norman JE, Asano M, Tokuoka S, Ezaki H, Nishimori I, Tsuji Y,** Malignant breast tumors among atomic bomb survivors, JNCI 62:1347, 1979.

42. **Boice JD, Monson RR,** Breast cancer in woman after repeated fluoroscopic examinations of the chest, JNCI 59:823, 1977.

43. **British Breast Group,** Steroid receptor assays in human breast cancer, Lancet 1:298, 1980.

44. **Henderson IC, Canellos GP,** Cancer of the breast: the past decade, N Engl J Med 302:78, 1980.

45. **McGuire WL, Horwitz KB, Zava DT, Garola RE, Chamness GC,** Hormones in cancer: update 1978, Metabolism 27:487, 1978.

46. **McGuire WL,** Hormone receptors: their role in predicting prognosis and response to endocrine therapy, Semin Oncol 5:428, 1978.

10 The Endocrinology of Pregnancy

One of the crucial aspects of intrauterine life is dependency upon the effective exchange of nutritive and metabolic products between fetus and mother. It is not surprising that there should exist mechanisms by which a growing fetus can exert some influence or control over the exchange process, and hence its environment. The methods by which a fetus can influence its own growth and development involve a variety of messages transmitted, in many cases, by hormones. Hormonal messages from the conceptus can affect metabolic processes, uteroplacental blood flow, and cellular differentiation. Furthermore, a fetus may signal its desire and readiness to leave the uterus by hormonal initiation of parturition. *This chapter will review steroid and protein hormones of pregnancy, as well as perinatal thyroid physiology, and fetal lung maturation.*

Steroid Hormones in Pregnancy

Steroidogenesis in the fetal-placental unit does not follow the conventional mechanisms of hormone production within a single organ. Rather, the final products result from critical interactions and interdependence of separate organ systems which individually do not possess the necessary enzymatic capabilities. It is helpful to view the process as consisting of a fetal compartment, a placental compartment, and a maternal compartment. Separately the fetal and placental compartments lack certain steroidogenic activities. Together, however, they are complementary and form a complete unit, which utilizes the maternal compartment as a source of basic building materials and as a resource for clearance of steroids.

271

Progesterone

In its key location as a way station between mother and fetus, the placenta can utilize precursors from either mother or fetus to circumvent its own deficiencies in enzyme activity. The placenta converts little, if any, acetate to cholesterol or its precursors. Cholesterol as well as pregnenolone are obtained from the maternal blood stream for progesterone synthesis. The fetal contribution is negligible since progesterone levels remain high after fetal demise. Thus, the massive amount of progesterone produced in pregnancy depends upon placental-maternal cooperation.

Progesterone is largely produced by the corpus luteum until about 10 weeks of gestation. Indeed, until approximately the 7th week, the pregnancy is dependent upon the presence of the corpus luteum. (1) After a transition period of shared function between the 7th week to the 12th week, the placenta emerges as the major source of progesterone. At term, progesterone levels range from 100 to 200 ng/ml, and the placenta produces about 250 mg per day.

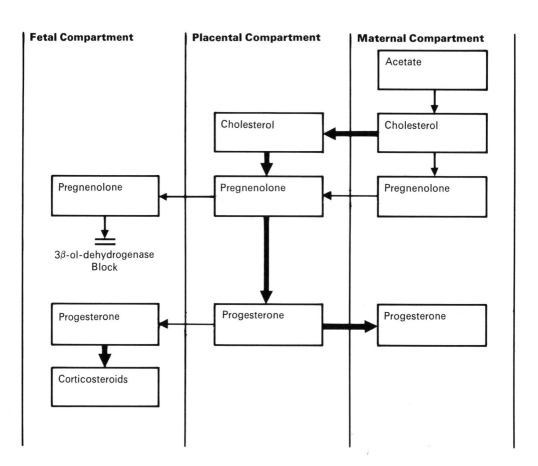

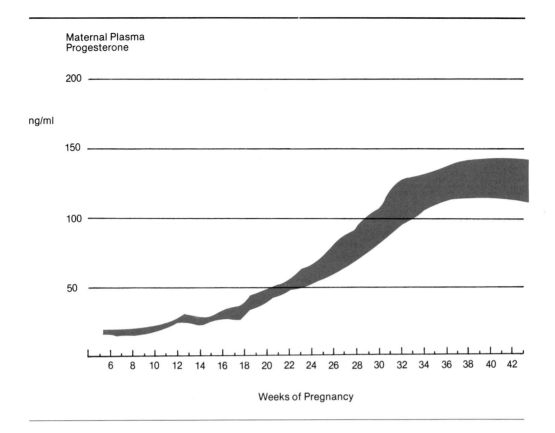

Maternal Plasma Progesterone

ng/ml

Weeks of Pregnancy

In contrast to estrogen, progesterone production by the placenta is largely independent of the quantity of precursor available, the uteroplacental perfusion, fetal well-being, or even the presence of a live fetus. This is because the fetus contributes essentially no precursor. The majority of placental progesterone is derived from maternal cholesterol which is readily available. At term a small portion (3%) is derived from maternal pregnenolone. The cholesterol utilized for progesterone synthesis enters the trophoblast as low density lipoprotein (LDL)-cholesterol, by means of the process of endocytosis (internalization) involving the LDL cell membrane receptors. (2) Hydrolysis of the protein component of LDL may yield amino acids for the fetus, and essential fatty acids may be derived from hydrolysis of the cholesterol esters.

Amniotic fluid progesterone concentration is maximal between 10 and 20 weeks, then decreases gradually. Myometrial levels are about 3 times higher than maternal plasma levels early in pregnancy, remain high, and are about equal to the maternal plasma concentration at term.

In early pregnancy the levels of 17-hydroxyprogesterone rise, marking the activity of the corpus luteum. By the 10th week of gestation this compound has returned to baseline levels, indicating that the placenta has little 17-hydroxylase activity. However, beginning about the 32nd week there is a second, more gradual rise in 17-hydroxyprogesterone, due to placental utilization of fetal precursors.

273

There are two active metabolites of progesterone which increase significantly during pregnancy. There is about a 10-fold increase of the 5α-reduced metabolite. (3) This compound contributes to the refractory state in pregnancy against the pressor action of angiotensin-II. The circulating level, however, is the same in normal and hypertensive pregnancies. The concentration at term of deoxycorticosterone (DOC) is 1200 times the nonpregnant levels. Some of this is due to the 3–4-fold increase in cortisol binding globulin during pregnancy, but a significant amount is due to 21-hydroxylation of circulating progesterone in the kidney. (4) This activity is significant during pregnancy because the rate is proportional to the plasma concentration of progesterone. The fetal kidney is also active in 21-hydroxylation of the progesterone secreted by the placenta into the fetal circulation. At the present time there is no physiologic role known for DOC during pregnancy.

Little is known about specific functions for the various steroids produced throughout pregnancy. Progesterone appears to have a role in parturition as will be discussed in Chapter 11. It also has been suggested that progesterone may be important in suppressing the maternal immunological response to fetal antigens, preventing maternal rejection of the trophoblast. (5) Progesterone clearly has an important role in allowing implantation. Whereas the human corpus luteum makes significant amounts of estradiol, it is progesterone and not estrogen that is required for successful implantation. (6) Since implantation normally occurs about 6–7 days after ovulation, and human chorionic gonadotropin (HCG) must appear by the 10th day after ovulation to rescue the corpus luteum, the blastocyst must successfully implant and secrete HCG within a narrow window of time. In the first 5–6 weeks of pregnancy, HCG stimulation of the corpus luteum results in the secretion of about 25 mg of progesterone and 0.5 mg of estradiol daily. While estrogen levels begin to increase at 4–5 weeks due to placental secretion, progesterone production by the placenta does not significantly increase until about 10–11 weeks after ovulation.

Perhaps the most important role for progesterone is to serve as the principal substrate pool for fetal adrenal gland production of gluco- and mineralocorticoids. The fetal adrenal gland is extremely active, but produces steroids with a 3β-hydroxy-Δ^5 configuration like pregnenolone and dehydroepiandrosterone, rather than 3-keto-Δ^4 products such as progesterone. The fetus therefore lacks significant activity of the 3β-hydroxysteroid dehydrogenase, Δ^{4-5} isomerase system. Thus the fetus must borrow progesterone from the placenta to circumvent this lack, in order to synthesize the biologically important corticosteroids. In return the fetus supplies what the placenta lacks, 19 carbon compounds to serve as precursors for estrogens.

Estrogens

The basic precursors of estrogens are 19 carbon androgens. However, there is a virtual absence of 17-hydroxylation and 17–20 desmolase activity in the human placenta. As a result, 21 carbon products (progesterone and pregnenolone) cannot be converted to 19 carbon steroids (androstenedione and dehydroepiandrosterone). Like progesterone, estrogen produced by the placenta must derive its precursors from outside of the placenta.

The androgen compounds utilized for estrogen synthesis in human pregnancy are, in the early months of gestation, derived from the maternal blood stream. By the 20th week of pregnancy, the vast majority of estrogen excreted in the maternal urine is derived from fetal androgens. In particular, approximately 90% of estriol excretion can be accounted for by dehydroepiandrosterone sulfate (DHAS) production by the fetal adrenal gland. (7)

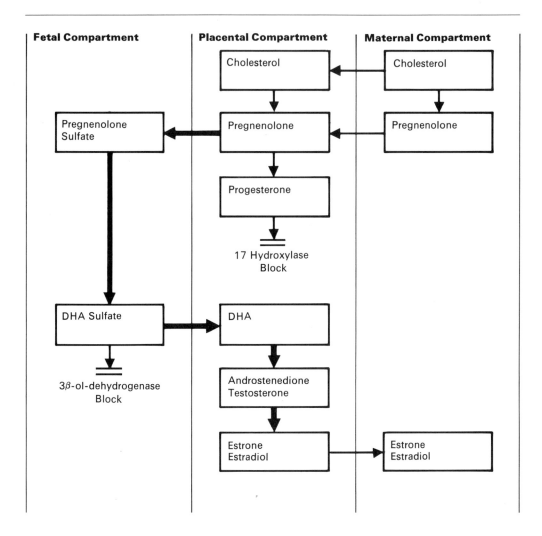

The fetal endocrine compartment is also characterized by rapid and extensive conjugation of steroids with sulfate. Perhaps this is a protective mechanism, blocking the biologic effects of potent steroids present in such great quantities. In order to utilize fetal precursors, the placenta must be extremely efficient in cleaving the sulfate conjugates brought to it via the fetal bloodstream. Indeed the sulfatase activity in the placenta is rapid and quantitatively very significant. It is recognized that a deficiency in placental sulfatase is associated with low estrogen excretion, giving clinical importance to this metabolic step. This syndrome will be discussed in greater detail later in this chapter.

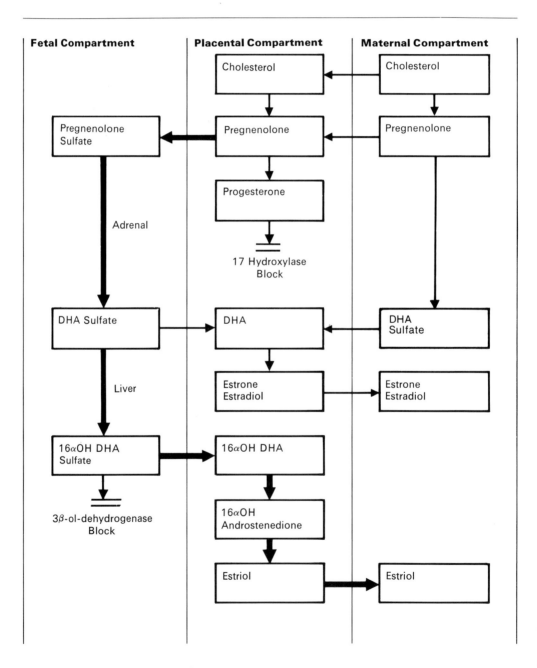

The placenta also lacks 16α-hydroxylation ability, and estriol with its 16α-hydroxyl group therefore must be derived from an immediate fetal precursor. The fetal liver is very active in 16α-hydroxylation. Therefore the fetal adrenal provides DHAS as precursor for placental production of estrone and estradiol, and the fetal adrenal, with the aid of 16α-hydroxylation in the fetal liver, provides the 16α-hydroxydehydroepiandrosterone sulfate for placental estriol formation. After birth, neonatal 16-hydroxylation activity rapidly disappears. The maternal contribution of DHAS to total estrogen synthesis must be negligible because in the absence of normal fetal adrenal glands (as in an anencephalic infant) maternal estrogen levels and excretion are extremely low. The fetal adrenals secrete more than 200 mg of DHAS daily, about 10 times more than the mother. (8)

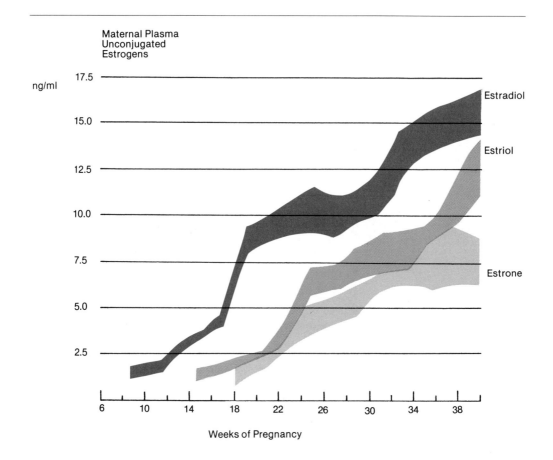

The concentrations of the unconjugated compounds in the maternal compartment for the three major estrogens in pregnancy are as follows:

1. The rise in estrone begins at 6–10 weeks and individual values range from 2 to 30 ng/ml at term. (9) This wide range in normal values precludes the use of estrone measurements in clinical applications.

2. Individual estradiol values vary between 6 and 40 ng/ml at 36 weeks of gestation, and then undergo an accelerated rate of increase. (9) At term, an equal amount of estradiol arises from maternal DHAS and fetal DHAS and its importance in fetal monitoring is minimal.

3. Estriol is first detectable at 9 weeks when the fetal adrenal gland secretion of precursor becomes active. Estriol concentrations plateau at 31–35 weeks, then increase again at 35–36 weeks. (10)

During pregnancy, estrone and estradiol excretion is increased about 100 times over nonpregnant levels. However, the increase in maternal estriol excretion is about a thousand-fold. This enormous rise coupled with its dependence on fetal precursor is the basis of its utility in fetal monitoring.

The estrogens presented to the maternal bloodstream are rapidly metabolized by the maternal liver prior to excretion into the maternal urine as a variety of more than 20 products. The bulk of these maternal urinary estrogens are composed of glucosiduronates conjugated at the 16-position. Significant amounts of the 3-glucosiduronate and the 3-sulfate-16-glucosiduronate are also excreted. Only approximately 8–10% of the maternal blood estriol is unconjugated.

The Fetal
Adrenal Cortex

The fetal adrenal cortex is differentiated by 7 weeks into a thick inner fetal zone and thin outer definitive zone. Early in pregnancy, adrenal growth and development are remarkable, and the gland achieves a size equal to or larger than that of the kidney by the end of the first trimester. After the first trimester the adrenal glands slowly decrease in size until a second spurt in growth begins at about 34–35 weeks. The glands remain proportionately larger than the adult adrenal glands. After delivery, the fetal zone (about 85% of the bulk of the gland) rapidly degenerates to be replaced by the adult definitive zone of the adrenal cortex. Thus the specific steroidogenic characteristics of the fetus are associated with a specific morphologic change of the adrenal gland which is limited in function to the time period of fetal life.

Fetal DHAS production rises steadily concomitant with the increase in fetal adrenal weight. (11) The well-known increase in maternal estrogen levels is significantly influenced by the increased availability of fetal DHAS as a precursor. Indeed, the accelerated rise in maternal estrogen levels near term can be explained in part by an increase in fetal DHAS. The stimulus for the substantial adrenal growth and steroid production has been a puzzle.

Early in pregnancy, the adrenal gland may function without ACTH, perhaps in response to HCG. After 20 weeks, fetal ACTH is required. During the last 12–14 weeks of pregnancy, however, when fetal ACTH levels are declining progressively, the adrenal quadruples in size. (12) Because pituitary prolactin is the only fetal pituitary hormone to increase throughout pregnancy, paralleling fetal adrenal gland size changes, it has been proposed that fetal prolactin is the critical tropic substance. (13) In experimental preparations, however, only ACTH exerts a steroidogenic effect. There is no fetal adrenal response to prolactin, HCG, growth hormone, or melanocyte-stimulating hormone (MSH). (14) Furthermore, in patients treated with bromocriptine, fetal blood prolactin levels are suppressed, but DHAS levels are unchanged. (15)

There is no question that ACTH is essential for the steroidogenic mechanism of the fetal adrenal gland. (16) ACTH activates adenylate cyclase, leading to steroidogenesis. Soon the supply of cholesterol becomes rate-limiting. Further ACTH action results in an increase in LDL receptors leading to an increased uptake of circulating LDL-cholesterol. With internalization of LDL-cholesterol, hydrolysis by lysosomal enzymes of the cholesterol ester makes cholesterol available for steroidogenesis. For this reason, fetal plasma levels of LDL are low, and after birth newborn levels of LDL rise as the fetal adrenal involutes.

The unique features of the fetal adrenal gland can be ascribed to its high estrogen environment. A series of tissue culture studies has demonstrated that hormonal peptides of pituitary or placental origin are not the factors which are responsible for the behavior of the fetal adrenal gland. (17–19) Estrogens at high concentration inhibit 3β-hydroxysteroid dehydrogenase-isomerase activity in the fetal adrenal gland, and in the presence of ACTH enhance the secretion of dehydroepiandrosterone (DHA). Estradiol concentrations of 10–100 ng/ml were required to inhibit cortisol secretion. (20) The total estrogen concentrations in the fetus are easily in this range. The hyperplasia of the fetal adrenal cortex is the result of the high ACTH due to the relatively low cortisol levels, a consequence of the enzyme inhibition. With birth and the loss of exposure to estrogen, the fetal adrenal gland quickly changes to the adult type of gland.

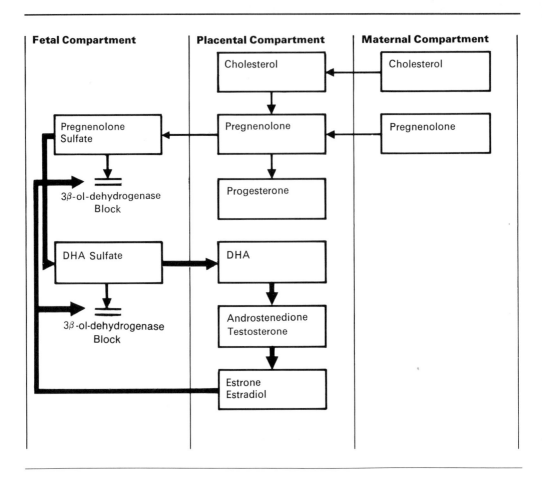

Fetal Compartment	Placental Compartment	Maternal Compartment
	Cholesterol	Cholesterol
Pregnenolone Sulfate	Pregnenolone	Pregnenolone
3β-ol-dehydrogenase Block	Progesterone	
DHA Sulfate	DHA	
3β-ol-dehydrogenase Block	Androstenedione Testosterone	
	Estrone Estradiol	

The principal mission of the fetal adrenal may be to provide DHAS as the basic precursor for placental estrogen production. Estrogen, in turn, feeds back to the adrenal to direct steroidogenesis along the Δ5 pathway to provide even more of its precursor, DHAS. Thus far this is the only known function for DHAS. It is still unclear, however, why there is an increase in activity in the last 4–5 weeks of pregnancy when fetal ACTH is decreasing. One explanation could be a change in sensitivity of the adrenal gland as term approaches, perhaps due to an increase in bioactive ACTH (not detected in the studies utilizing radioimmunoassay).

Measurement of Estrogen in Pregnancy

Because pregnancy is characterized by a great increase in maternal estrogen levels, and estrogen production is dependent upon fetal and placental steroidogenic cooperation, the amount of estrogen present in the maternal blood or urine reflects both fetal and placental enzymatic capability and hence, well-being. Attention has been focused on estriol because 90% of maternal estriol is derived from fetal precursors. The end product to be assayed in the maternal blood or urine is influenced by a multitude of factors. Availability of precursor from the fetal adrenal gland is a prime requisite as well as the ability of the placenta to carry out its conversion steps. Maternal metabolism of the product as well as the efficiency of maternal renal excretion of the product can modify the daily amount of estrogen in the urine. Blood flow to any of the key organs in the fetus, placenta, and mother becomes important. In addition, drugs or diseases can affect any level in the cascade of events leading up to assay of estrogen.

For years, measurement of estrogen in a 24-hour urine collection was the standard method of assessing fetal well-being. This has been replaced by radioimmunoassay of unconjugated estriol in the plasma. Assays which measure the total plasma estriol show the same large variations from day to day as seen with the old urinary assays. It is important that the clinical use of estrogen assay in pregnancy be limited to the measurement of unconjugated estriol. (21) Because of its short half-life (5–10 minutes) in the maternal circulation, unconjugated estriol shows less variation than urinary or total blood estriol.

Normal Values and Interpretation. There are two essential aspects to the clinical use of estriol assays. First, a single specimen is meaningless. Daily assays must be performed on morning blood samples to provide a serial assessment of sequential changes. Second, to be significant, there must be a decrease of approximately 40% from the mean of the three highest consecutive values. (21, 22) While estrogen levels in the mother are related to the size of the fetal adrenal gland and its production of precursor, there is a poor correlation between birth weight and plasma estriol levels. (21) Macrosomia is not always associated with high estriol levels. On the other hand, excessive adrenal activity as in congenital adrenal hyperplasia can be associated with unusually high levels. (23)

Problems. Drugs which affect the maternal estrogen level include corticosteroids and antibiotics. Corticosteroids administered to the mother cross the placenta poorly, and large amounts (the equivalent of 75 mg of cortisol daily) are required to suppress fetal adrenal production of estriol precursor. The synthetic steroids, dexamethasone and betamethasone, however, cross the placenta more easily, and maternal estriol assessment is not reliable for at least 1 week, and sometimes 2 weeks, after the last dose. (24) Antibiotics which affect the flora of the maternal gastrointestinal tract depress maternal total estriol levels by interfering with the enterohepatic circulation. Such antibiotics inhibit the hydrolysis of the biliary estriol conjugates in the gut, preventing their reabsorption and reconjugation, leading to loss of estriol in the feces. (25) Total blood and urinary estriol decline, but unconjugated estriol is unaffected. Falsely elevated blood total estriols will be encountered in the presence of renal disease or when a patient is receiving oxytocin for the induction of labor because of the antidiuretic action of oxytocin, but once again unconjugated estriol remains unchanged. The measurement of unconjugated estriol by a specific radioimmunoassay is, therefore, the method of choice.

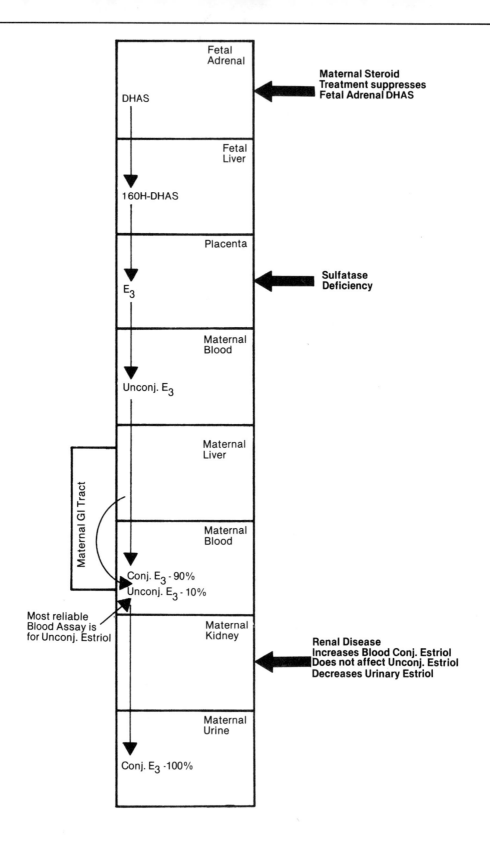

Amniotic Fluid Estrogen Measurements	Amniotic fluid estriol is correlated with the fetal estrogen pattern rather than the maternal. Most of the estriol in the amniotic fluid is present as 16-glucosiduronate or as 3-sulfate-16-glucosiduronate. A small amount exists as 3-sulfate. Very little unconjugated estriol is present in the amniotic fluid because free estriol is rapidly transferred across the placenta and membranes. Estriol sulfate is low in concentration because the placental and fetal membranes hydrolyze the sulfated conjugates, and the free estriol is then passed out of the fluid.

Because the membranes and the placenta have no glucuronidase activity, the glucosiduronate conjugates are removed slowly from the fetus. The glucosiduronates therefore predominate in the fetal urine and the amniotic fluid. Because of the slow changes in glucosiduronates, measurements of amniotic fluid estriol have wide variations in both normal and abnormal pregnancies. An important clinical use for amniotic fluid estrogen measurements has not emerged. |
| Estetrol | Estetrol (15α-hydroxyestriol) is formed from fetal precursors, and is very dependent upon 15-hydroxylation activity in the fetal liver. The capacity for 15-hydroxylation of estrogens increases during fetal life, reaching a maximum at term. This activity then declines during infancy and is low, absent, or undetectable in adults. The clinical use of maternal blood and urine estetrol measurements is of no advantage over the usual estriol assessment. |
| Clinical Uses of Estriol Assays | Assessment of maternal estriol levels has been superceded by various biophysical fetal monitoring techniques such as nonstress testing, stress testing, and measurement of fetal breathing and activity. Nevertheless, in certain clinical situations the addition of estriol assays is useful. The combination of a low estriol and a positive stress test is ominous. (21, 26) Certainly patients should not be managed by estriols alone. While a low estriol and a positive stress test indicate a fetus in jeopardy, a low estriol with a negative stress test allows postponement of intervention.

Diabetes Mellitus. The classic obstetric dilemma in diabetes has been when to deliver the patient. The risk of neonatal death when the infant is delivered before 38 weeks of gestation is significantly higher than in the normal population. On the other hand, the risk of sudden intrauterine fetal loss rises when the pregnant diabetic is allowed to go to term.

What is it that makes the diabetic pregnancy unique in that fetal jeopardy is heralded by a drop in maternal estriol levels? The answer to this question is not known. It is clinically recognized that the diabetic pregnancy is marked by the association between intrauterine fetal demise and a rapid decline in estriol. Fetal death can occur within 24 hours of a fall in estriol. The rapid change in estriol suggests a sudden failure of the fetal adrenal gland to provide precursors. |

283

Either daily estriol assays or frequent fetal heart rate monitoring is successful in testing fetal status in diabetic pregnancy. (22) Combining the two methods achieves the most effective means of avoiding unnecessary intervention. It is our clinical practice to follow diabetic pregnancies with fetal heart rate monitoring, adding daily estriol assays when the patient is a severe diabetic, if there is a history of previous poor fetal outcome, and when a diabetic patient is hospitalized.

Estriols and Hypertension. The use of serial estriol assays in patients with toxemia has a different orientation when compared to diabetic pregnancies. Whereas in diabetic pregnancies estriol is a means of detecting fetal distress and impending demise, in toxemia the obstetrician uses estriol measurements to be assured that the fetus is growing and doing well, and that the pregnancy may be allowed to continue until fetal maturity has been attained. Because unconjugated estriol is not excreted by the kidney, its concentration is not affected by changes in maternal renal function. A rising normal estriol excretion is very reassuring that the fetus is doing well.

Chronically low levels of estriol during pregnancy are a grave prognostic sign for the fetus. Low estriol values during a pregnancy with hypertension are associated with elevated perinatal mortality, (27) and in a small series, we reported that chronically low estriol excretion in toxemic pregnancy was associated with a high incidence of neurologic defects. (28)

The first-line assessment of fetal well-being in patients with hypertension is nonstress and stress testing. If a patient is hospitalized, daily estriol measurements provide additional useful information. Chronically low estriol levels indicate fetal jeopardy, while normal rising values indicate that conservative management is justified from the fetal point of view.

Erythroblastosis Fetalis. In pregnancies with erythroblastosis fetalis, the use of estriol assays has no proven value. Normal estriol values do not predict the condition of the fetus, and in particular, there is no correlation with the fetal hemoglobin at birth.

Prolonged Gestation. Approximately 10% of all pregnancies continue past the 42nd week, but not all of these post-term pregnancies result in the birth of a postmature baby. Postmature infants have a 2–3-fold increase in perinatal mortality, a higher rate of intrapartum asphyxia, a 20% incidence of neonatal hypoglycemia, and a greater tendency to develop health problems in the first 3 years of life. Interruption of the pregnancy would be a simple matter if every patient undelivered after the 42nd week of gestation could be easily delivered by induction of labor. Unfortunately, this is not the case, and some means of diagnosing the true postmature fetus is an important clinical issue.

In prolonged pregnancies, assessment of estriol levels may be rational, but it is usually not practical. One cannot predict which patients will carry their pregnancies to 42 weeks and beyond, therefore baseline serial assays are not available for comparison and proper judgment. The use of fetal heart rate monitoring is the most practical approach to the management of a post-term pregnancy.

Intrauterine Growth Retardation. In general, it can be stated that the failure to demonstrate a rising estriol level is consistent with a failure of the fetus to grow normally. As such, the estriol assessment is an adjunct in the evaluation of suspected intrauterine growth retardation.

Placental Sulfatase
Deficiency

Patients with the placental sulfatase disorder are unable to hydrolyze DHAS or 16α-hydroxy-DHAS, and, therefore, the placenta cannot form normal amounts of estrogen. A deficiency in placental sulfatase is usually discovered when patients go beyond term and are found to have extremely low estriol levels and no evidence of fetal distress. The patients usually fail to go into labor and require delivery by cesarean section. Through 1976, less than 20 cases had been reported. (29, 30) All newborn children have been male, suggesting that the disorder is due to an X-linked recessive gene. The characteristic steroid findings are as follows: extremely low estriol and estetrol in the mother with extremely high amniotic fluid DHAS and normal amniotic fluid DHA and androstenedione. The normal DHA and androstenedione with a high DHAS rule out the adreno-genital syndrome. The small amount of estriol which is present in these patients probably arises from 16-hydroxylation of DHAS in the maternal liver, thus providing 16-hydroxylated DHA to the placenta for aromatization to estriol. Measurement in maternal urine of steroids derived from fetal sulfated compounds is a simple and reliable means of prenatal diagnosis. This can be done by measuring just one steroid, 16α-hydroxy-DHA, which can be up to 20 times increased over the normal mean value. (31) Demonstration of a high level of DHAS in the amniotic fluid is also reliable.

**Protein Hormones
of the Placenta**

Human Chorionic
Gonadotropin (HCG)

Human chorionic gonadotropin is a glycoprotein, a peptide framework to which carbohydrate sidechains are attached. Alterations in the carbohydrate components (about one third of the molecular weight) change the biologic properties. For example, the long half-life of HCG is approximately 24 hours as compared to 2 hours for luteinizing hormone (LH), a 10-fold difference which is due mainly to the greater sialic acid content of HCG. As with the other glycoproteins, follicle-stimulating hormone (FSH), LH, and thyroid stimulating hormone (TSH), HCG consists of two noncovalently linked subunits, called alpha (α) and beta (β). The α subunits in these glycoprotein hormones are virtually identical, consisting of 89–92 amino acids. Unique biological activity as well as specificity in radioimmunoassays must be attributed to the molecular differences in the β subunits.

285

The 30 terminal amino acids of the β-HCG are unique and different from the sequence on LH. Despite this difference (which allows specific antisera to discriminate between HCG and LH in assays) HCG is biologically similar to LH. To this day, the only definitely known function for HCG is support of the corpus luteum, taking over for LH on about the 8th day after ovulation when β-HCG can be first detected in maternal blood.

Continued survival of the corpus luteum is totally dependent upon HCG, and, in turn, the survival of the pregnancy is dependent upon steroids from the corpus luteum until the 7th week of pregnancy. (1) From the 7th week to the 10th week, the corpus luteum is gradually replaced by the placenta, and by the 10th week, removal of the corpus luteum will not be followed by steroid withdrawal abortion.

It is very probable, but not conclusively proven, that HCG stimulates steroidogenesis in the early fetal testes, so that androgen production will ensue and masculine differentiation can be accomplished. (32) It also appears that the function of the inner fetal zone of the adrenal cortex may depend upon HCG for steroidogenesis early in pregnancy. The mechanism for control of placental steroidogenesis is unknown and it is not certain whether the presence of HCG is necessary.

HCG is secreted by the syncytiotrophoblast, reaching a maximum level of 50,000–100,000 mIU/ml at 10 weeks of gestation. The old bioassay tests for pregnancy have been replaced by immunological and receptor tests for the presence of HCG in maternal urine and blood. The tests are reliable with essentially no falsely positive reactions. Falsely negative results can occur prior to the 5th and 6th week of gestation because the sensitivity of the tests must be maintained at a level high enough to avoid crossreactions with LH.

Why does the corpus luteum involute at the time that HCG is reaching its highest levels? One possibility is that a specific inhibitory agent becomes active at this time. Another is down-regulation of receptors by the high levels of HCG. In early pregnancy, down-regulation may be avoided because HCG is secreted in an episodic fashion. (33)

HCG levels decrease to about 10,000–20,000 mIU/ml by 20 weeks and remain at that level to term. HCG levels close to term are higher in women bearing female fetuses. (34, 35) This is true of serum levels, placental content, urinary levels, and amniotic fluid concentrations. The mechanism and purpose of this difference are not known.

There are two clinical conditions in which blood HCG titers are very helpful, trophoblastic disease and ectopic pregnancies. Following molar pregnancies, in patients without persistent disease, the HCG titer should fall to a nondetectable level by 15 weeks. Patients with trophoblastic

286

disease show an abnormal curve (a titer greater than 500 mlU/ml) frequently by 3 weeks and usually by 6 weeks. (36)

Virtually 100% of patients suspected of an ectopic pregnancy, but not having the condition, will have a negative blood HCG assay. (37) A positive test can also be utilized in diagnosis. The HCG level increases at different rates in normal and ectopic pregnancies. In a normal pregnancy, the HCG should approximately double every 2 days. (38) An HCG above 6000 mlU/ml is almost always associated with an intrauterine pregnancy. When the HCG titer is below 6000 mlU/ml and ultrasound examination fails to identify an intrauterine pregnancy, a patient may be managed expectantly if the HCG titer doubles in 2 days. (39) If the titer does not double, laparoscopy is indicated. Laparoscopy is also indicated when the titer is above 6000 mlU/ml and ultrasound shows no evidence of an intrauterine pregnancy.

Human Placental Lactogen (HPL)

Human placental lactogen (HPL), also secreted by the syncytiotrophoblast, is a single chain polypeptide held together by two disulfide bonds. It is about 96% similar to human growth hormone (HGH), but has only 3% of HGH somatotropin activity. Although HPL has about 50% of the lactogenic activity of sheep prolactin in certain bioassays, it is probably not lactogenic in human pregnancy. Its half-life is short, about 15 minutes; hence its appeal as an index of placental problems. The level of HPL in the maternal circulation is correlated with fetal and placental weight, plateauing in the last 4 weeks of pregnancy. There is no circadian variation, and only minute amounts of HPL enter the fetal circulation. Very high maternal levels are found in association with multiple gestations; levels up to 40 μg/ml have been found with quadruplets and quintuplets. An abnormally low level is anything less than 4 μg/ml in the last trimester.

Physiologic Function. Experimentally, the maternal level of HPL can be altered by changing the circulating level of glucose. HPL is elevated with hypoglycemia and depressed with hyperglycemia. This information along with studies in fasted pregnant women have led to the following formulation for the physiologic function of HPL. (40–45)

The metabolic role of HPL is to mobilize lipids as free fatty acids. In the fed state, there is abundant glucose available, leading to increased insulin levels, lipogenesis, and glucose utilization. This is associated with decreased gluconeogenesis, and a decrease in the circulating free fatty acid levels, as the free fatty acids are utilized in the process of lipogenesis to deposit storage packets of triglycerides (see Chapter 14, "Obesity").

287

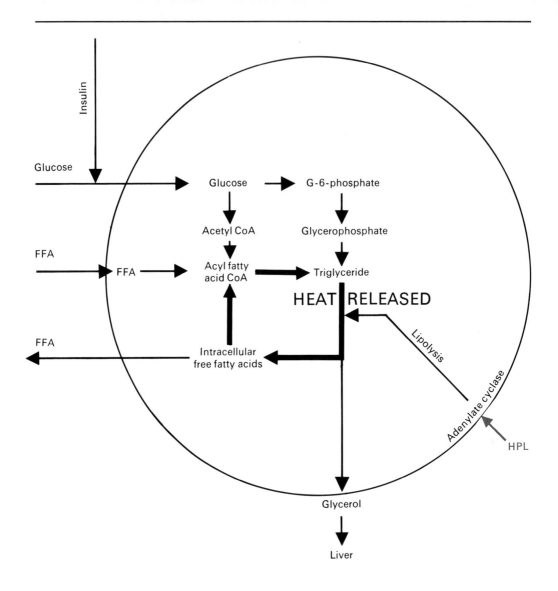

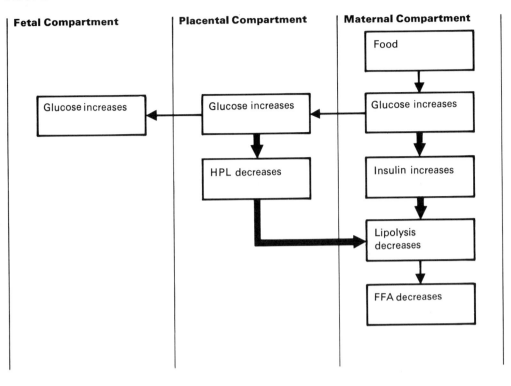

Pregnancy has been likened to a state of "accelerated starvation," (42) characterized by a relative hypoglycemia in the fasting state. This state is due to two major influences:

1. Glucose provides the major, although not the entire, fuel requirement for the fetus. A difference in gradient causes a constant transfer of glucose from the mother to the fetus.

2. Placental hormones, specifically estrogen and progesterone, and especially HPL, interfere with the action of maternal insulin. In the second half of pregnancy when HPL levels rise approximately 10-fold, HPL is a major force in the diabetogenic effects of pregnancy. The latter is characterized by increased levels of insulin associated with decreased cellular response.

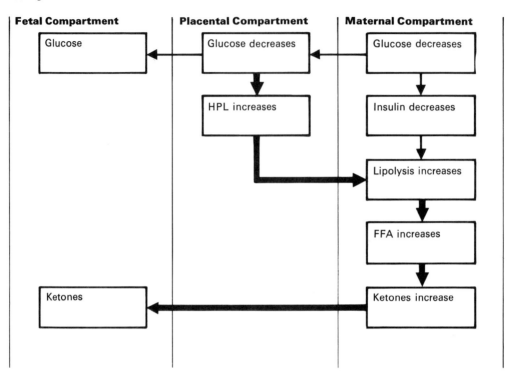

In the fasting state, as the supplies of glucose decrease, HPL levels rise, stimulating lipolysis leading to an increase in circulating free fatty acids in order to provide a different fuel for the mother so that glucose and amino acids can be conserved for the fetus. With sustained fasting, maternal fat is utilized for fuel to such an extent that maternal ketone levels rise. There is limited transport of free fatty acids across the placenta. Therefore, when glucose becomes scarce for the fetus, fetal tissues utilize the ketones which do cross the placenta. Thus, decreased glucose levels lead to decreased insulin and increased HPL, increasing lipolysis and ketone levels. HPL may also enhance the fetal uptake of ketones and amino acids. The mechanism for the insulin antagonism by HPL may be the HPL-stimulated increase in free fatty acid levels, which in turn directly interferes with insulin-directed entry of glucose into cells.

This mechanism can be viewed as an important means to provide fuel for the fetus between maternal meals. However, with a sustained state of inadequate glucose intake the subsequent ketosis may impair brain development and function. Pregnancy is not the time to severely restrict caloric intake.

HPL Clinical Uses. Blood levels of HPL are related to placental function. While some studies indicated that HPL was valuable in screening patients for potential fetal complications, others have not supported the use of antepartum HPL measurements. (46–48) Even though utilization of the HPL assay can have an impact on perinatal care, (49) fetal heart rate monitoring techniques are more reliably predictive and sensitive for assessing fetal well-being. Furthermore, a totally uneventful pregnancy has been reported despite undetectable HPL. (50)

Previous suggestions that a low or declining level of HPL and a high level of HCG are characteristic of trophoblastic disease were not accurate. Because of the rapid clearance of HPL, aborting molar pregnancies are likely to have low levels of HPL, while the level of HCG is still high. However, intact molar pregnancies may have elevated levels of both HPL and HCG. (51)

Human Chorionic Thyrotropin (HCT)

The human placenta contains two thyrotropic substances. One is called human chorionic thyrotropin (HCT), similar in size and action to pituitary TSH. The content in the normal placenta is very small. HCT differs from the other glycoproteins in that it does not appear to share the common α subunit. Antiserum generated to α-HCG does not neutralize the biologic activities of HCT, but it does that of HCG and pituitary TSH. Rarely, patients with trophoblastic disease may have hyperthyroidism. Studies indicate that HCG has intrinsic thyrotropic activity, and thus it is the second placental thyrotropic substance. (52) On a molecular basis it is calculated that HCG contains approximately 1/4000th of the thyrotropic activity of human TSH. (53) In conditions with very elevated HCG levels, the thyrotropic activity can be sufficient to produce hyperthyroidism.

Human Chorionic Adrenocorticotropin Hormone

The rise in free cortisol that takes place throughout pregnancy may be due to ACTH production by the placenta. (54) The placental content of ACTH is higher than can be accounted for by the contribution of sequestered blood. In addition, cortisol levels in pregnant women are resistant to dexamethasone suppression, suggesting that there is a component of maternal ACTH that does not originate in the maternal pituitary gland. One can speculate that placental ACTH raises maternal adrenal activity in order to provide the basic building blocks (cholesterol and pregnenolone) for placental steroidogenesis.

Other Placental Peptides

β-Endorphin and β-lipotropin are synthesized in the human placenta. Both fetal and maternal blood levels of β-endorphin increase during labor, probably originating from the pituitary glands and secreted in parallel with ACTH. (55) Fetal levels at delivery are higher than adult levels, and are inversely correlated with arterial pH and pO_2. (56) Whether measurement can be utilized clinically remains to be determined.

291

The human placenta contains a number of releasing and inhibiting hormones, including gonadotropin releasing hormone (GnRH), thyroid releasing hormone (TRH) and somatostatin. (57) Immunoreactive GnRH can be localized in the cytotrophoblast. It is not known whether chorionic GnRH plays a role in HCG synthesis or placental steroidogenesis.

The trophoblast secretes a pregnancy-specific β_1-globulin into the maternal circulation. It appears shortly after implantation and increases steadily until term. Its functions and importance are unknown, but it is already saddled with a difficult name, Schwangerschafts protein 1 (SP_1). The placenta pours a flood of proteins into the maternal circulation, and it remains to be seen whether their identity and function can be sorted out.

α-Fetoprotein

α-Fetoprotein (AFP) is a relatively unique glycoprotein derived largely from fetal liver, and partially from the yolk sac until it degenerates at about 12 weeks. Its function is unknown but it may serve as a protein carrier of steroid hormones in fetal blood. Peak levels are reached early in the second trimester (16–18 weeks), then levels decrease gradually until term. Because AFP is highly concentrated in the CNS, availability of CNS to the amniotic fluid (as with neural tube defects) results in elevated amniotic fluid and maternal blood levels. Other fetal abnormalities, such as intestinal obstruction, omphalocele, and congenital nephrosis, are also associated with high levels of AFP in the amniotic fluid. Maternal blood levels of AFP reflect the amniotic fluid level. Because of a high incidence of false positive results in maternal serum AFP screening programs, each patient with a high blood level requires ultrasound evaluation to detect anencephaly, multiple gestation, erroneous dating or intrauterine demise, and then, if necessary, amniocentesis to measure the amniotic fluid AFP. An elevated amniotic fluid AFP deserves further meticulous ultrasound examination, because not all of these cases are associated with an abnormal fetus.

Relaxin

Relaxin is a peptide hormone produced by the corpus luteum of pregnancy, and not detected in men or nonpregnant women. While it has been argued that the human corpus luteum is the sole source of relaxin in pregnancy, it has also been identified in human placenta. (58, 59) The maternal serum concentration rises during the first trimester and declines in the second trimester. (60) This suggests a role in maintaining early pregnancy, but its function is not really known. In animals relaxin softens the cervix, inhibits uterine contractions, and relaxes the pubic symphysis.

Prolactin

The decidual endometrium of pregnancy appears to have a specialized endocrine function, the secretion of prolactin. Prolactin is synthesized by endometrium during a normal menstrual cycle, but this synthesis is not initiated until histologic decidualization begins. (61) During pregnancy prolactin secretion is limited to the fetal pituitary, the maternal pituitary, and the uterus. Neither trophoblast nor fetal membranes synthesize prolactin, but both the myometrium and endometrium can produce prolactin. (62, 63) The endometrium requires the presence of progesterone to initiate prolactin, while progesterone suppresses prolactin synthesis in the myometrium. (63) Prolactin derived from the decidua is the source of the prolactin found in the amniotic fluid. (64)

Amniotic fluid concentrations of prolactin parallel maternal serum concentration until the 10th week of pregnancy, rise markedly until the 20th week, and then decrease. The maternal and fetal blood levels of prolactin are derived from the respective pituitary glands. Bromocriptine suppression of pituitary secretion of prolactin throughout pregnancy produces minimal maternal and fetal blood levels, yet there is normal fetal growth and development, and amniotic fluid levels are unchanged. (65) Fortunately decidual secretion of prolactin is unaffected by bromocriptine because decidual prolactin may be important for fluid and electrolyte regulation of the amniotic fluid.

No clinical significance can be attached to maternal and fetal blood levels of prolactin in abnormal pregnancies. Decidual and amniotic fluid prolactin levels are lower, however, in hypertensive pregnancies and in patients with polyhydramnios. (66) Prolactin receptors are present in the chorion laeve, and their concentration is lower in patients with polyhydramnios. (67).

Perinatal Thyroid Physiology

The human fetal thyroid gland develops the capacity to concentrate iodine and synthesize hormone between 10 and 13 weeks of gestation, the same time that the pituitary begins to synthesize TSH. (68) Some thyroid development and hormone synthesis are possible in the absence of the pituitary gland, but optimal function requires TSH. By 12–14 weeks, development of the pituitary-thyroid system is complete. Function is minimal, however, until an abrupt increase in fetal TSH occurs at 20 weeks. As with gonadotropin and other pituitary hormone secretion, this thyroid function correlates with the maturation of the hypothalamus and the development of the pituitary portal vascular system, which makes releasing hormone available to the pituitary gland.

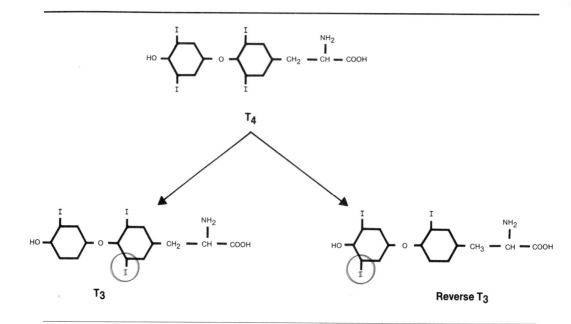

T_4

T_3

Reverse T_3

Fetal TSH levels reach a plateau at 28 weeks, and remain relatively high to term. The free thyroxine (T_4) concentration increases progressively. At term, fetal T_4 levels exceed maternal levels. Thus a state of fetal thyroidal hyperactivity exists near term.

Placental transfer of TSH, T_4, and 3,5,3'-triiodothryonine (T_3) is severely limited in both directions. Indeed, the placenta is essentially impermeable to these substances no matter whether the fetus is euthyroid or hypothyroid. Slight transfer may occur, however, at pharmacologic concentrations.

Removal of one iodine from the phenolic ring of T_4 yields T_3, while removal of an iodine from the nonphenolic ring yields reverse T_3 (RT_3) which is biologically inactive. In a normal adult, about one third of the T_4 secreted daily is deiodinated to T_3, while about 45% is converted to RT_3. About 83% of T_3 is produced from T_4 in peripheral tissues, while 17% is secreted by the thyroid. T_3 is 3–5 times more potent than T_4, and virtually all the biological activity of T_4 can be attributed to the T_3 generated from it. While T_4 may have some intrinsic activity of its own, it serves mainly as a prohormone of T_3. Carbohydrate calories appear to be the primary determinant of T_3 levels in adults. A reciprocal relationship exists between T_3 and RT_3. Low T_3 and elevated RT_3 are seen in a variety of illnesses such as febrile diseases, burn injuries, malnutrition, and anorexia nervosa.

294

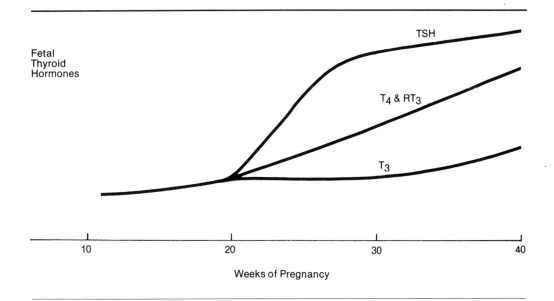

Fetal Thyroid Hormones

TSH

T_4 & RT_3

T_3

10   20   30   40

Weeks of Pregnancy

The major thyroid hormone secreted by the fetus is T_4. Total T_3 and free T_3 levels are low throughout gestation, however, levels of RT_3 are elevated, paralleling the rise in T_4. Like T_3, this compound is derived predominantly from conversion of T_4 in peripheral tissues. The increased production of T_4 in fetal life is compensated by rapid inactivation via conversion to the inactive RT_3.

Treatment of maternal hyperthyroidism with propylthiouricil, even with moderate doses of 100–200 mg daily, suppresses T_4 and increases TSH levels in the newborns. (69) The infants are clinically euthyroid, however, and their laboratory measurements are normal by the 4th to 5th day of life. In addition, follow-up assessment has indicated unimpaired intellectual development in children whose mothers received propylthiouricil during pregnancy. (70)

With delivery, the newborn moves from a state of relative T_3 deficiency to a state of T_3 thyrotoxicosis. Shortly after birth serum TSH concentrations increase rapidly to a peak at 30 minutes of age. They fall to baseline values by 48–72 hours. In response to this increase in TSH, total T_4 and free T_4 increase to peak values by 24–48 hours of age. T_3 levels increase even more, peaking by 24 hours of age. By 3–4 weeks, the thyroidal hyperactivity has disappeared.

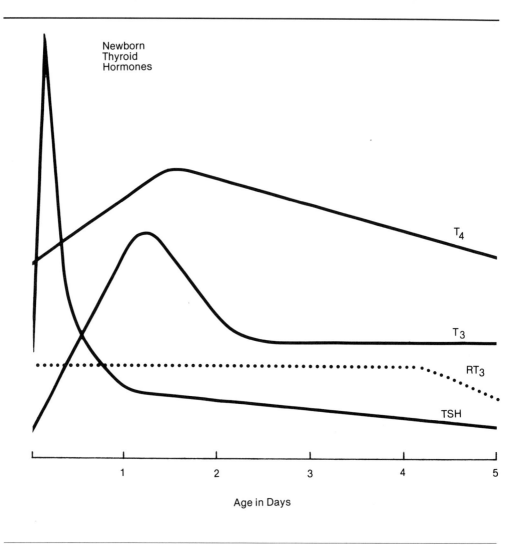

Newborn Thyroid Hormones

T_4

T_3

RT_3

TSH

1   2   3   4   5

Age in Days

The postnatal surge in TSH is accompanied by a prolactin surge, suggesting that both are increased in response to TRH. The TRH surge is thought to be a response to rapid neonatal cooling. A puzzle is the fact that the early increase in T_3 is independent of TSH and is tied in some way to cutting of the umbilical cord. Delaying cord cutting delays the increase in T_3, but TSH levels still reach their peak at 30 minutes. In some way cord cutting augments peripheral (largely liver) conversion of T_4 to T_3. The later increases in T_3 and T_4 (after 2 hours) are due to increased thyroid gland activity. These thyroid changes after birth probably represent defense mechanisms against the sudden entry into the cold world. The high RT_3 levels during pregnancy continue during the first 3–5 days of life, then fall gradually to normal adult levels by 2 weeks.

Summary of Fetal and Newborn Thyroid Changes:

1. TSH and T_4 appear in the fetus at 10–13 weeks. Levels are low until an abrupt rise at 20 weeks.

2. T_4 rises rapidly and exceeds maternal values at term.

3. T_3 levels rise, but concentrations are relatively low, similar to hypothyroid adults.

4. RT_3 levels exceed normal adult levels.

5. The fetal pattern of low T_3 and high RT_3 is similar to that seen with calorie malnutrition.

6. After delivery, TSH peaks at 30 minutes of age, followed by a T_3 peak at 24 hours and a T_4 peak at 24–48 hours. The T_3 increase is independent of the TSH change.

7. High RT_3 levels persist for 3–5 days, after delivery, then reach adult values by 2 weeks.

Newborn Screening for Hypothyroidism

The incidence of neonatal hypothyroidism is about 1/4000 live births. The problem is that congenital hypothyroidism is not apparent clinically at birth. Fortunately, infants with congenital hypothyroidism have low T_4 and high TSH concentrations easily detected in a blood spot, and early treatment before 3 months of age is associated with normal development. (71) There is a familial tendency for hypothyroidism, and if the diagnosis is made in the antepartum period, weekly intraamniotic injections of thyroxine can raise fetal levels of thyroid hormone. Furthermore, a T_4 analog is available which crosses the placenta and can prevent the clinical manifestations of experimental cretinism in the monkey fetus. (72) Amniotic fluid iodothyronines reflect fetal plasma levels. Normal values have been established which allow prenatal diagnosis of fetal hypothyroidism by amniocentesis. (73)

Fetal Lung Maturation

The respiratory distress syndrome consists of progressive atelectasis of the lungs of a newborn infant caused by an increase in surface tension. The pulmonary alveoli are lined with a surface-active phospholipid-protein complex called pulmonary surfactant synthesized in the type II pneumonocyte. It is this surfactant which decreases surface tension, thereby facilitating lung expansion and preventing atelectasis. In full-term fetuses, surfactant is present at birth in sufficient amounts to permit adequate lung expansion and normal breathing. In premature fetuses, however, surfactant is present in lesser amounts, and when insufficient, postnatal lung expansion and ventilation are frequently impaired, resulting in the clinical syndrome of respiratory distress.

297

Phosphatidylcholine (lecithin) has been identified as a major lipid of the surfactant complex. Beginning at 20–22 weeks of pregnancy, a less stable and less active lecithin, palmitoylmyristoyl lecithin is formed. Hence, a premature infant does not always develop respiratory distress syndrome; however, in addition to being less active, synthesis of this lecithin is more susceptible to stress and acidosis, making the premature infant more susceptible to respiratory distress. At about the 35th week of gestation, there is a sudden surge of dipalmitoyl lecithin, the major surfactant lecithin, which is stable and very active. Since the fetal lungs contribute to the formation of amniotic fluid and the sphingomyelin concentration of amniotic fluid changes relatively little throughout pregnancy, measurement of the lecithin/sphingomyelin (L/S) ratio indicates the change which occurs at approximately 34–36 weeks of pregnancy when the great increase in dipalmitoyl lecithin takes place, and the degree to which the lungs will adapt to newborn life.

Gluck et al. were the first to demonstrate that the L/S ratio correlates with pulmonary maturity of the fetal lung. (74) In normal development, sphingomyelin concentrations are greater than those of lecithin until about gestational week 26. Prior to 34 weeks, the L/S ratio is approximately 1:1. At 34–36 weeks, with the sudden increase in lecithin, the ratio rises acutely. In general, a ratio of 2.0 or greater indicates pulmonary maturity and that respiratory distress syndrome will not develop in the newborn. Respiratory distress syndrome associated with a ratio greater than 2.0 usually follows a difficult delivery with a low 5-minute Apgar score, suggesting that severe acidosis can inhibit surfactant production. A ratio in the transitional range (1.0 to 1.9) indicates that respiratory distress syndrome may develop, but that the fetal lung has entered the period of lecithin production, and a repeat amniocentesis in 1 or 2 weeks usually reveals a mature L/S ratio. The rise from low to high ratios may actually occur within 3–4 days.

Abnormalities of pregnancy may affect the rate of maturation of the fetal lung, resulting either in an early mature L/S ratio or a delayed rise in the ratio. Accelerated maturation of the ratio is associated with hypertension, advanced diabetes, hemoglobinopathies, heroin addiciton, and poor maternal nutrition. Delayed maturation is seen with diabetes without hypertension, and Rh-sensitization.

Previously it was believed that delivery by cesarean section was associated with a greater incidence of respiratory distress syndrome when groups were corrected for gestational age. Since respiratory distress syndrome is related to the maturity of the fetal lung, and the L/S ratio is an index of pulmonary maturity, comparison of mode of delivery with the L/S ratio has allowed a more accurate appraisal of this problem. Gabert et al. (75) and Donald et al. (76) demonstrated that the maturity of the lungs as indicated by the

L/S ratio determines the presence of respiratory distress syndrome regardless of the mode of delivery.

Since Liggins observed survival of premature lambs, despite premature labor, following the administration of cortisol to the fetus, the acceleration of pulmonary maturity with pharmacologic amounts of corticosteroids has become common clinical practice. At present, fetal lung maturation can be best viewed as not the result of just cortisol, but the synergistic action of cortisol, prolactin, T_4, and perhaps other yet unidentified agents. (77, 78) Insulin partially antagonizes this stimulatory effect, which explains the delay in L/S ratio maturation associated with hyperglycemia in pregnancy. (79, 80).

References

1. **Csapo AL, Pulkkinen MO, Wiest WG,** Effects of luteectomy and progesterone replacement in early pregnant patients, Am J Obstet Gynecol 115:759, 1973.

2. **Simpson ER, Bilheimer DW, MacDonald PC,** Uptake and degradation of plasma lipoproteins by human choriocarcinoma cells in culture, Endocrinology 104:8, 1979.

3. **Parker CR, Everett RB, Quirk JG, Whalley PJ, Gant NF,** Hormone production during pregnancy in the primigravid patient: I. Plasma levels of progesterone and 5α-pregnane-3,20-dione throughout pregnancy of normal women and women who developed pregnancy-induced hypertension. Am J Obstet Gynecol 135:778, 1979.

4. **Parker CR, Everett RB, Whalley PJ, Quirk JG, Gant NF, MacDonald PC,** Hormone production during pregnancy in the primigravid patient: II. Plasma levels of deoxycorticosterone throughout pregnancy of normal women and women who developed pregnancy-induced hypertension. Am J Obstet Gynecol 138:626, 1980.

5. **Siiteri PK, Febres F, Clemens LE,** Progesterone and maintenance of pregnancy: is progesterone nature's immunosuppressant? Ann NY Acad Sci 296:384, 1977.

6. **Aitken RJ,** The hormonal control of implantation, in *Maternal Recognition of Pregnancy, Ciba Foundation Symposium 64*, Excerpta Medica, New York, 1979, pp 53–83.

7. **Siiteri PK, MacDonald PC,** Placental estrogen biosynthesis during human pregnancy, J Clin Endocrinol Metab 26:751, 1966.

8. **Madden JD, Gant NF, MacDonald PC,** Study of the kinetics of conversion of maternal plasma dehydroisoandrosterone sulfate to 16α-hydroxydehydroisoandrosterone sulfate, estradiol, and estriol, Am J Obstet Gynecol 132:392, 1978.

9. **Buster JE, Abraham GE,** The applications of steroid hormone radioimmunoassays to clinical obstetrics, Obstet Gynecol 46:489, 1975.

10. **Buster JE, Sakakini J Jr, Killam AP, Scragg WH,** Serum unconjugated estriol levels in the third trimester and their relationship to gestational age, Am J Obstet Gynecol 125:672, 1975.

11. **Parker CR Jr, Leveno K, Carr BR, Hauth J, MacDonald PC,** Umbilical cord plasma levels of dehydroepiandrosterone sulfate during human gestation, J Clin Endocrinol Metab 54:1216, 1982.

12. **Winters AJ, Oliver C, Colston C, MacDonald PC, Porter JC,** Plasma ACTH levels in the human fetus and neonate as related to age and parturition, J Clin Endocrinol Metab 39:269, 1974.

13. **Winters AJ, Colston C, MacDonald PC, Porter JC,** Fetal plasma prolactin levels, J Clin Endocrinol Metab 41:626, 1975.

14. **Walsh SW, Norman RL, Novy MJ,** In utero regulation of rhesus monkey fetal adrenals: effects of dexamethasone, adrenocorticotropin, thyrotropin-releasing hormone, prolactin, human chorionic gonadotropin, and α-melanocyte-stimulating hormone on fetal and maternal plasma steroids, Endocrinology 104:1805, 1979.

15. **del Pozo E, Bigazzi M, Calaf J,** Induced human gestational hypoprolactinemia: lack of action on fetal adrenal androgen synthesis, J Clin Endocrinol Metab 51:936, 1980.

16. **Carr BR, Simpson ER,** Lipoprotein utilization and cholesterol synthesis by the human fetal adrenal gland, Endocr Rev 2:306, 1981.

17. **Fujieda K, Faiman C, Reyes FI, Winter JSD,** The control of steroidogenesis by human fetal adrenal cells in tissue culture: I. Responses to adrenocorticotropin, J Clin Endocrinol Metab 53:34, 1981.

18. **Fujieda K, Faiman C, Reyes FI, Thliveris J, Winter JSD,** The control of steroidogenesis by human fetal adrenal cells in tissue culture: II. Comparison of morphology and steroid production in cells of the fetal and definitive zones. J Clin Endocrinol Metab 53:401, 1981.

19. **Fujieda K, Faiman C, Reyes FI, Winter JSD,** The control of steroidogenesis by human fetal adrenal cells in tissue culture: III. The effects of various hormonal peptides. J Clin Endocrinol Metab, 53:690, 1981.

20. **Fujieda K, Faiman C, Reyes FI, and Winter JSD,** The control of steroidogenesis by human fetal adrenal cells in tissue culture: IV. The effects of exposure to placental steroids, J Clin Endocrinol Metab 54:89, 1982.

21. **Distler W, Gabbe SG, Freeman RK, Mestman JH, Goebelsmann U,** Estriol in pregnancy: V. Unconjugated and total plasma estriol in the management of pregnant diabetic patients, Am J Obstet Gynecol 130:424, 1978.

22. **Whittle MJ, Anderson D, Lowensohn RI, Mestman JH, Paul RH, Goebelsmann U,** Estriol in pregnancy: VI. Experience with unconjugated plasma estriol assays, Am J Obstet Gynecol 135:764, 1979.

23. **Cathro DM, Betrand J, Coyle MG,** Antenatal diagnosis of adrenocortical hyperplasia, Lancet 1:732, 1969.

24. **Ohrlander SAV, Gennser GM, Grennert L,** Impact of betamethasone load given to pregnant women on endocrine balance of fetoplacental unit, Am J Obstet Gynecol 123:228, 1975.

25. **Adlercreutz H, Martin F, Tikkanen MJ, Pulkkinen M,** Effect of ampicillin administration on the excretion of twelve estrogens in pregnancy urine, Acta Endocrinol 80:551, 1975.

26. **Curet LB, Olson RW,** Ocytocin challenge tests and urinary estriols in the management of high-risk pregnancies, Obstet Gynecol 55:296, 1980.

27. **MacLeod SC, Mitton DM, Avery CR,** Relationship between elevated blood pressure and urinary estriols during pregnancy, Am J Obstet Gynecol 109:375, 1971.

28. **Yogman MW, Speroff L, Huttenlocher PR, Kase NG,** Child development after pregnancies complicated by low urinary estriol excretion and pre-eclampsia, Am J Obstet Gynecol 115:1069, 1972.

29. **Osathanondh R, Canick J, Ryan KJ, Tulchinsky D,** Placental sulfatase deficiency: a case study, J Clin Endocrinol Metab 43:208, 1976.

30. **Tabei T, Heinrichs WL,** Diagnosis of placental sulfatase deficiency, Am J Obstet Gynecol 124:409, 1976.

31. **Taylor NF, Shackleton CHL,** Gas chromatographic steroid analysis for diagnosis of placental sulfatase deficiency: a study of nine patients, J Clin Endocrinol Metab 49:78, 1979.

32. **Kaplan SL, Grumbach MM,** Pituitary and placental gonadotropins and sex steroids in the human fetus and subhuman primate fetus, Clin Endocrinol Metab 7:480, 1978.

33. **Owens OM, Ryan KJ, Tulchinsky D,** Episodic secretion of human chorionic gonadotropin in early pregnancy, J Clin Endocrinol Metab 53:1307, 1981.

34. **Wide L, Hobson B,** Relationship between the sex of the foetus and the amount of human chorionic gonadotrophin in placentae from tbe 10th to the 20th week of pregnancy, J Endocrinol 61:75, 1974.

35. **Boroditsky RS, Reyes FI, Winter JSD, Faiman C,** Serum human chorionic gonadotropin and progesterone patterns in the last trimester of pregnancy: relationship to fetal sex, Am J Obstet Gynecol 121:238, 1975.

36. **Schlaerth JB, Morrow CP, Kletzky OA, Nalick RH, D'Ablaing GA,** Prognostic characteristics of serum human chorionic gonadotropin titer regression following molar pregnancy. Obstet Gynecol 58:478, 1981.

37. **Schwartz RO, DiPietro DL,** β-HCG as a diagnostic aid for suspected ectopic pregnancy, Obstet Gynecol 56:197, 1980.

38. **Kadar N, Caldwell BV, Romero R,** A method of screening for ectopic pregnancy and its indications. Obstet Gynecol 58:162, 1981.

39. **Kadar N, DeVore G, Romero R,** The discriminatory HCG zone: its use in the sonographic evaluation for ectopic pregnancy, Obstet Gynecol 58:156, 1981.

40. **Grumbach MM, Kaplan SL, Vinik A,** Chapter 2, HCS, in *Peptide Hormones, Vol 2B*, Berson SA, Yalow RS, eds, North-Holland, Amsterdam, 1973, pp 797–819.

41. **Spellacy WN, Buhi WC, Schram JC, Birk SA, McCreary SA,** Control of human chorionic somatomammotropin levels during pregnancy, Obstet Gynecol 37:567, 1971.

42. **Felig, P,** Maternal and fetal fluid homeostasis in human pregnancy, Am J Clin Nutr 26:998, 1973.

43. **Felig P, Lynch V,** Starvation in human pregnancy: hypoglycemia, hypoinsulinemia, and hyperketonemia, Science 170:990, 1970.

44. **Kim YJ, Felig P,** Plasma chorionic somatomammotropin levels during starvation in mid-pregnancy, J Clin Endocrinol Metab 32:864, 1971.

45. **Felig P, Kim YJ, Lynch V, Hendler R,** Amino acid metabolism during starvation in human pregnancy, J Clin Invest 51:1195, 1972.

46. **Letchworth AT, Chard T,** Placental lactogen levels as a screening test for fetal distress and neonatal asphyxia, Lancet 1:704, 1972.

47. **Ylikorkala O,** Maternal serum HPL levels in normal and complicated pregnancy as an index of placental function, Acta Obstet Gynecol Scand, Suppl 26, 1973.

48. **Zlatnik FJ, Varner MW, Hauser KS,** Human placental lactogen: a predictor of perinatal outcome? Obstet Gynecol 54:205, 1979.

49. **Spellacy WN, Buhi WC, Birk SA,** The effectiveness of human placental lactogen measurements as an adjunct in decreasing perinatal deaths, Am J Obstet Gynecol 121:835, 1975.

50. **Nielsen PV, Pedersen H, Kampmann E,** Absence of human placental lactogen in an otherwise uneventful pregnancy, Am J Obstet Gynecol 135:322, 1979.

51. **Dawood MY, Teoh ES,** Serum human chorionic somato-mammotropin in unaborted hydatidiform mole, Obstet Gynecol 47:183, 1976.

52. **Nisula BC, Morgan FJ, Canfield RE,** Evidence that chorionic gonadotropin has intrinsic thyrotropic activity, Biochem Biophys Res Commun 59:86, 1974.

53. **Kenimer JG, Hershman JM, Higgins HP,** The thyrotropin in hydatidiform moles is human chorionic gonadotropin, J Clin Endocrinol Metab 40:482, 1975.

54. **Rees LH, Buarke CW, Chard T, Evans SW, Letchorth AT,** Possible placental origin of ACTH in normal human pregnancy, Nature 254:620, 1975.

55. **Goland RS, Wardlaw SL, Stark RI, Frantz AG,** Human plasma β-endorphin during pregnancy, labor, and delivery, J Clin Endocrinol Metab 52:74, 1981.

56. **Wardlaw SL, Stark RI, Baxi L, Frantz AG,** Plasma β-endorphin and β-lipotropin in the human fetus at delivery: correlation with arterial pH and pO_2, J Clin Endocrinol Metab 49:888, 1979.

57. **Siler-Khodr TM, Khodr GS,** Production and activity of placental releasing hormones, in *Fetal Endocrinology*, Novy MJ, Resko JA, eds, Academic Press, New York, 1981, pp 183–210.

58. **Weiss G, O'Byrne EM, Hochman J, Steinetz BG, Goldsmith L, Flitcraft JG,** Distribution of relaxin in women during pregnancy, Obstet Gynecol 52:569, 1978.

59. **Fields PA, Larkin LH,** Purification and immunohistochemical localization of relaxin in the human term placenta, J Clin Endocrinol Metab 52:79, 1981.

60. **Quagliarello J, Steinetz BG, Weiss G,** Relaxin secretion in early pregnancy, Obstet Gynecol 53:62, 1979.

61. **Maslar IA, Riddick DH,** Prolactin production by human endometrium during the normal menstrual cycle, Am J Obstet Gynecol 135:751, 1979.

62. **Bigazzi M, Pollicino G, Nardi E,** Is human decidua a specialized endocrine organ? J Clin Endocrinol Metab 49:847, 1979.

63. **Walters CA, Daly DC, Kuskik WF, Kuslis ST, Riddick DH,** Hormonal control of myometrial prolactin production, Program, Annual Meeting of The Endocrine Society, Abstract 877, 1982.

64. **Riddick DH, Maslar IA,** The transport of prolactin by human fetal membranes, J Clin Endocrinol Metab 52:220, 1981.

65. **Ho Yuen B, Cannon W, Lewis J, Sy L, Woolley S,** A possible role for prolactin in the control of human chorionic gonadotropin and estrogen secretion by the fetoplacental unit, Am J Obstet Gynecol 136:286, 1980.

66. **Luciano AA, Varner MW,** Decidual, amniotic fluid, maternal, and fetal prolactin in normal and abnormal pregnancies, Program, Annual Meeting of The Endocrine Society, Abstract 880, 1982.

67. **Healy DL, Herington AC, O'Herlihy C,** Idiopathic polyhydramnios: evidence for a prolactin receptor abnormality, Program, Annual Meeting of The Endocrine Society, Abstract 23, 1982.

68. **Fisher DA, Dussault JH, Sack J, Chopra IJ,** Ontogenesis of hypothalamic-pituitary-thyroid function and metabolism in man, sheep, and rat, Recent Prog Horm Res, 33:59, 1977.

69. **Cheron RG, Kaplan MM, Larsen PR, Selenkow HA, Crigler JF Jr,** Neonatal thyroid function after propylthiouracil therapy for maternal Graves' disease, N Engl J Med 304:525, 1981.

70. **Burrow GN, Klatskin EH, Genel M,** Intellectual development in children whose mothers received proplythiouracil during pregnancy, Yale J Biol Med 51:151, 1978.

71. **Maenpaa J,** Congenital hypothyroidism, aetological and clinical aspects suggests a familial tendency for hypothyroidism, Arch Dis Child 47:914, 1972

72. **Bachrach LK, Burrow GN, Holland FJ,** Treatment of primate hypothyroidism in utero with s,f-dimethyl-3′-isopropyl-L-thyroxine (DIMIT), Program, Annual Meeting of The Endocrine Society, Abstract 978, 1982.

73. **Klein AH, Murphy BEP, Artal R, Oddie TH, Fisher DA,** Amniotic fluid thyroid hormone concentrations during human gestation, Am J Obstet Gynecol 136:626, 1980.

74. **Gluck L, Kulovich MV, Borer RC, Brenner PH, Anderson GG, Spellacy WN,** Diagnosis of respiratory distress syndrome by amniocentesis, Am J Obstet Gynecol 109:440, 1971.

75. **Gabert HA, Bryson MJ, Stenchever MA,** The effect of cesarean section on respiratory distress in the presence of a mature lecithin/sphingomyelin ratio, Am J Obstet Gynecol 116:366, 1973.

76. **Donald IR, Freeman RK, Goebelsmann U, Chan WH, Nakamura RM,** Clinical experience with the amniotic fluid lecithin/sphingomyelin ratio, Am J Obstet Gynecol 115:547, 1973.

77. **Hauth JC, Parker CR, MacDonald PC, Porter JC, Johnston JM,** A role of fetal prolactin in lung maturation, Obstet Gynecol 51:81, 1978.

78. **Mendelson CR, Johnston JM, MacDonald PC, Snyder JM,** Multihormonal regulation of surfactant synthesis by human fetal lung in vitro, J Clin Endocrinol Metab 53:307, 1981.

79. **Smith BT, Giroud CJP, Robert M, Avery ME,** Insulin antagonism of cortisol action on lecithin synthesis by cultured fetal lung cells, J Pediatr 87:953, 1975.

80. **Gross IA, Smith GJW, Wilson CM, Maniscalco WM, Ingleson LD, Brehier A, Rooney SA,** Insulin decreases the amount of surfactant phospholipid in fetal rat lung tissue explants: the influence of hormones on the biochemical development of fetal rat lung in organ culture: II Insulin, Pediatr Res 14:834, 1980.

11 Prostaglandins

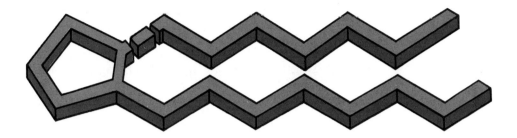

Prostaglandins play a fundamental role in the regulation of reproductive events. It is remarkable that most of the roles for prostaglandins predicted many years ago have come true. But what was once a relatively simple story has become exceedingly complex, especially from the biochemical point of view, as more and more members of the prostaglandin family are recognized.

This chapter will review the fundamental biochemistry of prostaglandins and focus on the roles prostaglandins play in pregnancy, specifically physiologic control mechanisms in luteal regression, the fetal circulation, parturition, uteroplacental blood flow, and maternal blood pressure.

Prostaglandin History

The historical evolution of the prostaglandin story is by now a familiar one. America can claim the first clue to the existence of prostaglandins because two New York gynecologists from Columbia, Kurzrok and Lieb, reported, in 1930, the effects of fresh human seminal fluid on strips of human uterus. This clue was overlooked, however, and the field was left for the pioneer work to come from Sweden and England, especially from the Karolinska Institute in Stockholm.

Goldblatt in England, in 1933, and von Euler in Sweden, in 1934, independently discovered that extracts of seminal vesicles stimulated smooth muscle preparations and also had vasodepressor activity. A year later, in 1935, von Euler reported that this biologic activity was due to an acidic lipid which he named prostaglandin. Nothing further was done until the late 1950s. World War II was certainly one reason for this hiatus, but also techniques were not sufficiently sensitive to measure and study prostaglandins which were available only in small amounts.

The supply problem was initially overcome by collecting large batches of sheep seminal vesicles and utilizing biosynthesis. This was an expensive and major logistic effort. The reward was the characterization and synthesis of prostaglandins in the early 1960s in the laboratory of Professor Sune Bergstrom, a student of von Euler's.

The discovery in 1970 that a coral (*Plexaura homomala*) off the coast of Florida contained large amounts of prostaglandin materials which could be used for the production of pure prostaglandins was a big boost for laboratory and clinical research. Shortly after, total synthesis of prostaglandins was achieved, and supply was no longer a problem.

During the 1970s the reproductive world was startled by the work of Sultan Karim. He was the first to use prostaglandins for the successful induction of labor and abortions, and this clinical application was responsible for a great surge of interest both clinically and in the laboratory. Recent history has centered on the exciting discoveries of the mechanism of action for aspirin, and of the new members of the prostaglandin family: thromboxane, prostacyclin, and the leukotrienes. Therefore, an appreciation for the makeup of this remarkable family is essential in order to understand the current prostaglandin world.

Prostaglandin Biochemistry

Biosynthesis

The family of prostaglandins with the greatest biologic activity is that having two double bonds, derived from arachidonic acid. (1) Arachidonic acid can be obtained from two sources, directly from the diet (from meats) or by formation from its precursor linoleic acid which is found in vegetables. In the plasma, 1–2% of the total free fatty acid content is free arachidonic acid. The majority of arachidonic acid is covalently bound in esterified form as a significant proportion of the fatty acids in phospholipids and in esterified cholesterol. Arachidonic acid is only a minor fatty acid in the triglycerides packaged in adipose tissue.

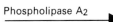

Phospholipase A$_2$ → Phospholipids | Arachidonic Acid

The rate-limiting step in the formation of the prostaglandin family is the release of free arachidonic acid. A variety of hydrolases may be involved in arachidonic acid release, but because of the abundance of arachidonate in the 2 position of phospholipids, phospholipase A$_2$ activation is an important initiator of prostaglandin synthesis. Types of stimuli that activate such lipases include: burns, infusions of hyper- and hypotonic solutions, thrombi and small particles, endotoxin, snake venom, mechanical stretching, catecholamines, bradykinin, angiotensin, and the sex steroids.

After the release of arachidonic acid the synthetic path can go in two different directions: the lipoxygenase pathway or the cyclooxygenase pathway. (1) The 5-lipoxygenase pathway has several leukotriene (LT) products, now designated LTA$_4$, LTB$_4$, LTC$_4$, LTD$_4$, and LTE$_4$. The leukotrienes are components of SRS, slow reacting substance. They are synthesized as a consequence of an anaphylactic challenge and are considered to be major agonists in producing bronchospasm during an asthmatic attack. Leukotrienes are 100–1000 times more potent than histamine or prostaglandins on the pulmonic airway. They stimulate an immediate vasoconstriction followed by leakage of fluid. Further roles are postulated for a variety of inflammatory responses, including arthritis. The future development of specific inhibitors has great potential for the treatment of immune and inflammatory responses and asthma. The 12-lipoxygenase pathway leads to 12-HETE. Little is known about 12-HETE, other than it functions as a leucostatic agent. The lipoxygenase products can also release lysosomal proteolytic enzymes.

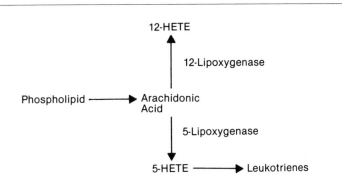

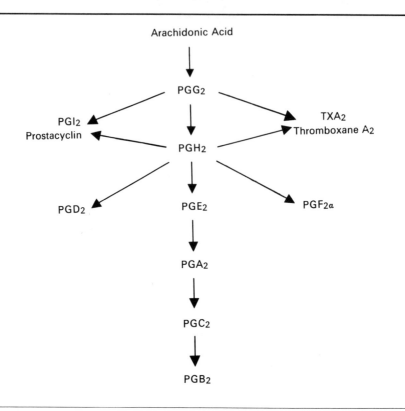

The cyclooxygenase pathway leads to the prostaglandins. The first true prostaglandin (PG) compounds formed are PGG_2 and PGH_2 (half-life of about 5 minutes), the mothers of all other prostaglandins. The numerical subscript refers to the number of double bonds. This number depends on which of the three precursor fatty acids has been utilized. Besides arachidonic acid, the other two precursor fatty acids are linoleic acid, which gives rise to the PG_1 series, and pentanoic acid, the PG_3 series. The latter two series are of less importance in physiology, hence the significance of the arachidonic acid family. The prostaglandins of original and continuing relevance to reproduction are PGE_2 and $PGF_{2\alpha}$ and possibly PGD_2. The A, B, and C prostaglandins either have little biological activity, or do not exist in significant concentrations in biological tissues.

Thromboxane and Prostacyclin	Thromboxanes are not true prostaglandins due to the absence of the pentane ring, but prostacyclin (PGI$_2$) is a legitimate prostaglandin. Thromboxane (TX) (half-life about 30 seconds) and PGI$_2$ (half-life about 2–3 minutes) can be viewed as opponents, each having powerful biologic activity which counters or balances the other. TXA$_2$ is the most powerful vasoconstrictor known, while PGI$_2$ is a potent vasodilator. These two agents also have opposing effects on platelet function. Platelets, lungs, and the spleen predominately synthesize TXA$_2$, while the heart, stomach, and blood vessels throughout the body synthesize PGI$_2$. The lungs are a major source of prostacyclin. Normal pulmonary endothelium makes prostacyclin while TXA$_2$ appears in response to pathological stimuli. (2) The pulmonary release of prostacyclin may contribute to the body's defense against platelet aggregation. (3)

Actually there is some controversy over whether prostacyclin is a circulatory hormone. Measured by indirect means (bioassay technique) prostacyclin appeared to undergo about 50% inactivation in one circulation through peripheral tissue. (4, 5) Direct measurement (gas chromatography), on the other hand, failed to detect prostacyclin in blood samples coming directly from lung arteries and veins. (6)

Let's take a closer look at platelets. The primary function of platelets is the preservation of the vascular system. Blood platelets stick to foreign surfaces or other tissues, a process called adhesion. They also stick to each other and form clumps; this process is called aggregation. Because platelets synthesize TXA$_2$, a potent stimulator of platelet aggregation, the natural tendency of platelets is to clump and plug defects and damaged spots. The endothelium, on the other hand, produces PGI$_2$, and its constant presence inhibits platelet aggregation and adherence, keeping blood vessels free of platelets and ultimately clots. Thus, prostacyclin has a defensive role in the body. It is 4–8 times more potent a vasodilator than the E prostaglandins, and it prevents the adherence of platelets to healthy vascular endothelium. However, when the endothelium is damaged, platelets gather, beginning the process of thrombus formation. Even in this abnormal situation, prostacyclin strives to fulfill its protective role as increased PGI$_2$ can be measured in injured endothelium, thrombosed vessels, and in the vascular tissues of hypertensive animals.

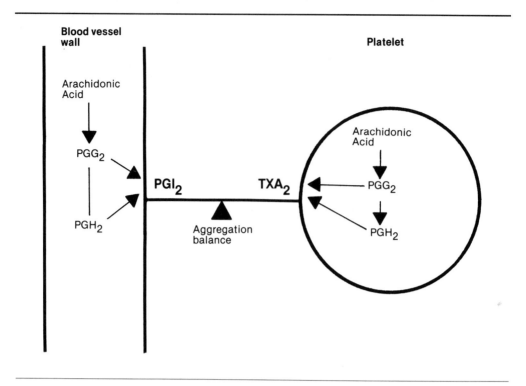

Blood vessel wall — Arachidonic Acid → PGG_2 → PGH_2 → PGI_2 — Aggregation balance — TXA_2 ← PGG_2 ← PGH_2 ← Arachidonic Acid — Platelet

Conditions associated with vascular disease can be understood through the prostacyclin-thromboxane mechanism. (4, 7–9) For example, atheromatous plaques and nicotine inhibit prostacyclin synthesis. Increasing the cholesterol content of human platelets increases the sensitivity to stimuli which cause platelet aggregation due to increased thromboxane production. (10) The well-known associations between low density and high density lipoproteins (LDL and HDL) and cardiovascular disease may also be explained in terms of PGI_2. LDL inhibits prostaglandin production and HDL overcomes the LDL inhibition. (8) Platelets from diabetics make more TXA_2. Platelets from Class A diabetic pregnant women make more TXA_2 than platelets from normal pregnant women. Platelets from women using oral contraceptives make more TXA_2 than controls. The same is true of smokers and people with strong family histories of cardiovascular disease. Incidentally, onion and garlic inhibit platelet aggregation and TXA_2 synthesis. (11). Perhaps the perfect contraceptive pill is a combination of progestin, estrogen, and some onion or garlic.

In some areas of the world there is a low incidence of cardiovascular disease. This can be directly attributed to diet and the protective action of prostacyclin. The diet of Eskimos and Japanese has a high content of pentanoic acid and low levels of linoleic and arachidonic acids. Pentanoic acid is the precursor of prostaglandin products with 3 double bonds, and as it happens, PGI_3 is an active agent while TXA_3 is either not formed, or it is inactive. The fat content of most common fish is 8–12% pentanoic acid, and more than 20% in the more exotic (and expensive) seafoods such as scallops, oysters, and caviar.

312

The balance between PGI_2 and TXA_2 may also be of importance in the body's defense against cancer. Experimental data in animals indicate that TXA_2 encourages and PGI_2 discourages metastatic tumor growth. In addition TXA_2 is a direct stimulator of metastatic activity and cell proliferation in tumor cell preparations. Thus, tumor cell production of TXA_2 appears to be related to tumor cell proliferation.

Metabolism

The metabolism of prostaglandins occurs primarily in the lungs, kidney, and liver. The lungs are important in the metabolism of E and F prostaglandins. Indeed, there is an active transport mechanism which specifically carries E and F prostaglandins from the circulation into the lungs. Therefore, members of the prostaglandin family have a short half-life, and in most instances, exert their action at the site of their synthesis. Because of the rapid half-lives, studies are often carried out by measuring the inactive end products, for example 6-keto-$PGF_{1\alpha}$, the metabolite of prostacyclin, and TXB_2, the metabolite of thromboxane A_2.

Prostaglandin Inhibition

A review of prostaglandin biochemistry is not complete without a look at the inhibition of the synthetic cascade of products. Corticosteroids were previously thought to inhibit the prostaglandin family by stabilizing membranes and preventing the release of phospholipase. It is now believed that corticosteroids induce the synthesis of a substance which blocks the action of phospholipase. (12) Thus far, steroids and some local anesthetic agents are the only substances known to work at this step.

Aspirin is an irreversible inhibitor, selectively acetylating the fatty acid dioxygenase involved in prostaglandin synthesis. The other inhibiting agents, such as indomethacin, are reversible agents, forming a reversible bond with the active site of the enzyme.

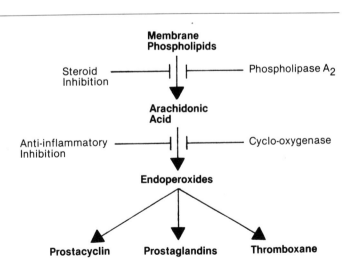

The analgesic, antipyretic, and anti-inflammatory actions of these agents are mediated by inhibition of the cylo-oxygenase enzyme. Because of the irreversible nature of the inhibition by aspirin, aspirin exerts a long lasting effect on platelets, effectively maintaining inhibition in the platelet for its life span (8–10 days). The sensitivity of the platelets to aspirin may explain the puzzling results in the early studies in which aspirin was given to prevent subsequent morbidity and mortality following thrombotic events. It takes only a little aspirin to effectively inhibit thromboxane synthesis in platelets. (3) Going beyond this dose will not only inhibit thromboxane synthesis in platelets, but also the protective prostacyclin production in blood vessel walls. Controversy continues as to what dose of aspirin and what frequency of administration are best. Some suggest that doses of 3.5 mg/kg (about half an aspirin tablet) given at 3-day intervals effectively induces maximum inhibition of platelet aggregation without affecting prostacyclin production by the vessel walls. (13) Others claim that the dose should be even lower, 40–50 mg daily. (14) The major handicap with the use of inhibitors of PG synthesis is that they strike blindly and with variable effect from tissue to tissue. Obviously drugs which selectively inhibit TXA_2 synthesis will be superior to aspirin in terms of antithrombotic effects.

Prostaglandins and Luteal Regression

Prostaglandin $F_{2\alpha}$ causes luteal regression in many species. It is the agent responsible for terminating the life span of the corpus luteum if fertilization fails to take place, so that a subsequent repeat ovulation can rapidly follow. The $PGF_{2\alpha}$ originates in the endometrium, and its synthesis is stimulated by the estrogen being produced in growing follicles. It is transported directly to the corpus luteum through the vasculature connecting the ovary and the uterus, thus achieving an effective concentration at the corpus luteum and avoiding a systemic level with widespread actions.

The mechanism of $PGF_{2\alpha}$-induced luteolysis is 2-fold: a rapid anti-LH action followed by a loss of luteinizing hormone (LH) receptors in the corpus luteum. (15) The rapid action is expressed only in intact cells and appears to be the result of some mediator that blocks LH receptor activation of adenylate cyclase. The slower response is an indirect action, interfering with prolactin maintenance of LH receptors.

Luteolysis has not been demonstrated in the primate, and it is well known that removal of the uterus does not interfere with normal ovulatory cycles. However, high doses of estrogen can induce luteolysis in the monkey and perhaps in the human. In monkey studies, estrogen induces a drop in progesterone during the luteal phase, mirrored by a rise in F prostaglandin. Furthermore, indomethacin can block this effect of estrogen. (16)

The human application of these findings can be found in the use of postcoital estrogen for contraception. High doses of estrogen can decrease progesterone levels in human cycles. (17) It is important to remember that the mechanism of estrogen is through $PGF_{2\alpha}$, and since the mechanism of $PGF_{2\alpha}$ is antagonism of LH action, human chorionic gonadotropin (HCG) can overcome this effect of estrogen. Hence, the effective action of estrogen when used for postcoital contraception is limited to the 7 days prior to implantation, before the corpus luteum is subject to rescue by HCG.

Prostaglandins and the Fetal Circulation

The predominant effect of prostaglandins on the fetal and maternal cardiovascular system is to maintain the ductus arteriosus, renal, mesenteric, uterine, placental, and probably the cerebral and coronary arteries in a relaxed or dilated state. The importance of the ductus arteriosus can be appreciated by considering that 59% of the cardiac output flows through this connection between the pulmonary artery and the descending aorta.

Control of ductal patency and closure is mediated through prostaglandins. The arterial concentration of oxygen is the key to the caliber of the ductus. With increasing gestational age, the ductus becomes increasingly responsive to increased oxygen. In this area, too, attention has turned to PGI_2 and TXA_2.

Fetal lamb ductus homogenates produce mainly PGI_2 when incubated with arachidonic acid. PGE_2 and $PGF_{2\alpha}$ are formed in small amounts and TXA_2 not at all. Although PGE_2 is less abundant than PGI_2 in the ductus, it is a more potent vasodilator of the ductus and is more responsive to oxygen (decreasing vasodilatation with increasing oxygen). (18) Thus, PGE_2 appears to be the most important prostaglandin in the ductus from a functional point of view, while PGI_2, the major product in the main pulmonary artery, appears to be the major factor in maintaining vasodilatation in the pulmonary bed. The ductus is dilated maximally in utero by production of prostaglandins, and a positive vasoconstrictor process is required to close it. The source of the vasoconstrictor is probably the lung. With increasing maturation, the lung shifts to TXA_2 formation. This fits with the association of ductal patency with prematurity. With the onset of pulmonary ventilation at birth leading to vascular changes which deliver blood to the duct directly from the lungs, TXA_2 can now serve as the vasoconstrictor stimulus. The major drawback to this hypothesis is the failure of inhibitors to affect the constriction response to oxygen.

Administration of vasodilating prostaglandins can maintain patency after birth, while preparing an infant for surgery to correct a congenital lesion causing pulmonary hyperfusion. Infants with persistent ductus patency may be spared thoracotomy by treatment with an inhibitor of prostaglandin synthesis. The use of indomethacin to close a persistent ductus in the premature infant is successful about 40% of the time. (18) The variable success so far cannot be attributed to any single factor, and further studies are clearly necessary. At least one important factor, however, is early diagnosis and treatment because with increasing postnatal age the ductus becomes less sensitive to prostaglandin inhibitors, probably because of more efficient clearance of the drug. (19)

This aspect of the use of prostaglandin inhibitors is of concern in considering the use of agents to inhibit premature labor. The drug half-life in the fetus and newborn is prolonged because the metabolic pathways are limited, and there is reduced drug clearance because of immature renal function. In utero constriction of the ductus can cause congestive heart failure and fetal pulmonary hypertension. (20, 21) Prolonged ductus constriction leads to subendocardial ischemia and fibrotic lesions in the tricuspid valve muscles. Infants with persistent pulmonary hypertension have hypoxemia, cardiomegaly and right to left shunting through the foramen ovale or the ductus. Infants of mothers given either indomethacin or salicylates chronically are frequently reported to have this syndrome. Duration of exposure and dosage are critical. It takes occlusion of the ductus for more than 2 weeks to produce fetal pulmonary hypertension and cardiac hypertrophy. Side effects appear to be minimized when administration is limited to mothers less than 34 weeks pregnant, and long-term use is avoided. (22)

Prostaglandins and Parturition

Perhaps the best example of the interplay among fetus, placenta, and the mother is the initiation and maintenance of parturition. Endocrine changes in the uteroplacental environment are the principal governing factors accounting for the eventual development of uterine contractions. The sequence of events has been recently reviewed in detail, where references to the original work are available. (23, 24)

Extensive work in tbe sheep has implicated the fetal pituitary-adrenal axis in normal parturition. The sequence of events in the sheep begins about 10 days prior to labor with elevation of fetal cortisol, probably in response to fetal pituitary ACTH. Fetal adrenalectomy or hypophysectomy prolongs pregnancy, while infusion of ACTH or glucocorticoids into the sheep fetus stimulates premature labor. Maternal stimulation of the fetal adrenal is not a factor because in sheep (and in human beings) there is little or no placental transfer of maternal ACTH into the fetal circulation.

Increased glucocorticoid secretion by the fetal adrenal gland presumably starts a chain of events associated with labor. The sequence of events continues in the sheep with a decline in progesterone. This change is brought about by the induction of 17α-hydroxylase enzyme activity in the sheep placenta.

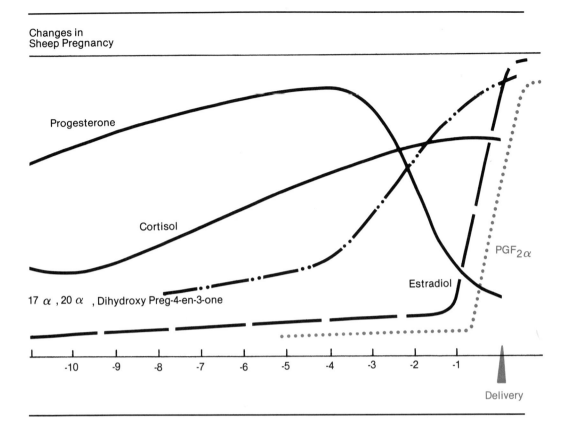

Glucocorticoid treatment of sheep placental tissue specifically increases the rate of production of $17\alpha,20\alpha$-dihydroxypregn-4-en-3-one. This dihydroxyprogesterone compound has also been identified in sheep placental tissue obtained after spontaneous labor. Thus direct synthesis of progesterone does not decline, but increased metabolism to a 17-hydroxylated product results in less available progesterone. Progesterone withdrawal is associated with a decrease in the resting potential of myometrium, i.e., an increased response to electric and oxytocic stimuli. Conduction of action potential through the muscle is increased, and the myometrial excitability is increased.

Dihydroxyprogesterone also serves as a precursor for the rise in estrogen levels which occurs a few days prior to parturition. Estrogens enhance rhythmic contractions as well as increasing vascularity and permeability, and the oxytocin response. Thus, progesterone withdrawal and estrogen increase lead to an enhancement of conduction and excitation.

The final event is a rise in $PGF_{2\alpha}$ production hours before the onset of uterine activity. A cause-and-effect relationship between the rise in estrogen and the appearance of $PGF_{2\alpha}$ has been demonstrated in the sheep. These events indicate that the decline in progesterone, the rise in estrogen, and the increase in $PGF_{2\alpha}$ are all secondary to direct induction of a placental enzyme by a glucocorticoid.

317

The steroid events in human pregnancy are somewhat similar to events in the ewe, with a very important difference: a more extended time scale. Steroid changes in the sheep occur over the course of several days, while in human pregnancy the changes begin at approximately 34–36 weeks and occur over the last 5 weeks of pregnancy.

Cortisol rises dramatically in amniotic fluid, beginning at 34–36 weeks, and correlates with pulmonic maturation. Cord blood cortisol concentrations are high in infants born vaginally or by cesarean section following spontaneous onset of labor. In contrast, cord blood cortisol levels are lower in infants born without spontaneous labor, whether delivery is vaginal (induced labor) or by cesarean section (elective repeat section). In keeping with the extended time scale of events, administration of glucocorticoids is not followed acutely by the onset of labor in pregnant women (unless the pregnancy is past due).

It is unlikely that the cortisol increments in the fetus represent changes due to increased adrenal activity in the mother in response to stress. Although maternal cortisol crosses the placenta readily, it is largely (85%) metabolized to cortisone in the process. This, in fact, may be the mechanism by which suppression of the fetal adrenal gland by maternal steroids is avoided. In contrast to the maternal liver, the fetal liver has a limited capacity for transforming the biologically inactive cortisone to the active cortisol. On the other hand, the fetal lung does possess the capability of changing cortisone to cortisol, and this may be an important source of cortisol for the lung. Cortisol itself induces this conversion in lung tissue. Increased fetal adrenal activity is followed by changes in steroid levels as well as important developmental accomplishments (e.g., increased pulmonary surfactant production and the accumulation of liver glycogen.)

But the increased levels of fetal cortisol associated with labor appear to be secondary to the stress of the process, and at the present time there is no evidence that fetal cortisol production triggers human parturition. In human parturition the important contribution of the fetal adrenal, rather than cortisol, is probably its effect on placental estrogen production. The common theme in human pregnancies associated with failure to begin labor on time is decreased estrogen production, e.g. anencephaly and placental sulfatase deficiency. In contrast, mothers bearing fetuses who cannot form normal amounts of cortisol, such as those with congenital adrenogenital syndrome, deliver on time. (25)

An increase in estrogen levels in maternal blood begins at 34–35 weeks of gestation, but a late increase just prior to parturition (as in the sheep) has not been observed in human pregnancy. Perhaps a critical level is the signal in human pregnancy rather than a triggering increase. Although not definitively demonstrated, increased or elevated estrogen levels are thought to play a key role in increasing prostaglandin production.

Progesterone maintenance of uterine quiescence and increased myometrial excitability associated with progesterone withdrawal appear to be firmly established as mechanisms of parturition in other species. In primates, the role of progesterone is less clear, largely because of the inability to demonstrate a definite decline in peripheral blood levels of progesterone prior to parturition. Recently, MacDonald's group has suggested that local regulation of progesterone levels may take place within the pregnant uterus by means of a binding protein in the fetal membranes. Decreased local levels of progesterone, combined with increased levels of estrogen, lead to prostaglandin synthesis and increased myometrial activity.

Evidence for a role of prostaglandins in parturition includes the following:

1. Prostaglandin levels in maternal blood and amniotic fluid increase in association with labor.

2. Arachidonic acid levels in the amniotic fluid also rise in labor, and arachidonate injected into the amniotic sac initiates parturition

3. Patients taking high doses of aspirin have a highly significant increase in the average length of gestation, incidence of postmaturity, and duration of labor.

4. Indomethacin prevents the normal onset of labor in monkeys and stops premature labor in human pregnancies.

5. Stimuli known to cause the release of prostaglandins (cervical manipulation, stripping of membranes, and rupture of membranes) augment or induce uterine contractions.

6. Prostaglandins induce labor.

Fetal respiratory movements are influenced by prostaglandins. The administration of indomethacin to fetal sheep increases, while infusion of PGE suppresses, fetal breathing movements. (21) This may be the explanation for the decrease in fetal breathing movements during labor.

The precursor fatty acid for prostaglandin production in part may be derived from storage pools in the fetal membranes, or the decidua, or both. Phospholipase A_2 has been demonstrated in both human chorioamnion and uterine decidua. Gustavii has suggested that progesterone withdrawal allows degeneration of decidual cells and release of lysosomal enzyme, leading to the activation of lipase enzyme. (26) Others believe the major source of arachidonic acid is the fetal membranes. (27, 28) However, the precise mechanism for initiating prostaglandin synthesis, presumably by activation of the enzyme phospholipase A_2, remains unknown.

319

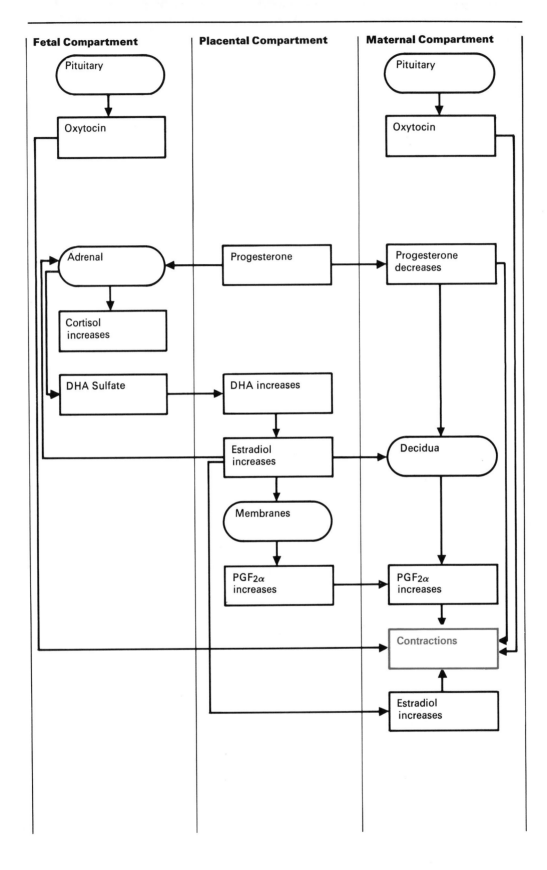

The Texas thesis is that availability of arachidonic acid for prostaglandin production during parturition is due to stimulation of hydrolysis of phosphatidylethanolamine and phosphatidylinositol in decidual, amnion, and chorion laeve tissues. (29–31) Microsomes from amnion, chorion laeve, and decidual vera tissues contain lipases that hydrolyze fatty acids esterified in the 2 position. Specific phospholipase activity combined with a diacylglycerol lipase which also has a specificity for arachidonic acid, provides a mechanism for the release of arachidonic acid. The activity of these enzymes in fetal membranes and decidual vera tissue increases with increasing length of gestation.

The key may be the increasing formation of estrogen (both estradiol and estriol) in the maternal circulation as well as amniotic fluid. The marked rise in amniotic fluid estrogen near term may affect the activity of the lipase enzymes, leading to the liberation of arachidonic acid. In addition, the rise in estrogen may stimulate the appearance of the progesterone binding protein.

New evidence regarding prostacyclin during parturition is of uncertain significance. Prostacyclin is produced (at least in vitro) by a variety of tissues involved in pregnancy: endometrium, myometrium, placenta, amnion, chorion, decidua. (32, 33) The level of prostacyclin, as reflected by its metabolite 6-keto-PGF$_{1\alpha}$, rises with the progression of labor; the maximum level occurs at placental expulsion. (34) By the second postpartum hour, the mean level is below the prelabor level. The levels in the umbilical artery and vein are not significantly different, but they are 3–4 times higher than maternal levels. The increases in the maternal circulation are much smaller than increases in the other prostaglandins. As will be discussed later, this prostacyclin is probably more important in the vascular responses of mother and fetus, and probably does not play a role in initiating or maintaining uterine contractions.

There is little evidence that increased maternal levels of oxytocin are responsible for initiating parturition, although a low fixed level may be an essential permissive factor. Once labor has begun, however, oxytocin levels do rise, especially during the second stage. Thus, oxytocin may be important for developing the more intense uterine contractions. Extremely high concentrations of oxytocin can be measured in the cord blood at delivery and, release of oxytocin from the fetal pituitary may also play a role during labor. Indeed, the magnitude of the fetal contribution to the maternal side is similar to the dose usually infused to induce labor.

Animal studies have implicated the formation of low resistance pathways in the myometrium, called gap junctions, as an important action of steroids and prostaglandins during labor. Gap junctions are thought to play a role in synchronizing the myometrium. Gap junction formation is related to the estrogen/progesterone ratio and to the presence of the stimulating prostaglandins, PGE_2 and $PGF_{2\alpha}$. The final contraction of uterine muscle results from increased free calcium concentrations in the myofibril, the result of prostaglandin action, an action opposed to that of progesterone which promotes calcium binding in the sarcoplasmic reticulum. (35)

Induction of Labor and Cervical Ripening

Pharmacologically and physiologically, prostaglandins have two direct actions associated with labor: ripening of the cervix and a direct oxytocic action. For ripening of the cervix, PGE_2 is very effective while $PGF_{2\alpha}$ has little effect. In English studies, a single instillation of 2 mg PGE_2 resulted in a shorter duration of labor, less oxytocin augmentation, and a reduced frequency of cesarean sections. (36)

A major clinical application for the induction of labor in the United States is the use of intravaginal PGE_2 in cases of fetal demise and anencephalic fetuses. (37) Based on our own experience, certain precautions have been developed. It is best to start slowly, using ¼–½ tablets every 2–4 hours. The patient should be well hydrated with an electrolyte solution to counteract the induced vasodilatation and decreased peripheral resistance. If satisfactory uterine activity is established, the next suppository should be withheld. And finally, because there is a synergistic effect when oxytocin is used shortly after prostaglandin administration, there should be a minimum of 12 hours between the last prostaglandin dose and beginning oxytocin augmentation.

Therapeutic Abortion

Prostaglandins are effective for postcoital contraception and first trimester abortion, but impractical due to the high incidence of side effects, including an unacceptable rate of incomplete abortions. For midtrimester abortions, intramniotic prostaglandin, intramuscular methyl esters, and vaginal PGE suppositories are available. The major clinical problems have been the efficacy in accomplishing complete expulsion and the high level of systemic side effects. Overall, there is a higher risk of hemorrhage, fever, infection, antibiotic administration, readmission to the hospital, and more operative procedures when compared to saline abortions. These complications can be minimized if care is paid to two aspects of the clinician's technique. First, laminaria should be used to reduce the incidence of cervical injury and the need for retreatment. Second, aggressive management of the third stage is necessary. Examination of the patient is necessary immediately after expulsion of the fetus, removing the placenta with ring forceps, inspecting the cervix, and exploring the uterine cavity. This aggressive management will minimize the most troublesome side effects, which are due to retained tissue. Prostaglandin E_2 and PGE analogs have proven to be most efficacious with the least side effects for the induction of labor, ripening of the cervix, and therapeutic abortion. The long-term instability of these compounds has been a major obstacle to commercial development. Attempts to solve this problem are focusing on improved gels as the physical base and on sustained release vaginal delivery systems.

322

Prostaglandins, Uteroplacental Blood Flow, and Maternal Blood Pressure

A change must take place in the maternal vascular system to accommodate the volume and flow changes during pregnancy. The maternal plasma volume begins to increase about the 6th week of pregnancy. It rapidly expands during the second trimester, but increases only slightly in the last trimester until term. There is a greater increment in plasma volume as compared to the red cell volume in normal pregnancy (mean plasma volume increase of 1074 ml vs. 350 ml increase in red cell volume). (38) In order to accommodate the increase in volume (and cardiac output) without a significant increase in the maternal blood pressure, there must be a decrease in the peripheral vascular resistance. There are two mechanisms for the decrease in resistance: one is the increasing fraction of the cardiac output which passes through the uteroplacental circulation; the other is vasodilatation in the maternal vascular tree. Maintenance of normal maternal blood pressure and also maintenance of uteroplacental blood flow (and therefore effective exchange functions across the placenta) depend upon vasodilatation, both in the systemic maternal circulation and locally within the uteroplacental unit. Prostacyclin may mediate this important function.

Toxemia of Pregnancy as a Chronic Disease

For the sake of nostalgia and for an economy of words, it continues to be useful to use "toxemia" of pregnancy interchangably with pregnancy-induced hypertension. A more important change in our thinking has been the acceptance of the concept of toxemia as a chronic problem throughout pregnancy, not an acute disease arising at the time of hypertension. Measuring the metabolic clearance rate of dehydroepiandrosterone sulfate (DHAS), Gant et al. demonstrated a decline in DHAS clearance prior to the development of clinically evident toxemia. (39) Subsequently, the same group showed that the pressor response to angiotensin II was different as early as 22 weeks in a group of primigravid women who went on to develop near term the typical clinical manifestations of toxemia. (40) Even the routine measurement of blood pressure, by a standardized technique that included a 5-minute rest period, was able to delineate a group of women who later became hypertensive, in that they had higher blood pressures throughout pregnancy. (41)

The above studies indicate that toxemia of pregnancy is caused by or associated with a disturbance in a homeostatic mechanism responsible for maintenance of blood pressure and uteroplacental blood flow. The metabolic requirements of the fetus are best served by maintaining an adequate blood flow. In pregnancy, there is a need beyond the ordinary organ's concern with cellular function, there is the obligation of meeting the demands of the growing fetus. Toxemia is associated with a 40–60% reduction in blood flow through the uteroplacental unit in women, but it has been impossible to determine whether this is a primary or secondary event. If toxemia is due to the development of impaired blood flow over a period of time, it would seem that the clinical symptoms of the disease would be a late occurrence, and subclinical abnormalities should be detectable earlier in pregnancy (as in the above studies). Indeed, it is generally accepted that clearance of DHAS reflects a decrease in uteroplacental blood flow and therefore, reduced uteroplacental blood flow precedes the appearance of hypertension.

Prostaglandins and Toxemia

Two properties of certain classes of prostaglandins are noteworthy in searching for the mechanism of vasodilatation and regulation of blood flow in pregnancy. First, E prostaglandins and prostacyclin are potent vasodilators, decreasing the peripheral resistance and systemic blood pressure by directly relaxing the smooth muscle of the arterial walls. Second, the majority of the activity of these prostaglandins appears to be limited to the immediate vicinity of the synthesizing tissue itself.

Initially, attention was focused on E and F prostaglandins. The important observations in the monkey (42–44), the sheep (45), the dog (46), and the rabbit (47), were as follows:

1. Angiotensin II increased uterine blood flow.

2. Angiotensin II increased PGE production by the pregnant uterus.

3. Inhibition of prostaglandin synthesis lowered basal blood flow, blocked the blood flow and PGE response to angiotensin II, and raised the systemic blood pressure.

These findings are consistent with a role for E prostaglandins in maintaining the resting uteroplacental and maternal vasomotor tone, and in moderating resistance to flow in response to vasoconstrictors. In the experiments in monkeys in the third trimester, angiotensin II-induced hypertension following indomethacin failed to increase uterine artery blood flow as had been noted after the initial infusion of angiotensin. A significant obstacle in the interpretation of these studies is the impact of surgical and anesthetic stress.

The entire renin-angiotensin-aldosterone system is increased in pregnancy, presumably due to a direct stimulation of substrate (angiotensinogen) synthesis by estrogen. It appears that this increase is the basic mechanism for producing the increased blood volume of pregnancy. The importance of the angiotensin-aldosterone system is underscored by the fetal death noted in sheep and rabbits when angiotensin II formation was prevented by inhibiting the converting enzyme. (48) The demonstration that blood vessels produce prostaglandins (49–51) led to the speculation that vascular prostaglandins were responsible for the concomitant vasodilatation associated with the increased renin-angiotensin-aldosterone activity. A pregnant woman's blood pressure at any point in time then reflected the balance of these various forces. A role for prostaglandins was supported by the demonstration that the administration of indomethacin or aspirin decreased the amount of angiotensin necessary to produce a pressor response in pregnant women. (52) This is consistent with the conclusion that pressor responsiveness to angiotensin II during pregnancy is determined by the degree of vascular resistance to the pressor agent. (53) A hypothesis was then suggested linking estrogen, the renin-angiotensin-system, and prostaglandins. (51)

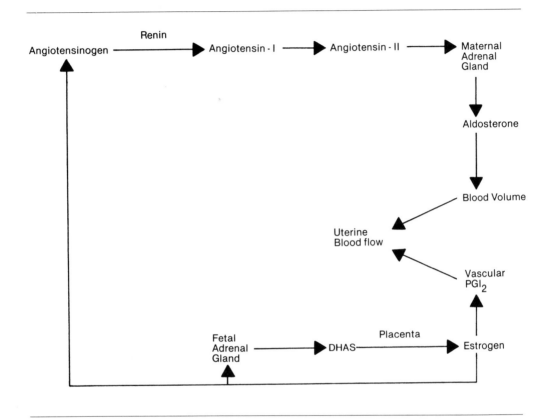

Estrogen can be viewed as a principal messenger for ensuring normal growth and development. Estrogen increases uterine blood flow, apparently via the mediation of a vasodilating prostaglandin (54). The major precursor for placental estrogen production is DHAS, secreted by the fetal adrenal gland. What regulates estrogen production has been an important question in placental physiology. This question appears to be answered, with the concept that the fetal adrenal-placental unit governs its own rate of estrogen production. (55) The amount of precursor available for estrogen production may be the major rate-limiting factor. Estrogen itself circulates back to the fetus to increase the production of its precursor by suppressing the activity of the enzyme, 3β-hydroxydehydrogenase, thus diverting the steroidogenic pathway to DHAS. This mechanism allows ever increasing levels of estrogen production. The rising levels of estrogen increase the activity of the aldosterone system to expand blood volume, and at the same time may stimulate prostacyclin production within fetal and maternal blood vessels to maintain vasodilatation and blood flow. Toxemia of pregnancy may represent defective prostacyclin production, increased degradation of prostacyclin, a loss of response to prostacyclin, or a combination of these factors.

Prostacyclin and Toxemia

The emergence of prostacyclin as a vasodilator even more potent than E prostaglandins directed attention to this new member of the prostaglandin family. In addition, it was appreciated that the prostacyclin metabolite migrates with E prostaglandins in separation systems. Therefore, previous studies implicating E prostaglandins may have been dealing with prostacyclin.

Many investigators have reported a general decrease in prostacyclin associated with preeclampsia. (56–62) Lower levels of this potent vasodilator and inhibitor of platelet activity could explain three of the most significant clinical consequences of toxemia: hypertension, platelet consumption, and reduced uteroplacental blood flow.

For years, investigators have implicated disseminated intravascular coagulation (DIC) as an important component of the symptom complex associated with toxemia. Pritchard has argued strongly that thrombocytopenia in toxemia is not an etiological factor, but a consequence of the disease, most consistent with platelet adherence at sites of vascular endothelial damage. (63) A closer analysis reveals that the thrombocytopenia associated with toxemia is most similar to that seen with various microangiopathies, a consequence of abnormal platelet-endothelial interaction. (64) Such a mechanism for the thrombocytopenia of toxemia is consistent with a problem in prostacyclin production or function.

	Disseminated Intravascular Coagulation	Microangiopathy
Etiology	Thromboplastins, thrombin, fibrin	Endothelial cell damage, platelet activation
Pathology	Intravascular fibrin	Intravascular platelet deposition
Fibrinogen levels	Low	Normal or high
Platelet count	Mild to moderately decreased	Moderate to markedly decreased
Red cells	Slight to moderate fragmentation	Moderate to marked fragmentation

As with blood pressure measurement, DHAS clearance, and angiotensin II pressor response, decreased platelet counts, when studied in a carefully controlled manner, may also precede the development of hypertension. Early platelet consumption may be seen with preeclampsia before deterioration of urate clearance or elevation of blood pressure. The failure of heparin therapy to affect the clinical course of preeclampsia supports the fact that DIC is not the mechanism of the thrombocytopenia. Indeed, the reason that hypertension does not accompany coagulation disorders associated with intrauterine fetal demise and abruption placentae, may be that these classic problems are due to infusion of thromboplastin and DIC, and not due to an endothelial prostacyclin disorder.

The pathologic appearance of blood vessels in the placental bed in toxemic pregnancies bears significant resemblance to the blood vessels associated with microangiopathic syndromes. (65) Patients with the hemolytic uremic syndrome and thrombotic thrombocytopenic purpura share a common problem: defective prostacyclin activity. (66–70) Another similar syndrome has been reported recently, a problem with a "lupus" anticoagulant. (71) "Lupus" anticoagulant is a spontaneously acquired inhibitor of blood coagulation that interferes with activation of prothrombin. It is an immunoglobulin that is associated with an inhibition of prostacyclin synthesis in a variety of tissues. Although first recognized in patients with systemic lupus erythematosus, it has been detected in other clinical conditions as well. Lesions in the placenta and the placental vessels in this syndrome resembled those formerly believed to be only associated with hypertension in pregnancy. These lesions (fibrinoid necrosis, acute atherosis, and intraluminal thrombosis) have now been described in idiopathic intrauterine growth retardation, diabetic pregnancies, systemic lupus erythematosus, and toxemia. Are these examples of diseases of different mechanisms, but all having the same target: prostacyclin?

Inadequate prostacyclin activity may be due to a deficient stimulating factor in plasma, or increased degradation by plasma. Introduction of normal plasma could restore the normal state. Plasmapheresis or plasma transfusions have markedly improved the survival rate of patients with thrombotic thrombocytopenic purpura. Plasma exchange has been reported in 3 cases of severe toxemia. (69) In all 3, renal function improved, and 2 of the 3 achieved healthy infants. A 3-hour 4-liter plasma exchange using a 5% protein solution (86% albumin and 14% globulins) was given daily for 4–6 days, then every other day. Less hypotensive medications were required, although eventually hypertension became progressive.

Because of the problems of dosage and the unknown intensity of effect on prostacyclin and thromboxane, respectively, treatment with aspirin does not seem logical. Yet, Crandon and Isherwood (70) reported a lower incidence of toxemia in patients taking aspirin compared to patients with no drug intake, and Goodlin et al. (72) reported a case of severe toxemia in whom platelet counts improved with the administration of aspirin. Selective inhibition of TXA_2 might yield even more impressive results.

Evidence is accumulating to link prostacyclin to the clinical and pathological manifestations of toxemia. Having recognized and accepted the concept that toxemia is a chronic disease, the challenge of the 1980s is to discover a practical method for early diagnosis, long before the irreversible end stage represented by the classical triad of hypertension, proteinura and edema develops. Accurate early diagnosis would open the door for pharmacologic intervention.

References

1. **Ramwell PW, Foegh M, Loeb R, Leovey EMK,** Synthesis and metabolism of prostaglandins, prostacyclin, and thromboxanes: the arachidonic acid cascade, Semin Perinatol 4:3, 1980.

2. **Gryglewski RJ, Korbut R, Oetkiewicz A, Splawinski J, Wojtaszek B, Swies J,** Lungs as a generator of prostacyclin-hypothesis on physiological significance, Arch Pharmacol 304:45, 1979.

3. **Moncada S, Korbut R,** Dipyridamole and other phosphodiesterase inhibitors act as antithrombotic agents by potentiating endogenous prostacyclin, Lancet 1:1286, 1978.

4. **Moncada S, Korbut R, Bunting S, Vane JR,** Prostacyclin is a circulating hormone, Nature 273:767, 1978.

5. **Moncada S, Vane JR,** Prostacyclin: homeostatic regulator or biological curiosity? Clin Sci 61:369, 1981.

6. **Christ-Hazelhof E, Nugteren DH,** Prostacyclin is not a circulating hormone, Prostaglandins 22:739, 1981.

7. **Moncada S, Vane JR,** Arachidonic acid metabolites and the interactions between platelets and blood vessel walls, N Engl J Med 300:1142, 1979.

8. **Nordoy A, Svensson B, Wiebe D, Hoak JC,** Lipoproteins and the inhibitory effect of human endothelial cells on platelet function, Circ Res 43:527, 1978.

9. **Ziboh VA, Maruta H, Lord J, Cagle WD, Lucky W,** Increased biosynthesis of thromboxane A_2 by diabetic platelets, Eur J Clin Invest 9:223, 1979.

10. **Stuart MJ, Gerrard JM, White JG,** Effect of cholesterol on production of thromboxane B_2 by platelets in vitro, N Engl J Med 302:6, 1980.

11. **Makheja A, Vanderhoek JY, Bailey JM,** Inhibition of platelet aggregation and thromboxane synthesis by onion and garlic, Lancet 1:781, 1979.

12. **Flower RJ, Blackwell GJ,** Anti-inflammatory steroids induce biosynthesis of the phospholipase A_2 inhibitor which prevents prostaglandin generation, Nature 278:456, 1979.

13. **Masotti G, Poggesi L, Galanti G, Abbate R, Neri Srneri GG,** Differential inhibition of prostacyclin production and platelet aggregation by aspirin, Lancet 2:1213, 1979.

14. **Hanley SP, Bevan J, Cockbill SR, Heptinstall S,** Differential inhibition by low-dose aspirin of human venous prostacyclin synthesis and platelet thromboxane synthesis, Lancet 1:969, 1981.

15. **Behrman HR,** Prostaglandins in hypothalmo-pituitary and ovarian function, Annu Rev Physiol 41:685, 1979.

16. **Auletta FJ, Agins H, Scommegna A,** Prostaglandin $F_{2\alpha}$ mediation of the inhibitory effect of estrogen on the corpus luteum of the rhesus monkey, Endocrinology 103:1183, 1978.

17. **Gore BC, Caldwell BV, Speroff L,** Estrogen-induced human luteolysis, J Clin Endocrin Metab 36:615, 1973.

18. **Coceani F, Olley PM, Lock JE,** Prostaglandins, ductus arteriosus, pulmonary circulation: current concepts and clinical potential, Eur J Clin Pharmacol 18:75, 1980.

19. **Brash AR, Hickey DE, Graham TP, Stahlman MT, Oates JA, Cotton RB,** Pharmacokinetics of indomethacin in the neonate: relation of plasma indomethacin levels to response of the ductus arteriosus, N Engl J Med 305:67, 1981.

20. **Levin DL,** Effects of inhibition of prostaglandin synthesis on fetal development, oxygenation, and the fetal circulation, Semin Perinatol 4:35, 1980.

21. **Rudolph AM,** The effects of nonsteroidal antiinflammatory compounds on fetal circulation and pulmonary function, Obstet Gynecol 58:635, 1981.

22. **Niebyl JR,** Prostaglandin synthetase inhibitors, Semin Perinatol 5:274, 1981.

23. **Novy MJ, Liggins GC,** Role of prostaglandins, prostacyclin, and thromboxanes in the physiologic control of the uterus and in parturition, Semin Perinatol 4:45, 1980.

24. **Challis JRG, Mitchell BF,** Hormonal control of pre-term and term parturition, Semin Perinatol 5:192, 1981.

25. **Price HV, Cone BA, Keogh M,** Length of gestation in congenital adrenal hyperplasia, J Obstet Gynaecol Br Comm 78:430, 1971.

26. **Gustavii B,** Release of lysosomal acid phosphatase into the cytoplasm of decidual cells before the onset of labor in human, Br J Obstet Gynaecol 82:177, 1975.

27. **Schwarz BE, Schultz FM, MacDonald PC, Johnston JM,** Initiation of human parturition: III. Fetal membrane content of prostaglandin E_2 and $F_{2\alpha}$ precursor, Obstet Gynecol 46:564, 1975.

28. **Curbelo V, Bejar R, Benirschke K, Gluck L,** Premature labor: 1. Prostaglandin precursors in human placental membranes, Obstet Gynecol 57:473, 1981.

29. **Ozazaki T, Sagawa N, Okita JR, Bleasdale JE, MacDonald PC, Johnston JM,** Diacylglycerol metabolism and arachidonic acid release in human fetal membranes and decidua vera, J Biol Chem 256:7316, 1981.

30. **Okazaki T, Sagawa N, Bleasdale JE, Okita JR, MacDonald PC, Johnston JM,** Initiation of human parturition: XIII. Phospholipase C, phospholipase A_2, and diacylglycerol lipase activities in fetal membranes and decidual vera tissues from early and late gestation, Biol Reprod 25:103, 1981.

31. **DiRenzo GC, Johnston JM, Okazaki T, Okita JR, MacDonald PC, Bleasdale JE,** Phosphatidylinositol specific phospholipase C in fetal membranes and uterine decidua, J Clin Invest 67:847, 1981.

32. **Abel MH, Kelly RW,** Differential production of prostaglandins within the human uterus, Prostaglandins 18:821, 1979.

33. **Mitchell MD, Bibby JG, Hicks BR, Turnbull AC,** Possible role for prostacyclin in human parturition, Prostaglandins 16:931, 1978.

34. **Ylikorkala O, Makarainen L, Viinikka L,** Prostacyclin production increases during human parturition, Br J Obstet Gynaecol 88:513, 1981.

35. **Carsten MF,** Calcium accumulation by human uterine microsomal preparations: effects of progesterone and ocytocin, Am J Obstet Gynecol 133:598, 1979.

36. **MacKenzie IZ, Embrey MP,** A comparison of PGE_2 and $PGF_{2\alpha}$ vaginal gel for ripening the cervix before induction of labour, Br J Obstet Gynaecol 86:167, 1979.

37. **Southern EM, Gutknecht GD, Mohberg NR, Edelman DA,** Vaginal prostaglandin E_2 in the management of fetal intrauterine death, Br J Obstet Gynaecol 85:437, 1978.

38. **Brinkman CR,** Physiology and pathophysiology of maternal adjustments to pregnancy, in *Clinical Perinatology,* Aladjem S, Brown AK, eds, C. V. Mosby, St. Louis, 1975.

39. **Gant NP, Hutchinson HT, Siiteri PK, MacDonald PC,** Study of the metabolic clearance of dehydroisoandrosterone sulfate in pregnancy, Am J Obstet Gynecol 111:555, 1971.

40. **Gant NF, Daley GL, Chand S, Whalley PJ, MacDonald PC,** A study of angiotensin II pressor response throughout primigravid pregnancy, J Clin Invest 52:2682, 1973.

41. **Gallery EDM, Ross M, Hunyor SN, Gyory AX,** Predicting the development of pregnancy-associated hypertension, the place of standardized blood-pressure measurement, Lancet 1:1273, 1977.

42. **Franklin GO, Dowd AJ, Caldwell BV, Speroff L,** The effect of angiotensin II intravenous infusion on plasma renin activity and prostaglandins A, E, and F levels in the uterine vein of the pregnant monkey, Prostaglandins, 6:271, 1974.

43. **Speroff L, Haning RV Jr, Ewaschuk EJ, Alberino SL, Kieliszek FX,** Uterine artery blood flow studies in the pregnant monkey, in *Hypertension in Pregnancy*, Lindheimer MD, Katz AL, Zuspan FP, eds, John Wiley, New York, 1976, pp 315–327.

44. **Speroff L, Haning RV Jr, Levin RM,** The effect of angiotensin II and indomethacin on uterine artery blood flow in pregnant monkeys, Obstet Gynecol 50:611, 1977.

45. **McLaughlin MK, Brennan SC, Chez RA,** Effects of indomethacin on sheep uteroplacental circulations and sensitivity to angiotensin II, Am J Obstet Gynecol 132:430, 1978.

46. **Terragno NA, Terragno DA, Pacholxzyk D, McGiff JC,** Prostaglandins and the regulation of uterine blood flow in pregnancy, Nature 249:57, 1974.

47. **Venuto RC, O'Dorisio T, Stein JH, Ferris TF,** Uterine prostaglandin E secretion and uterine blood flow in the pregnant rabbit, J Clin Invest 55:193, 1975.

48. **Broughton Pipkin F, Turner SR, Symonds EM,** Possible risk with captopril in pregnancy: some animal data, Lancet 1:1256, 1980.

49. **Alexander RW, Gimbrone MA Jr,** Stimulation of prostaglandin E synthesis in cultured human umbilical vein smooth muscle cells, Proc Natl Acad Sci 73:1617, 1976.

50. **Gimbrone MA Jr, Alexander RW,** Angiotensin II stimulation of prostaglandin production in cultured human vascular endothelium, Science 189:219, 1975.

51. **Speroff L, Dorfman GS,** Prostaglandins and pregnancy hypertension, Clin Obstet Gynecol 4:635, 1977.

52. **Everett RB, Worley RJ, MacDonald PC, Gant NF,** Effect of prostaglandin synthetase inhibitors on pressor response to angiotensin II in human pregnancy, J Clin Endocrinol Metab 46:1007, 1978.

53. **Gant NF, Chand S, Whalley PJ, MacDonald PC,** The nature of pressor responsiveness to angiotensin II in human pregnancy, Obstet Gynecol 43:854, 1974.

54. **Resnik R,** The endocrine regulation of uterine blood flow in the non-pregnant uterus: a review, Am J Obstet Gynecol 140:151, 1981.

55. **Fujieda K, Faiman C, Feyes FL, Winter JSD,** The control of steroidogenesis by human fetal adrenal cells in tissue culture: IV. The effects of exposure to placental steroids, J Clin Endocrinol Metab 54:89, 1982.

56. **Downing I, Shepherd GL, Lewis PJ,** Reduced prostacyclin production in pre-eclampsia, Lancet 2:1374, 1980.

57. **Bodzenta A, Thomson JM, Poller L,** Prostacyclin activity in amniotic fluid in pre-eclampsia, Lancet 2:650, 1980.

58. **Carreras LO, Defreyn G, Van Houtte E, Vermylen J, Van Assche A,** Prostacyclin and pre-eclampsia, Lancet 1:442, 1981.

59. **Remuzzi G, Marchesi D, Zoja C, Muratore D, Mecca G, Misiani R, Rossi E, Barbato M, Capetta P, Donati MB, de Gaetano G,** Reduced umbilical and placental vascular prostacyclin in severe pre-eclampsia, Prostaglandins 20:105, 1980.

60. **Bussolino F, Benedetto C, Massobrio M, Camussi G,** Maternal vascular prostacyclin activity in pre-eclampsia, Lancet 2:702, 1980.

61. **Ylikorkala O, Makila UM, Viinikka L,** Amniotic fluid prostacyclin and thromboxane in normal, pre-eclamptic, and some other complicated pregnancies, Am J Obstet Gynecol 141:487, 1981.

62. **Goodman RP, Killam AP, Brash AR, Branch RA,** Prostacyclin production during pregnancy: comparison of production during normal pregnancy and pregnancy complicated by hypertension, Am J Obstet Gynecol 142:817, 1982.

63. **Pritchard JA, Cunningham FG, Mason RA,** Coagulation changes in eclampsia: their frequency and pathogenesis, Am J Obstet Gynecol 124:855, 1976.

64. **Bern MM, Driscoll SG, Leavitt T Jr,** Thrombocytopenia complicating pre-eclampsia, Obstet Gynecol 57:28S, 1981.

65. **De Wolf F, Robertson WB, Brosens I,** The ultrastructure of acute atherosis in hypertensive pregnancy, Am J Obstet Gynecol 123:154, 1975.

66. **Jorgensen KA, Pedersen RS,** Familial deficiency of prostacyclin production stimulating factor in the hemolytic uremic syndrome of childhood, Thromb Res 21:311, 1981.

67. **Machin SJ, Defreyn G, Chamone DAF, Vermylen J,** Plasma 6-keto-PGF$_{1\alpha}$ levels after plasma exchange in thrombotic thrombocytopenic purpura, Lancet 1:661, 1980.

68. **Remuzzi G, Imperti L, DeGaetano G,** Prostacyclin deficiency in thrombotic microangiopathy, Lancet 2:1422, 1981.

69. **d'Apice AJF, Reti LL, Pepperell RJ, Fairley KF, Kincaid-Smith P,** Treatment of severe pre-eclampsia by plasma exchange, Aust NZ J Obstet Gynaecol 20:231, 1980.

70. **Crandon AJ, Isherwood DM,** Effect of aspirin on incidence of pre-eclampsia, Lancet 1:1356, 1979.

71. **Carreras LO, Defreyn G, Machin SJ, Vermylen J, Deman R, Spitz B, Assche AV,** Arterial thrombosis, intrauterine death and "lupus" anti-coagulant: detection of immunoglobulin interfering with prostacyclin formation, Lancet 1:244, 1981.

72. **Goodlin RC, Haesslein HO, Gleming J,** Aspirin for the treatment of recurrent toxemia, Lancet 2:51, 1978.

12 Normal and Abnormal Sexual Development

Abnormalities of sexual differentiation are seen infrequently in an individual gynecologist's practice. There are, however, few practitioners who have not been challenged at least once by a newborn with ambiguous genitalia or by a young woman with primary amenorrhea on a genetic basis. The categorization of the various syndromes in this area is confusing, and constant reference to multiple textbooks is essential for informed practice.

This chapter will present a catalogue of the major problems and our clinical approach to diagnosis. Normal sexual differentiation will be considered in order to provide a basis of understanding for the various types of abnormal development. This is followed by a section on the diagnosis and management of ambiguous genitalia. Some subjects are discussed in other chapters, but brief descriptions will be repeated here in order to present a complete picture. The text by Jones and Scott is recommended for greater detail, including descriptions of operative techniques used for the surgical repair of genital abnormalities.

Normal Sexual Differentiation

The gender identity of a person (whether an individual identifies himself as a male or a female) is the end result of genetic, hormonal, and morphologic sex as influenced by the environment of the individual. It includes all behavior with any sexual connotation, such as body gestures and mannerisms, habits of speech, recreational preferences, and content of dreams. Sexual expression, both homosexual and heterosexual, can be regarded as the result of all influences on the individual, both prenatal and postnatal.

Prenatally, sexual differentiation follows a specific sequence of events. First is the establishment of the genetic sex. Second, under the control of the genetic sex the gonads differentiate, determining the hormonal environment of the embryo, the differentiation of internal duct systems, and the formation of the external genitalia. It has become apparent that the embryonic brain is also sexually differentiated, probably via a control mechanism very similar to that which determines the sexual development of the external genitalia. The inductive influences of hormones on the central nervous system may have an effect on the patterns of hormone secretion and sexual behavior in the adult.

Gonadal Differentiation

In human embryos, the gonads begin development during the 5th and 6th weeks of gestation. The complete differentiation of normal gonads depends upon the arrival at the genital ridges of the dorsal mesentery of sufficient numbers of viable primordial germ cells. The germ cells arise extragonadally and, therefore, must migrate into the sites of gonadal differentiation. If they fail to arrive, gonads do not develop (gonadal agenesis) and only a fibrous streak will exist. At 6 weeks of fetal life, the indifferent gonad is bipotential, possessing both cortical and medullary areas, and composed of germ cells, epithelia (potential granulosa-Sertoli cells), mesenchyme (potential theca-Leydig cells), and the mesonephric duct system. (1)

Differentiation of a testis (medullary dominance, cortical regression) depends on the active influence of one or more genes located in the pericentromeric region of the short arm of the Y chromosome. These genes are either identical with, or closely linked, to a gene that codes for a cell surface protein which appears to be the director of testicular organization, the "inducer" substance interacting between germ and somatic cells. This antigen is known as Y-induced histocompatibility antigen, H-Y antigen for short. White blood cells can be tested for the presence of H-Y antigen (H-Y assay), a somewhat, but not totally, reliable indicator for the presence of testicular tissue. It has been detected as early as the 8-cell stage embryo.

In the human, autosomal genes are also essential for gonadal development. (2) These autosomal genes regulate migration of the germ cells, the processing or functioning of the H-Y antigen system, and coding of the steroidogenic enzymes. In the absence of a Y chromosome, the cortical

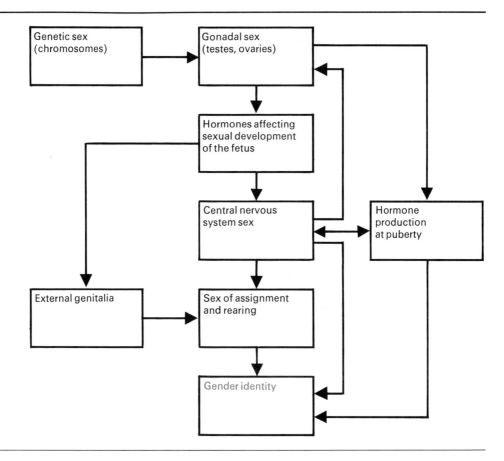

zone develops and contains the germ cells, while the medullary portion regresses with its remnant being the rete ovarii, a compressed nest of tubules and Leydig cells in the hilus of the ovary. The formation of the testicle precedes any other sexual development in time, and a functionally active testis controls subsequent sexual development.

Testicular differentiation begins at 7 weeks; first with spermatogenic cords, then seminiferous tubules, followed by Leydig cell formation a week later. Human chorionic gonadotropin (HCG) stimulation produces Leydig cell hypertrophy, and peak fetal testosterone levels are seen at 12 weeks. (2)

In an XX individual, without the active influence of a Y chromosome, the bipotential gonad develops into an ovary about 2 weeks later than testicular development. The cortical zone differentiates and enlarges, and the germ cells proliferate by mitosis, reaching a peak of 5–7 million by 20 weeks. Medullary components regress to a hilar aggregation of rete tubules and residual nests of Leydig-like hilar cells. By 20 weeks, the fetal ovary achieves mature compartmentalization with primordial follicles containing oocytes, initial evidence of follicle maturation and atresia, and an incipient stroma. Degeneration (atresia) begins even earlier, and by birth, approximately 1–2 million germ cells remain. These have become surrounded by a layer of follicular cells, forming primordial follicles with oocytes which have entered the first meiotic division. Meiosis is arrested in the prophase of the first meiotic division until reactivation of follicular growth which may not occur until years later.

Excessively rapid atresia in gonadal dysgenesis (45,X) accounts for the streak gonad seen in these cases. A complete 46,XX chromosomal complement is necessary for normal ovarian development. Deletion of any portion of an X chromosome results in streak gonads. The short arm of the Y appears to contain loci similar to the short arm of the X chromosome. The absence of either results in short stature and gonadal dysgenesis.

Duct System Differentiation

The Wolffian and Müllerian ducts are discrete primordia which temporarily coexist in all embryos during the ambisexual period of development. One type of duct system persists normally and gives rise to special ducts and glands, whereas the other disappears during the 3rd fetal month, except for nonfunctional vestiges.

The elaboration of androgens by the medullary cells (forerunners of the Leydig cells) in the early testicle stimulates development of the Wolffian duct system into epididymis, vas deferens, and seminal vesicles. Another substance (known as Müllerian inhibiting factor, MIF) is responsible for regression of the Müllerian duct system in the male. MIF is an incompletely characterized protein hormone which is the initial endocrine product of the testis. This influence from the fetal testis is unilateral. Duct system differentiation will proceed, therefore, according to the nature of the adjacent gonad.

The internal genitalia possess the intrinsic tendency to feminize. In the absence of a Y chromosome and a functional testis, the lack of MIF allows retention of the Müllerian system and development of Fallopian tubes, uterus, and upper vagina. In the absence of testosterone, the Wolffian system regresses. In the presence of a normal ovary or the absence of any gonad, Müllerian duct development takes place.

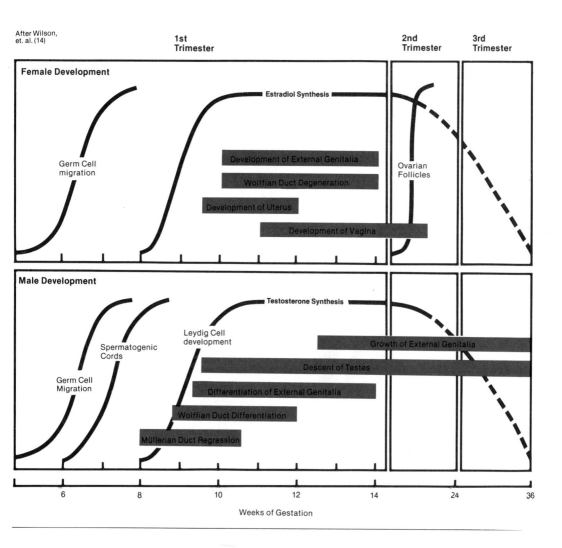

After Wilson, et. al. (14)

1st Trimester   2nd Trimester   3rd Trimester

Female Development

Estradiol Synthesis

Germ Cell migration

Development of External Genitalia

Wolffian Duct Degeneration

Development of Uterus

Development of Vagina

Ovarian Follicles

Male Development

Testosterone Synthesis

Leydig Cell development

Spermatogenic Cords

Germ Cell Migration

Growth of External Genitalia

Descent of Testes

Differentiation of External Genitalia

Wolffian Duct Differentiation

Müllerian Duct Regression

6   8   10   12   14   24   36

Weeks of Gestation

External Genitalia Differentiation

In the bipotential state (8th fetal week), the external genitalia consist of a urogenital sinus, two lateral labioscrotal swellings, and a genital tubercle. Unlike the internal genitalia where both duct systems initially coexist, the external genitalia are neutral primordia able to develop into either male or female structures depending on gonadal steroid hormone signals. Normally, this differentiation is under the active influence of androgen from the Leydig cells of the testis. The genital tubercle forms the penis, labioscrotal folds fuse to form a scrotum, and folds of the urogenital sinus form the penile urethra. The testis begins androgen secretion by 8–9 weeks; masculinization of the external genitalia is manifest 1 week later and is completed by 17 weeks. To achieve this morphologic change, external genitalia target tissue cells must convert testosterone (T) to dihydrotestosterone (DHT) by the intracellular enzyme 5α-reductase. In the male, DHT mediates the following androgen events: temporal hairline recession, growth of facial and body hairs, development of acne, and development of the external genitalia and prostate.

Genital tubercle

Urogenital slit

Anal pit

Tail

Urethral folds

Labioscrotal swelling

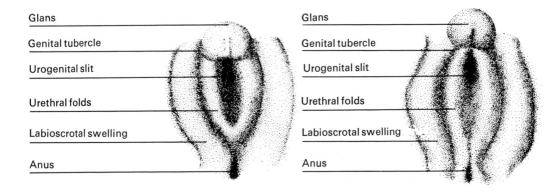

Bipotential Stage

Glans

Genital tubercle

Urogenital slit

Urethral folds

Labioscrotal swelling

Anus

Glans

Genital tubercle

Urogenital slit

Urethral folds

Labioscrotal swelling

Anus

Glans penis

Meatus

Clitoris

Urethral meatus

Labia minora

Vaginal orifice

Labia majora

Scrotum

Raphe

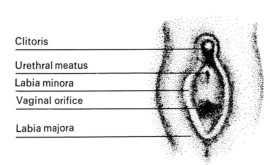

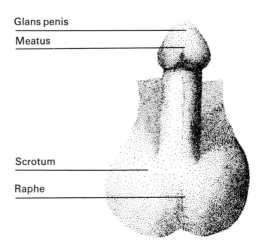

In the absence of this androgen effect (the absence of a Y chromosome, the presence of an ovary, the absence of a gonad, abnormalities in androgen receptor or postreceptor events, or defects of the 5α-reductase enzyme), the folds of the urogenital sinus remain open, forming the labia minora, the labioscrotal folds form the labia majora, the genital tubercle forms the clitoris, and the urogenital sinus differentiates into the vagina and the urethra. Thus, the lower vagina is formed as part of the external genitalia.

Exposure to androgens at critical time periods leads to variable masculinization. Androgen superimposes variable external ambiguity on the basic female phenotype (clitoral hypertrophy, hypospadias, scrotalization of nonfused labia). By the same token, if sufficient local androgen concentration or activity is not achieved by the 12th week in the male, incompletely masculinized genitalia will result. Because of shared common tissue origin, male-female external genital structural ambiguities reflect abnormal androgen impact—males too little, females too much.

Central Nervous System Differentiation

At the same time as the presence or absence of androgens is playing a critical role in genitalia development, the neuroendocrine mechanism of the central nervous system is also being influenced. Androgens present in sufficient amounts during the appropriate critical stage of development may program the CNS to induce the potential for male sexual behavior. (3) Experimental and analytical evidence suggests that a behavioral effect can be traced to this early androgen influence. Inappropriate fetal hormonal programming may contribute, therefore, to the spectrum of psychosexual behavior seen in humans.

Abnormal Sexual Differentiation

The standard classification of individuals with intersexuality (hermaphroditism) proceeds according to gonadal morphology. In this terminology, a *true hermaphrodite* possesses both ovarian and testicular tissue. A *male pseudohermaphrodite* has testes, but external and sometimes internal genitalia take on female phenotypic aspects. A *female pseudohermaphrodite* has ovaries, but genital development displays masculine characteristics. These classifications are modified to reflect gonadal abnormalities due to abnormal sex chromosome constitution or abnormalities of phenotype attributable to an inappropriate fetal hormone environment. Hypospadias in the absence of any other deformity is not included in this classification:

Disorders of Fetal Endocrinology

1. ***Female pseudohermaphroditism (partial virilization)***
    a. Congenital adrenal hyperplasia
        i.   21-Hydroxylase deficiency
        ii. 11-Hydroxylase deficiency
        iii. 3β-ol-Dehydrogenase deficiency
    b. Nonadrenal androgenization
        i.   Drug intake
        ii. Maternal disease

2. ***Male pseudohermaphroditism (inadequate virilization)***
    a. Müllerian duct inhibitory factor defect
    b. Impaired androgenization
        i.   Complete testicular feminization
        ii. Incomplete testicular feminization
        iii. 5α-Reductase deficiency
    c. Testosterone biosynthesis defects
        i.   20–22-Desmolase defect
        ii. 3β-ol-Dehydrogenase deficiency
        iii. 17α-Hydroxylase deficiency
        iv. 17–20-Desmolase deficiency
        v.   17-Hydroxysteroid dehydrogenase deficiency

Disorders of Gonadal Development

1. ***Male Pseudohermaphroditism***
    a. Primary gonadal defect
    b. Y Chromosome defect

2. ***True Hermaphroditism***

3. ***Gonadal dysgenesis***
    a. Turner's syndrome
    b. Mosaicism
    c. Structural abnormality—X chromosome
    d. Normal karyotype

Masculinized Females
(Female
Pseudohermaprhrodites)

Masculinized females possess ovaries and are female by genetic sex (XX), but the external genitalia are not those of a normal female. Of all infants with ambiguous genitalia, 40–45% have adrenal hyperplasia. Rarer causes of female pseudohermaphroditism are excess maternal androgen caused by drug ingestion or tumor secretion.

The Adrenogenital Syndrome. The adrenogenital syndrome in females is characterized by masculinized external genitalia, and is diagnosed by demonstrating excessive androgen production by the adrenal cortex, due either to tumor or hyperplasia. The syndrome may appear at birth or develop postnatally. If present at birth, it is invariably due to virilizing adrenal hyperplasia, while if first noted in an older child it is usually due to an adrenal tumor.

The presence of excessive androgens is manifested by varying degrees of fusion of the labioscrotal folds, clitoral enlargement, and anatomical changes of the urethra and vagina. Generally, the urethra and vagina share a urogenital sinus formed by the fusion of labial folds. This sinus opens at the base of the clitoris which is usually enlarged. The degree of urogenital sinus deformity is related to the timing in prenatal development of the onset of masculinizing androgen effect. Only the external genitalia are affected because internal genitalia differentiation is completed by the 10th week of gestation while the adrenal cortex begins function by the 12th week. Since the female external genitalia phenotype is not completed until 140 days of fetal age, early androgen excess (7–12 weeks) may fully masculinize, whereas late (18–20 weeks) androgen may create limited ambiguity of the basically female appearance of the urogenital sinus and genital folds. The size of the clitoris depends on the quantity rather than timing of androgen excess. Cases of incorrect sex assignment in the female are due to the similarity between these external genitalia and hypospadias and bilateral cryptorchidism in a male infant.

If untreated, the female with adrenal hyperplasia will develop signs of progressive virilization. Pubic hair will appear by age 2–4, followed by axillary hair, then body hair and beard. Bone age is advanced by age 2, and because of early epiphyseal closure, height in childhood is achieved at the expense of shortened stature in adulthood. Progressive masculinization continues with the development of the male habitus, acne, deepened voice, and primary amenorrhea and infertility.

In addition to sexual changes, patients may present with metabolic disorders such as salt-wasting, hypertension, or rarely, hypoglycemia. An electrolyte imbalance of the salt-losing type is usually apparent within a few days of birth and occurs in approximately one third of patients with virilizing adrenal hyperplasia. Beginning with a refusal to feed, failure to thrive, apathy, and vomiting, the infant goes on to an Addisonian-like crisis with hyponatremia, hyperkalemia, and acidosis. Rapid diagnosis and treatment are necessary to save these infants. Less frequent is hypertension, which occurs in approximately 5% of patients with virilizing adrenal hyperplasia.

Pathophysiology. Virilizing adrenal hyperplasia is the result of an inherited abnormality of steroid biosynthesis which results in an inability to synthesize glucocorticoids. The hypothalamic-pituitary axis reacts to the low level of cortisol by elevated ACTH secretion in a homeostatic response to achieve normal levels of cortisol production. This stimulation causes a hyperplastic adrenal cortex which produces androgens as well as corticoid precursors in abnormal quantities. Therefore, one can see a well-compensated infant who has achieved normal cortisol levels, but at the expense of extensive masculinization.

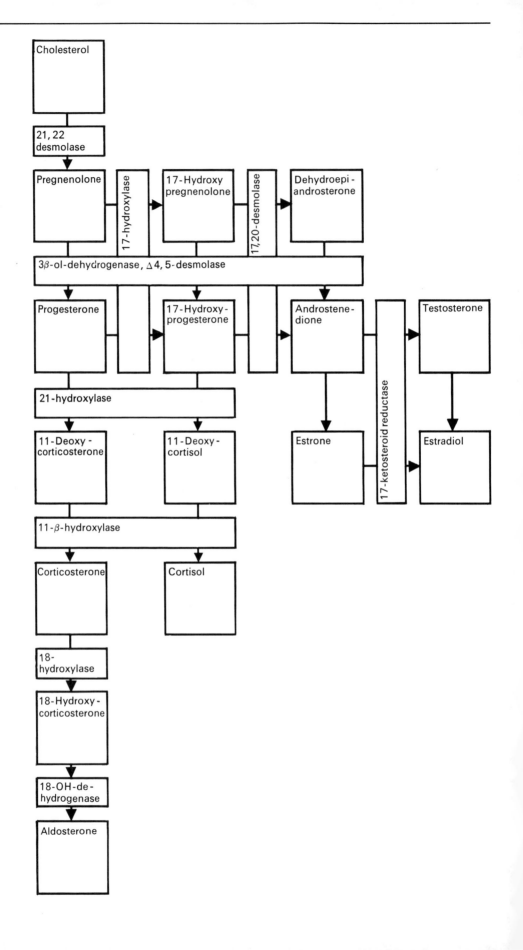

Although the most common defects are the 21-hydroxylase and 11β-hydroxylase types, each of the enzymatic steps from cholesterol to cortisol can be expressed in specific clinical disease. (4) Some affect the adrenal only, while others affect adrenal and ovarian steroid synthesis. It should be noted here that similar defects occur in males as well as females. Both excessive and insufficient androgenization can be seen in affected males.

Enzyme Defect in Adrenal Only: Deficient 21-Hydroxylase. The 21-hydroxylase block is the most common form of congenital adrenal hyperplasia, the most frequent cause of sexual ambiguity, and the most frequent endocrine cause of neonatal death. With severe uncompensated blocks of this type, salt wasting and shock accompany significant virilization. In less severe variations, when sufficient cortisol can be produced, virilization due to excess androgen is still present. Therefore, two different clinical forms are recognized, the salt wasting and the simple virilizing forms. The difference between the two forms has been explained by the completeness of the defect or the presence of defects in both 17-hydroxy and 11-deoxy pathways in salt wasters. A new proposal suggests that simple virilizers have a 21-hydroxylation defect confined to the fasiculata, while salt wasters have the defect in both fasiculata and glomerulosa, the glomerulosa defect leading to reduced aldosterone synthesis. (4) Endocrine studies show elevated 17-ketosteroid and pregnanetriol urinary excretion, and high levels of 17-hydroxyprogesterone (17-OHP) in serum.

Enzyme Defect in Adrenal Only: Deficient 11β-Hydroxylase. The final step in cortisol synthesis is blocked in this condition. The adrenal fasiculata and glomerulosa function as two separate glands, with the fasiculata regulated by ACTH and the glomerulosa regulated by the renin-angiotensin system. In this defect, the 11β-hydroxylase deficiency is present only in the fasiculata, and is accompanied by a fasiculata deficiency in 18-hydroxylase. (4) The glomerulosa capability of these two enzymes is not impaired. As a result, metabolically active precursors of corticosterone and cortisol add to excess androgen synthesis as liabilities of ACTH-induced hyperplasia. Hypertension is induced by elevated dexoycorticosterone (DOC) with reduced renin and aldosterone, and virilization by androgens of the "deoxy" type (dehydroepiandrosterone (DHA), dehydroepiandrosterone sulfate, and androstenedione). The diagnosis is confirmed by high plasma DOC and compound S (11-deoxycortisol) levels and increased urinary excretion of their tetrahydro derivatives.

345

Enzyme Defect in Adrenal and Ovary: Deficient 17α-Hydroxylase. With block of the 17α-hydroxylase enzyme, synthesis of cortisol, androgens, and estrogens is curtailed. Only the non-17-hydroxylated corticoids, DOC and corticosterone, are formed. (5) The resulting syndrome is composed of hypertension, infantile female external genitalia, which do not mature at puberty, and primary amenorrhea with elevated follicle-stimulating hormone (FSH) and luteinizing hormone (LH). Genital ambiguity is not a problem at birth.

Enzyme Defects in Adrenal and Ovary: Deficient 3β-ol-Dehydrogenase. Lack of this essential step in the formation of all biologically active steroids affects both the adrenal cortex and the ovary. Thus, there is decreased synthesis of corticoids, androgens, and estrogens. These infants are severely ill at birth and rarely survive. The external genitalia ambiguity presumably results from the massive increase in DHA and androstenediol which are androgenic when available in excess.

Enzyme Defects in Adrenal and Ovary: Deficient 20–22-Desmolase. A block in this step prevents conversion of cholesterol to pregnenolone, the necessary precursor to all biologically active steroids. The adrenals are enlarged and filled with cholesterol esters. Predictably, the internal and external genitalia are female, and death occurs.

Genetic Aspects. The genetic defect in virilizing adrenal hyperplasia is an autosomal recessive gene. Within families, the clinical picture is uniform, the type of syndrome (simple, salt-losing, hypertensive) is always the same in affected siblings. The ratio in offspring of unaffected parents is one affected to three nonaffected individuals. Treated patients have a 1:100 to 1:200 chance of producing an affected infant. Males and females are at equal risk. The overall incidence of the 21-hydroxylase deficiency is between 1:5,000 and 1:15,000.

New and her colleagues have recently reported a new and cryptic form of 21-hydroxylase deficiency in family members of patients with classic overt disease. (4, 6) These were discovered as a result of HLA studies, the gene for the hydroxylase deficiency having been linked to this locus. As a result of extensive hormonal studies (using ACTH), this group has proposed that allelic variants at the steroid 21-hydroxylase locus produce different degrees of 21-hydroxylase deficiency, resulting in the diversity of phenotypes such as overt classical disease, late onset deficiency, and asymptomatic cryptic types. (4) The phenotypic variability displayed in other enzyme defects of steroid biosynthesis (11β-hydroxylase, 17-hydroxysteroid dehydrogenase) may also be the result of genetic heterogeneity.

The diagnosis of congenital adrenal hyperplasia due to 21-hydroxylase deficiency may be obtained prenatally by demonstrating elevated levels of 17-OHP and androstenedione in the amniotic fluid. HLA genotyping of amniotic cells may yield confirmation by showing that the fetus is HLA identical to an affected sibling. The 11β-hydroxylase deficiency is associated with elevated levels of 11-deoxycortisol in amniotic fluid, but this defect is not linked to HLA.

Diagnosis. Since the genetic sex is XX, the sex chromatin will be positive. For years the demonstration of a metabolic defect and its location depended upon the study of urinary steroid excretion. The table shows the normal and abnormal values of 17-ketosteroids. Notice that, in the first few days of life, the excretion of 17-ketosteroids is normally slightly higher; however, pregnanetriol excretion is not elevated.

Urinary 17-Ketosteroid Excretion (mg per 24 hours)

Age	Normal Values	Values in Virilizing Adrenal Hyperplasia
1–10 days	0.5–5.0	
2–3 weeks	0.5–1.0	2–6
1–6 months	0.5	1–10
7–12 months	0.5	3–10
1–5 years	1.0	4–30
6–9 years	2.0	11–40
10–15 years	4–10	16–50
Over 15 years	7–13	21–80

Further study of the urine will reveal abnormal levels of pregnanetriol with 21- and 11β-hydroxylase blocks, elevated levels of tetrahydro-S and DOC in the hypertensive type (11β-hydroxylase block), and elevated levels of DHA in the 3β-ol-dehydrogenase defect. Total excretion of 17-ketosteroids may not be impressively elevated with the 3β-ol-dehydrogenase block.

In recent years, the radioimmunoassay of blood 17-OHP has proved useful in the diagnosis and management of congenital adrenal hyperplasia. With the 21- and 11β-hydroxylase blocks, the 17-OHP level may be 50–400-fold above normal (normal is less than 1 ng/ml).

During delivery of affected infants, the concentration of 17-OHP is elevated in cord blood (1000–3000 ng/dl), but it rapidly decreases to 100–200 ng/dl after 24 hours. A delay in measurement gains accuracy. In contrast to 17-ketosteroids where the delay must be several days, with 17-OHP the delay need be only a day or two. In affected patients, 17-OHP levels range from 3000 to 40,000 ng/dl. Of course, in patients with 3β-dehydrogenase or 17-hydroxylase blocks the 17-OHP level will not be elevated. With the 3β-dehydrogenase block, the blood levels of DHA and DHA sulfate (DHAS) will be markedly increased.

347

Treatment. Treatment of adrenal hyperplasia is to supply the deficient hormone, cortisol. This decreases ACTH secretion and lowers production of androgenic precursors. The addition of salt-retaining hormone to glucocorticoid therapy has improved the control of the disease. When the plasma renin activity is normalized, ACTH and androgen levels are further decreased, and a decrease in the glucocorticoid dose is also possible. Therefore, the modern management of hormonal control requires the measurement of the blood levels of 17-OHP, androstenedione, testosterone, and plasma renin activity. (4) The drugs of choice are hydrocortisone and 9-fluorohydrocortisone. This method of treatment and monitoring applies to all forms of adrenal hyperplasia. Minor stresses will cause brief elevations of adrenal androgens, but usually do not require readjustment of dosage. With major stress, such as surgery, additional hormonal support is necessary.

The surgical treatment of the anatomical abnormalities should be carried out in the first few years of life, when the patient is still too young to remember the procedure and too young to have developed psychological problems centered about the abnormal external genitalia. If clitoridectomy is necessary, it is important to know that women who undergo total clitoral amputations have no subsequent impairment of erotic responsiveness or capacity for orgasm.

Normal reproduction is possible with replacement therapy of the cortisol deficiency. Many cases come to cesarean section because normal anatomy of the perineum may be obscured by scar tissue from earlier plastic surgery; therefore, greater blood loss and the risk of a hematoma with a vaginal delivery are significant factors. A masculine pelvis is not expected since the adult form and size of the inlet of the pelvis are assumed largely during the growth spurt in puberty. However, a small pelvis might be anticipated if the bone age is up to age 13–14 when treatment is initiated.

The maintenance steroid dose usually does not need to be changed during pregnancy. Urinary 17-ketosteroids do not alter appreciably during pregnancy, and may be used for monitoring the patient. The dosage of steroids used in the treatment of this syndrome replaces the approximate amount normally produced, and, therefore, is a physiologic dose. At these low doses, teratogenic effects would be unlikely, and none have been noted.

The need for additional steroids during the stress of labor and delivery is obvious, and is usually met by the administration of cortisone acetate intramuscularly and cortisol intravenously. Infection and impaired wound healing have not been problems. Aside from the liability associated with genetic transmission of this syndrome, the children born to patients with adrenal hyperplasia have been normal. The newborn should be closely observed for adrenal insufficiency due to steroid crossover and suppression of the fetal adrenal in utero.

Masculinization Due to Elevated Androgens in Maternal Circulation	Masculinization of the female fetus, while in most cases due to fetal virilizing adrenal hyperplasia, may be produced by an androgen-secreting maternal tumor, or may be due to the intake of exogenous androgenic substances. When not caused by an error in the metabolism of the fetal adrenal gland, virilization is not progressive, urinary 17-ketosteroids and blood 17-OHP are not elevated, and no hormonal therapy is needed. Subsequent development will be normal. Therefore, surgical correction of abnormalities in the external genitalia is the only indicated treatment.

The occurrence of an androgen-secreting tumor in a mother during pregnancy is rarely seen. On the other hand, the iatrogenic cause of masculinization is a well-known story. The majority of these cases resulted from antenatal maternal treatment of threatened or recurrent abortion with various progestin compounds. In view of the lack of evidence for positive results with such therapy, the use of progestin compounds in pregnancy is contraindicated.

Incompletely Masculinized Males; (Male Pseudohermaphrodites)	Incompletely masculinized males are male by genetic sex (XY) and possess testicles, but the external genitalia are not normally male. Male pseudohermaophrodites may arise in one of three ways:

1. An insensitivity to androgen,

2. Abnormal androgen synthesis,

3. Absent or defective Müllerian inhibiting factor.

Syndromes of Androgen Insensitivity

Complete Androgen Insensitivity—Testicular Feminization. The phenotype of this condition (also discussed in Chapter 5) is female because there is a congenital insensitivity to androgens, transmitted by means of a maternal X-linked recessive gene responsible for the androgen intracellular receptor. (7) Therefore, androgen induction of Wolffian duct development does not occur. However, MIF activity is present, and the individual does not have Müllerian development (a natural experiment which indicates the presence of an MIF). The vagina is short (derived from the urogenital sinus only) and ends blindly. The uterus and tubes are absent. There is no problem of sex assignment as there is no trace of androgen activity. This syndrome accounts for about 10% of all cases of primary amenorrhea.

The "complete" form indicates that there is no androgen response; therefore, normal external female development occurs, and these infants should be reared as females. The gonads may be present in the inguinal canals, and children with inguinal hernias and/or inguinal masses should be suspected of testicular feminization. There is no virilization at puberty because of the lack of androgen response. In contrast to dysgenetic gonads with a Y chromosome, the occurrence of gonadal tumors is relatively late. (7, 8) Therefore, gonadectomy should be performed at approximately age 16–18, to allow endogenous hormonal changes and a smooth transition through puberty.

Because of the importance of prophylactic gonadectomy, detection of this syndrome demands careful investigation for other affected family members. Future apparent sisters of affected individuals have a 1 in 3 chance of being XY; female offspring of a normal sister of an affected individual have a 1 in 6 chance of being XY. About a third of the patients have negative family histories and presumably represent new mutations.

Incomplete Androgen Insensitivity. A spectrum of disorders, all due to an X-linked recessive trait, are known as incomplete forms of testicular feminization. (9) The clinical presentation ranges from almost complete failure of virilization to essentially complete phenotypic masculinization. Toward the feminine end of the spectrum is Lub's syndrome, while toward the masculine end is Reifenstein's syndrome. Recently, males have been described whose only indication of androgen insensitivity was azospermic or severe oligospermic infertility. Indeed the incidence may approach 40% or more of men with infertility due to azospermia or severe oligospermia. (10) The diversity of presentation represents variable manifestations of the same mutant gene. The biochemical abnormality lies in the degree of function of the androgen receptor or postreceptor events. (11)

Sex assignment may be a problem when ambiguous genitalia exist because of a partial response of the receptor. If sex assignment is female, early gonadectomy is performed to avoid neoplasia. In the Reifenstein syndrome, the phallus may be large enough to allow a male sex assignment at birth, despite the perineal hypospadias. After puberty, however, the inadequate androgen receptor resource becomes evident and feminization with gynecomastia occurs. The receptor function is inadequate to respond to the surge of androgen at puberty; without androgen effect, estrogen activity prevails. These individuals are infertile and cannot react to exogenous androgen, the karyotype is male XY, distinguishing it from other feminizing syndromes of puberty in phenotypic males (e.g. Klinefelter's syndrome).

The endocrine profiles of both the complete and incomplete forms are similar: high blood levels of testosterone, LH, and estradiol.

5α-Reductase Deficiency. This form of familial incomplete male pseudohermaphroditism is due to an autosomal recessive trait characterized by severe perineal hypospadias and underdevelopment of the vagina. (12) In the past it was known as pseudovaginal perineoscrotal hypospadias (PPH). It differs from the incomplete forms of testicular feminization because, at puberty, masculinization occurs. Normal testicular function occurs, and there is no lack of response

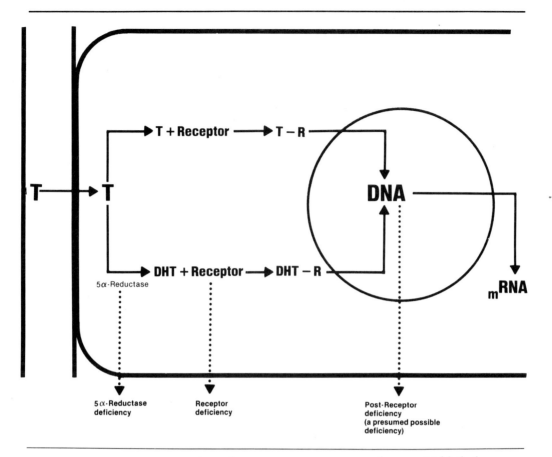

T

T + Receptor → T – R

DNA

5α-Reductase

DHT + Receptor → DHT – R

mRNA

5 α-Reductase
deficiency

Receptor
deficiency

Post-Receptor
deficiency
(a presumed possible
deficiency)

to endogenous or exogenous androgen. At birth, however, the external genitalia are similar to that of incomplete testicular feminization; i.e. hypospadias, varying failure of fusion of laboiscrotal folds and a urogenital opening, or separate urethral and vaginal openings. The cleft in the scrotum appears to be a vagina (there are no Müllerian ducts), and these patients have been reared as girls with an enlarged clitoris. At birth, steroid levels are normal, ruling out adrenal disorders. Diagnosis can be established by demonstrating an elevated T/DHT ratio based upon the blood levels of testosterone and dihydrotestosterone, especially after HCG stimulation. The karyotype is XY, and, as with other incompletely masculinized males, the sex assignment is female if the phallus is inadequate. Gonadectomy is necessary to avoid not only neoplasia but the virilization that is certain to appear at puberty. The deficiency is believed to be due to the homozygous state, manifest clinically only in males. Homozygous 46,XX females have normal fertility.

Study of this syndrome points out three important lessons in intersexuality. (13) In this condition, the Wolffian duct virilizes in a normal male fashion, but the urogenital sinus and genital tubercle persist as female structures. The failure is due to inadequate DHT formation intracellularly in these external genitalia tissues at the time the normal male fetus virilizes. In the 5α-reductase deficiencies, the seminal vesicles, ejaculatory ducts, epididymis, and vas deferens which

351

are all testosterone-dependent are present, whereas the DHT-dependent structures, external genitalia, urethra, and prostate do not develop along male lines. Affected men have less facial and body hair, less temporal hairline recession and no problems with acne. DHT presence is a requirement only in the fetus, as indicated by the significant genital virilization these patients undergo at puberty and thereafter. (14) Whereas the conversion from male to female role is exceedingly traumatic psychologically, the reversal of sex identity (female to male) these patients undergo at puberty is apparently uncomplicated. (3) In one such case, a "double-life" was conducted. Although functioning in all public respects as a female, one 5α-reductase individual conducted numerous and prolonged heterosexual affairs, which were quite satisfactory, albeit clandestine. He had known of his male sexual identity since puberty, but delayed medical assistance for fear that exposure would bring shame and guilt to his religously devout elderly "old world" mother. He decided to keep his secret until his mother died. He finally sought diagnostic help at age 65, however, because his mother at age 93 continued to enjoy good health.

Abnormal Androgen Synthesis.

Defects in testosterone synthesis can be at any one of the five required enzymatic reactions which lead from cholesterol to testosterone; 21,22-desmolase; 3β-ol-dehydrogenase; 17α-hydroxylase, 17,20-desmolase; and 17-ketosteroid reductase. These defects are inherited as autosomal recessive traits, and the phenotypes range from partial to complete male pseudohermaphroditism.

Patients with male pseudohermaphroditism who are considered variants of testicular feminization upon partial virilization at puberty may actually have a defect in androgen synthesis. The diagnosis is made by demonstrating elevated 17-ketosteroids, and elevated blood levels of androstenedione and estrogens, while the blood level of testosterone is low or low-normal. (15) When the enzyme involves a reaction which is active in the adrenal gland (all but the 17-ketosteoid reductase), the adrenal blocks are usually severe with adrenal failure and death in the newborn period.

The male pseudohermaphrodite due to deficient testicular 17-ketosteroid reductase activity has male internal genitalia and no Müllerian structures. Masculinization, however, is incomplete. These individuals may develop gynecomastia at puberty due to elevated estrogen levels arising from peripheral conversion of the increased androstenedione. Early gonadectomy is required to avoid virilization at puberty and testicular neoplasia.

Abnormal Müllerian Inhibiting Factor

Hernia Uterine Inguinale (Uterine Hernia Syndrome). Individuals with this syndrome appear to be normal males, but relatively well-differentiated Müllerian duct structures are found, usually a uterus and tubes in an inguinal hernia sac. This is apparently an isolated failure of MIF and Müllerian regression, inherited as a recessive trait, either X-linked or autosomal. Fertility is usually preserved.

Abnormal
Gonadogenesis

The proper development and eventual function of the gonad depends on the presence of germ cells, the appropriate sex chromosome constitution, and appropriate gonadal ridge somatic cells. Errors in meiotic division can cause aneuploidy and abnormal sex chromosomes. These occur by nondisjunction, anaphase lag, translocation, breakage, rearrangements, or deletions. Mitosis can also be marred by nondisjunction and anaphase lag leading to mosaicism. Two or more different cell lines can persist and appear in different tissues. Finally, abnormal gonadogenesis may occur as a result of structural or disease related catastrophies leading to loss of fetal gonadal function.

Bilateral Dysgenesis of the Testes (Swyer Syndrome). Affected individuals have an XY karyotype but normal (infantile) female external and internal genitalia. (16) There are fibrous bands in place of the gonads yielding primary amenorrhea and lack of secondary sexual development at puberty. It is a matter of prudent practice to avoid the possibility of virilization or neoplasm; therefore, laparotomy and removal of these band areas are advocated. Presumably, testes failed to develop or were eliminated (testicular regression) before internal or external genital differentiation in this syndrome. Estrogen and progestin sequential therapy supports female secondary sex development. Menstruation occurs from endometrial cells with an XY chromosome.

True Agonadism. The pathogenesis of this condition, in view of a normal XY sex chromosome complement, must be complete testicular degeneration sometime between 6 and 12 weeks of pregnancy. If testicular loss is early, there is inadequate androgen stimulation (minimal Wolffian development and female external genitalia), and Müllerian ducts are preserved. The presence of a normal vagina, uterus, and tubes distinguishes this syndrome from testicular feminization variants. However, if testes loss occurs late, no gonads will be present, external genitalia will be ambiguous (but primarily female), and rudimentary components of both Müllerian and Wolffian internal ducts present. Laparotomy (removal of bands) is required as a precaution against neoplasia.

353

Event	Time of Event (Days after Fertiliz- ation)	Nomenclature	Müllerian Duct	Wolffian Duct	External Genitalia
Early embryonic testicular regression	Before 43	Pure gonadal dysgenesis	Present	Absent	Female
Late embryonic testic- ular regression	43–59	Swyer syn- drome	Present	Absent	Female
Early fetal testicular regression	60–69	Agonadism	Present	Absent	Ambiguous
	70–75	Testicular dys- genesis	Present	Present	Ambiguous
	75–84	Testicular regression	Absent	Present	Ambiguous
Midfetal testicular regression	90–120	Rudimentary testis	Absent	Present	Male infantile
Late fetal testicular regression	After 140	Vanishing tes- tis, Anorchia	Absent	Present	Male infantile

Anorchia. Affected XY individuals have infantile unambiguous male external genitalia, male Wolffian ducts, and lack Müllerian ducts. There are, however, no detectable testes. Early testis function did occur (Wolffian presence, MIF function), but was not sustained in sufficient amounts or duration to develop a normal size phallus. It is frequently called "the disappearing testis syndrome." Sex of assignment depends on the extent of external genitalia development.

True Hermaphrodites

Abnormal sexual differentiation can occur as a result of a mixture of gonadal sex (true hermaphroditism) or complete uncertainty of gonadal sex (gonadal dysgenesis with some virilization). (17) A true hermaphrodite possesses both ovarian and testicular tissue. Both types may be contained in one gonad (ovotestis) or one side may be an ovary, the other a testis. The internal structures correspond to the adjacent gonad. In the majority, external genitalia are ambiguous with sufficient male character to allow male sex assignment. However, three-fourths develop gynecomastia and half menstruate post-puberty. Fifty percent are genetic females (XX), few are XY, the rest are mosaics with at least one cell line XX.

Gonadal Dysgenesis

Gonadal dysgenesis due to the presence of only one X chromosome in all cell lines (X chromosome monosomy) is Turner's syndrome. The individual is 45,X or as written in the past, XO. In the absence of gonadal development, the individuals are phenotypic females. The well-known characteristics are short stature (48–58 inches), sexual infantilism, and streak gonads. The streak gonad is composed of fibrous tissue, containing no ova or follicular derivatives. Other congenital problems in this syndrome are: a webbed neck, coarctation of the aorta, a high arched palate, cubitus valgus, a broad shield-like chest with widely spaced nipples, a low hairline on the neck, short fourth metacarpal bones, and renal abnormalities. Usually the diagnosis is not made until puberty when amenorrhea and lack of sexual development become apparent. At birth, however, lymphedema of the extremities may indicate the condition. About 98% of conceptuses with only one X chromosome abort. The remaining 2% account for an incidence of 45,X in about 1 in 10,000 liveborn girls.

A large variety of mosaic patterns is seen with gonadal dysgenesis. From analysis of the various combinations, it is apparent that short stature is related to loss of the short arm of one X chromosome. Thus X, XXp-, and XXqi are all short. Xqi designates an isochromosome for the long arms, and Xp-, deletion of the short arm. The loss of the long arm of one of the X chromosomes (XXq-) is associated with amenorrhea and streak gonads, but the patients are not short and do not have the other malformations. Thus, loss of material from the short arms of the X chromosome leads to short stature and the other stigmata of Turner's syndrome. Streak gonads result if any part of an X chromosome is missing. This suggests that normal ovarian development requires two loci, one on the long arm and one on the short arm; loss of either results in gonadal failure. Thyroid autoimmunity is common in Turner's syndrome, but Hashimoto's thyroiditis may be specific to the 46,XXqi cases.

The presence of menstrual function and reproduction in a patient with Turner's phenotype must be due to a mosaic complement, such as a 46,XX line in addition to 45,X. Multiple X females (47,XXX) have normal development and reproductive function, although mental retardation may be more frequent. Secondary amenorrhea and/or eunuchoidism may be seen.

Just as X chromosome monosomy, with deletion of the second X chromosome, results in Turner's phenotype— female phenotype, sexual infantilism, and dysgenetic gonads—the same will apply to loss of the Y chromosome. The 45,X karyotype derived from leukocyte culture does not guarantee that a mosaic does not exist with a gonadal cell line containing XY. For this reason, repeated pelvic examinations are required to detect incipient signs of gonadal neoplasia as an adnexal mass. If a presumed 45,X (based on white cell culture karyotype) develops breasts or sexual hair *without* exogenous therapy, a gonadoblastoma or dysgerminoma should be considered and ruled out. Heterosexual signs require the same scrutiny in all 45,X individuals. The hope that clinical decisions could be eased by detection of the H-Y antigen has not been fulfilled thus far.

Pure Gonadal Dysgenesis

A normal XY karyotype can be found in a phenotypic female with sexual infantilism and streak gonads. Clearly, the genetic content of the Y chromosome is abnormal despite its morphologic presence in these cases. Removal of streaks is required.

Noonan's Syndrome

Both affected males and females have apparently normal chromosome complements and normal gonadal function. The phenotypic appearance of the female is that of a patient with Turner's syndrome: short stature, webbed neck, shield chest, and cardiac malformations. The cardiac lesions, however, are different. Pulmonic stenosis is most frequent in Noonan's syndrome as opposed to aortic coarctation in Turner's. Apparently this syndrome results from a mutant gene or genes (9). In the past these patients have been referred to as male Turner's or Turner's with normal chromosomes.

Summary

In gonadal dysgenesis, the gonadal structures are streak gonads, and the external genitalia are of infantile female type. In mixed gonadal dysgenesis, testicular tissue may be present on one side and a streak gonad on the other. Mosaicism is the likely underlying abnormality, though it may not be detected in the cell line studied. The external genitalia may be female, ambiguous, or almost normal male. Ambiguous genitalia are produced if testicular tissue is present, from clitoral hypertrophy to basically male with hypospadias. Internal genitalia are basically female with some Müllerian regression (absent tube) expressed adjacent to the gonad with testicular components. Virilization and neoplasia dictate timely gonadectomy.

Diagnosis of Ambiguous Genitalia

Ambiguous external genitalia in a newborn infant represents a major diagnostic challenge. The physician may find himself in a pressure-filled situation because of the necessity for making such an influential decision as the sex of rearing. Diagnostic procedures may delay the decision, and it is well-recognized that a period of delay is far better than later reversal of the sex assignment. Parental education and guidance are essential in this anxiety-ridden situation.

The most important point to remember when confronted with a newborn infant with ambiguous genitalia or an apparently male infant with bilateral cryptorchidism, is that the prime diagnosis until ruled out is congenital adrenal hyperplasia. The reason is clear: adrenal hyperplasia is the only condition which is life-threatening. Signs of adrenal failure such as vomiting, diarrhea, dehydration, and shock may develop rapidly.

The history of a previously affected relative may aid in the diagnosis of testicular feminization or any of its variants. Similarly, the history of a sibling with genital ambiguity or the history of a previous neonatal death in a sibling strongly suggest the possibility of adrenal hyperplasia. A history of maternal exposure to androgenic compounds may be difficult to elicit. The mother may be unaware of the nature of her medications, and the obstetrician should be consulted.

Palpation of the genital and inguinal regions is the most important part of the physical examination. Careful examination of the phallus may differentiate between a clitoris and a penis. The penis has a midline ventral frenulum, while the clitoris has two folds which extend from the lateral aspects of the clitoris to the labia minora. The position of the urethral meatus may range from a mild hypospadias to an opening in the perineal area into a urogenital sinus.

Ovaries are not found in scrotal folds or in the inguinal regions. Therefore, palpable masses in these locations represent testicles. The testicles, however, may be intraabdominal. If testicles are not palpable, the infant should be considered to have virilizing adrenal hyperplasia until demonstrated otherwise. A uterus may be palpable on rectal examination, especially shortly after birth when the uterus is a little enlarged in response to maternal estrogen.

The buccal smear for the sex chromatin pattern along with serum electrolytes, serum 17-OHP, urinary 17-ketosteroids should be ordered immediately in all newborns with ambiguous genitalia. The Lyon hypothesis states that in females, one of the two normal X chromosomes is functionally inactive in all somatic cells. This inactivation occurs at an early embryonic age, is irreversible, and is random and independent. Thus, the normal female is a mosaic made of two cell populations, one consisting of cells in which the X chromosome inherited from the mother is active, and the other in which the paternal X is active. During interphase the inactive X is detected as the nuclear chromatin or Barr body. In the normal female, the percentage of buccal smear cells which contain a sex chromatin mass should be greater than 20%. The sex chromatin percentage may be low in females until the third day of life.

Because both masculinized females and incompletely masculinized males can result from enzyme blocks in the adrenal, urinary 17-ketosteroids, and 17-OHP are necessary regardless of the sex chromatin pattern. In 3β-dehydrogenase and 17-hydroxylase enzyme blocks, the urinary pregnanetriol and 17-OHP will not be elevated. 21-Hydroxylase and 11β-hydroxylase blocks will be associated with pregnanetriol excretion of 2 mg or more per 24 hours (in some laboratories, up to 4 mg is normal) but massive elevations of 17-OHP in blood. The 17-ketosteroids may not be im-

357

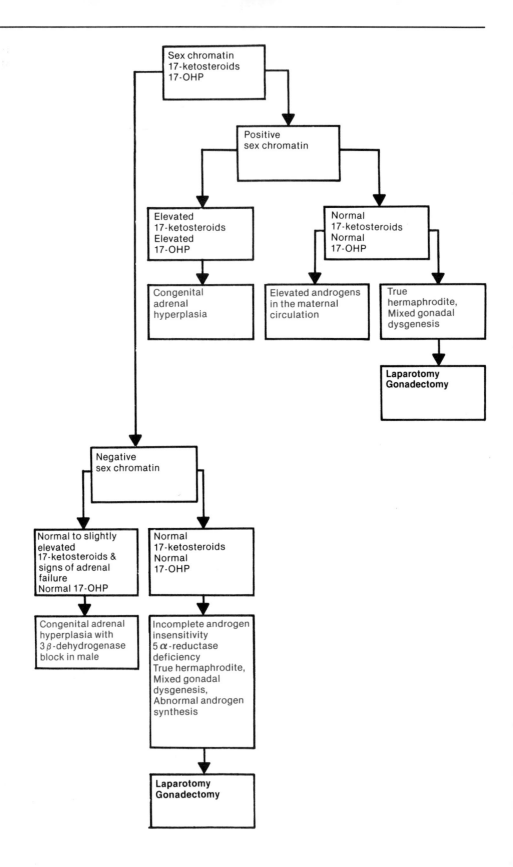

pressively increased with a 3β-dehydrogenase block. *Clinical signs of adrenal failure indicate that the newborn has adrenal hyperplasia regardless of the urinary steroid excretion pattern.* The diagnosis is certain if such an infant is hyperkalemic and hyponatremic.

Endoscopy and special x-ray studies are not necessary for assigning sex; however, the information gained will be helpful in delineating the exact structures and abnormalities present.

Although laparotomy is not necessary for assignment of sex, it may be the only way to arrive at a definitive diagnosis. Laparotomy is indicated in the following situations (laparoscopic evaluation is inadequate because gonads may be small and hidden in the inguinal canal):

1. The sex chromatin-positive infant with ambiguous genitalia, normal 17-ketosteroid excretion, in apparent good health, and no history of maternal androgen exposure. This is either a true hermaphrodite or a variant of mixed gonadal dysgenesis, and gonadectomy is indicated.

2. The sex chromatin-negative patient with ambiguous genitalia, without palpable gonads, and normal 17-ketosteroid excretion. The possibilities are incompletely masculinized males (variants of testicular feminization), a true hermaphrodite, mixed gonadal dysgenesis, and 5α-reductase deficiency. Sex of rearing will be female, and gonadectomy is necessary to avoid virilization at puberty and the propensity to develop gonadal neoplasia.

Chromosome analysis is not necessary for the assignment of sex, and indeed, may require much time. For the purposes of documentation, and confirmation, however, a karyotype is indicated except in patients with adrenal hyperplasia.

Assignment of Sex of Rearing

In a newborn who presents a problem of correct sex assignment, it is better to delay than to reverse the sex assignment at a later date. Generally, the decision can be made within a few days, at most a few weeks. In dealing with the parents, terms with unfortunate connotations, such as hermaphrodite, should be avoided. An easy way to explain ambiguous genital development to parents is to indicate that the genitals are unfinished, rather than abnormal from a sexual point of view. Chromosome discrepancies are probably best left unmentioned.

The future fertility in all masculinized females is unaffected. With proper treatment, reproduction is possible, since the internal genitalia and gonads are those of a normal female. Therefore, all masculinized females should be reared as females.

The only other category of patients with ambiguous genitalia with reproductive capability consists of males with 1) isolated hypospadias, 2) the male with repaired isolated cryptorchidism, and 3) the male with the uterine hernia syndrome.

All other patients with ambiguous genitalia will be sterile. Except for salt-losing adrenal hyperplasia, the physician's prime concern is not with physical survival, but to enable the patient to grow into a psychologically normal, healthy, and well-adjusted adult. The sex of assignment depends upon only one judgment: can the phallus ultimately develop into a penis adequate for intercourse. The success of a penis is dependent upon erectile tissue, and the genitalia should not only be serviceable, but also erotically sensitive. Technically, the construction of female genitalia is easier, and therefore, the physician must be convinced that a functional penis is possible.

All decisions regarding sex of rearing and the overall treatment program should be made early in life. If a case has been neglected, sex reassignments must be made according to the gender identity in which a child has developed. Reassignment of sex can probably be made safely up to age 18 months.

It is recommended that older individuals requesting sexual changes be referred to research-oriented clinical programs established in university medical centers.

References

1. **Van Wagenen G, Simpson ME,** *Embryology of the Ovary and Testis, Homo Sapiens and Mucaca Mulatta,* Yale University Press, 1965.

2. **Wilson JD, Griffin JE, George FW, Leshin M,** The role of gonadal steroids in sexual differentiation, Recent Prog Horm Res 37:1, 1981.

3. **Imperato-McGinley J, Peterson RE, Gaultier T, Sturla E,** Androgens and the evolution of male gender identity among male pseudohermaphrodites with 5α-reductase deficiency. N Engl J Med 300:1233, 1979.

4. **New MI, Dupont B, Pang S, Pollack M, Levine LS,** An update of congenital adrenal hyperplasia, Recent Prog Horm Res 37:105, 1981.

5. **Biglieri EG, Herron MA, Brust N,** 17-Hydroxylation deficiency in man. J Clin Invest 45:1946, 1966.

6. **Levine LS, Dupont B, Lorenzen F, Pang S, Pollack M, Oberfield SE, Kohn B, Lerner A, Cacciari E, Mantero F, Cassio A, Scaroni C, Chiumells G, Rondanini GF, Gargantini L, Giovannelli G, Virdis R, Bartolotta E, Migliori C, Pintor C, Tato L, Barboni F, New MI,** Genetic and hormonal characterization of cryptic 21-hydroxylase deficiency. J Clin Endocrinol Metab 53:1192, 1981.

7. **Morris J, McL,** Gonadal anomalies and dysgenesis, in *Progress in Infertility*, Behrman SJ, Kistner RW, eds, Little Brown, Boston, 1975, pp 265–279.

8. **Manuel M, Katayama KP, Jones Jr HW,** The age of occurrence of gonadal tumors in intersex patients with a Y chromosome. Am J Obstet Gynecol 124:293, 1976.

9. **Wilson JD, Harrod MJ, Goldstein JL, Hemsell DL, MacDonald PC,** Familial incomplete male pseudohermaphroditism, type 1. N Engl J Med 290:1097, 1974.

10. **Aiman J, Griffin JE,** The frequency of androgen receptor deficiency in infertile men. J Clin Endocrinol Metab 54:725, 1982.

11. **Griffin JE, Wilson JD,** The syndromes of androgen resistance. N Engl J Med 302:198, 1980.

12. **Walsh PC, Madden JD, Harrod MJ, Goldstein JL, MacDonald PC, Wilson JD,** Familial incomplete male pseudohermaphroditism, type 2. N Engl J Med 291:949, 1974.

13. **Haseltine FP, Ohno S,** Mechanism of gonadal differentiation. Science 211:1272, 1981.

14. **Wilson JD, George FW, Griffin JE,** The hormonal control of sexual development. Science 211:1278, 1981.

15. **Givens JR, Wiser WL, Summitt RI, Kerber IF, Anderson RN, Pittaway DE, Fish SA,** Familial pseudohermaphroditism without gynecomastia due to deficient testicular 17-ketosteroid reductase activity. N Engl J Med 291:938, 1974.

16. **Coulam CB,** Testicular regression syndrome. Obstet Gynecol 53:44, 1979.

17. **Simpson JL,** True hermaphroditism: etiology and phenotypic considerations. Birth Defects 14(6c):9, 1978.

Abnormal Puberty and Growth Problems

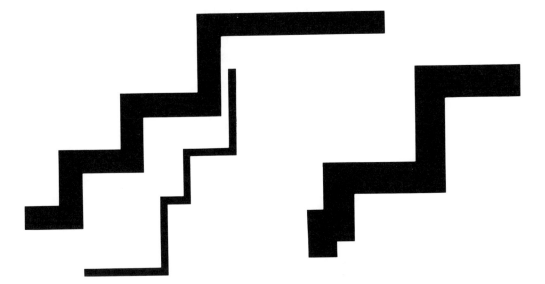

The ability to diagnose and manage disorders of female pubescence requires a thorough understanding of the physical and hormonal events which mark the evolution of the child into a sexually mature adult capable of reproduction. Abnormalities in this process of developmental endocrinology either lead to premature or retarded (delayed) puberty. *This chapter reviews the important landmarks and mechanism of normal female maturation as well as the abnormalities which lead to precocious or delayed puberty.*

The Period of Infancy and Childhood

The mechanism of puberty is discussed in Chapter 2 (Neuroendocrinology). A review of the changing sensitivity of hypothalamic centers to gonadal steroids is also presented here.

Separation of the newborn from its sources of maternal and placental estrogen and progesterone at birth releases newborn follicle-stimulating hormone (FSH) and luteinizing hormone (LH) from negative feedback. A prompt rise in gonadotropin secretion follows which, in female neonates, may reach adult castrate level by 3 months of life. As a result, transient estradiol secretion associated with waves of ovarian follicle maturation and atresia are induced. Negative feedback is reasserted, and gonadotropins decline at age 2 years and remain at very low levels to at least 8 years of age. During this period, the hypothalamopituitary system controlling gonadotropins (the "gonadostat") is highly sensitive to negative feedback of estrogen (estradiol concentration in these years remains low at 10 pg/ml). Studies on gonadal dysgenesis and other hypogonadal infants indicate that the "gonadostat" is 6–15 times more sensitive to negative feedback at this period than in the adult. (1) Gonadotropin secretion is, therefore, restrained by low levels of estrogen.

The reduction in gonadotropin is not related entirely to exquisite sensitivity to negative feedback. The low levels of FSH and LH seen in hypogonadal children (primarily gonadal dysgenesis) between the ages of 5 and 11 years are the same as the low levels in normal infants of this age. (2) Because gonadotropin releasing hormone (GnRH) infusion stimulates moderate LH and FSH secretion in these agonadal subjects, a central nonsteroidal suppressor of endogenous GnRH and gonadotropin synthesis appears operative. Endogenous opiates may be this influence.

The Prepubertal Period

As puberty approaches, three critical changes in the low level endocrine homeostatic function of childhood appear:

1. "Adrenarche."

2. Decreasing repression of the "gonadostat."

3. Gradual amplification of the peptide-peptide and peptide-steroid interactions leading to "gonadarche."

Adrenarche

The growth of pubic and axillary hair is due to an increased production of adrenal androgens at puberty. Thus, this phase of puberty is often referred to as adrenarche or pubarche. Premature pubarche by itself is occasionally seen, i.e., pubic and axillary hair without any other sign of sexual development. Premature thelarche (breast development) without any other signs of puberty is very rare, but does occur. Increased adrenal cortical function, expressed by a rise in circulating dehydroepiandrosterone (DHA), dehydroepiandrosterone sulfate (DHAS), and androstenedione occurs progressively in late childhood from about age 6 to adolescence (13–15 years of age). (3) It is associated with an increase in the size and differentiation of the inner zone of the cortex (zona reticularis). Generally, the beginning of adrenarche precedes by 2 years the growth spurt, the rise in estrogens and gonadotropins in prepuberty, and menarche of midpuberty. Because of this temporal relationship, activation of adrenal androgen secretion has been viewed as a possible initiating event in the ontogeny of the pubertal transition.

Considerable evidence, however, supports a dissociation of the control mechanisms which initiate adrenarche and those governing GnRH-pituitary-ovary maturation ("gonadarche"). (4) Premature adrenarche (precocious appearance of pubic and axillary hair before age 8 years) is not associated with a parallel abnormal advancement of gonadarche. In hypergonadotropic hypogonadism (gonadal dysgenesis) with increased FSH and LH or in hypogonadotropic states such as Kallmann's syndrome, adrenarche occurs despite the absence of gonadarche. When adrenarche is absent, as in children with cortisol-treated Addison's disease (hypoadrenalism), gonadarche still occurs. Finally, in true precocious puberty occurring before 6 years of age, gonadarche precedes adrenarche.

Adrenarche does not appear to be under direct control of gonadotropin, ACTH, or prolactin; cortisol and DHAS vary independently with age, in anorexia, and in chronic disease, as well as adrenarche. A pituitary-adrenal androgen stimulating factor, formed by cleavage of a high molecular weight precursor which also contains ACTH and β-lipotropin, acting on an ACTH prepared and maintained adrenal, has been suggested as the agent stimulating adrenarche. (5) The name for this material is CASH, corticotropin androgen stimulating hormone.

Regardless of its relation to adrenarche, factors which induce gonadarche in late prepuberty involve de-repression of the CNS-pituitary gonadostat, progressive responsiveness of the anterior pituitary to exogenous (and presumably endogenous) GnRH, and follicle reactivity to FSH and LH.

Decreasing Repression of the "Gonadostat"

For approximately 8 years, from early infancy to the prepubertal period, LH and FSH are suppressed to very low nonpulsatile levels. Two mechanisms for this restraint on gonadotropin secretion are thought to exist: (a) a highly sensitive negative feedback of low level gonadal estrogen on hypothalamic and pituitary sites, and (b) an intrinsic central inhibitory influence which reduces basal gonadotropin concentrations and limits their response to exogenous GnRH, even in agonadal children. Gonadal dysgenesis patients display marked elevations of gonadotropins for the first 2–3 years of life. Thereafter, a striking decline in concentrations of FSH and LH occurs, reaching a nadir at 6–8 years. By age 10–11 (at the time puberty would have occurred), however, gonadotropins are elevated once again to the castrate range. The overall pattern of basal gonadotropin secretion in agonadal children is qualitatively similar to that observed in normal females. Whereas negative feedback inhibition may play the more important role in early childhood, the central intrinsic inhibitor becomes functionally dominant in midchildhood and persists up to prepuberty. Suppression of, or damage to, the neural source of this inhibition has been postulated in the pathogenesis of precocious puberty due to hypothalamic lesions compressing or destroying posterior hypothalamic areas. Normal pubertal timing of gonadarche, with the reactivation of gonadotropin synthesis and secretion, would result from a combined reduction in intrinsic suppression of GnRH and decreased sensitivity to the negative feedback of estrogen. The decrease in inhibitory feedback of estrogen has been well documented in animals. (6) The reversal of intrinsic suppression may be related to endogenous opiates or the observed decrease in melatonin noted in boys. (7).

Alteration and Amplification of GnRH-Gonadotropin and Gonadotropin-Ovarian Steroid Interactions

Normal pubertal maturation in girls is accompanied by marked changes in the pattern of gonadotropin responses to the hypothalamic releasing hormone GnRH. FSH responses to GnRH are initially very pronounced but decrease steadily throughout the first decade and are further reduced after the onset of puberty. In contrast, LH responses are low in prepubertal girls and increase strikingly during puberty. (8) The appearance and increased amplitude and frequency of pulsatile GnRH is believed to provoke progressively enhanced responses of FSH and LH secretion. It is assumed that GnRH, released from intrinsic restraint and hypersensitive negative feedback, acts as a self-primer on the gonadotrope cells of the anterior pituitary by inducing cell surface receptors specific for GnRH and necessary for its action (up-regulation). Thus, gonadotrope cells increase their capacity to respond to GnRH first by synthesis and later by secretion of gonadotropins. As gonadotropin secretion appears, ovarian follicle steroid synthesis is stimulated and estrogen secretion rises. Elsewhere (see Chapter 2), the evidence for the dichotomous effects of estrogen feedback on the anterior pituitary has been reviewed. Suffice to say at this point, by midpuberty, estrogen enhances LH secretion responses to GnRH (positive feedback) while maintaining relative inhibition (negative feedback) of FSH response.

The onset of GnRH pulses first occurs during sleep. There is sleep-associated release of LH in both sexes which correlates with the timing (early puberty) of LH responses to exogenous GnRH. Sleep-related LH pulses also are seen in children with idiopathic precocious puberty, in anorexia nervosa patients during intermediate stages of exacerbation and recovery, and also in agonadal patients during the pubertal age period when their gonadotropins are returning from midchildhood reductions. (9)

GnRH pulses appear and are maintained independent of steroid feedback. Positive estrogen feedback is established only in midpuberty just prior to menarche. (10)

Rhythmic pulses of GnRH given to immature rhesus monkeys can initiate activity of the pituitary gonadal apparatus, supporting the primacy of endogenous GnRH in the establishment and maintenance of puberty. Similar effects have been demonstrated in prepubertal girls. (11)

Puberty

The cascade of events initiated by the release of pulsatile GnRH from prepubertal feedback and central negative inhibition results in increased levels of gonadotropins and steroids with appearance of secondary sexual characteristics and eventual adult function (menarche and later, ovulation). Between the ages of 10 and 16, the endocrine sequence observed includes first, pulsatile patterns of LH during sleep, followed by similar pulses of less amplitude occurring throughout the 24-hour day. Episodic peaks of estradiol result and menarche appears. By mid to late puberty, maturation of the positive feedback relationship between estradiol and LH is established leading to ovulatory cycles.

Timing of Puberty

Although the major determinant of the timing of puberty is genetic, other factors such as nutrition, physical health, social and psychologic factors all influence the age of onset and the rate of progression of the pubertal change. The decline in the age of menarche displayed by children in developed countries undoubtedly reflects improved nutritional status. Frisch believes that a critical body weight (48 kg) must be reached by a girl to achieve menarche. (12) Possibly more important than total weight may be the shift in body composition toward a greater percent fat. Indeed, moderately obese girls (20–30% over normal weight) have earlier menarche than normal weight girls. Conversely, anorectics and intense exercisers (low weight or low percent fat component of weight) have delayed menarche or secondary amenorrhea. That other factors are involved is indicated by the delayed menarche experienced by morbidly obese girls (greater than 30% overweight), diabetics, and intense exercisers of normal weight. Intriguingly, blind girls experience earlier menarche. There is a fairly good correlation between the times of menarche of mothers and daughters and between sisters. (13)

Stages of Pubertal
Development

On the average, the pubertal sequence of accelerated growth, breast development, pubarche, and menarche requires a period of 4½ years (range 1½–6 years). The largest body of data has been accumulated in healthy European girls; however, current North American standards are approximately 6 months earlier for each stage. (14, 15)

In general, the first sign of puberty is an acceleration of growth followed by breast budding (thelarche) (median 9.8 years). Although the sequence may be reversed, pubic hair appears after the breast bud (median 10.5 years) with axillary hair growth 2 years later. Menarche is a late event (median 12.8 years), occurring after the peak of growth has passed.

Height Gain in Centimeters

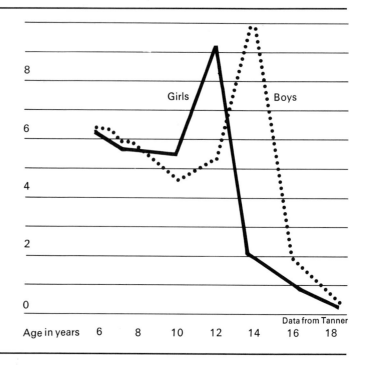

Data from Tanner

Age in years   6   8   10   12   14   16   18

Growth

An adolescent girl's growth spurt occurs 2 years earlier than that of a boy, and in 1 year, her rate of growth doubles, yielding a height increment of between 6 and 11 cm (2 and 4 inches). (16) The average girl reaches this growth peak about 2 years after breast budding and 1 year prior to menarche. Hormonal requirements for this increased growth velocity include growth hormone (GH) and gonadal estrogen. Adrenal androgens are not involved because cortisol-repleted Addisonian patients display normal pubertal growth patterns.

In general, it can be said that environmental factors are important in the onset of puberty. Children have been maturing progressively earlier in most of the world in the last century, and improved living standards and nutrition in the mother antenatally and in children postnatally have played a significant role in producing taller, heavier children with earlier maturation. Studies of identical twins and nonidentical twins show that the age at menarche is chiefly controlled by genetic factors when the environment is optimum. In affluent cultures, the trend toward lowering of the menarcheal age and puberty has now been halted. (15)

Age at Menarche

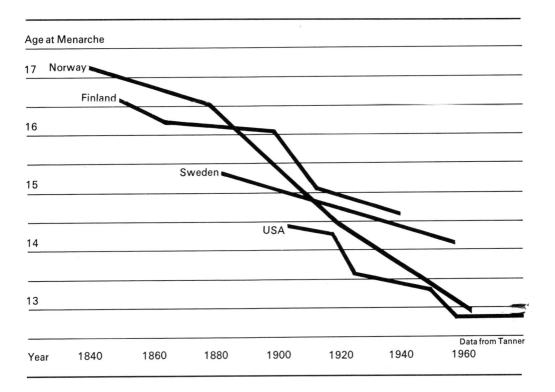

Data from Tanner

| Menarche | The relationship between menarche and the growth spurt is relatively fixed: menarche occurs after the peak in growth velocity has passed. Slower growth (totaling no more than about 6 cm (2.5 inches)) is noted after initiation of menses. |

The relationship between menarche and the growth spurt is relatively fixed: menarche occurs after the peak in growth velocity has passed. Slower growth (totaling no more than about 6 cm (2.5 inches)) is noted after initiation of menses.

The normal range of menarche in American girls is 9.1–17.7 years with a median of 12.8. (15) Early cycles are usually anovulatory, irregular, and occasionally heavy. Anovulation usually lasts 12–18 months after menarche, but there are reports of pregnancy before menarche.

Summary of Pubertal Events

1. FSH and LH levels rise moderately before the age of 10 and are followed by a rise in estradiol. Early gonadotropin LH pulses are seen only in sleep, but gradually extend throughout the day. In the adult, they occur at roughly 1.5–2 hourly intervals.

2. As gonadal estrogen increases (gonadarche), breast development, female fat distribution, and vaginal and uterine growth occur. Skeletal growth rapidly increases as a result of gonadal estrogen secretion. Sex hormone binding globulin (SHBG) rises.

3. Adrenal androgen (adrenarche) and, to a lesser degree, gonadal androgen secretion cause pubic and axillary hair growth. Adrenarche plays little if any part in skeletal growth. While temporally related to gonadarche, adrenarche is an independent, functionally unrelated biological event.

369

4. At midpuberty, sufficient gonadal estrogen secretion proliferates the endometrium, and the first menses (menarche) occurs. Estradiol positive feedback on LH secretion is demonstrable thereafter.

5. Postmenarchal cycles are anovulatory. Sustained, predictable positive gonadotropin responses to estradiol or Clomid are late pubertal events.

Grumbach has summarized all these events. (17) The onset of puberty is an evolving sequence of maturational steps. The hypothalamic-pituitary gonadotrope-gonadal system differentiates and functions during fetal life and early infancy. Thereafter, it is suppressed to low activity levels during childhood by a combination of hypersensitivity of the "gonadostat" to estrogen negative feedback and an intrinsic CNS inhibitor. All the components located below GnRH (below the CNS) are competent to respond at all ages (as will be seen in the pathogenesis of precocious puberty). After a decade of functional GnRH insufficiency (between late infancy and the onset of puberty), GnRH secretion is resumed and gonadarche (the reactivation of the CNS-pituitary-ovarian apparatus) appears. Prolongation of intrinsic CNS suppression or disability in any of the components of the gonadarche cascade leads to delayed or absent pubescence.

Precocious Puberty

Puberty is the biologic transition between immature and adult reproductive function. Its timing, endocrine milieu, and physical expressions have been characterized sufficiently to set clinically reasonable time limits for the normal appearance of female maturity and to allow recognition of the pathogenesis and pathophysiology of most of the causes of premature or delayed pubescence.

Pubertal changes before the age of 8 are regarded as precocious. Increased growth is often the first change in precocious puberty. This is usually followed by breast development and growth of pubic hair. On occasion, pubarche, thelarche, and linear growth occur simultaneously. Menarche, however, may be the very first sign.

Classically, precocious puberty has been divided into true sexual precocity in which the hormones are secreted by maturing gonads, and precocious pseudopuberty in which maturing normal gonads are not the source of the sex steroids. These classifications are of little practical use since the physician is obligated to rule out a serious disease process in the face of precocious development, and the above classification can only be made after full evaluation.

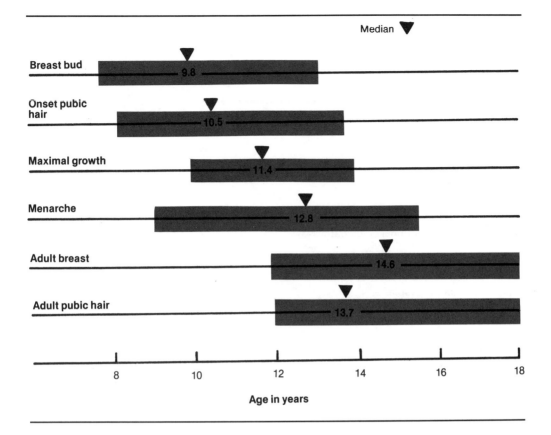

Sexual development does not require ovulatory capability. Evaluation of a patient's possible fertility, for example, with basal body temperatures or progesterone assays, is an unnecessary procedure. More importantly, true sexual precocity with potential fertility and adult levels of gonadotropins does not rule out the possibility of a serious disease process (e.g. a CNS tumor). While it is true that the most common form of sexual precocity in females is idiopathic or constitutional precocity (true sexual precocity), this must be a diagnosis by exclusion with prolonged follow-up in an effort to detect slowly developing lesions of the brain, ovary, or adrenal gland.

Classification of Sexual Precocity	Total numbers of cases of three series		Approximate numbers described in literature	
True sexual precocity:	Girls	Boys	Girls	Boys
Cerebral	19	14		
Pineal gland			0	50
Hamartoma			8	22
Neurofibromatosis				6
Cryptogenic, constitutional or idiopathic	114	18		
Hypothyroid sexual precocity			9	2
Polyostotic fibrous dysplasia	5	1		
Gonadotropin-producing tumors:				
Chorionepithelioma			8	3
Hepatoma		1		5
Presacral tumor				3
Precocious pseudopuberty:				
Ovarian tumors (excluding chorionepithelioma)	3		80	
Scrotal tumors		3		30
Congenital virilizing adrenal hyperplasia in boy		31		
Adrenal adenoma	2	2		
Adrenal carcinoma	1	2		
Incomplete sexual precocity:				
Premature adrenarche or pubarche	12	5		
Premature Thelarche	11			
Total	167	77		

Diagnosis of Precocious Puberty	A classification of sexual precocity is presented in the table to provide a guide to the possible conditions and their relative incidence encountered in a large series of cases. (18) The cause of precocious development may be immediately suggested by the history and physical examination. A familial occurrence renders unlikely a variety of causes, mainly tumors.

A classification of sexual precocity is presented in the table to provide a guide to the possible conditions and their relative incidence encountered in a large series of cases. (18) The cause of precocious development may be immediately suggested by the history and physical examination. A familial occurrence renders unlikely a variety of causes, mainly tumors.

Particular attention should be given to the following possibilities: drug ingestion, cerebral problems such as cranial trauma or encephalitis, retarded growth with symptoms of hypothyroidism, and a pelvic or abdominal mass. A left hand-wrist film (for use with atlases) should be obtained for bone age. Determination of thyroid function is indicated, and the urinary excretion of 17-ketosteroids or a blood assay of DHAS should be measured. An electroencephalogram and brain scan are probably indicated in patients with premature precocious puberty, even in the face of a normal overall evaluation, including normal routine skull x-rays. Other procedures should be dictated by the clinical findings. Virilization, of course, demands a full adrenal evaluation.

Precocious Development Due to Stimulation of Gonadotropin Secretion

The signs of constitutional sexual precocity are due to premature maturation of the hypothalamic-pituitary-ovarian axis, resulting in production of gonadotropins and sex steroids. This diagnosis should be made only by exclusion and deserves long-term follow-up, as cerebral abnormalities may not become apparent until adulthood. Despite the precocious sexual development, these children fortunately resemble children of their own chronologic age in other parameters. Adult fertility and time of menopause are not affected.

A number of cerebral problems including abnormal skull development due to rickets can cause precocious development. The various tumors include: craniopharyngioma, optic glioma, astrocytoma, and supraseller teratomas—all usually near the hypothalamus. Pineal tumors, for unknown reasons, are associated with precocious puberty only in boys. Nontumorous causes include encephalitis, meningitis, hydrocephalus, and von Recklinghausen's disease. An injury to the skull may stimulate sexual development. The mechanism is unknown, and a latent period of 1–2 months is usually seen. A hamartoma is a hyperplastic malformation at the base of the hypothalamus which usually produces precocity in the first few years of life.

Albright's syndrome (polyostotic fibrous dysplasia) consists of multiple disseminated cystic bone lesions which easily fracture, café au lait skin areas of various sizes and shapes, and sexual precocity. Premature menarche may be the first sign of the syndrome. The etiology is unknown. Skeletal abnormalities may become evident following the onset of puberty. The combination of multiple bone fractures, café au lait patches, and premature development should lead to the diagnosis.

373

Sexual precocity occurs in a small number of children with long-standing hypothyroidism. While reported cases have been severe and therefore clinically obvious, laboratory evaluation of thyroid function is probably indicated in all cases of sexual precocity.

Precocious Development Due to Availability of Sex Steroids

Only 1–2% of girls with precocious puberty have an ovarian tumor. The tumor is usually an estrogen-producing neoplasm or cyst. To emphasize again the rarity of this condition, only 5% of granulosa cell tumors and 1% of theca cell tumors occur before puberty. (19) Teratomas, dysgerminomas, and choriocarcinomas can produce gonadotropin which, by its high local concentration, stimulates ovarian hormone production. The production of gonadotropin may be so great that a pregnancy test will be positive. Palpation of a pelvic or abdominal mass demands surgical exploration. Increasing use has been made of pelvic ultrasonography and whole body (abdominal) CT scan for the work-up of precocious puberty.

A feminizing adrenal tumor is very rare and is associated with increased excretion of 17-ketosteroids and increased blood levels of DHAS.

Drug ingestion should be suspected when there is dark pigmentation of the nipples and breast areola, an effect of certain synthetic estrogens such as stilbestrol.

Special Cases of Precocious Development

Special cases of precocious development include the isolated appearance of one sexual characteristic: premature adrenarche or pubarche (pubic hair), or premature thelarche (breast development). Sparse hair growth on the vulva does not represent precocious pubarche. Little is known about these conditions other than that they are associated with an increased incidence of central nervous system abnormalities, such as mental deficiency. The usual effort should be made to exclude a serious disease process. If the bone age is advanced, treatment is indicated.

Diagnosis of Precocious Puberty

The cause of precocious development may be obvious by findings in the history or physical examination. Familial occurrence helps to exclude certain disease processes (tumors). Clinically, the nature of precocity dictates certain diagnostic priorities:

1. Rule out life-threatening disease. These include neoplasms of the CNS, ovary, adrenal.

2. Define the velocity of the process. Is it progressing or stabilized? Management decisions hinge on this determination. Isolated, nonendocrine causes of vaginal bleeding (trauma, foreign body, vaginitis, genital neoplasm) must be excluded.

The differential diagnosis is derived from the physical and laboratory findings as noted:

Differential Diagnostic Steps

Physical Diagnosis:
    Record of growth, Tanner stages.
    External genitalia changes.
    Abdominal, pelvic, neurologic examination.
    Signs of androgenization.
    Special findings: McCune-Albright, hypothyroidism.

Laboratory Diagnosis:
    Serial bone age.
    Skull film, CT scan, EEG.
    FSH, LH, HCG subunit assay.
    Thyroid function tests (TSH and free T_4).
    Androgens (serum DHAS, testosterone).

Serial bone age studies are useful. If retarded, hypothyroidism may be present. In advanced bone age accompanied by adult gonadotropin levels, constitutional or organic brain disease is likely. If gonadotropins are low, but bone age is accelerated, various forms of precocious pseudopuberty are the likely diagnoses.

Treatment of
Precocious
Development

For treatment of precocious development when no cause can be found, or when a cause cannot be removed, the use of a potent progestational agent to inhibit gonadotropin production has been the standard. The agent of choice is medroxyprogesterone acetate in depot form (Depo-Provera) given in large doses, 400 mg intramuscularly every 3 months. The antigonadotropic, antiestrogenic action of danazol may be an effective (but mildly androgenic) alternative. Recently, pituitary and gonadal desensitization (down-regulation of receptors), with long-acting GnRH agonists has been suggested as therapy for precocity. (20)

Pubic hair will not disappear, but further menstruation, breast development, and growth may be inhibited. It is important to inhibit growth until the chronologic age can catch up with the bone age, otherwise the prematurely tall child will be a short adult due to accelerated bone growth and early epiphyseal closure. The response to progestin therapy is not uniformly good. However, it is impossible to determine which child will respond favorably; therefore, all children should be treated. The psychologic management of the sexually precocious child is a serious matter deserving of time and attention, and one must be careful to consider the family dynamics and parental attitudes.

Even if the only achievement is inhibition of menses, this is useful. Precocious menses can be a psychologic and a social problem, both of which are easily avoided with the use of progestin therapy. Treatment should be continued until the chronologic age matches the bone age or until age 12. Hand-wrist films should be obtained every 6 months

375

until epiphyseal closure is demonstrated. Breakthrough bleeding can be stopped by the use of an estrogen (e.g. conjugated estrogens 2.5 mg or ethinyl estradiol 20 μg daily for 7 days). Recurrence of bleeding is unusual.

Treatment with a long-acting GnRH agonists has several advantages. The effect is reversible and significant regression of development occurs. But best of all, normal adult height achievement is possible because bone maturation halts until adrenarche, when it resumes.

Delayed Puberty

Since there is such a wide variation in normal development, it is difficult to define the patient with abnormally delayed sexual maturation. Only 1% of all girls will not have had menarche by the age of 18, and complete absence of breast budding by the age of 13 is probably abnormal. However, whenever a patient or parents are concerned enough to seek a physician's advice, some evaluation is indicated.

Delayed puberty is a rare condition in girls, and a genetic problem or hypothalamic-pituitary disorder must be suspected.

The following is a list of the causes of delayed puberty:

Constitutional delay.

Hypergonadotropic hypogonadism:
Gonadal dysgenesis.
Nondysgenesis gonadal failure.
Anorchia, agonadism.
Pure gonadal dysgenesis.

Defective steroid synthesis.

Hypogonadotropic hypogonadism:
CNS disease:
    Tumors (craniopharyngioma, histocytosis X).
    Malformation (vascular, bony deformities, cerebrospinal fluid dynamics).
    Infection (meningitis, encephalitis).
Gonadotropin deficiency:
    Anosmia—Kallmann's syndrome.
    Isolated and multiple pituitary deficiencies.
    Chronic disease (nephritis, juvenile diabetes mellitus).
    Malnutrition (starvation, regional ileitis, anorexia nervosa).

The major disorders include gonadal failure, hypothalamic pituitary disorders, disorders of steroid synthesis, and chronic illness of nonendocrine type. Simple (constitutional) delay in adolescence is more common in boys than girls. It tends to occur repeatedly in families. Despite late appearance, the eventual pubertal sequence and ultimate fertility is normal.

Differential Diagnosis of Delayed Puberty and Primary Amenorrhea

The history and physical examination is very useful in the diagnostic work-up of delayed puberty. In the history, special note should be taken of past general health, height and weight records, and the pubertal milestone experience of older siblings and parents. On physical examination, in addition to body measurements, Tanner staging of any secondary sexual characteristics present, and a search for signs of hypothyroidism, gonadal dysgenesis, hypopituitarism or chronic illness should be made.

The failure of growth in stature suggests several possibilities. Isolated growth hormone deficiency is associated with somewhat delayed sexual maturity. Menarche may eventually occur, albeit delayed, but with bone age still discrepantly several years below chronologic age. More global pituitary hormone deficiency will result in total pubertal delay. Finally, gonadal dysgenesis (45,X) will be associated with decreased height and sexual infantilism with normal to slightly reduced bone age and hypergonadotropism.

Neurologic examination is important; evidence of intracranial disease, restricted visual fields, or absent sense of smell are key findings. Anatomic defects of the Müllerian ducts must be sought, especially when a disparity between normal puberty and absent menses is encountered.

Tanner Staging

	Breast	Pubic Hair
Stage I (prepubertal)	Elevation of papilla only	No pubic hair
Stage 2	Elevation of breast and papilla as small mound, Areola diameter enlarged. Median age: 9.8 years	Sparce, long, pigmented hair chiefly along labia majora. Median age: 10.5 years
Stage 3	Further enlargement without separation of breast and areola. Median age: 11.2 years	Dark, coarse, curled hair sparsely spread over mons. Median age: 11.4 years
Stage 4	Secondary mound of areola and papilla above the breast. Median age: 12.1 years	Adult-type hair, abundant but limited to the mons. Median age: 12.0 years
Stage 5	Recession of areola to contour of breast. Median age: 14.6 years	Adult type spread in quantity and distribution. Median age: 13.7 years

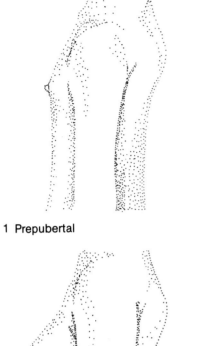

1 Prepubertal

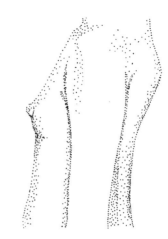

2 Breast Bud

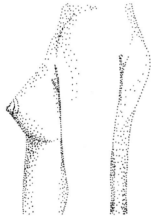

3 Breast Elevation

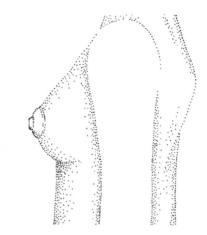

4 Areolar Mound

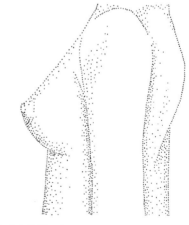

5 Adult Contour

378

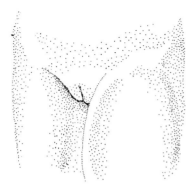

1 Prepubertal

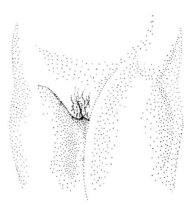

2 Presexual hair

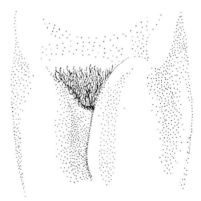

3 Sexual hair

4 Mid-escutcheon

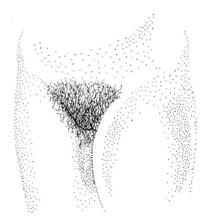

5 Female escutcheon

Laboratory work-up of delayed puberty usually includes x-rays for bone age, skull films, and serum gonadotropin levels. If short stature (5 feet) exists, evaluation according to the program outlined in Chapter 5, "Amenorrhea," will lead to the proper diagnosis.

If gonadotropins are increased into the postmenopausal range (hypergonadotropic hypogonadism), then some type of gonadal deficiency usually is the basis of delayed maturation. However, in sickle cell disease, approximately 20% of patients have delayed puberty and hypergonadotropism. Also 17α-hydroxylase deficiency in steroid synthesis (affecting both adrenals and ovaries) will cause hypergonadotropic delayed puberty.

Hypergonadotropic Hypogonadism. The most common disorder of this type is gonadal dysgenesis. In the 45,X patient, the typical phenotypic stigmata of Turner's syndrome will be displayed. However, these may be minimal or absent in sex chromosome mosaicism or structural deletions of the X chromosome. A Y-bearing cell line requires laparotomy and gonadal excision as prophylaxis against the risk of gonadal malignancy.

A hypergonadotropic 46,XX individual presents interesting possibilities. If hypertension, sexual infantilism, and an elevated serum progesterone are found, 17α-hydroxylase deficiency in steroid synthesis is likely. Acquired ovarian damage from torsion or inflammation should be ruled out. Finally, the 46,XX patient may have pure gonadal dysgenesis (gonadal streaks) or the resistant ovary syndrome.

Hypogonadotropic Hypogonadism. Decreased secretion of LH (less than 6 mIU/ml), associated with depressed FSH, is seen in hypothalamic (anosmia—Kallmann's syndrome), pituitary (tumor) disorders, or nonpathologic constitutional delay in development. Whereas Kallmann's syndrome presents with tall eunuchoidal stature, in the latter instances the typical patient is short with appropriate bone maturation delay. As previously noted, constitutional delay is frequently seen in a familial pattern, with the expectation of a late but otherwise normal growth pattern and adult reproductive function.

Poor nutrition (anorexia nervosa, malabsorption, chronic illness, regional ileitis, renal disease) may also lead to hypogonadotropic delayed growth and development.

In the presence of normal olfaction, exclusion of pituitary or parapituitary tumor by specialized neuroradiologic procedures is necessary. If tumor or vascular malformation is not found, the possibility of pituitary insufficiency can be evaluated with GnRH stimulation.

Müllerian tube segmental discontinuities, Müllerian agenesis, or testicular feminization will present as delayed menarche despite normal development of an adult female phenotype. Müllerian agenesis accounts for about one-fifth of cases of prolonged primary amenorrhea. Other obstructive anomalies of the Müllerian ducts are less frequently seen (1%). Anovulation and the polycystic ovary, and androgen-producing adrenal disease, can present as primary amenorrhea.

Treatment of Sexual Infantilism (Delayed Puberty)

The first priority in therapy is removal or correction of the primary etiology when possible. In this regard, thyroid therapy for hypothyroisidm, growth hormone for isolated GH deficiency, treatment of ileitis, are examples of specific therapy. In hypogonadism, cyclic estrogen and progestin therapy will initiate and sustain maturation and function of secondary sexual characteristics. In XY individuals, properly timed gonadectomy followed by sex hormone replacement is required. In constitutional delay, reassurance that the anticipated development will occur is the only management step needed.

Growth Problems in Normal Adolescents

Perhaps the worst thing about an adolescent growth problem is that it makes the individual "different." It is probably true that more than anyone else the adolescent does not like to be different. Therefore, excessive or insufficient growth is not a problem to be dismissed lightly, and psychologic support and reassurance are key features in the management of such problems. A willingness to listen to problems, together with an adult-to-adult attitude, will place the adolescent-physician relationship at the proper level of mutual respect.

The basic and essential laboratory procedure is a left hand-wrist x-ray for bone age. The Bayley-Pinneau tables predict future adult height, utilizing the bone age and present height. (21) To use the tables, one needs a measurement of height, the patient's age, and an x-ray of the left hand and wrist for bone age. All of the hand epiphyses and those of the distal end of the arm are used to determine the skeletal age. The Bayley-Pinneau tables begin on page 386.

To estimate a patient's adult height, use the tables as follows: Go down the left hand column to the patient's present height, follow this horizontal row to the column under the bone age which is given by 6-month intervals across the top. The number at the intersection represents the predicted adult height. If figures do not fall at the 1-inch or 6-month intervals used on the tables, the predicted height can be easily extrapolated.

It is important to use the table suitable for the rate of maturing. If the bone age is within 1 year of the chronologic age, use the table for average girls; if the bone age is accelerated 1 year or more, use the table for accelerated girls; if the bone age is retarded 1 year or more, use the table for retarded girls.

The tables are for use with bone age films of the hand and wrist only in conjunction with the Greulich-Pyle *Atlas*. (22) Use with bone age determined by any other method is less accurate.

Short Stature. Thorough medical history and physical examination will eliminate the usual disorders associated with short stature: malnutrition, chronic urinary tract disease, chronic infectious disease, hypothyroidism, mental illness, panhypopituitarism, and gonadal dysgenesis. In the history, the heights and weights of parents, siblings, and relatives should be obtained along with timing of growth in the family, dietary history, daily activities, and sleep habits. Normal history and examination in an individual with a bone age only 1 year behind the chronologic age suggests a constitutional pattern which does not require treatment.

Generally, endocrine disease is an uncommon basis for impairment of growth. Congenital hypothyroidism is the most frequent problem of this type, followed by hypopituitarism, hypothyroidism with onset during childhood, and excess cortisol.

It is unlikely that a patient with congenital hypothyroidism will present undiagnosed and untreated to a gynecologist. However, juvenile hypothyroidism must be suspected in an adolescent with obesity and short stature and a normal early childhood development. Similarly, an adolescent with hypopituitarism due to a slow growing pituitary tumor may present with a failure to develop secondary sexual characteristics and a failure to grow. Cortisol excess may be due to Cushing's disease (rare in childhood) or to therapy with corticosteroids. Excess endogenous or exogeneous corticosteroids suppress skeletal maturation and growth. Moderate overdoseage of cortisol, for example, when treating children with adrenal hyperplasia may suppress growth.

Treatment of Short Stature. If the physician concludes that an adolescent suffers from a delay of normal growth and no disease process is present, support and observation are indicated. If the bone age is more than 1 year below the chronologic age, but the family history reveals a consistent pattern of retarded but eventual normal growth, reassurance is essential. It is helpful to point out the x-ray, indicating that the individual has 1 year or more of unused potential in which to catch up with her friends.

When continued failure to grow is evident in the absence of disease, hormone treatment can be considered. Presently the use of growth hormone is restricted by short supplies, and is limited to use in growth hormone-deficient dwarfs. Fortunately, it is rare to see a female adolescent with this problem. More commonly it is an adolescent boy who is sensitive to reduced growth, and in whom the use of testosterone may be indicated. In cases of gonadal failure, estrogen may be used in a female to stimulate epiphyseal growth, bringing the bone age to match the chronologic age. Conjugated estrogen can be given in a dose of 1.25 mg daily for the 1st through the 25th of each month, and medroxyprogesterone acetate (Provera), 10 mg, is added on the 16th through the 25th to ensure consistent and predictable menstrual bleeding. Patients should be observed at 6-month intervals to document the pattern of growth and development. Hormone treatment may be discontinued when the bone age matches the chronologic age.

Tall Stature. This is rarely a problem in boys (basketball provides a ready outlet), but girls who are the daughters of very tall parents may come to the gynecologist for help. A predicted height greater than 6 feet probably deserves treatment. The Bayley-Pinneau tables are accurate in predicting the height of tall girls. (23)

If a family history for tallness is not elicited, an earnest search for a problem is indicated, although little more than a thorough history, examination, and routine laboratory tests are necessary.

A hand-wrist x-ray for bone age is also necessary. The degree of development of secondary sexual characteristics is important, since the more mature a girl is, the less effective treatment is in influencing her eventual height.

Treatment of Tall Stature. It is difficult to make a decision for treatment, and parental participation in the decision is essential. In a case where some success can be achieved, the patient is relatively young and may find it hard to know what to think about the future problem.

Since the adolescent growth spurt precedes menarche, treatment must begin before menarche in order to be optimally successfully. This would be as early as 8 or 9 years, and certainly before the age of 12. However, treatment begun after menarche may still achieve up to an inch of growth reduction. (24) Once begun, treatment must continue until epiphyses are fused. If treatment is stopped earlier, further growth will occur. The parents and patient must be informed of possible problems with menorrhagia, breast symptoms, water retention, etc.

Conjugated estrogen can be given in a dose of 10 mg daily from the 1st through the 25th of each month, and medroxyprogesterone acetate (Provera), 10 mg, is added on the 16th through the 25th to ensure consistent and predictable menstrual bleeding. Hand-wrist films should be taken every 6 months until epiphyseal closure is demonstrated.

References

1. **Winter JSD, Faiman, C,** The development of cyclic pituitary-gonadal function in adolescent females, J Clin Endocrinol Metab 37:714, 1973.

2. **Conte FA, Grumbach MM, Kaplan SL, Reiter EO,** Correlation of LHRF induced LH and FSH release from infancy to 19 years with the changing pattern of gonadotropin secretion in agonadal patients: relation to restraint of puberty, J Clin Endocrinol Metab 50:163, 1980.

383

3. **Sizonenko PC, Paunier L, Carmignac D,** Hormonal changes during puberty: IV. Longitudinal study of adrenal androgen secretion, Horm Res 7:288, 1976.

4. **Sklar CA, Kaplan SL, Grumbach MM,** Evidence for dissociation between adrenarche and gonadarche: studies in patients with idiopathic precocious puberty, gonadal dysgenesis, isolated gonadotropin deficiency, and constitutionally delayed growtth and adolescence, J Clin Endocrinol Metab 51:548, 1980.

5. **Pederson RC, Brownie AC, Ling N,** Pro-adrenocorticotropin/endorphin derived peptides: coordinate action on adrenal steroidogenesis, Science 208:1044, 1980.

6. **Foster DL, Ryan KD,** Endocrine mechanisms governing transaction into adulthood: a marked decreased in inhibitory feedback action of estradiol on tonic secretion of LH in the lamb during puberty, J Clin Endocrinology 105:896, 1979.

7. **Silman RE, Leone RM, Hooper RJ,** Melatonin, the pineal gland and human puberty, Nature 282:301, 1979.

8. **Job JC, Garnier PE, Chaussain JL, Milhaud G,** Elevation of serum gonadotropins (LH and FSH) after releasing hormone (LH-RH) injection in normal children and in patients with disorders of puberty, J Clin Endocrinol Metab 35:473, 1972.

9. **Kapen S, Boyan RM, Hellman L, Weltzman ED,** 24-Hour patterns of LH secretion in humans: ontogenic and sexual considerations, Prog Brain Res 42:103, 1975.

10. **Reiter EL, Kulen HE, Hamwood SM,** The absence of positive feedback between estrogen and LH in sexually immature girls, Pediatr Res 8:740, 1974.

11. **Marshall JC, Kilch RP,** Low dose pulsatile GnRH in anorexia nervosa: a model of human pubertal development, J Clin Endocrinol Metab 49:712, 1979.

12. **Frisch RE, McArthur JW,** Menstrual cycles: fatness as a determinant of minimum weight for height necessary for their maintenance or onset, Science 185:949, 1974.

13. **Tanner JM,** *Growth at Adolescence,* Ed 2, Blackwell Scientific Publications, Oxford, 1962.

14. **Marshall WA, Tanner JM,** Variations in the pattern of pubertal changes in girls, Arch Dis Child 44:291, 1969.

15. **Zacharias L, Rand WM, Wurtman RJ,** A prospective study of sexual development and growth in American girls: the statistics of menarche, Obstet Gynecol Surv 31:325, 1976.

16. **Fried RI, Smith EE,** Postmenarcheal growth patterns, J Pediatr 61:562, 1962.

17. **Grumbach MM,** The neuroendocrinology of puberty, in *Neuroendocrinology*, Krieger CT, Hughes JC, eds, Sinauer, Inc., Sunderland, Mass., 1980, p 249.

18. **Van Der Werff Ten Bosch JJ,** Isosexual precocity, in *Endocrine and Genetic Diseases of Childhood*, Gardner LI, ed, W. B. Saunders, Philadelphia, 1969.

19. **Pedowitz P, Felmus LB, Mackles A,** Precocious pseudo-puberty due to ovarian tumors, Obstet Gynecol Surv 10:633, 1955.

20. **Crowley WF, Comite F, Vale W, Rivier J, Loriaux DL, Cutler GB,** Therapeutic use of pituitary desensitization with a long-acting LHRH agonist: a potential new treatment for idiopathic precocious puberty, J Clin Endocrinol Metab 52:370, 1981.

21. **Bayley N, Pinneau SR,** Tables for predicting adult height from skeletal age: revised for use with the Greulich-Pyle hand standards, J Pediatr 40:423, 1952.

22. **Greulich WW, Pyle SL,** *Radiographic Atlas of Skeletal Development of the Hand and Wrist*, Stanford University Press, Stanford, Calif., 1950.

23. **Schoen EJ, Solomon IL, Warner D, Wingerd J,** Estrogen treatment of tall girls, Am J Dis Child 125:71, 1973.

24. **Norman H, Wettenhall B, Cahill C, Roche AF,** Tall girls: a survey of 15 years of management and treatment, Adolesc Med 86:602, 1975.

385

To predict height, find vertical column corresponding to skeletal age and horizontal row for the present height. The number at the intersection is the predicted height in inches. If figures do not fall at the whole inch or 6-month intervals, the predicted height must be extrapolated.

Skeletal age	6/0	6/6	7/0	7/6	8/0	8/6	9/0	9/6	10/0	10/6	11/0	11/6	12/0
Height 37	51.4												
in inches 38	52.8	51.5											
39	54.2	52.8	51.5										
40	55.6	54.2	52.8	51.8									
41	56.9	55.6	54.2	53.1	51.9								
42	58.3	56.9	55.5	54.4	53.2	51.9							
43	59.7	58.3	56.8	55.7	54.4	53.1	52.0						
44	61.1	59.6	58.1	57.0	55.7	54.3	53.2	52.1	51.0				
45	62.5	61.0	59.4	58.3	57.0	55.6	54.4	53.3	52.2				
46	63.9	62.3	60.8	59.6	58.2	56.8	55.6	54.5	53.4	52.0			
47	65.8	63.7	62.1	60.9	59.5	58.0	56.8	55.7	54.5	53.2	51.9	51.4	51.0
48	66.7	65.0	63.4	62.2	60.8	59.3	58.0	56.9	55.7	54.3	53.0	52.5	52.1
49	68.1	66.4	64.7	63.5	62.0	60.5	59.3	58.1	56.8	55.4	54.1	53.6	53.1
50	69.4	67.8	66.1	64.8	63.3	61.7	60.5	59.2	58.0	56.6	55.2	54.7	54.2
51	70.8	69.1	67.4	66.1	64.6	63.0	61.7	60.4	59.2	57.7	56.3	55.8	55.3
52	72.2	70.5	68.7	67.4	65.8	64.2	62.9	61.6	60.3	58.8	57.4	56.9	56.4
53	73.6	71.8	70.0	68.7	67.1	65.4	64.1	62.8	61.5	60.0	58.5	58.0	57.5
54		73.2	71.3	69.9	68.4	66.7	65.3	64.0	62.6	61.1	59.6	59.1	58.6
55		74.5	72.7	71.2	69.6	67.9	66.5	65.2	63.8	62.2	60.7	60.2	59.7
56			74.0	72.5	70.9	69.1	67.7	66.4	65.0	63.3	61.8	61.3	60.7
57				73.8	72.2	70.4	68.9	67.5	66.1	64.5	62.9	62.4	61.8
58					73.4	71.6	70.1	68.7	67.3	65.6	64.0	63.5	62.9
59					74.7	72.8	71.3	69.9	68.4	66.7	65.1	64.6	64.0
60						74.1	72.6	71.1	69.6	67.9	66.2	65.6	65.1
61							73.8	72.3	70.8	69.0	67.3	66.7	66.2
62								73.5	71.9	70.1	68.4	67.8	67.2
63								74.6	73.1	71.3	69.5	68.9	68.3
64									74.2	72.4	70.6	70.0	69.4
65										73.5	71.7	71.1	70.5
66										74.7	72.9	72.2	71.6
67											74.0	73.3	72.7
68												74.4	73.8
69													74.8
70													
71													
72													
73													
74													

12/6	13/0	13/6	14/0	14/6	15/0	15/6	16/0	16/6	17/0	17/6	18/0	
												37
												38
												39
												40
												41
												42
												43
												44
												45
												46
												47
51.0												48
52.1	51.1											49
53.1	52.2	51.3	51.0									50
54.2	53.2	52.4	52.0	51.7	51.5	51.4	51.2	51.2	51.1	51.0	51.0	51
55.3	54.3	53.4	53.1	52.7	52.5	52.4	52.2	52.2	52.1	52.0	52.0	52
56.3	55.3	54.4	54.1	53.8	53.5	53.4	53.2	53.2	53.1	53.0	53.0	53
57.4	56.4	55.4	55.1	54.8	54.5	54.4	54.2	54.2	54.1	54.0	54.0	54
58.4	57.4	56.5	56.1	55.8	55.6	55.4	55.2	55.2	55.1	55.0	55.0	55
59.5	58.5	57.5	57.1	56.8	56.6	56.4	56.2	56.2	56.1	56.0	56.0	56
60.6	59.5	58.5	58.2	57.8	57.6	57.4	57.2	57.2	57.1	57.0	57.0	57
61.6	60.5	59.5	59.2	58.8	58.6	58.4	58.2	58.2	58.1	58.0	58.0	58
62.7	61.6	60.6	60.2	59.8	59.6	59.4	59.2	59.2	59.1	59.0	59.0	59
63.8	62.6	61.6	61.2	60.9	60.6	60.4	60.2	60.2	60.1	60.0	60.0	60
64.8	63.7	62.6	62.2	61.9	61.6	61.4	61.2	61.2	61.1	61.0	61.0	61
65.9	64.7	63.7	63.3	62.9	62.6	62.4	62.2	62.2	62.1	62.0	62.0	62
67.0	65.8	64.7	64.3	63.9	63.6	63.4	63.3	63.2	63.1	63.0	63.0	63
68.0	66.8	65.7	65.3	64.9	64.6	64.4	64.3	64.2	64.1	64.0	64.0	64
69.1	67.8	66.7	66.3	65.9	65.7	65.5	65.3	65.2	65.1	65.0	65.0	65
70.1	68.9	67.8	67.3	66.9	66.7	66.5	66.3	66.2	66.1	66.0	66.0	66
71.2	69.9	68.8	68.4	68.0	67.7	67.5	67.3	67.2	67.1	67.0	67.0	67
72.3	71.0	69.8	69.4	69.0	68.7	68.5	68.3	68.2	68.1	68.0	68.0	68
73.3	72.0	70.8	70.4	70.0	69.7	69.5	69.3	69.2	69.1	69.0	69.0	69
74.4	73.1	71.9	71.4	71.0	70.7	70.5	70.3	70.2	70.1	70.0	70.0	70
	74.1	72.9	72.4	72.0	71.7	71.5	71.3	71.2	71.1	71.0	71.0	71
		73.9	73.5	73.0	72.7	72.5	72.3	72.2	72.1	72.0	72.0	72
		74.9	74.5	74.0	73.7	73.5	73.3	73.2	73.1	73.0	73.0	73
					74.7	74.5	74.3	74.2	74.1	74.0	74.0	74

Bayley-Pinneau Table for Accelerated Girls

To predict height, find vertical column corresponding to skeletal age and horizontal row for the present height. The number at the intersection is the predicted height in inches. If figures do not fall at the whole inch or 6-month intervals, the predicted height must be extrapolated.

Skeletal age		7/0	7/6	8/0	8/6	9/0	9/6	10/0	10/6	11/0	11/6	12/0
Height in inches	37	52.0										
	38	53.4	51.9									
	39	54.8	53.3	52.0								
	40	56.2	54.6	53.3	51.9							
	41	57.6	56.0	54.7	53.2	51.9						
	42	59.0	57.4	56.0	54.5	53.2	51.9					
	43	60.4	58.7	57.3	55.8	54.4	53.2	51.9				
	44	61.8	60.1	58.7	57.1	55.7	54.4	53.1	51.4			
	45	63.2	61.5	60.0	58.4	57.0	55.6	54.3	52.6	54.0		
	46	64.6	62.8	61.3	59.7	58.2	56.9	55.6	53.7	52.1	51.6	51.1
	47	66.0	64.2	62.7	61.0	59.5	58.1	56.8	54.9	53.2	52.7	52.2
	48	67.4	65.6	64.0	62.3	60.8	59.3	58.0	56.1	54.4	53.9	53.3
	49	68.8	66.9	65.3	63.6	62.0	60.6	59.2	57.2	55.5	55.0	54.4
	50	70.2	68.3	66.7	64.9	63.3	61.8	60.4	58.4	56.6	56.1	55.5
	51	71.6	69.7	68.0	66.1	64.6	63.0	61.6	59.6	57.8	57.2	56.6
	52	73.0	71.0	69.3	67.4	65.8	64.3	62.8	60.7	58.9	58.4	57.7
	53	74.4	72.4	70.7	68.7	67.1	65.5	64.0	61.9	60.0	59.5	58.8
	54		73.8	72.0	70.0	68.4	66.7	65.2	63.1	61.2	60.6	59.9
	55			73.3	71.3	69.6	68.0	66.4	64.3	62.3	61.7	61.0
	56			74.7	72.6	70.9	69.2	67.6	65.4	63.4	62.8	62.2
	57				73.9	72.2	70.5	68.8	66.6	64.6	64.0	63.3
	58					73.4	71.7	70.0	67.8	65.7	65.1	64.4
	59					74.7	72.9	71.3	68.9	66.8	66.2	65.5
	60						74.2	72.5	70.1	68.0	67.3	66.6
	61							73.7	71.3	69.1	68.5	67.7
	62							74.9	72.4	70.2	69.6	68.8
	63								73.6	71.3	70.7	69.9
	64								74.8	72.5	71.8	71.0
	65									73.6	72.9	72.1
	66									74.7	74.1	73.3
	67											74.4
	68											
	69											
	70											
	71											
	72											
	73											
	74											

12/6	13/0	13/6	14/0	14/6	15/0	15/6	16/0	16/6	17/0	17/6	
											37
											38
											39
											40
											41
											42
											43
											44
											45
											46
											47
51.9											48
53.0	51.9	50.9									49
54.1	52.9	51.9	51.4	51.0							50
55.2	54.0	53.0	52.5	52.0	51.7	51.5	51.4	51.3	51.1	51.0	51
56.3	55.0	54.0	53.5	53.1	52.7	52.5	52.4	52.3	52.1	52.0	52
57.4	56.1	55.0	54.5	54.1	53.8	53.5	53.4	53.3	53.1	53.0	53
58.4	57.1	56.1	55.6	55.1	54.8	54.5	54.4	54.3	54.1	54.0	54
59.5	58.2	57.1	56.6	56.1	55.8	55.5	55.4	55.3	55.1	55.0	55
60.6	59.3	58.2	57.6	57.1	56.8	56.5	56.4	56.3	56.1	56.0	56
61.7	60.3	59.2	58.6	58.2	57.8	57.6	57.4	57.3	57.1	57.0	57
62.8	61.4	60.2	59.7	59.2	58.8	58.6	58.4	58.3	58.1	58.0	58
63.9	62.4	61.3	60.7	60.2	59.8	59.6	59.4	59.3	59.1	59.0	59
64.9	63.5	62.3	61.7	61.2	60.9	60.6	60.4	60.3	60.1	60.0	60
66.0	64.6	63.3	62.8	62.2	61.9	61.6	61.4	61.3	61.1	61.0	61
67.1	65.6	64.4	63.8	63.3	62.9	62.6	62.4	62.3	62.1	62.0	62
68.2	66.7	65.4	64.8	64.3	63.9	63.6	63.4	63.3	63.1	63.0	63
69.3	67.7	66.5	65.8	65.3	64.9	64.6	64.4	64.3	64.1	64.0	64
70.3	68.8	67.5	66.9	66.3	65.9	65.7	65.5	65.3	65.1	65.0	65
71.4	69.8	68.5	67.9	67.3	66.9	66.7	66.5	66.3	66.1	66.0	66
72.5	70.9	69.6	68.9	68.4	68.0	67.7	67.5	67.3	67.1	67.0	67
73.6	72.0	70.6	70.0	69.4	69.0	68.7	68.5	68.3	68.1	68.0	68
74.7	73.0	71.7	71.0	70.4	70.0	69.7	69.5	69.3	69.1	69.0	69
	74.1	72.7	72.0	71.4	71.0	70.7	70.5	70.3	70.1	70.0	70
		73.7	73.0	72.4	72.0	71.7	71.5	71.4	71.1	71.0	71
		74.8	74.1	73.5	73.0	72.7	72.5	72.4	72.1	72.0	72
				74.5	74.0	73.7	73.5	73.4	73.1	73.0	73
						74.4	74.5	74.4	74.1	74.0	74

Bayley-Pinneau Table for Retarded Girls

To predict height, find vertical column corresponding to skeletal age and horizontal row for the present height. The number at the intersection is the predicted height in inches. If figures do not fall at the whole inch or 6-month intervals, the predicted height must be extrapolated.

Skeletal age	6/0	6/6	7/0	7/6	8/0	8/6	9/0	9/6	10/0	10/6	11/0	11/6
Height in inches 38	51.8											
39	53.2	51.9										
40	54.6	53.3	51.9									
41	55.9	54.6	53.2	52.0								
42	57.3	55.9	54.5	53.3	52.2	51.0						
43	58.7	57.3	55.8	54.6	53.5	52.2	51.1					
44	60.0	58.6	57.1	55.8	54.7	53.5	52.3	51.3				
45	61.4	59.9	58.4	57.1	56.0	54.7	53.5	52.4	51.5			
46	62.8	61.3	59.7	58.4	57.2	55.9	54.7	53.6	52.6	51.3		
47	64.1	62.6	61.0	59.6	58.5	57.1	55.9	54.8	53.8	52.5	51.2	
48	65.5	63.9	62.3	60.9	59.7	58.3	57.1	55.9	54.9	63.6	52.3	51.8
49	66.9	65.2	63.6	62.2	60.9	59.5	58.3	57.1	56.1	54.7	53.4	52.9
50	68.2	66.6	64.9	63.5	62.2	60.8	59.5	58.3	57.2	55.8	54.5	54.0
51	69.6	67.9	66.2	64.7	63.4	62.0	60.6	59.4	58.4	56.9	55.6	55.1
52	70.9	69.2	67.5	66.0	64.7	63.2	61.8	60.6	59.5	58.0	56.6	56.2
53	72.3	70.6	68.8	67.3	65.9	64.4	63.0	61.8	60.6	59.2	57.7	57.2
54	73.7	71.9	70.1	68.5	67.2	65.6	64.2	62.9	61.8	60.3	58.8	58.3
55		73.2	71.4	69.8	68.4	66.8	65.4	64.1	62.9	61.4	59.9	59.4
56		74.6	72.7	71.1	69.7	68.0	66.6	65.3	64.1	62.5	61.0	60.5
57			74.0	72.3	70.9	69.3	67.8	66.4	65.2	63.6	62.1	61.6
58				73.6	72.1	70.5	69.0	67.6	66.4	64.7	63.2	62.6
59				74.9	73.4	71.7	70.2	68.8	67.5	65.8	64.3	63.7
60					74.6	72.9	71.3	69.9	68.7	67.0	65.4	64.8
61						74.1	72.5	71.1	69.8	68.1	66.4	65.9
62							73.7	72.3	70.9	69.2	67.5	67.0
63							74.7	73.4	72.1	70.3	68.6	68.0
64								74.6	73.2	71.4	69.7	69.1
65									74.4	72.5	70.8	70.2
66										73.7	71.9	71.3
67										74.8	73.0	72.4
68											74.1	73.4
69												74.5
70												
71												
72												
73												
74												

12/0	12/6	13/0	13/6	14/0	14/6	15/0	15/6	16/0	16/6	17/0	
											40
											41
											42
											43
											44
											45
											46
											47
51.5											48
52.6	51.6										49
53.6	52.7	51.9	51.2								50
54.7	53.7	52.9	52.2	51.9	51.6	51.3	51.2	51.1	51.1	51.0	51
55.8	54.8	53.9	53.2	52.9	52.6	52.3	52.2	52.1	52.1	52.0	52
56.9	55.8	55.0	54.2	53.9	53.6	53.3	53.2	53.1	53.1	53.0	53
57.9	56.9	56.0	55.3	54.9	54.6	54.3	54.2	54.1	54.1	54.0	54
59.0	58.0	57.1	56.3	56.0	55.6	55.3	55.2	55.1	55.1	55.0	55
60.1	59.0	58.1	57.3	57.0	56.6	56.3	56.2	56.1	56.1	56.0	56
61.2	60.1	59.1	58.3	58.0	57.6	57.3	57.2	57.1	57.1	57.0	57
62.2	61.1	60.2	59.4	59.0	58.6	58.3	58.2	58.1	58.1	58.0	58
63.3	62.2	61.2	60.4	60.0	59.7	59.4	59.2	59.1	59.1	59.0	59
64.4	63.2	62.2	61.4	61.0	60.7	60.4	60.2	60.1	60.1	60.0	60
65.5	64.3	63.3	62.4	62.1	61.7	61.4	61.2	61.1	61.1	61.0	61
66.5	65.3	64.3	63.5	63.1	62.7	62.4	62.2	62.1	62.1	62.0	62
67.6	66.4	65.3	64.5	64.1	63.7	63.4	63.3	63.1	63.1	63.0	63
68.7	67.4	66.4	65.5	65.1	64.7	64.4	64.3	64.1	64.1	64.0	64
69.7	68.5	67.4	66.5	66.1	65.7	65.4	65.3	65.1	65.1	65.0	65
70.8	69.5	68.5	67.6	67.1	66.7	66.4	66.3	66.1	66.1	66.0	66
71.9	70.6	69.5	68.6	68.2	67.7	67.4	67.3	67.1	67.1	67.0	67
73.0	71.7	70.5	69.6	69.2	68.8	68.4	68.3	68.1	68.1	68.0	68
74.0	72.7	71.6	70.6	70.2	69.8	69.4	69.3	69.1	69.1	69.0	69
	73.8	72.6	71.6	71.2	70.8	70.4	70.3	70.1	70.1	70.0	70
	74.8	73.6	72.7	72.2	71.8	71.4	71.3	71.1	71.1	71.0	71
		74.7	73.7	73.3	72.8	72.4	72.3	72.1	72.1	72.0	72
			74.7	74.3	73.8	73.4	73.3	73.1	73.1	73.0	73
					74.8	74.4	74.3	74.1	74.1	74.0	74

14   Obesity

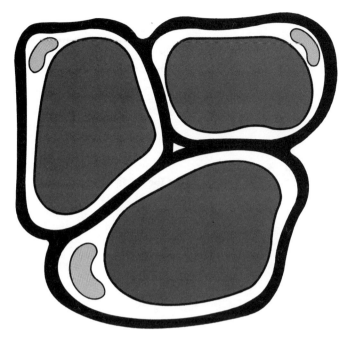

One of the least rewarding experiences in clinical medicine is treating obesity. Because from 25 to 45% of American adults over 30 years old are more than 20% overweight, the unrewarding fight against obesity is all too common, not only with our patients, but also with ourselves. Unfortunately, for over 100 years the incidence of obesity has been increasing in the United States, a reflection of an increasingly sedentary life in an affluent society. (1)

The lack of success in treating obesity is not due to an unawareness of the implications of obesity; there is a clear-cut relationship between mortality and weight. The death rate from diabetes mellitus, for example, is approximately 4 times higher among obese diabetics than among those who control their weight. Also higher among obese individuals is the incidence of gallbladder disease, cardiovascular disease, renal disease, and cirrhosis of the liver. The death rate from appendicitis is double, presumably from anesthetic and surgical complications. Even the rate of accidents is higher, perhaps because fat people are awkward or because their view of the ground or floor is obstructed. When the personal and social problems encountered by obese persons are also considered, it is no wonder that a physician without a weight problem cannot comprehend why fat individuals remain overweight.

The frequency with which a practitioner encounters the obese patient whose weight does not decrease despite a sworn adherence to a limited-calorie diet makes one question if there is something physiologically different about this patient. Is the problem due to lack of discipline and cheating on a diet, or does it also involve a pathophysiologic factor? Is the physiology of obese people unusual, or are they simply gluttons?

As a basis for a more understanding approach to obesity this chapter reviews the physiology of adipose tissue, discusses differences between normal and obese people, and comments on treatment.

Definition of Obesity

There is a difference between obesity and overweight. (2) Obesity is an excess of body fat. Overweight is a body weight in excess of some standard or ideal weight. The ideal weight for any adult is believed to correspond to his or her ideal weight from age 20 to 30. The following formulas give ideal weight in pounds:

Women: **100 + (4 × (height in inches minus 60))**

Men: **120 + (4 × (height in inches minus 60))**

At a weight close to ideal weight, individuals may be overweight, but not overfat. This is especially true of individuals engaged in regular exercise. An estimate of body fat, therefore, rather than a measurement of height and weight, is more significant.

The most accurate method of determining body fat is to determine the density of the body by underwater measurement. It certainly is not practical to measure density by submerging individuals in water in our offices, therefore skinfold measurements with calipers have become popular as an index of body fat. The skinfold measurement is also not necessary for clinical practice. It is far simpler to utilize the body mass index nomogram, a method which has been found to correspond closely to densitometry measurements. (3)

The body mass index is the ratio of weight divided by the weight squared (in metric units). To read the central scale, align a straight edge between height and body weight. A body mass index of about 30 is roughly equivalent to 30% excess body weight, the point at which excess mortality begins. Above 40, the risk from obesity itself is comparable to that associated with major health problems such as hypertension and heavy smoking.

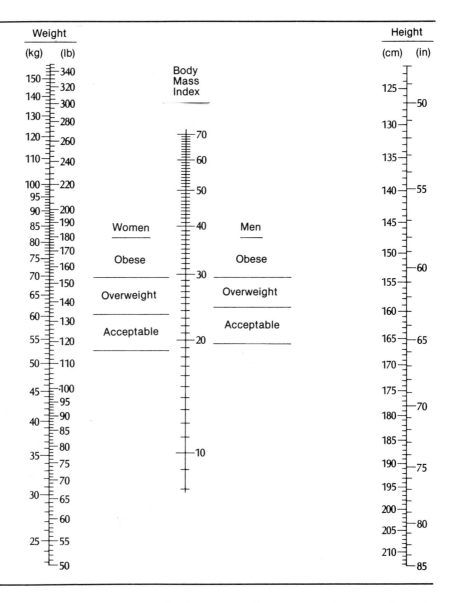

Weight | Body Mass Index | Height

Weight (kg) (lb): 150—340, 140—320, 300, 130—280, 120—260, 110—240, 100—220, 95, 90—200, 85—190, 180, 80—170, 75—160, 70—150, 65—140, 60—130, 55—120, 50—110, 45—100, 95, 40—90, 85, 80, 35—75, 70, 30—65, 60, 25—55, 50

Body Mass Index: 70, 60, 50, 40, 30, 20, 10

Women — Obese — Overweight — Acceptable

Men — Obese — Overweight — Acceptable

Height (cm) (in): 125, 50, 130, 135, 140—55, 145, 150—60, 155, 160, 165—65, 170, 175, 180—70, 185, 190—75, 195, 200, 205—80, 210—85

A person is obese when the amount of adipose tissue is sufficiently high (20% or more over ideal weight) to detrimentally alter biochemical and physiologic functions and to shorten life expectancy. Obesity is associated with four major risk factors for atherosclerosis: hypertension, diabetes, hypercholesterolemia, and hypertriglyceridemia. Overweight individuals have a higher prevalence of hypertension at every age, and the risk of developing hypertension is related to the amount of weight gain after age 25. (4) The two in combination (hypertension and obesity) increase the risk of heart disease, cerebrovascular disease, and death.

Unfortunately the basal metabolic rate decreases with age. A 30-year-old individual will inevitably gain weight if there is no change in caloric intake or exercise level over the years. The middle aged spread is both a biological and a psychosociological phenomenon. It is therefore important for both our patients and ourselves to understand adipose tissue and the problem of obesity.

Physiology of Adipose Tissue

Adipose tissue serves three general functions:

1. Adipose tissue is a storehouse of energy.

2. Fat serves as a cushion from trauma.

3. Adipose tissue plays a role in the regulation of body heat.

Each cell of adipose tissue may be regarded as a package of triglyceride, the most concentrated form of stored energy. There are 8 calories per gram of triglyceride as opposed to 1 calorie per gram of glycogen. The total store of tissue and fluid carbohydrate in adults (about 300 calories) is inadequate to meet between-meal demands. The storage of energy in fat tissue allows us to do other things beside eating.

The mechanism for mobilizing energy from fat involves various enzymes and neurohormonal agents. Following ingestion of fat and its breakdown by gastric and pancreatic lipases, absorption of long-chain triglycerides and free fatty acids take place in the small bowel. Chylomicrons (microscopic particles of fat) transferred through lymph channels into the systemic venous circulation are normally removed by hepatic parenchymal cells where a new lipoprotein is released into the circulation. When this lipoprotein is exposed to adipose tissue, lipolysis takes place through the action of lipoprotein lipase, an enzyme derived from the fat cells themselves. The fatty acids that are released then enter the fat cells where they are reesterified with glycerophosphate into triglycerides.

Glucose serves three important functions:

1. Glucose supplies carbon atoms in the form of acetyl coenzyme A (acetyl CoA).

2. Glucose provides hydrogen for reductive steps.

3. Glucose is the main source of glycerophosphate.

The production and availability of glycerophosphate (required for reesterification of fatty acids and their storage as triglycerides) are considered rate-limiting in lipogenesis, and this process depends on the presence of glucose.

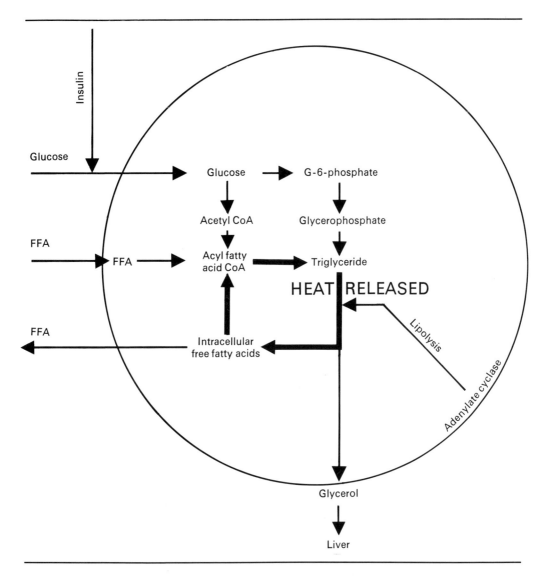

After esterification, subsequent lipolysis results in the release of fatty acids and glycerol. In the cycle of lipolysis and reesterification, energy is freed as heat. A low variable level of lipolysis takes place continuously; its basic function may be to provide body heat.

The chief metabolic products produced from fat are the circulating free fatty acids. Their availability is controlled by adipose tissue cells. When carbohydrate is in short supply, a flood of free fatty acids can be released. The free fatty acids in the peripheral circulation are almost wholly derived from endogenous triglyceride that undergoes rapid hydrolysis to yield free fatty acid and glycerol. The glycerol is returned to the liver for resynthesis of glycogen.

Free fatty acid release from adipose tissue is stimulated by physical exercise, fasting, exposure to cold, nervous tension, and anxiety. The release of fatty acids by lipolysis varies from one anatomic site to another. Omental, mesenteric, and subcutaneous fat are more labile and easily mobilized than fat from other sources. Areas from which energy is not easily mobilized are retrobulbar and perirenal fat where the tissue serves a structural function. Adipose tissue lipase is sensitive to stimulation by both epinephrine and norepinephrine. Other hormones that activate lipase are ACTH, thyroid stimulating hormone (TSH), growth hormone, thyroxine (T_4), 3,5,3'-triiodothryonine (T_3), cortisol, glucagon, as well as vasopressin and human placental lactogen (HPL).

Lipase enzyme activity is inhibited by insulin, which appears to be alone as the major physiologic antagonist to the array of stimulating agents. When both glucose and insulin are abundant, transport of glucose into fat cells is high, and glycerophosphate production increases to esterify fatty acids.

The carbohydrate and fat composition of the fuel supply is constantly changing, depending upon stresses and demands. Since the central nervous system and some other tissues can utilize only glucose for energy, a homeostatic mechanism for conserving carbohydrate is essential. When glucose is abundant and easily available, it is utilized in adipose tissue for producing glycerophosphate to immobilize fatty acids as triglycerides. The circulating level of free fatty acids in muscle will, therefore, be low, and glucose will be used by all of the tissues.

When carbohydrate is scarce, the amount of glucose reaching the fat cells declines and glycerophosphate production is reduced. The fat cell releases fatty acids, and their circulating levels rise to a point where glycolysis is inhibited. Thus, carbohydrate is spared in those tissues capable of using lipid substrates. If the rise of fatty acids is great enough, the liver is flooded with acetyl CoA. This is converted into ketone bodies, and clinical ketosis results.

In the simplest terms, when a person eats, glucose is available, insulin is secreted, and fat is stored. In starvation, the glucose level falls, insulin secretion decreases, and fat is mobilized.

If only single large meals are consumed, the body learns to convert carbohydrate to fat very quickly. Epidemiologic studies on school children demonstrate a positive correlation between fewer meals and a greater tendency toward obesity. (5) The person who does not eat all day and then stocks up at night is perhaps doing the worst possible thing.

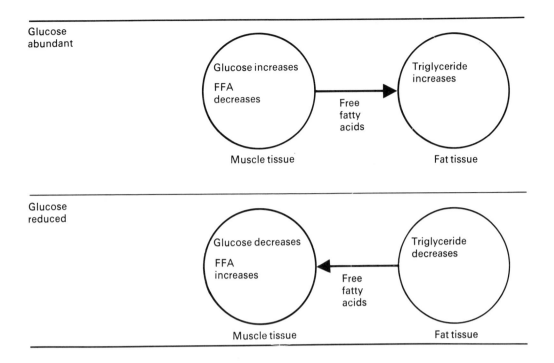

Glucose
abundant

Glucose increases

FFA decreases

Free fatty acids

Triglyceride increases

Muscle tissue

Fat tissue

Glucose
reduced

Glucose decreases

FFA increases

Free fatty acids

Triglyceride decreases

Muscle tissue

Fat tissue

Clinical Obesity
Obesity and the Brain

The hypothalamic location of the appetite center was established in 1940 by the demonstration that bilateral lesions of the ventromedial nucleus produce experimental obesity in rats. Such lesions lead to hyperphagia and decreased physical activity. Interestingly, this pattern is similar to that seen in human beings—the pressure to eat is reinforced by the desire to be physically inactive. The ventromedial nucleus was thought to represent an integrating center for appetite and hunger information. Destruction of the ventromedial nucleus was believed to result in a loss of satiety signals, leading to hyperphagia.

Overeating and obesity, however, may not be due to ventromedial nucleus damage but rather to destruction of the nearby ventral noradrenergic bundle. (6) Hypothalamic noradrenergic terminals are derived from long fibers ascending from hindbrain cell bodies. Lesions of the ventromedial nucleus produced by radiofrequency current fail to cause obesity. These lesions lead to overeating and obesity only when they extend beyond the ventromedial nucleus. Selective destruction of the ventral noradrenergic bundle results in hyperphagia. The lesions that produce hyperphagia also reduce the potency of amphetamine as an appetite suppressant. This noradrenergic bundle may function as a satiety system and be the site of amphetamine action.

There may be two kinds of obesity: obesity stemming from a CNS regulatory defect, or obesity due to a metabolic problem occurring despite a normal central mechanism.

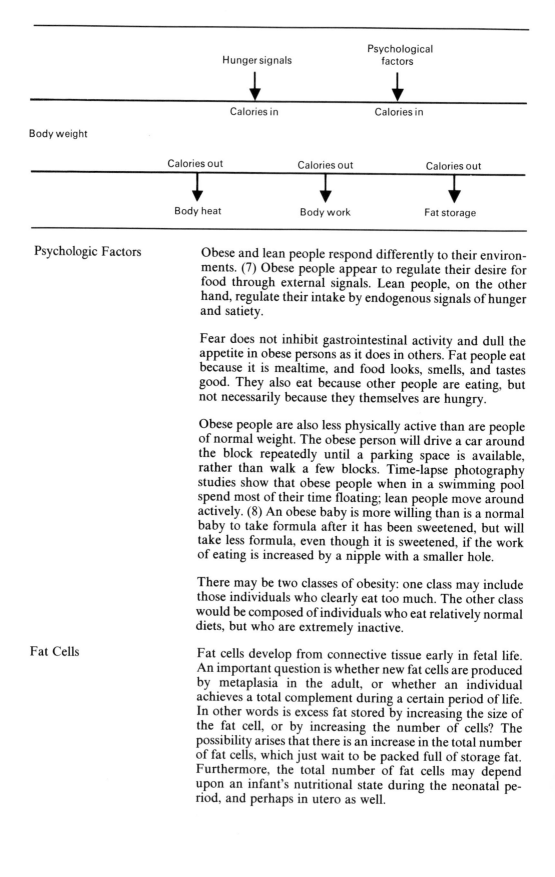

Hunger signals → Calories in

Psychological factors → Calories in

Body weight

Calories out → Body heat

Calories out → Body work

Calories out → Fat storage

Psychologic Factors

Obese and lean people respond differently to their environments. (7) Obese people appear to regulate their desire for food through external signals. Lean people, on the other hand, regulate their intake by endogenous signals of hunger and satiety.

Fear does not inhibit gastrointestinal activity and dull the appetite in obese persons as it does in others. Fat people eat because it is mealtime, and food looks, smells, and tastes good. They also eat because other people are eating, but not necessarily because they themselves are hungry.

Obese people are also less physically active than are people of normal weight. The obese person will drive a car around the block repeatedly until a parking space is available, rather than walk a few blocks. Time-lapse photography studies show that obese people when in a swimming pool spend most of their time floating; lean people move around actively. (8) An obese baby is more willing than is a normal baby to take formula after it has been sweetened, but will take less formula, even though it is sweetened, if the work of eating is increased by a nipple with a smaller hole.

There may be two classes of obesity: one class may include those individuals who clearly eat too much. The other class would be composed of individuals who eat relatively normal diets, but who are extremely inactive.

Fat Cells

Fat cells develop from connective tissue early in fetal life. An important question is whether new fat cells are produced by metaplasia in the adult, or whether an individual achieves a total complement during a certain period of life. In other words is excess fat stored by increasing the size of the fat cell, or by increasing the number of cells? The possibility arises that there is an increase in the total number of fat cells, which just wait to be packed full of storage fat. Furthermore, the total number of fat cells may depend upon an infant's nutritional state during the neonatal period, and perhaps in utero as well.

Studies of fat obtained at surgery indicate that the mean fat cell volume is increased threefold in obese people, but an increase in the number of fat cells is seen only in the grossly obese. (9) When patients diet, the fat cells decrease in size, but not in number. Hypercellular obesity may be a more difficult problem to overcome, since an individual may be saddled with a permanent increase in fat cells.

Some researchers think that, at some period in a person's life, a fixed number of fat cells is obtained. Adolescence, infancy, and intrauterine life seem particularly critical. (10, 11) This premise is not solidly established, because there is no certain way to identify an empty fat cell, and potential fat cells cannot be recognized. Nevertheless, a hyperplastic type of obesity (more fat cells) may be associated with childhood and have a poor prognosis; a hypertrophic type (enlarged fat cells) that is responsive to dieting may occur in adults. It is best to recognize that an obese individual who has suffered with the problem lifelong does have a disorder, but we do not understand it.

Endocrine Changes

The most important endocrine change in obesity is elevation of the basal blood insulin level. Increases in body fat change the body's secretion and sensitivity to insulin. There is a decrease in the number of insulin receptor sites at a cellular level, most significantly in fat, liver, and muscle tissue. The key factors which affect insulin resistance are the amount of fat tissue in the body, the caloric intake per day, the amount of carbohydrates in the diet, and the amount of daily exercise. The mechanism for the increased resistance to insulin observed with increasing weight may be down-regulation of insulin receptors brought about by the increase in insulin secretion. The increase in insulin resistance affects the metabolism of carbohydrate, fat and protein. Circulating levels of free fatty acids increase as a result of inadequate insulin suppression of the fat cell.

Genetics plays a greater role in the development of maturity onset diabetes than juvenile onset. (12) It is impossible to predict exactly who eventually will develop diabetes as the tendency is recessive and it will not develop in every generation in a family. But weight is a good tipoff. As weight increases, the frequency of occurrence of diabetes increases. Both gestational diabetes and insulin-dependent diabetes are more common in overweight pregnant patients.

Contrary to popular misconception, hypothyroidism does not cause obesity. Weight gain due to hypothyroidism is confined to the fluid accumulation of myxedema. There is no place, therefore, for thyroid hormone administration in the treatment of obesity when the patient is euthyroid.

Other endocrine changes associated with obesity include decreased growth hormone secretion, and increased cortisol production and metabolic clearance rates (thus, plasma and urinary cortisol are relatively normal). The fasting level of growth hormone is decreased as well as the response to

401

insulin, arginine, starvation, and sleep. There is evidence of decreased pancreatic alpha (α) cell function in obese non-diabetic people. (13) Glucagon secreted by the α cells acutely raises blood glucose levels by stimulating hepatic glycogenolysis and the production of new glucose from amino acids in the liver. Glucagon also activates lipolysis in the fat cell and stimulates insulin secretion. The basal levels of glucagon are equal in obese and nonobese patients, but the glucagon response to alanine is reduced by 50% in the obese group.

Obese people are relatively unable to excrete both salt and water, especially while dieting. During dieting this seems to be mediated by increased output of aldosterone and vasopressin. Since water produced from fat outweighs the fat, people on diets often show little initial weight loss. The early use of a diuretic may encourage a patient to persist with dieting.

The basic question is whether metabolic changes observed in obesity represent adaptive responses to a markedly enlarged fat organ, or whether they are representative of a metabolic or hormonal defect. It appears that the former is true. These changes are secondary responses; they are totally reversible with weight loss. Four-year follow-up in a group of patients who did not regain their weight after dieting revealed persistently normal insulin and glucose responses; patients who regained their weight showed further deterioration in these metabolic factors. (14)

Experimental Obesity

In a Vermont study, 28 male volunteers in the state prison underwent induced weight gain to about 20% above their basal weights. (15) Subjective changes were noted that correlate with the behavior of obese patients. The volunteers experienced increased appetite late in the day and decreased desire for physical activity. Once the weight gain was achieved, these normal people required about twice as many calories to maintain their obesity as did spontaneously obese people; there was no difficulty in returning to normal weight. These results suggest that there is something different about obese people.

With the gain in weight, the subjects showed an increase in fasting plasma insulin levels, decreased glucose tolerance, and decreased responses of adipose tissue to insulin stimulation of lipolysis. There was no increase in adipose cell number. These metabolic changes reverted to normal when the gained weight was lost. Hence, the hyperinsulinemia of obesity does not seem to be an etiologic, primary response, but rather a secondary change.

Aside from not smoking cigarettes, weight reduction is the most important health measure available for reducing the risk of cardiovascular disease. (16) For most patients, after a routine evaluation to rule out pathology such as diabetes mellitus, the physician is left with the frustrating task of prescribing a diet. But it is not enough to just prescribe a diet or prescribe an anorectic drug. An effective weight loss program requires commitment from both patient and physician.

Physican and patient should agree on the goal of a diet program. While the physician may wish the patient to reach ideal weight, the patient may be satisfied with less. Motivation is improved when the goals meet both personal and medical objectives. It is realistic to lose 4–5 pounds in the first month and 20–30 pounds in 4–5 months.

Despite various fads and diet books, the best diet continues to be a limitation of calories to between 900 and 1200 calories per day, the actual amount depending on what the individual patient will accept and pursue.

Ideal Diet:
- Carbohydrates — 40–45%
- Protein — 20%
- Fat — 35–40%

The discouraging aspect is that to lose a pound of fat, the equivalent to a 3500-calorie intake must be expended. Dieting has to be slow and steady to be effective. Successful programs include behavior modification, frequent visits to the physician, and involvement of family members. Behavior modification starts with daily recording of activity and behavior related to food intake, followed by the elimination of inappropriate cues (other than hunger) which lead to eating.

Careful studies (performed in hospitalized subjects on metabolic wards) have indicated that the carbohydrate and fat composition of the diet has no effect on the rate of weight loss. (7) Restriction of calories remains the important principle. Substituting one of the liquid formulas for meals has been successful in many individuals. Unbalanced formulations, however, have the same side effects as seen with total starvation (carbohydrate-deprived regimens). Adequate carbohydrate is necessary for utilization of amino acids. In addition, electrolyte problems have been encountered, and there is an initial diuretic phase that can lead to postural hypotension.

The protein sparing modified fast is a ketogenic regimen providing approximately 800 calories per day. The problems of the liquid protein diet are largely overcome with high quality protein and the provision of necessary vitamins and minerals. However, it is thought that these programs still carry considerable risk and should not be conducted without medical supervision. (17) The other disadvantage to the semistarvation diet is that short-term success does not guarantee long-term weight maintenance. It is reported that at best only one fourth to one third of individuals who lose weight by a semistarvation ketogenic regimen plus behavior modification therapy will have significant long-term weight reduction. (18) On the other hand, for that one fourth to one third, this represents a major accomplishment and is worth doing.

As an index of the general lack of success with diets, a summary of 10 studies (approximately 1200 patients) revealed that only 30% lose 20 pounds or more, only 4% lose 40 pounds or more. (9) Commercial organizations are no more successful than physician-directed programs or non-profit self-help groups. (19) Thus, it is obvious why gimmicks abound in this area of patient management.

Anorectics are useful as short-term therapy to control hunger, especially at the beginning of a diet and at a plateau or relapse stage. Compared to amphetamines, there is less abuse associated with nonamphetamine anorectics (diethylpropion, fenfluramine, mazindol, and phentermine). All of these agents act on the central nervous system to depress appetite.

Surgical treatment and starvation should be reserved for patients who are morbidly obese. Both methods involve many potential problems and require close monitoring.

Controlled studies have not demonstrated the effectiveness of thyroid preparations or human chorionic gonadotropin (HCG). (20) Indeed, adding thyroid hormone increases the loss of lean body mass rather than fat tissue. It is clear that adjunctive drug measures are not successful unless the patient is also motivated either to limit caloric intake or to increase the exercise level in what will be a lifelong battle.

A regular pattern of physical exercise reduces the risk of myocardial infarction in all people. (21) Both weight loss and increased physical activity, through an unknown mechanism, lower the level of low density lipoprotein (LDL), and increase the level of high density lipoprotein (HDL). A further benefit of moderate exercise is an inhibition of appetite which lasts many hours. There is one study, however, that indicates a rebound increase in appetite 1–2 days after exercise. (22) The optimum program includes, therefore, a *daily* period of exercise.

Unfortunately one cannot burn up significant calories quickly; it takes 18 minutes of running to compensate for the average hamburger. (23)

Activity	Calories per Hour
Sleeping	90
Office work	240
Walking	240
Golf	300
Housework	300
Bicycling	360
Swimming	360
Tennis	480
Bowling	510
Running slowly	750 (ca. 120/mile)
Cross country skiing	840
Running fast	960 (ca. 160/mile)

Most frustrating is the problem of some patients who limit caloric intake, yet do not lose weight. In fact, as the weights of certain patients increase, the number of calories required to remain in equilibrium decreases, probably due to a combination of reduced activity and a change in metabolism. The Vermont study demonstrated that the normal person with induced obesity requires 2700 calories to remain in equilibrium; spontaneously obese patients require only about 1300 calories. (15) The physician must be careful to avoid a condemning or punitive attitude, and understand that it is possible to significantly restrict caloric intake and not lose weight.

Patients appear doomed to frustration and despair unless the physician can motivate them to increase physical activity. In all individuals dieting is more effective when combined with physical exercise, but this is especially true in chronically obese patients. In other words, the life-style of an obese person must be changed to overcome the desire to be inactive (walk instead of riding). Only by significantly increasing caloric expenditure will the input-output equilibrium be disturbed.

The obese person feels trapped. Obesity leads to characteristic behavioral manifestations, including passive personality, frequent periods of depression, decreased self-respect, and a sense of being hopelessly overwhelmed by problems. But just as the endocrine and metabolic changes seem to be secondary to obesity, many of the psychosocial attributes surrounding obesity may also be secondary. (24)

Motivation to change and emotional support during the change are important. They can be provided by friends, relatives, physicians, or self-help organizations. If the vicious circle of failed diets, resignation to fate, guilt, and shame can be broken, a more effective, happier person will emerge.

References

1. **Van Itallie JB, Hirsch J,** Appraisal of excess calories as a factor in causation of disease, Am J Clin Nutr 32:2648, 1979.

2. **Powers PS,** *Obesity, the Regulation of Weight,* Williams & Wilkins, Baltimore, 1980.

3. **Thomas AE, McKay DA, Cutlip MB,** A nomograph method for assessing body weight, Am J Clin Nutr 29:302, 1976.

4. **Stamler R, Stamler J, Riedlinger WF, Algera G, Roberts RH,** Weight and blood pressure: findings in hypertension screening of 1 million Americans, JAMA 240:1607, 1978.

5. **Fabry P, Hejda S, Cerny K,** Effect of meal frequency in school children. Changes in weight-height proportion and skinfold thickness, Am J Clin Nutr 18:358, 1966.

6. **Gold RM,** Hypothalamic obesity: the myth of the ventro-medial nucleus, Science 182:488, 1973.

7. **Gordon ES,** Metabolic aspects of obesity, Adv Metab Disord 4:229, 1970.

8. **Mayer J,** Inactivity as a major factor in adolescent obesity, Ann NY Acad Sci 131:502, 1965.

9. **Bray GA, Davidson MB, Drenick EJ,** Obesity: a serious symptom, Ann Intern Med 77:787, 1972.

10. **Ravelli G, Stein ZA, Susser MW,** Obesity in young men after famine exposure in utero and early infancy, N Engl J Med 295:349, 1976.

11. **Charney E, Goodman HC, McBride M, Lyon B, Pratt R,** Childhood antecedents of adult obesity, N Engl J Med 295:6, 1976.

12. **Fanda OP, Soeldner SS,** Genetic, acquired, and related factors in the etiology of diabetes mellitus, Arch Intern Med 137:461, 1977.

13. **Wise JK, Hendler R, Felig P,** Obesity: evidence of decreased secretion of glucagon, Science 178:513, 1972.

14. **Hewing R, Liebermeister H, Daweke H, Gries FA, Gruneklee D,** Weight regain after low calories diet: long term pattern of blood sugar, serum lipids, ketone bodies, and serum insulin levels, Diabetologia 9:197, 1973.

15. **Sims EAH, Danforth E Jr, Horton ES, Bray GA, Glennon JA, Salans LB,** Endocrine and metabolic effects of experimental obesity in man, Recent Prog Horm Res 29:457, 1973.

16. **Gordon T, Kannel WB,** Obesity and cardiovascular disease: the Framingham study, Clin Endocrinol Metab 5:367, 1976.

17. **Bistrian BR,** The medical treatment of obesity, Arch Intern Med 141:429, 1981.

18. **Bistrian BR, Sherman M,** Results of the treatment of obesity with a protein-sparing modified fast, Int J Obes 2:143, 1978.

19. **Volkmar FR, Stunkard AJ, Woolston J, Bailey RA,** High attrition rates in commercial weight reduction programs, Arch Intern Med 141:426, 1981.

20. **Rivlin RS,** Drug therapy: therapy of obesity with hormones, N Engl J Med 292:26, 1975.

21. **Paffenbarger RS Jr, Wing AL, Hyde RT,** Physical activity as an index of heart attack risk in college alumni, Am J Epidemiol 108:161, 1978.

22. **Edholm OG, Fletcher JG, Widdowson EM, McCance RA,** The energy expenditure and food intake of individual men, Br J Nutr 9:286, 1955.

23. **Konishi F,** Food energy equivalents of various activities, J Am Diet Assoc 46:186, 1965.

24. **Solow C, Siberfarb PM, Swift K,** Psychosocial effects of intestinal bypass surgery for severe obesity, N Engl J Med 290:300, 1974.

15   Steroid Contraception

The steroid contraception message for the decade of the 1980s should be a positive one. The message during the 1970s was negative, emphasizing problems and side effects. As a result, in 1980, 12% of the women in the childbearing age in America were using oral contraception compared to 20% in 1975. This decline was due, in significant part, not only to legitimate concerns about side effects, but also to unjustified fears brought about by our warnings which were publicized and often exaggerated by the media. (1)

It is time to change our approach. The new birth control pills are extremely safe. Information from four on-going large epidemiologic studies is now available, which allows us to emphasize with confidence the safety of the pill.

The clinical trials with steroids for contraception started with combination pills in 1952 (they were first commercially available in 1960). However, it was not until 1968 that the first reliable prospective studies were initiated, and it was not until the late 1970s that a dose-response relationship between problems and the amount of steroids in the pill was appreciated. The clinical impact of the data from the prospective studies has been very significant, and clinicians should continue to carefully scan the literature for reliable information from the following four studies:

In England:
1. The Study of the Royal College of General Practitioners
2. The Study of the Oxford Family Planning Association

In America:
3. The Kaiser Permanente Study (Walnut Creek)
4. The Women's Health Study

Contraceptive steroids are not natural hormones and should not be so considered, i.e. a woman on the pill is not the same as a pregnant woman in more ways than the obvious one, nor can the effects be equated with phases of the menstrual cycle. Contraceptive steroids induce a pharmacologic state, not a physiologic one. *This chapter will survey those physiologic mechanisms under stress in the woman taking oral contraception, and review our methods for patient management. The major theme of this chapter is the relationshp between steroid dose and side effects, emphasizing the safety of the low dose birth control pills (containing less than 50 µg estrogen).*

Pharmacology of Steroid Contraception

The Estrogen Component

The major obstacle to the use of steroids for contraception was inactivity of the compounds when given orally. A major breakthrough occurred in 1938 when it was discovered that the addition of an ethinyl group at the 17 position made estradiol orally active. Ethinyl estradiol is a very potent oral estrogen and is one of the two forms of estrogen in every oral contraceptive. The other estrogen is the 3-methyl ether of ethinyl estradiol, mestranol.

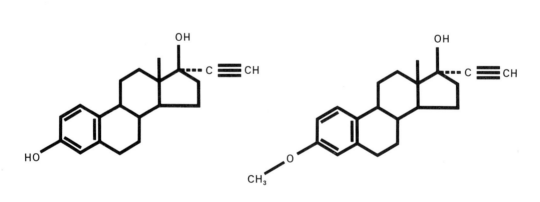

Ethinyl estradiol   Mestranol

Mestranol and ethinyl estradiol are different from natural estradiol and must be regarded as pharmacologic drugs. A variety of animal studies have suggested that mestranol is weaker than ethinyl estradiol, because mestranol must first be converted to ethinyl estradiol in the body. Indeed, mestranol will not bind to the cytoplasmic estrogen receptor. Therefore, unconjugated ethinyl estradiol is the active estrogen in the blood for both mestranol and ethinyl estradiol. In the human body, differences in potency between ethinyl estradiol and mestranol do not appear to be significant, certainly not as great as indicated by assays in rodents. This is not an important clinical point anymore since all of the new dose pills contain ethinyl estradiol.

The estrogen content (dosage) of the pill is of major clinical importance. Thrombosis is the most serious side effect of the pill, playing a key role in the increased risk of death from a variety of circulatory problems such as myocardial infarction, pulmonary embolism, and stroke. This side effect is related to estrogen, and it is dose related. Therefore, the dose of estrogen becomes a critical issue in selecting a birth control pill.

The Progestin Component

The discovery of ethinyl substitution and oral potency led to the preparation of ethisterone, an orally active derivative of testosterone. In 1951, it was found that removal of the 19 carbon from ethisterone to form norethindrone did not destroy the oral activity, and most importantly, it changed the major hormonal effect from that of an androgen to that of a progestational agent. Accordingly, the progestational derivatives of testosterone were designated as 19-nortestosterones (denoting the missing 19 carbon). The androgenic properties of these compounds, however, were not totally eliminated and minimal anabolic and androgenic potential remains within the structure.

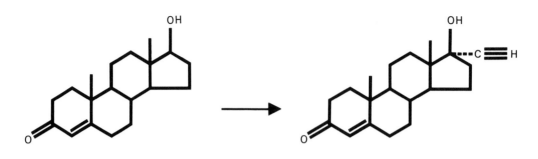

Testosterone → Ethisterone

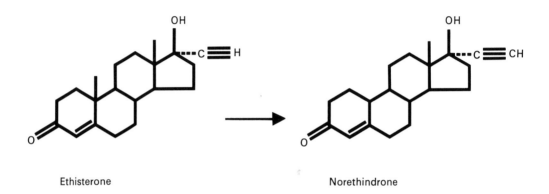

Ethisterone → Norethindrone

The "impurity" of the 19-nortestosterone, i.e. androgenic as well as progestational effects, was further complicated in the past by a mistaken belief that they were metabolized within the body to estrogenic compounds. This question was restudied, and it was found that the previous evidence for metabolism to estrogenic compounds was due to an artifactual result in the laboratory analysis. In animal and human studies, only norethindrone, norethynodrel, and ethynodiol diacetate have weak estrogen activity due to weak binding to the estrogen receptor. (2) Clinically, androgenic and estrogenic activities of the progestin component appear to be insignificant in the new low dose pills.

Norethindrone is the prototype of this family of compounds, and for many years the patent (now expired) for norethindrone was held by the Syntex Corporation. The formation of the Syntex Corporation, a significant force in American steroid pharmacology, is a fascinating story. This episode in steroid history begins with Russell Marker, a chemist who never received his Ph.D. degree. After leaving school, Marker worked with the Ethyl Gasoline Corporation, and in 1926, developed the process of octane rating, based on the discovery that knocking in gasoline was due to hydrocarbons with an uneven number of carbons.

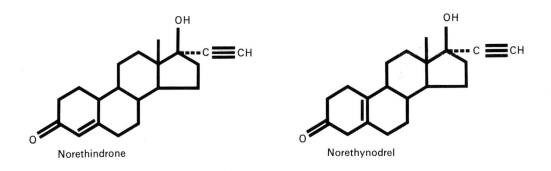

Norethindrone

Norethynodrel

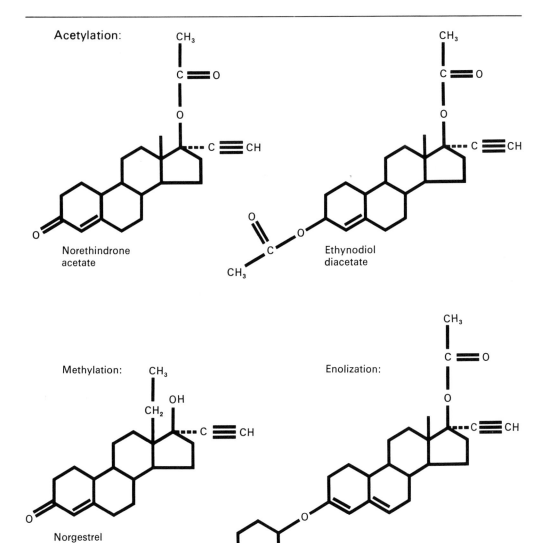

Acetylation:

Norethindrone
acetate

Ethynodiol
diacetate

Methylation:

Norgestrel

Enolization:

Quingestanol acetate

413

From 1927 to 1935, Marker worked at the Rockefeller Institute publishing a total of 32 papers on configuration and optical rotation as methods of identifying compounds. In 1935, he moved to Pennsylvania State University where he trained himself in steroid chemistry and became interested in solving the problem of producing abundant and cheap amounts of progesterone. At that time it required the ovaries from 2,500 pregnant pigs to produce 1 mg of progesterone. In 1939, Marker became convinced that the solution to the problem of obtaining large quantities of steroid hormones was to find plants which contained sufficient amounts of sapogenin, a plant steroid which could be used as a starting point for steroid hormone synthesis. This conviction was strengthened with the discovery that a species of *Trillium*, known locally as Beth's root, was collected in North Carolina and used in the preparation of Lydia Pinkham's Compound, popular at the time to relieve menstrual troubles. The active compound in Beth's root was diosgenin, a plant steroid.

Marker organized extensive botanical expeditions. In 1942, he collected the roots of the Mexican yam, and back in Pennsylvania, he worked out the degradation of diosgenin to progesterone. United States pharmaceutical companies refused to back Marker, and even refused to patent the process at Marker's urging.

In 1943 he resigned from Pennsylvania State University and went to Mexico where he prepared several pounds of progesterone (worth $600,000). This progesterone gained him entry to Hormone Laboratories in Mexico City. The two partners in Hormone Laboratories and Marker formed a company which they called Syntex. The price of progesterone fell from $200 to $2 a gram.

In 1947, the three partners had a falling out, and Marker sold his share of the company and retired on the Pennsylvania State University campus. However, he took his know-how with him. Fortunately for Syntex, he had published a scientific description of his process and there still was no patent on his discoveries. Syntex recruited Dr. George Rosenkranze to reinstitute the commercial manufacture of progesterone, a deed which took him 2 years.

In 1949, it was discovered that cortisone relieved arthritis and the race was on to develop an easy and cheap method to synthesize cortisone. Dr. Carl Djerassi joined Syntex to work on this synthesis using the Mexican yam plant steroid diosgenin as the starting point. This accomplishment was reported in 1951, but soon after an even better method of cortisone production was discovered at Upjohn, using microbiologic fermentation. This latter method used progesterone as the starting point and therefore Syntex found itself as the key supplier to other companies for this important process, at the rate of 10 tons of progesterone per year and a price of 48 cents per gram.

The Syntex chemists then turned their attention to the sex steroids. They discovered that the removal of the 19 carbon from progesterone increased the progestational activity of the molecule. Ethisterone, prepared a dozen years earlier, was available, and the Syntex chemists reasoned that removal of the 19 carbon would increase the progestational activity of this orally active compound. In 1951, norethindrone was synthesized, and the patent for this drug is the only patent for a drug listed in the National Inventors Hall of Fame in Washington. Shortly after, the Searle Company filed a patent for norethynodrel.

Both the Syntex and Searle compounds were tested by Gregory Pincus and colleagues in 1953–1954. Pincus had been a consultant for Searle for quite some time, and, therefore, he picked the Searle compound for extended use. Syntex, a wholesale drug supplier, was without marketing expertise and organization. Pincus convinced Searle that the commercial potential of an oral contraceptive warranted the risk of potential consumer reaction. By the time Syntex had secured arrangements with Ortho for a marketing outlet, Searle marketed Enovid in 1960. Ortho-Novum using norethindrone from Syntex appeared in 1962.

A second group of progestins became available for use when it was discovered that acetylation of the 17-hydroxy group of 17-hydroxyprogesterone produced oral potency.

Acetylation at the 17 position gives oral potency, but an addition at the 6 position is necessary to give sufficient progestational strength for human use, probably by inhibiting metabolism.

Mechanism of Action

The combination pill consisting of the estrogen and progestin components is given daily for 3 out of every 4 weeks. The combination pill prevents ovulation by inhibiting gonadotropin secretion, exerting its principal effect on pituitary or hypothalamic centers, and probably both. The progestational agent in the pill appears to suppress primarily luteinizing hormone (LH) secretion, while the estrogenic agent suppresses follicle-stimulating hormone (FSH) secretion. Therefore, the estrogenic component significantly contributes to the contraceptive efficacy. The estrogen in the pill serves two other important purposes. It provides stability to the endometrium so that irregular shedding and unwanted breakthrough bleeding can be avoided; and the presence of estrogen is required to potentiate the action of the progestational agents. The latter function of estrogen has allowed reduction of the progestational dose in the pill. The mechanism for this action may be an increase in the concentration of intracellular progestin receptors by estrogen. Therefore, a certain pharmacologic level of estrogen is necessary to maintain the potency of the combination pill.

415

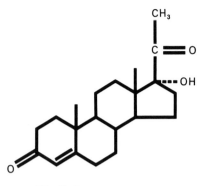

17α-Hydroxyprogesterone

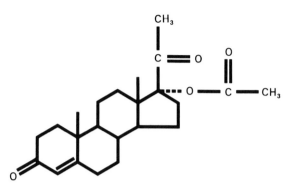

17-Acetoxy progesterone

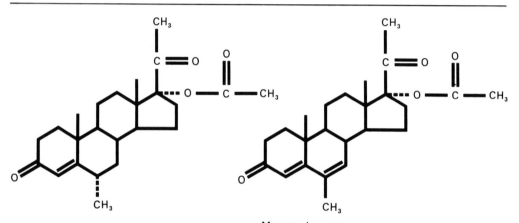

Medroxyprogesterone acetate
(Provera)

Megestrol acetate

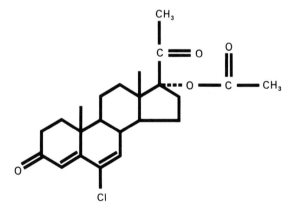

Chlormadinone acetate

Since the effect of a progestational agent will always take precedence over estrogen (unless the dose of estrogen is increased many, many fold), the endometrium, cervical mucus, and perhaps tubal function reflect progestational stimulation. The progestin in the combination pill produces an endometrium which is not receptive to ovum implantation, a decidualized bed with exhausted and atrophied glands. The cervical mucus becomes thick and impervious to sperm transport. It is possible that further contraceptive effects are obtained by progestational influences on secretion and peristalsis within the Fallopian tube.

With this variety of contraceptive actions, it is hard to understand how the omission of a pill or two can result in a pregnancy. Indeed, careful review of pill failures reveals that pregnancies usually occur because initiation of the next cycle is delayed a few days allowing escape from ovarian suppression. It is very important that the 7-day interval between 21-day pill cycles be strictly observed in order to obtain reliable, effective contraception.

Failure Rates per Year:

	Theoretical	Actual Use
Oral contraceptives	0.1%	2.0%
IUD	2.0%	5.0%
Condoms	3.0%	10.0%
Diaphragm	3.0%	19.0%
Foam/Cream/Jelly	10.0%	18.0%
Rhythm	13.0%	24.0%

Metabolic Effects

Thrombosis and Cardiovascular Disease

Data from the two British prospective studies have provided solid clinical information upon which reasonable decisions can be based. (3–6) The risk of deep thrombosis in the leg is 4 times greater in oral contraceptive users than nonusers, that of superficial thrombosis in the leg, 2 times greater. There is no evidence that varicose veins have any influence on deep thrombosis associated with pill use.

The difference between a retrospective study and prospective study should be emphasized. In a retrospective study, the percent of women using the pill is analyzed in patients who already have thrombosis. In a prospective study, the percent of women who develop thrombosis is compared between a group on the pill and a control group. The prospective data are more reliable because they represent actual events and do not depend upon statistical manipulation. The clinical significance of the British prospective studies is that, for the first time, reliable data provided risk estimates which supported the previous retrospective reports.

In December, 1969, the British Committee on the Safety of Drugs issued a recommendation that only the lowest estrogen dose brands should be used (at that time, 50 μg estrogen). Hence, data from the early part of the prospective studies were derived from pills containing more than 50 μg of estrogen, whereas data after 1969 reflected usage of brands containing 50 μg estrogen. Thus, the dose effect of estrogen could be analyzed.

The attributable risk of deep thrombosis was 80/100,000 users per year with the 50-μg dose. This incidence of 1:1200 compared remarkably well with that estimated previously in retrospective studies. The attributable risk of deep thrombosis with estrogen doses greater than 50 μg was 112/100,000 per year. Therefore, the attributable risk decreased by 28% upon using a lower estrogen dose. (3) Although previous retrospective studies had suggested that risk was lower for users of lower estrogen doses, these data were the first solid evidence that reducing the estrogen dose can significantly affect the incidence of what is probably the most serious side effect of the pill, thrombosis.

In Sweden, the incidence of thromboembolic disease with doses of 75 μg of estrogen or more has been compared to the incidence with 50- and 30-μg estrogen pills. (7) The average incidence for thromboembolism fell from 25.9 to 7.2 cases per 100,000 users per year. The reduction was due to a decrease in venous complications; there was no change in the frequency of arterial complications. This is not necessarily a negative observation in that it could mean that the arterial thrombosis would have occurred even without the use of oral contraceptives. The two most significant arterial events are myocardial infarction and neurovascular accidents. Indeed, according to the prospective studies, there is no significant increase in risk for any cause of death other than circulatory diseases.

Myocardial Infarction

The first public awareness of an increased risk for myocardial infarction followed the reports of two retrospective studies in England. (8, 9) In a group of women admitted to hospitals with nonfatal myocardial infarction, the risk in pill users 30–39 years of age was increased 2.7 times, while the relative risk in women 40–44 was 5.7. The other study analyzed women who did not survive myocardial infarction and revealed relative risks of 2.8 for women 30–39 and 4.8 for women 40–44. Consideration of other risk factors (hypertension, hypercholesterolemia, cigarette smoking, obesity, diabetes mellitus) indicated that oral contraceptives acted synergistically with these factors, rather than additively. (10–13) Indeed, it now appears that the majority of women who develop myocardial infarction are smokers. Very few young (under 35) nonsmoking women have heart attacks. It is probable that a smoker who stops smoking returns to the category of a nonsmoker, but it is unknown how long this may take.

A dose-effect relationship indicates that the incidence of thrombosis decreases as the dose of estrogen is lowered.

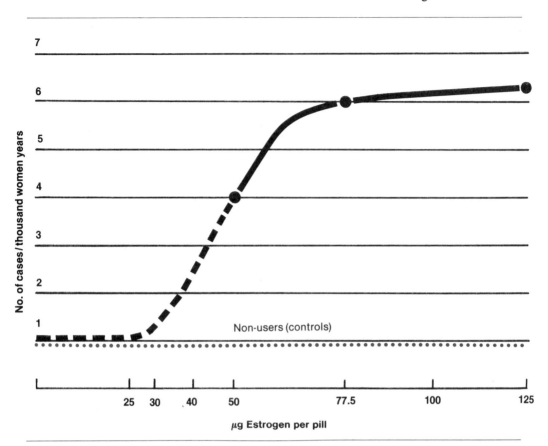

A possible explanation for the synergism between smoking and birth control pills is the effect of the pills and smoking on levels of lipoprotein used for cholesterol transport. (14) The significant lipoproteins are the following:

VLDL: Very low density lipoproteins, which carry tri-glycerides (mainly) and cholesterol.

LDL: Low density lipoproteins, which carry cholesterol in plasma; the levels of LDL are directly associated with the incidence of coronary heart disease.

HDL: High density lipoproteins, which also carry cho-lesterol in plasma and are inversely associated with the risk of coronary heart disease. Weight reduction and exercise increase HDL levels.

Regular pills (50 μg and more estrogen) and cigarette smoking increase LDL and VLDL with little change in HDL, an adverse effect in terms of coronary heart disease. Low dose pills (less than 50 μg estrogen) increase or have no effect on HDL and decrease LDL, a protective effect which is not necessarily an estrogen effect alone, but could reflect the decrease in progestin content as well. Indeed, in a very recent study of low dose oral contraceptives, effects on plasma lipids were proportional to the dose of both

419

steroidal components, and the lowest dose formulation produced the smallest changes. (15) The higher progestin doses decreased HDL levels.

The latest reports from the British prospective studies support a relationship between progestin levels and the risk of cardiovascular disease. A positive association has been noted between norethindrone acetate (in 50-µg pills) and deaths from arterial stroke and ischemic heart disease (16). A positive association was also noted between *d*-norgestrel dosage and stroke (in a 30-µg pill). The Royal College of General Practitioners' study found an increased rate of all arterial diseases with increasing doses of norethindrone acetate in 50-µg pills, and a 50% higher rate with 0.25 mg of *d*-norgestrel compared to 0.15 mg in a 30-µg pill. (17)

Fortunately, the highest dose of norethindrone acetate on the American market is 2.5 mg (Norlestrin 2.5/50, with 50 µg ethinyl estradiol). All others are 1.0 and 1.5 mg. At this lower dose range the British studies found no increased risk. Furthermore there were no cases of arterial disease in 30-µg pills using 0.15 mg of *d*-norgestrel. The norgestrel used in America has been a racemic mixture of equal parts of *l*-norgestrel which is inactive and the active *d*-norgestrel. Therefore, the dose of norgestrel in the 30-µg American pill is the lower dose, not found to be associated with arterial disease in the British studies.

In summary, the relationship between myocardial infarction and pill use is significantly affected by risk factors (especially smoking) and age. The risk for a young (under 35) healthy woman may be negligible with the new low dose pills. Beginning at age 35 and certainly after age 40, the risk becomes significant, but mortality is largely confined to smokers over 35.

Stroke

Clinical reports are consistent with an association between the use of oral contraceptives and neurovascular accidents in otherwise healthy young women. According to the retrospective studies, pill use increases the risk of thrombotic stroke 3-fold, and that of hemorrhagic stroke, 2-fold. (18)

No significant potentiation of hypertension among pill users was noted. Smoking and migraine headaches had variable effects on the risk of stroke. Heavy smoking by pill users was associated with an increased risk of hemorrhagic stroke while thrombotic stroke was not influenced. Migraine headache was not associated wth a change in the incidence of hemorrhagic stroke, but the incidence of thrombotic stroke was increased.

The prospective studies have corroborated the above risks and have found that the increased risk is highest in smokers and persists for an unknown length of time after past pill use. (19) The incidence of this problem with the new low dose pills is unknown. The prospective studies substantiate the contributory role of smoking and emphasize the importance of headaches as a warning sign. However, even the risk of subarachnoid hemorrhage has been challenged because an examination of British vital statistics data produced no evidence of increased mortality from this condition. (20).

Because of the seriousness of this potential complication, the onset of visual symptoms or severe headaches should be considered as indications for discontinuation of the pill. Rather than immediately discontinuing the pill, however, the physician and patient should consider switching to another brand within the same low dose range (less than 50 μg), or, if at a higher dose, a move to the low dose pill. Often this relieves the symptoms.

Clues to vascular headaches:

Headaches which last a long time.
Dizzyness, nausea, or vomiting with headaches.
Scotomata or blurred vision.
Episodes of blindness
Unilateral headaches.
Headaches which continue despite medication.

The Risk for Cardiovascular Death

The British prospective studies indicated in the 1970s that women who took the pill increased their risk of dying from cardiovascular disease (mainly heart attack, stroke, and thromboembolism) by 4–5 times. The risk increased significantly with other factors such as increasing age, smoking, obesity and conditions such as diabetes mellitus, hypertension, and hyperlipidemia. The risk was not confined to current users, but also appeared to affect former users, and in women over 35 there was an association with duration of usage. Since about 60% of American women in the reproductive age are current or former pill users, these reports provoked significant concern, leading many women to reconsider their decision to begin or maintain oral contraception.

If the British findings were correct, one would expect to detect the deaths attributable to pill use in an evaluation of vital statistics data. Analyses of the United States and of 21 countries in Europe, Asia, and North America have failed to reveal the high levels of death from cardiovascular diseases associated with pill use which the British data appeared to indicate. (21, 22) That is not to say that there is no risk, but it does suggest that the level of the risk is less than predicted by the British. It is likely that the British prediction was an exaggeration due to the small number of deaths in the study.

It is important to note that in the Royal College of General Practitioners' study, the risk levels for all age groups under 35 were not elevated. It should also be emphasized that the data were largely derived from pills containing 50 μg and higher doses of estrogen. Even by the British data, oral contraception is a very safe means of fertility control for healthy women under age 35, and the real risk of serious thrombotic side effects is probably even less with the new low dose pills.

In recent reports from England, it has been documented that the 30-μg estrogen pill is associated with significantly less death from venous and arterial events, including coronary heart disease, than the 50-μg pills. (16) Indeed, the Royal College of General Practitioners' study shows NO cases of arterial disease among users of brands containing 30 μg of estrogen and 0.15 mg of d-norgestrel. (17) In addition there is now evidence that there is a positive association between the progestin dose and deaths from arterial disease. (16) Therefore, a rationale for the utilization of the new low dose pills includes minimizing the progestin dose as well as the estrogen dose.

The case for the safety of the pill is further enhanced by the most recent American data from the Walnut Creek study. (23) In a population of young, healthy, middle-class women, the risk of death from circulatory disease in oral contraceptive users was negligible. There was no increased risk of myocardial infarction, cerebral thrombosis, ischemic cerebrovascular disease, arterial thrombosis and embolism, venous thrombosis or pumonary embolism. There was no significant difference in the overall death rate between ever users and never users. Any increased risks of circulatory diseases noted were attributable to smoking. The Walnut Creek study could not relate effects to type and dose of pills (because the information was not recorded).

These encouraging results surely were derived from experience with higher dose pills, because the 16,638 women in the study were followed from 1969 through 1977. Furthermore, the great majority of the women in both American and the British studies were age 25 or older when enrolled and thus the risks for women in their teens and early 20s, and for women in the 1980s on lower dose pills, probably have been overstated.

The Walnut Creek study came under some attack, being criticized mainly for a relatively small number of woman-years of current use. However, confidence in the Walnut Creek study was bolstered by the 1981 reports from the Royal College of General Practitioners and the Oxford Family Planning Study (24, 25). The Royal College Report was based on data up to December 1979, and included approximately 184,000 woman-years of experience for users and up to 139,000 woman-years for controls.

These up-to-date analyses of the British experience, derived largely from pills containing 50 μg of estrogen, confirmed a 40% higher death rate among ever users, a relative risk of 4.2 with an incidence of excess deaths of 22.7 per 100,000 woman-years. These deaths were virtually all due to diseases of the circulatory system; only about 10% of the excess deaths were due to venous events, most being due to ischemic heart disease and, at least in the Royal College study, subarachnoid hemorrhage. The Oxford Family Planning study did not find a pill-related increase in subarachnoid hemorrhage. There was no significant increase in risk for any cause of death other than circulatory diseases.

Contrary to previous findings, the latest information provides no evidence that risk is associated with duration of oral contraceptive use, independent of the increasing risk with age. **BUT MOST SIGNIFICANTLY, UNDER THE AGE OF 35, THE REPORTED DIFFERENCES IN DEATH RATES AMONG EVER USERS AND NONUSERS COULD HAVE ARISEN BY CHANCE. IN OTHER WORDS, RISK IS PRIMARILY CONCENTRATED IN WOMEN OVER 35 WHO SMOKE AND ARE USING THE PILL.**

Observations that the risk of death is higher among former users do not establish that this is due to a residual effect of oral contraception (26). The women reported to have the greatest residual effect are women who smoked heavily and used oral contraception while they were in their 30s. Former users may have stopped taking the pill because of health problems which later led to circulatory death. In addition, these results are derived from women who took pills of high estrogen content (50 μg and more), and they indicate a greater relative risk, which, in terms of actual numbers of cases attributable to use of the pill, is very small. For all of these reasons, there should be only limited concern over any lingering risks to past users of oral contraceptives, especially to past users of the new low dose pills.

In conclusion, the new low dose pill (less than 50 μg) is safer than the pills previously used. The overall risk is very close to minimal in healthy women under the age of 40 who do not smoke, and under the age of 35 the synergistic effect of smoking may be negligible. Only smokers 35 and older have a significantly increased risk of dying from circulatory diseases.

Oncogenic Potential

A major concern about the impact of the pill on human health is whether steroid contraception causes cancer. The concern in this area has been directed toward the uterus (corpus and cervix) and the breast. It must be acknowledged that the duration of use of steroids has not been long enough to permit absolute statements on this critical issue. Nevertheless, reasonably secure judgments can be made on the basis of a large body of epidemiologic work.

Estrogen not only supports normal endometrium, but prolonged unopposed estrogen is associated with a progression of histologic change from hyperplasia to adenomatous hyperplasia to atypia. The chemotherapeutic use of progestational agents for endometrial cancer would suggest that periodic progestin can prevent or hinder these estrogen-induced changes. As currently constituted, the combined

423

progestin and estrogen pill does have a protective effect, and there have been no abnormal endometrial changes associated with this form of oral contraception. Indeed, endometrial cancer develops at a rate of about 50% less in women who have used combination oral contraceptives. This protection increases with duration of use and persists for 10 or more years after discontinuation (the actual length of duration of protection is unknown). (23, 27) Endometrial neoplasia developing with sequential therapy points out the delicate balance of hormones required to sustain the protective effects. Too much estrogen or too little progestin would not confer the safety seen with current formulations.

Recent studies have found that the number of partners a woman has had is the most important sex-related risk factor for dysplasia and carcinoma in situ of the uterine cervix. But the overall risk, even after controlling for sexual activity, roughly doubles with use of the pill for 5 or more years. (28, 29) A causal relationship is still not established, however, in that other explanations must be considered. For example, pill use may cause changes in the cervix which allow earlier and easier detection of abnormalities, or women with preexisting dysplasia may favor the pill among the various methods of contraception. Steroid contraceptives do not mask abnormal cervical changes, and the necessity for prescription renewals offers the opportunity for improved screening for cervical disease.

While there does not seem to be major concern in regard to uterine cancer, there are fears of the effects of estrogen on breast tissue. The prospective studies have yielded no indication of an association of breast cancer with pill usage, either current or former use. (30, 31) This has also been a consistent finding in retrospective studies. Worth noting is a protective effect toward benign disease of the breast (fibroadenoma and chronic cystic disease) associated with the progestin component of the pill, an effect which becomes apparent after 2 years of continuous usage. After 2 years of usage there is an increasing reduction in the incidence of fibrocystic disease of the breast with increasing duration of use. Women who take the pill are one fourth as likely to develop benign breast disease as nonusers. One case-control study first indicated that women with already established benign breast disease may have an increased incidence of breast cancer with long-term use of the pill. (32) This could not be substantiated by the same investigators in a larger analysis. (33)

In women with past or present breast cancer, hormonal treatment, of course, should be avoided. Although there are no apparent positive associations, more information is needed on the relationship between pill use, benign disease, and a family history of breast cancer. Concern still remains over the as yet undetermined effects of duration of use, the delay in obtaining statistics due to a prolonged latent period for cancer, and the risk among young women who have postponed their first pregnancy by using oral contraceptives. It is well recognized that delayed childbearing increases the risk of breast cancer.

The data derived from the British prospective studies are from women, the majority of whom started to use the pill in their 20s after at least one pregnancy. Therefore, a reasonable and important concern focuses on young women who are using or have used the pill in their teens or early 20s before their first pregnancy. A case-control study in California found an increased risk of breast cancer among women who had been long-term users of the pill prior to their first full-term pregnancy, a relative risk of 2.25 for up to 96 months of use, and 3.5 with 97 or more months of use. (34) Interestingly, there was no significantly increased risk if pill use began after the first full-term pregnancy. The numbers were small in this study and the data were gathered by telephone interviews; therefore, it is appropriate to consider the conclusions with caution.

Another case-control study concluded that women with breast cancer who had used the pill survived longer having smaller tumors of a lower grade of invasiveness. (35) Thus, pill use may have a beneficial effect on tumor growth and progression. Hopefully, these confusing aspects of pill use and breast cancer will be clarified by a large study currently in progress in America under the direction of the Centers for Disease Control. Complete results should be available in the mid 1980s. Preliminary results are very encouraging. No increased risk has been noted with long-term use, the presence of benign breast disease, a positive family history of breast cancer, and with pill use before the birth of a first child. An English study has found no association between breast cancer risk and either pill use or abortion before a first birth. (36)

The Walnut Creek study suggested that the only other cancer linked to pill usage is melanoma. (37) However, the major risk factor for melanoma is exposure to sunlight, and this was not controlled. At least one other cancer reflects a protective effect. Oral contraceptive use is associated with a 30% reduction in the risk of ovarian cancer. (38) This protective effect increases with duration of use and persists for 10 or more years after discontinuation.

Progestational agents have been implicated as causal factors for breast cancer. The situation is a very special one, being limited only to experiments with Beagle dogs. Mammary tumors in the Beagle dog are increased as a result of prolonged stimulation with large doses (up to 25 times human luteal phase levels) of progesterone or 17-hydroxy progesterone derivatives (such as Provera). (39) This has not been reported in any other species, and there is no clinical evidence for a relationship between progestin use and breast cancer in women.

| Adrenal Gland | For some time it has been known that estrogen increases cortisol-binding globulin, transcortin. It had been thought that the increase in plasma cortisol while on the pill was due to increased binding by the globulin and not an increase in free active cortisol. Now it is apparent that free and active cortisol levels are also elevated. In addition, progesterone and related compounds may displace cortisol from transcortin, and thus contribute to the elevation of unbound cortisol. Estrogen decreases the ability of the liver to metabolize cortisol, and this also may contribute to elevated levels. The effects of these elevated levels over prolonged periods of time are unknown. To put this in perspective, the increase is not as great as that which occurs in pregnancy, and in fact, it is within the normal range for nonpregnant women. |

The adrenal gland responds to ACTH normally, therefore there is no suppression of the adrenal gland itself. Initial studies showed that the response to metyrapone (a 11β-hydroxylase blocker) was abnormal, suggesting that the pituitary was suppressed. It has now been shown that estrogen accelerates the conjugation of metyrapone by the liver, and therefore the drug has less effect, thus explaining the subnormal responses initially reported. The pituitary-adrenal reaction to stress is normal in women on oral contraceptive pills.

Thyroid

As with transcortin, estrogen increases thyroxine-binding globulin, and prior to the new methods of calculating the free thyroxine levels, evaluation of thyroid function was a problem. Estimation of the free thyroxine level utilizes the measurement of thyroid binding globulin levels, the total thyroxine level, and the percentage of thyroxine saturation of the binding globulin. The free thyroxine level is an accurate assessment of a patient's thyroid state. Birth control pills affect the total thyroxine level in the blood as well as the amount of binding globulin, but the free thyroxine level is unchanged.

Carbohydrate Metabolism

There is an impaired glucose tolerance test in 15–40% of women on the pill, and in these women plasma levels of insulin as well as the blood sugar are elevated. Generally, the effect of the pill is to produce an increase in peripheral resistance to insulin action, probably by lowering concentrations of insulin receptors. This decrease in insulin binding is no greater than that seen during the luteal phase; however, extending this change over a greater duration may provide a significant challenge. (40) Most women can meet this challenge by increasing insulin secretion, and there is no change in the glucose tolerance test. Individuals who cannot respond with an appropriate increase in insulin may have an abnormal glucose tolerance.

Carbohydrate metabolism is affected by both the progestin and estrogen components of the pill. Compounds with a positive charge at the 5 carbon (3-keto structures and estrogens) have insulinogenic and insulin antagonistic effects. Not all progestins, however are diabetogenic. 6-Dehydro derivatives, such as megestrol, actually may improve glucose tolerance because they increase insulin response but have no antagonistic effects. The derangement of carbohydrate metabolism may also be affected by estrogen influences on lipid metabolism, hepatic enzymes, and elevation of free cortisol. The glucose intolerance appears to be dose-related, and once again the effect is less with the new low dose formulations.

The clinical significance of the elevated blood sugar remains uncertain. The elevation may be a functional change which is not deleterious and is completely reversible. It can be stated definitively that pill use does not produce an increase in diabetes mellitus. (41) Even patients who have risk factors for diabetes in their history do not seem to be affected.

In clinical practice it may, at times, be necessary to prescribe oral contraception for the overt diabetic. Although one would expect the insulin requirement to increase, close follow-up is indicated for the effect is neither consistent nor predictable. The use of oral contraceptives increases the risk of thrombosis in women with insulin-dependent diabetes mellitus; therefore, women with diabetes should be advised to use other forms of contraception.

Lipid
Metabolism

Various changes in the levels of lipids and lipoproteins have been reported, and not all studies are in agreement. The report from the Lipid Research Clinic Program which summarizes findings from women attending ten North American Lipid Research Clinics, seems to be the most extensive and reliable. (14) Oral contraceptive use (as noted earlier in this chapter) has been associated with a consistent increase in LDL, VLDL, cholesterol, and triglyceride levels. There was little change in HDL levels. It was noted that these changes were positively associated with the quantity of the estrogen component of the pills. It is not surprising, therefore, that the new lower dose pills (less than 50 μg) are associated with different results: higher HDL levels and lesser effects on LDL and VLDL (overall a protective response with regard to coronary heart disease). These responses are not solely due to the estrogen component because there is variation due to the progestin component as well. Indeed a recent study found significant decreases in HDL with high progestin doses. (15) Although these findings are consistent with the growing appreciation for the increased safety of the new lower dose pills, their exact clinical significance remains to be established.

Raised cholesterol, triglyceride, LDL, and VLDL levels are positively associated with coronary heart disease. Therefore, in women with strong family histories of coronary disease, women who are heavy smokers, women who are over 35, women with xanthomatosis, and perhaps women who have been on the pill for more than 5 years, it would be wise to evaluate lipid and lipoprotein levels periodically. Those who have high levels should not be on the pill.

427

Liver	The liver is affected in more ways and with more regularity and intensity by the sex steroids than any other extragenital organ. Estrogen influences the synthesis of hepatic DNA and RNA, hepatic cell enzymes, serum enzymes formed in the liver, and plasma proteins. Estrogenic hormones also affect hepatic lipid and lipoprotein formation, the intermediary metabolism of carbohydrates, and intracellular enzyme activity. The active transport of biliary components is impaired by a large number of estrogens as well as some progestins. The mechanism is unclear, but cholestatic jaundice and pruritus are occasional complications of the pill, and are similar to the recurrent jaundice of pregnancy, i.e. benign and reversible. Bromosulfophthalein (BSP) retention is abnormal in approximately 20% of patients and alkaline phosphatase is increased in 2%, but serum glutamic-oxaloacetic transaminase (SGOT) elevation, if persistent, is not due to the pill.

The only absolute hepatic contraindication to pill use is acute or chronic cholestatic liver disease. Cirrhosis and previous hepatitis do not seem to be aggravated. With the incidence of hepatitis increasing, it is important to know that, once recovered from the acute phase of the disease. a patient may take oral contraceptive pills.

Liver Adenomas

Hepatocellular adenomas can be produced by steroids of both the estrogen and androgen families. Actually, there are two different lesions, peliosis and adenomas. Peliosis is characterized by dilated vascular spaces without endothelial lining, and may occur in the absence of adenomatous changes. The adenomas are not malignant; their significance lies in the potential for hemorrhage. The most common presentation is acute right upper quadrant or epigastric pain. The tumors may be asymptomatic, however, or they may present suddenly with hematoperitoneum. There is some evidence that the tumors may regress when the pill is stopped.

The risk appears to be related to duration of pill use and to the steroid dose in the pills, and this is another argument in favor of the lowest dose pills. Recent data have not supported the contention that mestranol increased the risk more than ethinyl estradiol. It has been estimated that the risk of liver tumors is as low as 1 per 250,000 users. Moreover, the on-going prospective studies have accumulated that many women years of use and have not identified a single case of such a tumor. Perhaps informed consent regarding the problem should be limited to women who have been on the pill more than 5 years.

No reliable screening test or procedure is currently available. Routine liver function tests are normal. CT scanning may be the best means of diagnosis; angiography and ultrasonography are not reliable. Palpation of the liver should be part of the periodic evaluation in pill users. If an enlarged liver is found, the pills should be stopped, and regression should be evaluated and followed by CT scan.

428

| Gallbladder Disease | The relative risk of gallbladder disease in pill users is 2.0 with an estimated annual incidence of 158 per 100,000 users. A similar increase in risk has been noted with the use of replacement estrogen therapy in postmenopausal women. The incidence of gallstones in the British prospective studies rose after the first 2 years of use, and plateaued after 4–5 years at a rate twice that of the control group. The mechanism for this problem appears to be induced alterations in the composition of gallbladder bile, specifically a rise in cholesterol saturation that is presumably an estrogen effect. (42) Therefore, a decreased relative risk may become apparent in the forthcoming reports from the prospective studies as the effects of decreased dosage are ascertained. The Walnut Creek study failed to confirm an association between pill use and gallbladder disease. (23) |

| Hypertension | The first mention of hypertension and oral contraceptive pills was a brief paragraph in 1962 in the *Canadian Medical Association Journal* by Brownrigg, reporting a patient who had the onset of hypertension while being treated for endometriosis. (43) The first well-documented cases are in a classic paper by Laragh et al. in 1967. (44) |

The mechanism is thought to involve the renin-angiotensin system. The most consistent finding is a marked increase in plasma angiotensinogen, up to 8 times normal values. In the majority of women, excessive vasoconstriction is prevented by a compensatory decrease in plasma renin concentration. It had been thought that this mechanism was largely influenced by the estrogen in the pill. However, the Royal College of General Practitioners' study correlated hypertension with the dose of the progestin component. (17) This relationship is not totally clear; another English report found no association between hypertension and the progestin component. (16)

Here again the safety effect of reduced dosage is becoming apparent. In the first reports from the British prospective studies, significant hypertension developed after 5 years of pill usage in approximately 5% of users. Recent studies, however, have found no association between oral contraception and hypertension. Perhaps younger women using lower dose pills have a negligible risk of hypertension.

Variables such as previous toxemia of pregnancy, previous renal disease, or unsuspected renal disease do not predict whether a woman will develop hypertension on the pill. In addition, women who have developed hypertension on the pill are not more predisposed to develop toxemia of pregnancy. If hypertension does develop, the renin-angiotensinogen changes take 3–6 months to disappear after stopping the pill.

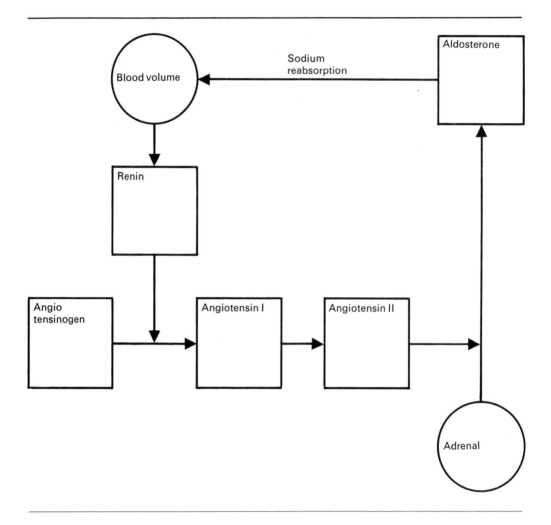

One must also consider the effects of oral contraceptives in patients with preexisting hypertension or cardiac disease. Again a judgment is necessary as to the importance of 100% contraception. Preexisting hypertension does increase the risk of thrombosis, but with medical control of the blood pressure and close follow-up, the patient and her physician may choose the new low dose pill for contraception. Close follow-up is also indicated in women with a history of preexisting renal disease, hypertension during pregnancy, and a family history of hypertension and its consequences. One consideration is the effect of the oral contraceptive on cardiac work. Significant increases in cardiac output, systolic blood pressure, and plasma volume have been recorded, probably a result of fluid retention. On the other hand, a recent study utilizing echocardiography failed to find any significant changes in left ventricular volume or contraction. (45) Nevertheless, it seems prudent to suggest that patients with marginal cardiac reserve should utilize other means of contraception.

Gastrointestinal disorders, breast discomfort, and weight gain remain the most common disturbing effects. Fortunately, these are most intense in the first few months of use, and in most cases, gradually disappear. It should be emphasized that the weight gain which takes place usually responds to dietary restriction. But for some patients, the weight gain is an anabolic response to the sex steroids, and discontinuation of oral contraception is the only way that weight loss can be achieved.

Chloasma, an increase in facial pigment, was at one time found to occur in approximately 5% of pill users. It is our clinical impression that chloasma is now an infrequent problem, perhaps due to the increasing use of low dose oral contraceptives. Unfortunately, once chloasma appears, it fades gradually following discontinuation of the pill, and may never disappear completely. Skin blanching medications may be useful.

In the British prospective studies, urinary tract infections were increased by 20%, and a correlation was noted with estrogen dose. An increased incidence of cervicitis also was reported, an effect related to the progestin dose. The incidence of cervicitis increased with the length of time the pill was used, from no higher after 6 months to 3 times higher by the 6th year of use. A significant increase in a variety of viral diseases, e.g. chickenpox, was observed, suggesting steroid effects on the immune system.

Hematologic effects include an increased sedimentation rate due to increased levels of fibrinogen, increased total iron-binding capacity due to the increase in globulins, and a decrease in prothrombin time. The cyclic use of the pill may prevent the appearance of symptoms in porphyria precipitated by menses. On the other hand, porphyria may be worsened. Decreases in blood levels of vitamins have been noted, including pyridoxine (B_6), B_2, B_{12}, folic acid, and ascorbic acid. Despite these changes, routine vitamin supplements have not been shown to be of benefit for women eating adequate, normal diets.

In well-controlled studies, no increases in eye abnormalities have been detected in pill users. Rarely, mental depression is associated with oral contraceptives. In some cases, the effect is due to estrogen interference with the synthesis of tryptophan and can be reversed with pyridoxine treatment. It seems wiser, however, to discontinue the pill if depression is encountered. Though infrequent, a reduction in libido is occasionally a problem, and may be a cause for seeking an alternative method of contraception.

Useful side effects include relief of dysmenorrhea, improvement of premenstrual tension, a decrease (two-thirds less) in menstrual bleeding and iron deficiency anemia, and improvement in hirsutism. Pill users have 50% less rheumatoid arthritis, but former users do not retain this protection. (46) Oral contraceptive users have a decreased risk of

431

gonorrhea, and women with gonorrhea who take oral contraceptives are only half as likely to develop salpingitis as women using no method of contraception. (47) Women on the pill are one-fourteenth as likely to develop ovarian cysts as nonusers.

A multicenter study is in progress to determine whether there is an association between the use of oral contraception and the occurrence of pituitary adenomas. At least one statistical analysis has found no such relationship.

Postpill Amenorrhea

The approximate incidence of "postpill amenorrhea" is 0.7–0.8%, but there is no evidence to support the idea that oral contraception causes secondary amenorrhea. Most women (80%) resume normal function in 3 months after discontinuing the pill, and 95–98% are ovulating in 1 year. If a cause and effect relationship exists between the pill and subsequent amenorrhea, one would expect the incidence of infertility to be increased after a given population discontinues use of the pill. In those women who discontinue the pill in order to get pregnant, 50% conceive by 3 months, and after 2 years a maximum of 15% of nonparous women and 7% of parous women fail to conceive, (6, 48) figures comparable to those quoted as the prevalence of spontaneous infertility. Attempts to document a cause and effect relationship between pill use and secondary amenorrhea have failed. (49) While patients with this problem come more quickly to our attention because of the previous pill use and physician follow-up, there is no cause and effect relationship. Patients who have not resumed menstrual function within 12 months should be evaluated as any other patient with secondary amenorrhea.

An important question is: should birth control pills be advised for a young woman with irregular menses and oligoovulation or anovulation? The fear of subsequent infertility should not be a deterrent to providing appropriate contraception. Women who have irregular menstrual periods are more likely to develop secondary amenorrhea whether they take the pill or not. Our clinical experience is that subsequent secondary amenorrhea is less of a risk and a less urgent problem for a young woman than leaving her unprotected. The need for contraception should take precedence.

**ABSOLUTE CONTRAINDICATIONS TO THE USE
OF THE PILL**

1. Thrombophlebitis, thromboembolic disorders, cerebral vascular disease, coronary occlusion, or a past history of these conditions, or conditions predisposing to these problems.

2. Markedly impaired liver function. Steroids are contraindicated in patients with acute hepatitis and until liver function tests return to normal.

3. Known or suspected carcinoma of the breast. The use of receptor assays on breast tumor tissue may allow the use of steroid contraception in the future, but currently the predictive ability for hormone sensitivity is not absolutely reliable.

4. Known or suspected estrogen-dependent neoplasia, especially carcinoma of the endometrium.

5. Undiagnosed abnormal genital bleeding (requires diagnostic evaluation).

6. Known or suspected pregnancy.

7. Obstructive jaundice in pregnancy (although not all patients with this history will develop jaundice on the pill).

8. Congenital hyperlipidemia because estrogen increases the risk of cardiovascular death in these patients.

9. Obese women who are smokers and over age 35.

**RELATIVE CONTRAINDICATIONS REQUIRING
CLINICAL JUDGMENT AND INFORMED
CONSENT BY THE PATIENT**

1. Migraine headaches. In retrospective studies, migraine headaches have been associated with an increased risk of stroke. However, some younger (under 30) women report an improvement in their headaches.

2. Hypertension. A woman under 30 who is otherwise healthy and whose blood pressure is controlled by medication can elect to use the pill.

3. Uterine leiomyoma. This does not seem to be a problem with the new low dose formulations.

4. Gestational diabetes. There is no evidence that pill use increases the incidence of overt diabetes mellitus, but these patients should have periodic tests of glucose tolerance.

5. Elective surgery. The pill should be discontinued, if possible, 1 month prior to elective surgery to avoid an increased risk for postoperative thrombosis.

6. Epilepsy. The frequency of seizures may be increased in women with epilepsy.

433

7.   Sickle cell disease or sickle C disease, but not sickle cell trait.

8.   Women over 35 who smoke.

9.   Diabetes mellitus.

Previously, patients have been monitored every 6 months while on oral contraception. In view of the increased safety of the new low dose pills for healthy young women with no risk factors, patients now need be seen only every 12 months for exclusion of problems by history, palpation of the liver, urinalysis, measurement of blood pressure, breast examination, and pelvic examination with Pap smear. Women with risk factors (such as smoking) can be seen every 6 months by appropriately trained paramedical personnel for screening of problems by history and blood pressure measurement (breast and pelvic examinations are necessary only yearly).

Laboratory surveillance should be used only when indicated. Routine biochemical measurements fail to yield sufficient information to warrant the expense. The following is a useful guide as to who should be monitored with blood screening tests for glucose, lipids and lipoproteins:

Women 35 years or older.
Women with a strong family history of heart disease, diabetes mellitus, or hyperlipidemia.
Women with gestational diabetes mellitus.
Women who have used the pill for more than 5 years (but it is probably not necessary to screen annually).
Women who develop hypertension on the pill.
Women with xanthomatosis.
Obese women.
Diabetic women.

The therapeutic principle remains: utilize the pill which gives effective contraception and the greatest margin of safety. The major side effects, those which are responsible for significant morbidity and mortality, are related to the estrogen component of the combination pill. The recent information reviewed in this chapter is a compelling argument for a dose-related response between the incidence of thrombosis and the estrogen content of the pill. Data linking cardiovascular complications to the progestin component are limited to high doses which are not used in the new low dose pills.

The current evidence supports the view that there is greater safety with pills containing less than 50 μg of estrogen. In the first half of 1980, the new low dose pills comprised only 30% of the oral contraceptive market in the United States, a disappointingly low percentage. The arguments in this chapter indicate that all patients should begin oral contraception with the new low dose combination pills, and that patients on higher dose pills (50 μg and higher of estrogen) should be switched to the new pills. The switch to a lower dose estrogen can be made immediately with no adverse reactions such as increased bleeding or failure of contraception.

In our clinical experience the 20-μg estrogen pill is associated with excessive breakthrough bleeding and, according to the literature, there is a slightly increased rate of failure. The 30- and 35-μg estrogen pills combine the safety of reduced estrogen with a tolerable level of problems. The breakthrough bleeding is not excessive and can be handled as outlined below. Contraceptive efficacy is not diminished by the 30- and 35-μg formulations. In general, there is compensation for potency in the new pills in that the more potent of the progestins are used in doses lower than those of the weaker progestins. The new pills all contain a minimum of both the estrogen and progestin components.

There is no clear-cut advantage demonstrated for one brand over another. The overriding principle is to utilize a new low dose brand for its safety margin. The pharmacologic effects in animals of various birth control pills have been used as a basis for therapeutic recommendations in selecting the optimal oral contraceptive pill. (50, 51) All too often this leads to the prescribing of a pill of excessive dosage with its attendant increased risk of serious side effects. In addition, it is by no means established that you can project potency data in animals to the clinical situation. The validity of this approach, tailor-making the pill to the patient, is not supported by appropriately controlled clinical trials. It is far more prudent to be guided by the principles of effectiveness and safety.

Effective contraception is present during the first cycle, providing the pills are started on the 5th day of the cycle, and no pills are missed. After a pregnancy of 12 or more weeks, oral contraception should not be started until 2 weeks after delivery to avoid the increased risk of thrombosis during the postpartum period. This is an important reason to change the obstetrical tradition of scheduling the postpartum visit at 6 weeks. A 2-week visit would be more productive in avoiding postpartum surprises, since the first ovulation essentially never occurs prior to the 3rd postpartum week. There is one exception: if bromocriptine is used to suppress prolactin and lactation promptly after delivery, ovulation may occur before 2 weeks. After the termination of a pregnancy of less than 12 weeks, oral contraception can be started immediately.

Combination pill contraception has been shown to diminish the quantity and quality of lactation in postpartum women, leading to decreased growth in the newborn. This has not been studied, however, with the new low dose pills. Also of concern is the potential hazard of crossover of steroids to the infant (although less than 1% is found in breast milk). For these reasons oral contraception is best deferred until lactation is discontinued.

If a woman misses one pill she should take that pill as soon as she remembers and take the next pill as usual. If she misses two pills, she should immediately begin using another form of contraception, stop taking the pills, wait 7 days and start a new cycle. The 7-day interval between pill cycles is crucial; extending this duration of time is probably the most important factor for contraceptive failure during pill usage. This is the major reason for the growing popularity among patients and physicians of the 28-day package which contains a terminal 7 days of inactive pills to enhance accurate adherence to the schedule.

There is no rationale for recommending a pill-free interval of a few months. The serious side effects of greatest frequency are not eliminated by pill-free intervals. In addition, this practice all too often results in unwanted pregnancies.

There is no evidence that the use of oral contraceptives in the pubertal, sexually active girl in anyway impairs growth of the reproductive system. Again, the most important concern is and should be the prevention of an unwanted pregnancy. For most teenagers the pill is the contraceptive method of choice, dispensed in the 28-day package for better compliance.

There are many anecdotal reports of patients who conceived on oral contraceptives while taking antibiotics. There is good reason to believe that rifampin decreases the efficacy of oral contraceptives by stimulating the liver's metabolic capacity. There is little evidence, however, that antibiotics such as ampicillin and tetracycline, which reduce the bacterial flora of the gastrointestinal tract, affect pill efficacy. To be cautious, patients on medications that affect liver metabolism (rifampin, coumadin, phenobarbital) should choose an alternative contraceptive, and patients requiring antibiotics for an acute illness should be advised to practice additional contraception.

Major Problems with the New Low Dose Pills
Amenorrhea on the Pill

The new low estrogen content is not of sufficient potency in some women to allow endometrial growth. The progestational effect dominates to such a degree that a shallow atrophic endometrium is produced, lacking sufficient tissue to yield withdrawal bleeding. It should be emphasized that permanent atrophy of the endometrium does not occur, and resumption of normal ovarian function will restore endometrial growth and development.

The major problem with amenorrhea while on the pill is the anxiety produced in both patient and physician because the lack of bleeding may be an early sign of pregnancy. The patient is anxious because of the uncertainty regarding pregnancy, and the clinician is anxious because of the medical-legal concerns stemming from the retrospective studies which indicated an increased risk of congenital malformations of the limbs and a small risk of congenital heart disease among the offspring of women who inadvertently used oral contraception in early pregnancy. This risk appears to be very low and may be limited to heart defects. The link between oral contraceptives and congenital limb reduction is based on one study which was not statistically definitive and which has not been confirmed. (52) In some studies there has been a small positive association between sex steroids and heart defects when hormones are taken during the early part of fetal development. (the relative risk is at most 2.0 which would increase the incidence from 8 to 16 per 1000 live births) (53, 54) In other studies no increased risk has been apparent. (55) The issue appears to be limited to pill use early in pregnancy, since no adverse effects on subsequent births have been noted in women who discontinue oral contraception, including no increase in chromosomal anomalies and no increase in the spontaneous abortion rate. (48)

The only noteworthy association is a greater frequency of dizygous twinning when oral contraceptives are used within 1 month of conception. (56) No other effects on fetal health or on the gender of the offspring have been noted. (57) Indeed, the only reason to recommend that women defer attempts to conceive for a month or two after stopping the pill is to improve the accuracy of gestational dating.

Fortunately, the incidence of amenorrhea while on the pill is low, less than 1%. Nevertheless, it is a difficult management problem. The use of a sensitive pregnancy test for the β subunit of human chorionic gonadotropin (HCG) will allow reliable testing for pregnancy even at this early stage. However, routine repeated use of such testing is expensive and annoying, and may lead to discontinuation of oral contraception. Some patients are reassured with an understanding of why there is no bleeding and are able to continue on the pill despite the amenorrhea. It is important to alert patients upon starting the pill that diminished bleeding and possibly no bleeding may ensue. Some women cannot reconcile themselves to a lack of bleeding, and this is an indication for trying other formulations.

The major deterrent to the use of the lower dose estrogen pills is breakthrough bleeding. It is not surprising that the incidence of this problem should increase as the estrogen dose of the pill is decreased. There are two characteristic breakthrough bleeding problems: irregular bleeding in the first few months after starting the pills, and unexpected bleeding after many months on the pill. Effort should be made to manage the bleeding problem in a way that allows the patient to remain on the low dose pill.

Breakthrough bleeding which occurs in the first few months of use is best managed by encouragement and reassurance. This bleeding usually disappears by the third cycle in the majority of women. If necessary, even this early pattern of breakthrough bleeding can be treated as outlined below. It is helpful to explain to the patient that this bleeding represents tissue breakdown as the endometrium adjusts from its usual thick state to the relatively thin state allowed by the hormones in the pill.

Breakthrough bleeding which occurs after many months of pill use is a consequence of the progestin-induced decidualization. This endometrium is shallow and tends to be fragile and prone to breakdown and asynchronous bleeding.

If bleeding occurs just before the end of the pill cycle, it can be managed by having the patient stop the pills, wait 7 days and start a new cycle. If breakthrough bleeding is prolonged or if it is aggravating to the patient, regardless of the point in the pill cycle, control of the bleeding can be achieved with a short course of exogenous estrogen. Conjugated estrogens, 2.5 mg, or ethinyl estradiol, 20 μg, are administered daily for 7 days when the bleeding is present, no matter where the patient is in her pill cycle. The patient continues to adhere to the schedule of pill taking. Usually one course of estrogen solves the problem, and reoccurrence of breakthrough bleeding is unusual (but if it does reoccur, another 7-day course of estrogen is effective).

Responding to irregular bleeding by having the patient take 2 or 3 pills daily is not effective. The progestin component of the pill will always dominate, hence doubling the number of pills will also double the progestational impact with its decidualizing, atrophic effect on the endometrium. The addition of extra estrogen while keeping the progestin dose unchanged is logical and effective. This allows the patient to remain on the lowest dose estrogen pill with its advantage of greater safety. Any bleeding which is not handled by this routine requires investigation for the presence of pathology.

**Should the Older
Woman Use the Pill?**

Since the average age of menopause is 51.5, some means of contraception may be necessary in most women until the age of 50. If an older woman elects to utilize oral contraception, she should be aware of the higher risk involved with increasing age; however it is appropriate to emphasize several considerations:

1. The risk of death for a woman in good health is less than what we have been led to believe by the early British reports. With the new low dose pills, the risk may be very acceptable for many healthy women.

2. Even though the risk increases with age, the risk of death is still lower than that associated with pregnancy itself (especially after the age of 40).

3. The risk to life increases rapidly for pill users who smoke and are over the age of 35. In addition to smoking, predisposing risk factors include: hypertension, diabetes mellitus, obesity, elevated lipids and lipoproteins, and a strong family history of coronary heart disease.

Women over the age of 35 who smoke or have any of the above risk factors should use contraceptive methods other than the pill, and rely upon therapeutic abortion for the occasional method failure.

For the older woman who is in good health and without risk factors, the new low dose pill may be an appropriate choice, if she is willing to undertake a slightly increased risk of circulatory death (knowing that the exact size of this risk cannot be accurately estimated at this time). An alternative and reasonable approach is to urge surgical sterilization for one of the partners.

An Alternative to the Pill

A useful alternative to the pill, especially in those women in whom estrogen is contraindicated, is Depo-Provera. (58, 59) Two observations are important: first, it requires 6–8 months for the drug to totally clear from the average woman, and second, the effective contraception level is maintained for 4 months. Therefore, 150 mg given intramuscularly every 3 months assures 100% contraception.

The progestin in depot form effectively blocks the LH surge, and in addition, affects the endometrium and cervical mucus. The suppression of gonadotropins is not as complete as with the pill. This is an advantage, since follicular growth is maintained at a sufficient level to produce estrogen levels comparable to those in the follicular phase of a normal cycle. In other words, Depo-Provera does not produce a hypoestrogenic state.

This progestin, in large continuous doses, produced breast tumors in Beagle dogs. This appears to be an effect unique to the Beagle dog, and has not appeared in other animals, or in women after years of use. (39) Major problems with Depo-Provera are breakthrough bleeding, weight gain, and depression. (58, 59) Breakthrough bleeding can be treated with exogenous estrogen as noted above. The incidence of breakthrough bleeding is 30% in the first year, and 10% thereafter. The majority of women become totally amenorrheic. Serious weight gain and depression (less than 5% incidence) are not relieved until the drug clears 6–8 months after the last injection.

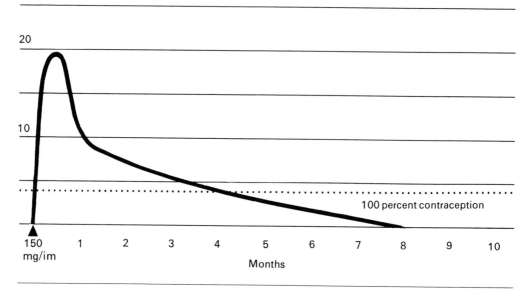

Provera Blood Level
ng/ml

20

10

100 percent contraception

150 mg/im   1   2   3   4   5   6   7   8   9   10

Months

Depo-Provera has cortisol-like effects, and in large doses, suppresses adrenal function. This does not appear to be a significant clinical problem in contraceptive doses.

The major advantage to the use of Depo-Provera is its freedom from the side effects of estrogen. (58, 59) Hence, it can be considered for patients with congenital heart disease, sickle cell anemia, patients with a previous history of thromboembolism, and women over 30, especially those who smoke or have other risk factors. However, the absolute safety in regard to thrombosis has not been proven in a controlled study. A further advantage in patients with sickle-cell disease is evidence indicating an inhibition of in vivo sickling with hematological improvement during treatment with Depo-Provera. (60) Depo-Provera is also useful for cases where compliance is a problem, e.g. mentally retarded young women. Another advantage is the finding that Depo-Provera increases the quantity of milk in nursing mothers, a direct contrast to the effect seen with combination pills. Although the concentration of the drug in the breast milk is relatively small, the effects of the drug on the child are unknown.

The belief that infertility with suppressed menstrual function may be caused by Depo-Provera is not borne out by the available data. The pregnancy rate in women discontinuing the injections because of a desire to become pregnant is normal. The median delay to conception is about 9 months after the last injection, and the delay does not increase with increasing duration of use. (61) Thus, it

440

appears that suppressed menstrual function persisting beyond 12 months after the last injection is not due to the drug and deserves evaluation.

Other Methods

While the pill provides almost 100% contraception, many women still find even minor side effects intolerable. Even more important are some of the unanswered questions concerning long-term use. For these reasons, a search for better contraception continues.

The minipill is the continuous daily use of a low dose of a potent progestational agent. The contraceptive effect is more dependent upon endometrial and cervical mucus effects, since LH is not consistently suppressed. Tubal physiology may also be affected, but ectopic pregnancy is not prevented as effectively as intrauterine pregnancy. The main disadvantages are incomplete contraception and breakthrough bleeding. The use-pregnancy rate is 2–8%. Breakthrough bleeding (30–40% incidence) is so unexpected, irregular, and heavy that extreme patient dissatisfaction is common. Certain clinical situations may warrant the use of the minipill: older women, hypertensive patients, postpartum lactating women—in general, those women in whom estrogen is hazardous.

Available minipills:

Micronor	Norethindrone	0.35 mg
Nor-Q.D.	Norethindrone	0.35 mg
Ovrette	Norgestrel	0.075 mg

Steroids diffuse through the walls of Silastic capsules at a rate controlled by the thickness of the walls and the surface area. A large dose of a potent progestin inside of a Silastic capsule implanted under the skin will give contraception for 1–2 years. However, the capsules must be removed through an incision. Bleeding problems are similar to the use of the minipill, since the principle is the same. Another approach is the use of vaginal Silastic rings impregnated with progestational compounds. One advantage is the possibility for patient insertion and removal on a monthly basis. The problem of side effects can be further reduced using low dose progestin-impregnated Silastic devices in the cervix. These could be contraceptive by changing cervical mucus and blocking sperm transport.

Clinical trials began in 1980 for a long-acting system of injectable biodegradeable microspheres. The advantages of this system include constant and accurate maintenance of steroid levels for up to 6 months, and the elimination of the necessity to remove operatively the injected containers because the microspheres are biodegradeable.

A new oral contraceptive formulation, the so-called triphasic product, has been developed with the aim to minimize breakthrough bleeding problems. This preparation has also been found to have no significant effects on glucose tolerance curves or HDL-cholesterol levels. (15) Its formulation and administration are as follows:

First 6 days: 0.050 mg *d*-norgestrel + 30 μg ethinyl estradiol

Middle 5 days: 0.075 mg *d*-norgestrel + 40 μg ethinyl estradiol

Last 11 days: 0.125 mg *d*-norgestrel + 30 μg ethinyl estradiol

A similar approach (Ortho-Novum 10/11), referred to as a biphasic method, keeps the estrogen level constant (35 μg ethinyl estradiol) but varies the progestin (0.5 mg norethindrone daily for the first 10 days and 1.0 mg the next 11 days).

Short of variations on the steroid theme, there is no new chemical method of contraception on the immediate horizon. (62) The time and monetary effort required to produce a safe, acceptable method means long delays from discovery to testing to general availability. Unfortunately, at this time, funding for research and development in contraception is decreasing, further diminishing hopes for new products.

Postcoital Contraception

Estrogen in large doses is effective in preventing conception after midcycle coital exposure. (63) Diethylstilbestrol, 25 mg b.i.d., is given for 5 days, within 72 hours after exposure, and preferably within 24 hours, along with an antiemetic for control of gastrointestinal symptoms.

The mechanism for this "morning after" technique remains to be determined, but its effectiveness has been confirmed in large clinical studies. Other estrogens can be used, and even a combination birth control pill, as follows:

Conjugated estrogens, 30 mg per day for 5 days.
Ethinyl estradiol, 5 mg per day for 5 days.
Oral, 4 tablets (2 given 12 hours apart). (64)

Because of possible harmful effects to a fetus, an already existing pregnancy should be ruled out prior to use of postcoital hormones. Furthermore, the patient should be offered therapeutic abortion if the drug fails.

The Medicated IUD

The intrauterine device (IUD) is relatively inexpensive, does not require continued motivation, and is easily reversible. There are significant drawbacks, however, including bleeding, pain, expulsion of the device, perforation, increased risk of pelvic infection, and unplanned pregnancies either with the device in situ or after unnoticed expulsion or perforation. In addition, the IUD does not protect against ectopic pregnancies. The number of ectopic pregnancies is not absolutely increased in IUD wearers. In fact, the risk of ectopic pregnancy is increased only in comparison to users of oral contraceptives, but is actually less when compared to noncontraceptors.

If pregnancy occurs with an IUD in place, the greatest risk of spontaneous or septic abortion is in the second trimester. If the IUD is not removed, there is, in addition, a greater risk for premature labor. An IUD should be removed as soon as possible when pregnancy occurs.

The newer IUDs have utilized hormones, copper, and different sizes and shapes in an effort to conform better to the endometrial cavity, thus causing minimal mechanical effects and reducing the incidence of side effects. It is likely that the contraceptive effect of copper involves a direct metabolic effect upon endometrial cells. The copper devices have pregnancy rates from 1.5 to 3.0 per 100 women per year. Such devices are approved for up to 3 years of use, but studies have indicated reliability up to 4 years. It appears that adding more copper reduces the pregnancy rate, although proper insertion with placement high in the fundus continues to be essential for effective contraceptive action.

The combination of progesterone with the T device is the only hormonal IUD available in the United States. The continuous release of small amounts of the hormone is associated with a local effect on the uterus without systemic effects. Sustained continuous release allows the use of progesterone itself rather than one of the synthetic progestins. Even though progesterone has a short half-life, the steady release allows maintenance of a constant and effective local level of the hormone.

The mechanism of action is unknown, although it is believed that it is the local effect of the progesterone on the endometrium which renders it incapable of sustaining implantation. The local progesterone also affects the cervical mucus, thus making passage of sperm difficult. There is a reduction in the incidence of cramping and bleeding due to a decrease in endometrial production of prostaglandins. For the same reason there is a beneficial effect of the local progesterone on dysmenorrhea and menorrhagia. The pregnancy rates are approximately 1.9 and 2.5 per 100 women-years in parous and nulliparous women, respectively. Currently, the device must be replaced every 1–2 years.

The risk of salpingitis is increased in women using IUDs. All types of currently available IUDs are equally likely to result in pelvic inflammatory disease (PID). The incidence rate of PID in women not using IUDs is 1:100 to 1:1000 per year. In IUD users, the incidence is 2–5 times increased. (47, 65) It has been estimated that 10,000 of 500,000 cases of acute PID each year in the United States are attributable to IUDs. (47) Because of these factors, we do not recommend an IUD until the patient understands that future fertility can be compromised. Indeed, IUD use should be actively discouraged in women who have not had any children.

Contraception and GnRH Agonists

A daily intranasal application of a gonadotropin releasing hormone (GnRH) agonist has been shown to have a contraceptive effect by lowering gonadotropins and ovarian steroid production. (66) Injections of a GnRH agonist during the menstrual cycle can induce sufficient impairment of gonadotropin support that the emerging follicle and subsequent corpus luteum function are defective. (67) The key to this action is the administration of GnRH (by a long-acting agonist) in a dose sufficient to overwhelm the usual pulsatile pattern and achieve a down regulation of GnRH receptors in the anterior pituitary gland. GnRH long-acting agonists when given shortly after the LH surge can also act directly on the gonad, shortening the luteal life span and decreasing luteal progesterone production. (68) Here the mechanism is a functional uncoupling of the LH receptor-adenylate cyclase complex.

At first glance these applications of the GnRH agonists offer hope for a specific method of contraception which would be effective but free of side effects. However, the application of such a method carries with it many practical problems. Any method which depends upon luteolysis requires accurate timing in order to thwart the reproductive process when it is vulnerable and to avoid rescue by the timely appearance of human chorionic gonadotropin (HCG). Interference with the menstrual cycle either at the pituitary or the ovary may lead to a hypoestrogenic state, or to irregular, unacceptable patterns of bleeding. Clinical trials to demonstrate contraceptive effectiveness would be a long process. For all of these reasons, this method is not around the corner.

To Keep Up-To-Date

A monthly newsletter is available which reviews the latest information, and highlights current problems and questions:

Contraceptive Technology Update
67 Peachtree Drive N.E.
Atlanta, GA 30309

References

1. **Jones EF, Beniger JR, Westoff CF,** Pill and IUD discontinuation in the United States, 1970–1975: the influence of the media, Fam Plan Perspect 12:293, 1980.

2. **Edgren RA,** Progestagens, in *Clinical Uses of Sex Steroids*, Givens Jr, ed, Yearbook, Chicago, 1980, pp 1–29.

3. **Royal College of General Practitioners,** *Oral Contraceptives and Health*, Pitman Publishing, New York, 1974.

4. **Royal College of General Practitioners,** Oral contraception study: mortality among oral contraceptive users, Lancet 2:727, 1977.

5. **Royal College of General Practitioners,** Oral Contraceptive study: oral contraceptives, venous thrombosis, and varicose veins, J R Coll Gen Pract 28:393, 1978.

6. **Vessey MP, McPherson K, Johnson B,** Mortality among women participating in the Oxford/Family Planning Association contraceptive study, Lancet 2:731, 1977.

7. **Bottinger LE, Boman G, Eklund G, Westerholm B,** Oral contraceptives and thromboembolic disease: effects of lowering oestrogen content, Lancet 1:1097, 1980.

8. **Mann JI, Vessey MP, Thorogood M, Doll R,** Myocardial infarction in young women with special reference to oral contraceptive practice, Br Med J 2:245, 1975.

9. **Mann JI, Inman WHW,** Oral contraceptives and death from myocardial infarction, Br Med J 2:245, 1975.

10. **Ory HW,** Association between oral contraceptives and myocardial infarction, JAMA 237:2619, 1977.

11. **Shapiro S, Slone D, Rosenberg L, Kaufman DW, Stolley PD, Miettinen OS,** Oral contraceptive use in relation to myocardial infarction, Lancet 1:743, 1979.

12. **Hennekens CH, Evans D, Peto R,** Oral contraceptive use, cigarette smoking and myocardial infarction, Br J Fam Plann 5:66, 1979.

13. **Rosenberg L, Hennekens CH, Rosner B, Belanger C, Rothman KH, Speizer FE,** Oral contraceptive use in relation to nonfatal myocardial infarction, Am J Epidemiol 11:59, 1980.

14. **Wallace RB, Hoover J, Barrett-Connor E, Rifkind BM, Hunninghake DB, Mackenthun A, Heiss G,** Altered plasma lipid and lipoprotein levels associated with oral contraceptive and oestrogen use, Lancet 2:111, 1979.

15. **Briggs MH, Briggs M,** Randomized prospective studies on metabolic effects of oral contraceptives, Acta Obstet Gynecol Suppl 105:25, 1982.

16. **Meade TW, Greenberg G, Thompson SG,** Progestogens and cardiovascular reactions associated with oral contraceptives and a comparison of the safety of 50 and 30 μg oestrogen preparations, Br Med J 1:1157, 1980.

17. **Kay CR,** The happiness pill, J R Coll Gen Pract 30:8, 1980.

18. **Collaborative Group for the Study of Stroke in Young Women,** Oral contraceptives and stroke in young women, JAMA 231:718, 1975.

19. **Petittie DB, Wingerd J,** Use of oral contraceptives, cigarette smoking and risk of subarachnoid hemorrhage, Lancet 2:234, 1978.

20. **Inman WHW,** Oral contraceptives and fatal subarachnoid hemorrhage, Br Med J 2:468, 1979.

21. **Tietze C,** The pill and mortality from cardiovascular disease: another look, Fam Plann Pespect 11:80, 1979.

22. **Belsey MA, Russel Y, Kinnear K,** Cardiovascular disease and oral contraceptives: a reappraisal of vital statistics data, Fam Plann Perspect 11:84, 1979.

23. **Ramcharan S, Pellegrin FA, Ray RM, Hsu J,** The Walnut Creek contraceptive drug study. Vol III. An interim report: a comparison of disease occurrence leading to hospitalization or death in users and nonusers of oral contraceptives, J Reprod Med 25:346, 1980.

24. **Royal College of General Practitioners,** Further analyses of mortality in oral contraceptive uses, Lancet 1:541, 1981.

25. **Vessey MP, McPherson K, Yeates D,** Mortality in oral contraceptive users, Lancet 1:549, 1981.

26. **Slone D, Shapiro S, Kaufman DW, Rosenberg L, Miettinen OS, Stolley PD,** Risk of myocardial infarction in relation to current and discontinued use of oral contraceptives, N Engl J Med 305:420, 1981.

27. **Kaufman DW, Shapiro S, Slone D, Rosenberg L, Miettinen OS, Stolley PD, Knapp RC, Leavitt T Jr, Watson WG, Rosenshein NB, Lewis JL Jr, Schottenfeld D, Engle RL Jr,** Decreased risk of endometrial cancer among oral contraceptive users, N Engl J Med 303:1045, 1980.

28. **Harris RWC, Brinton LA, Cowdell RH, Skegg DCG, Smith PG, Vessey MP, Doll R,** Characteristics of women with dysplasia or carcinoma in situ of the cervix uteri, Br J Cancer 42:359, 1980.

29. **Swan SH, Brown WL,** Oral contraceptive use, sexual activity, and cervical carcinoma, Am J Obstet Gynecol 139:52, 1980.

30. **Kay CR,** Breast cancer and oral contraceptives: findings in Royal College of General Practitioners' study, Br Med J 282:2089, 1981.

31. **Vessey MP, McPherson K, Doll R,** Breast cancer and oral contraceptives: findings in Oxford-Family Planning Association contraceptive study, Br Med J 282:2093, 1981.

32. **Fasal E, Paffenbarger RS Jr,** Oral contraceptives as related to cancer and benign lesions of the breast, JNCI 55:767, 1975.

33. **Paffenbarger RS Jr, Fasal E, Simmons ME, Kampert JB,** Cancer risk as related to use of oral contraceptives during fertile years, Cancer 39:1887, 1977.

34. **Pike MC, Henderson BE, Casagrande JT, Rosario I, Gray GE,** Oral contraceptive use and early abortion as risk factors for breast cancer in young women, Br J Cancer 43:72, 1981.

35. **Matthews PN, Millis RR, Hayward JL,** Breast cancer in women who have taken contraceptive steroids, Br Med J 282:774, 1981.

36. **Vessey MP, McPherson K, Yeates D, Doll R,** Oral contraceptive use and abortion before first term pregnancy in relation to breast cancer, Br J Cancer 45:327, 1982.

37. **Beral V, Ramcharan S, Faris R,** Malignant melanoma and oral contraceptive use among women in California, Br J Cancer 36:804, 1977.

38. **Rosenberg L, Shapiro S, Slone D, Kaufman DW, Helmrich SP, Miettinen OS, Stolley PD, Rosenshein NB, Schottenfeld D, Engle RL Jr,** Epithelial ovarian cancer and combination oral contraceptives, JAMA 247:3210, 1982.

39. **Frank DW, Kirton KET, Murchison TE, Quinlan WJ, Coleman ME, Gilbertson TJ, Feenstra ES, Kimball FA,** Mammary tumors and serum hormones in the bitch treated with medroxyprogesterone acetate or progesterone for four years, Fertil Steril 31:340, 1979.

40. **DePirro R, Forte F, Bertoli A, Greco AV, Lauro R,** Changes in insulin receptors during oral contraception, J Clin Endocrinol Metab 52:29, 1981.

41. **Wingrave SJ, Kay CR, Vessey MP,** Oral contraceptives and diabetes mellitus, Br Med J 1:23, 1979.

42. **Bennion LJ, Ginsberg RL, Garnick MB, Bennett PH,** Effects of oral contraceptives on the gallbladder bile of normal women, N Engl J Med 294:189, 1976.

43. **Brownrigg GM,** Toxemia in hormone-induced pseudopregnancy, Can Med Assoc J 87:408, 1962.

447

44. **Laragh JH, Sealey JE, Ledingham JGG, Newton MA,** Oral contraceptives, renin, aldosterone, and high blood pressure, JAMA 201, 918, 1967.

45. **Kessler KM, Warde DAL, Ledis JE, Kessler RM,** Left ventricular size and function in women receiving oral contraceptives, Obstet Gynecol 55:211, 1980.

46. **Royal College of General Practitioners,** Reduction in incidence of rheumatoid arthritis associated with oral contraceptives, Lancet 1:569, 1978.

47. **Eschenbach DA, Harnisch JP, Holmes KK,** Pathogenesis of acute pelvic inflammatory disease: role of contraception and other risk factors, Am J Obstet Gynecol 128:838, 1977.

48. **Royal College of General Practitiones,** Oral contraception study, the outcome of pregnancy in former oral contraceptive users, Br J Obstet Gynecol 83:608, 1976.

49. **Jacobs HS, Knuth UA, Hull MGR, Franks S,** Post-"pill" amenorrhea—cause or coincidence? Br Med J 2:940, 1977.

50. **Dickey RP, Stone SC,** Progestational potency of oral contraceptives, Obstet Gynecol 47:106, 1976.

51. **Chihal HJW, Peppler RD, Dickey RP,** Estrogen potency of oral contraceptive pills, Am J Obstet Gynecol 121:75, 1975.

52. **Rothman KJ, Louik C,** Oral contraceptives and birth defects, N Engl J Med 299:522, 1978.

53. **Rothman KJ, Fyler DC, Goldblatt A, Kreidberg MB,** Exogenous hormones and other drug exposures of children with cogenital heart disease, Am J Epidemiol 109:433, 1979.

54. **Heinonen OP, Slone D, Monson RR, Hook EB, Shapiro S,** Cardiovascular birth defects and antenatal exposure to female sex hormones, N Engl J Med 296:67, 1977.

55. **Ferencz C, Matanoski GM, Wilson PD, Rubin JD, Neill CA, Gutberlet R,** Maternal hormone therapy and congenital heart disease, Teratology 21:225, 1980.

56. **Rothman K,** Fetal loss, twinning, and birth weight after oral contraceptive use, N Engl J Med 297:468, 1977.

57. **Rothman K, Liess J,** Gender of offspring after oral contraceptive use, N Engl J Med 295:859, 1976.

58. **Beck LR, Dowsar DR, Pope VZ,** Long-acting steroidal contraceptive systems, Res Front Fertil Regul 1:1, 1980.

59. **Fraser IS, Weisberg E,** A comprehensive review of injectable contraception with special emphasis on depot-medroxyprogesterone acetate, Med J Aust 1:3, 1981.

60. **DeCeular K, Gruber C, Hayes R, Serjeant GR,** Medroxyprogesterone acetate and homozygous sickle-cell disease, Lancet 2:229, 1982.

61. **Pardthaisong T, Gray RH, McDaniel LB,** Return of fertility after discontinuation of depo medroxyprogesterone acetate and intra-uterine devices in northern Thailand, Lancet 1:509, 1980.

62. **Atkinson L, Schearer SB, Harkavy O, Lincoln R,** Prospects for improved contraception, Fam Plann Perspect 12:173, 1980.

63. **Dixon GW, Chlesselman JJ, Ory HW, Blye RP,** Ethinyl estradiol and conjugated estrogens as postcoital contraceptives, JAMA 244:1336, 1980.

64. **Yuzpe AA, Smith RP, Rademaker AW,** A multicenter clinical investigation employing ethinyl estradiol combined with *dl*-norgestrel as a postcoital contraceptive agent, Fertil Steril 37:508, 1982.

65. **Kaufman DW, Shapiro S, Rosenberg L, Monson RR, Miettinen OS, Stolley PD, Slone D,** Intrauterine contraceptive device use and pelvic inflammatory disease, Am J Obstet Gynecol 136:159, 1980.

66. **Bergquist C, Nillius SJ, Wide L,** Intranasal GnRH agonist as a contraceptive, Lancet 2:215, 1979.

67. **Sheehan KL, Casper RF, Yen SSC,** Luteal phase defects induced by an agonist of luteinizing hormone-releasing factor: a model for fertility control, Science 215:170, 1982.

68. **Casper RF, Yen SSC,** Induction of luteolysis in the human with a long acting analog of LHRH, Science 205:408, 1979.

16 Sperm and Egg Transport, Fertilization, and Implantation

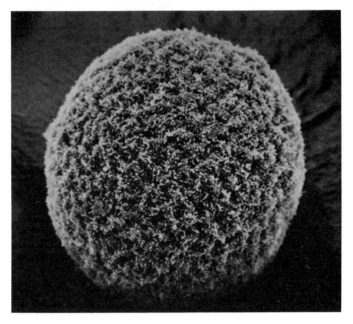

Knowledge of the interactions that take place between sperm and the female reproductive tract can aid the physician in making rational clinical judgments. *Therefore, prior to reviewing the clinical problem of infertility, this chapter will briefly examine the mechanisms involved in sperm and egg transport, fertilization, and implantation.*

Sperm Transport

Semen forms a gel almost immediately following ejaculation, but then is liquefied in 20–30 minutes by enzymes derived from the prostate gland. The alkaline pH of semen provides protection for the sperm from the acid environment of the vagina. This protection is transient, and most sperm left in the vagina are immobilized within 2 hours. The more fortunate sperm, by their own motility, gain entrance into the tongues of cervical mucus that layer over the ectocervix. It is the sperm that enter the uterus; the seminal plasma is left behind in the vagina. This entry is rapid, and sperm have been found in mucus within 90 seconds of ejaculation. (1) Bedford demonstrated that destruction of all sperm in the vagina 5 minutes after ejaculation does not interfere with fertilization in the rabbit, further attesting to the rapidity of transport. (2)

451

Uterine contractions propel the sperm upward, and in the human they can be found in the tube 5 minutes after insemination. (3) It is possible that the first sperm to enter the tube are at a disadvantage. In the rabbit these early sperm have only poor motility, and there is frequent disruption of the head membranes. (4) The sperm in this vanguard are unlikely to achieve fertilization. Other sperm that have colonized the cervical mucus, the cervical crypts, and the portion of the tubal isthmus nearest the uterus then make their way more slowly to the ampulla of the tube in order to meet the egg. Human sperm have been found in the Fallopian tube as long as 85 hours after intercourse, but it is not known whether these sperm have retained their fertilizing ability. (5) In animals, the fertilizable life span is usually one-half the motile life span.

The attrition in sperm numbers from vagina to tube is substantial. Of an average of 200 million to 300 million sperm deposited in the vagina, less than 200 achieve proximity to the egg. The major loss occurs in the vagina, with expulsion of semen from the introitus playing an important role. Other causes for loss are digestion of sperm by vaginal enzymes, phagocytosis of sperm all along the reproductive tract, and, to a limited extent, movement of sperm through the Fallopian tube into the peritoneal cavity. There are also reports of sperm burrowing into or being engulfed by endometrial cells.

Capacitation

The discovery in 1951 that rat and rabbit spermatozoa must spend some hours in the female tract before acquiring the capacity to penetrate ova stimulated intensive research efforts to delineate the environmental conditions required for this change in the sperm to occur. The process by which the sperm were transformed was called capacitation. Attention was focused upon the hormonal and time requirements, the potential for in vitro capacitation, and the identification of a substance in seminal fluid which, when added to capacitated sperm, rendered them decapacitated. (6)

An important finding was that capacitation changes the surface characteristics of sperm, as exemplified by removal of seminal plasma antigens, modification of their surface charge, and restriction of receptor mobility. This is associated with decreased stability of the plasma membrane and the membrane lying immediately under it, the outer acrosomal membrane. The membranes undergo further, more striking, modifications when capacitated sperm reach the vicinity of an ovum or when they are incubated in follicular fluid. There is a breakdown and merging of the plasma membrane and the outer acrosomal membrane. (7) This allows egress of the enzyme contents of the acrosome, the cap-like structure that covers the sperm nucleus. These enzymes, which include hyaluronidase, a neuraminidase-like factor, corona-dispersing enzyme, and a protease called acrosin, are all thought to play roles in sperm penetration of the egg investments.

Although capacitation classically has been defined as the change sperm undergo in the female reproductive tract, it is now apparent that sperm of some species, including the human, can acquire the ability to fertilize after a short incubation in defined media and without residence in the female reproductive tract. (8) Therefore, in vitro fertilization is possible.

Speculation concerning the use of the seminal fluid constituent that decapacitates sperm as a contraceptive agent was stimulated by its successful use in rabbits. Consideration of the amounts of material needed and the requirements for a delivery system indicate that, at least for the human, decapacitation factor is not a realistic contraceptive.

Egg Transport

Egg transport encompasses the period of time from ovulation to the entry of the egg into the uterus. The egg can be fertilized only during the early stages of its sojourn in the Fallopian tube.

In rats and mice the ovary and distal portion of the tube are covered by a common fluid-filled sac. Ovulated eggs are carried by fluid currents to the fimbriated end of the tube. By contrast, in primates, including humans, the ovulated eggs adhere with their cumulus mass of follicular cells to the surface of the ovary. The fimbriated end of the tube sweeps over the ovary in order to pick up the egg. Entry into the tube is facilitated by muscular movements that bring the fimbriae into contact with the surface of the ovary. Variations in this pattern surely exist, as evidenced by women who achieve pregnancy despite having only one ovary, and a single tube located on the contralateral side.

Although there can be a small negative pressure in the tube in association with muscle contractions, ovum pickup is not dependent upon a suction effect secondary to this negative pressure. Ligation of the tube just proximal to the fimbriae does not interfere with pickup. (9) The cilia on the surface of the fimbriae have adhesive sites, and these seem to have prime responsibility for the initial movement of the egg into the tube. This movement is dependent upon the presence of follicular cells surrounding the egg, because removal of these cells prior to egg pickup prevents effective egg transport. In the ampulla of the tube the cilia beat in the direction of the uterus. In man and monkey this unidirectional beat is also found in the isthmus of the tube, whereas in the rabbit there are additional rows of cilia that beat in the direction of the ovary. The specific contribution of the cilia to egg transport in the ampulla and isthmus is an unresolved question. Most investigators have credited muscular contractions of the tubes as the primary force for moving the egg. Halbert et al. showed in the rabbit, however, that interference with muscle contractility did not block egg transport. (10) They concluded that, in this species, cilia play a major role. Reversing a segment of the ampulla of the tube so that the cilia in this segment beat toward the ovary interferes with pregnancy in the rabbit without blocking fertilization. The fertilized ova are arrested when they come into contact with the transposed area. (11) This again suggests that ciliary beat is crucial for egg transport. Cilia play, in all likelihood, a less important role in the human. There are *fertile* women who have Kartagener's syndrome in which there is a congenital absence of dynein arms in cilia and, thus, the cilia do not beat. This deficiency in the cilia is found in the Fallopian tubes as well as in the respiratory tract. (12)

Muscular contractions of the tube are associated with a to-and-fro movement of the eggs rather than with a continuous forward progression. In most species transport of the ovum through the tube requires approximately 3 days. (13). The time spent within the various parts of the tube varies from one species to another. Transport through the ampulla is rapid in the rabbit, whereas in women it requires 30 hours for the egg to reach the ampullary-isthmic junction. The egg remains at this point another 30 hours, at which time it begins rapid transport through the isthmus of the tube.

Attempts to modify tubal function as a method for understanding its physiology have involved three major pharmacologic approaches. These are: 1) altering levels of steroid hormones, 2) the interference with or supplementation of adrenergic stimuli, and 3) treatment with prostaglandins. Although there is an abundant literature on the effects of estrogen and progesterone on tubal function, it is clouded by the use of different hormones, different doses, and different timing of injections. Because of these variations it is difficult to obtain a coherent picture and to relate the experimental results to the in vivo situation. In general, pharmacologic doses of estrogen favor retention of eggs in the tube. This "tube locking" effect of estrogen can be partially reversed by treatment with progesterone.

The isthmus of the tube has an extensive adrenergic innervation. Surgical denervation of the tube, however, does not disrupt ovum transport. Prostaglandins (PG) of the E series relax tubal muscle, whereas those of the F series stimulate muscle activity of the tube. Although $PGF_{2\alpha}$ and methylergonovine both stimulate human oviductal motility in vivo, they do not cause acceleration of ovum transport.

The effect on fertility of removal of different segments of the tube has been reviewed by Pauerstein and Eddy, who noted that excision of the ampullary-isthmic junction in rabbits did not block fertility. (14) This is equally true if small segments of the ampulla are removed, and pregnancy can occur even if the entire isthmus and uterotubal junction are excised. Although the fimbriae are thought to play a crucial role in fertility, spontaneous pregnancies have been reported following sterilization by fimbriectomy or following surgical repair of tubes whose fimbriated ends had been excised. (15, 16)

In most species, a period of residence in the tube appears to be a prerequisite for full development. Rabbit eggs can be fertilized in the uterus, but they do not develop unless transferred to the tubes within 3 hours of fertilization. (17) This and other work implies that there may be a component in uterine fluid during the first 48 hours following ovulation that is toxic to the egg. (18) Indirect evidence of an inhospitable environment is also provided by studies indicating that there must be synchrony between development of the endometrium and the egg for successful pregnancy to occur. (18) If the endometrium is in a more advanced stage of development than the egg, fertility is compromised. These studies were done in animals and may not be relevant to the human.

Successful pregnancies have occurred in the human following the Estes procedure, in which the ovary is transposed to the uterine cornua. (19) Eggs are ovulated directly into the uterus, completely bypassing the tube. This crucial difference between animal and human physiology is of more than academic importance. There has been considerable speculation concerning the use of drugs that could accelerate tubal transport, as a means of providing contraception by ensuring that the egg would reach the uterus when it was in an unreceptive state. Although this may work in animals, it would be of doubtful value in the human because even the limited success with the Estes procedure indicates that perfect synchrony is not required.

Animal and human reproduction also differ in the occurrence of ectopic pregnancy. Ectopic pregnancies are rare in animals, and in rodents they are not induced even if the uterotubal junction is occluded immediately following fertilization. The embryos reach the blastocyst stage and then degenerate.

Fertilization

Following ovulation, the fertilizable life span of the rabbit egg is between 6 and 8 hours. The fertilizable life of the human ova is unknown, but most estimates range between 12 and 24 hours. Equally uncertain is knowledge of the fertilizable life span of human sperm. The most common estimate is 48 hours, although motility can be maintained after the sperm have lost the ability to fertilize. Contact of sperm with the egg, which occurs in the ampulla of this tube, appears to be random, and there is no current evidence that the egg lures sperm to its surface.

The acellular zona pellucida that surrounds the egg at ovulation and remains in place until implantation, has two major functions in the fertilization process: 1) It contains receptors for sperm which are, with some exceptions, relatively species-specific; and 2) the zona becomes impervious to other sperm once the fertilizing sperm penetrates, and thus it provides a bar to polyploidy. (20) Penetration through the zona is rapid and, in all likelihood, is mediated by acrosin, which is bound to the inner acrosomal membrane of the sperm. (21) The pivotal role assigned to acrosin

455

has been disputed. For example, manipulations that increase the resistance of the zona to acrosin do not interfere with sperm penetration. The initiation of the block to penetration of the zone (and the vitellus) by other sperm is mediated by release of materials from the cortical granules, organelles which are found just below the egg surface. (22)

The second polar body is released at the time of fertilization, which leaves the egg with a haploid complement of chromosomes. The addition of chromosomes from the sperm restores the diploid number to the now fertilized egg.

The postacrosomal region of the sperm head makes initial contact with the vitelline membrane. At first the egg membrane engulfs the sperm head, and subsequently there is fusion of egg and sperm membranes. The chromatin material of the sperm head decondenses and the male pronucleus is formed. The male and the female pronuclei migrate toward each other, and as they move into close proximity the limiting membranes break down, and a spindle is formed on which the chromosomes become arranged. Thus, the stage is set for the first cell division.

The clinician is interested not only in how normal fertilization takes place, but also in the occurrence of abnormal events that can interfere with pregnancy. It is worthwhile, therefore, to consider the failures that occur in association with in vivo fertilization. This information also may provide an estimate of problems that can be anticipated with in vitro fertilization. Studies in the nonhuman primate have involved monkeys and baboons. A surgical method was used to flush the uterus of regularly cycling rhesus monkeys, and 9 preimplantation embryos and 2 unfertilized eggs were recovered from 22 flushes. Two of the 9 embryos were morphologically abnormal and probably would not have implanted. (23) Hendrickx and Kraemer used a similar technique in the baboon and recovered 23 embryos, of which 10 were morphologically abnormal. (24) This suggests that in nonhuman primates some ovulated eggs are not fertilized and that many early embryos are abnormal and, in all likelihood, will be aborted. Similar findings have been reported in the human in the classic study of Hertig et al. (25) They examined 34 early embryos recovered by flushing and examination of pathologic reproductive organs removed at surgery. Ten of these embryos were morphologically abnormal, including 4 of the 8 preimplantation embryos. Because the 4 preimplantation losses would not have been recognized clinically, there would have been 6 losses recorded in the remaining 30 pregnancies.

Using sensitive pregnancy tests, it has been suggested that approximately 25–40% of conceptions may be lost before they are clinically perceived. Given the high rate of abnormality, there is evidence for biologic selection against abnormal gametes and embryos throughout the reproductive process. Morphologically abnormal sperm are less successful than normal sperm in penetrating cervical mucus and in negotiating the uterotubal junction. (26) This selection does not seem to be operative against chromosomally abnormal sperm that are morphologically normal. Another protective mechanism is the attrition of sperm numbers that occurs between the vagina and the area of the tube that contains the egg. With only a small number of sperm making contact with the egg, there may be a decreased chance for penetration of the egg by more than one sperm.

There is no direct information on whether or not there is selection against chromosomally abnormal preimplantation embryos. There is, however, evidence that damaged preimplantation embryos are subject to selection. For example, brief treatment of preimplantation embryos in vitro with actinomycin D, a powerful teratogen when given to mothers after implantation, decreases the number of embryos that survive to term after reimplantation. Among those that do survive, there is no greater incidence of abnormalities compared to control embryos. (27) This indicates that the preimplantation embryo reacts in an all-or-none fashion to exogenous insults.

In the postimplantation period, if only clinically diagnosed pregnancies are considered, the generally accepted figure for spontaneous abortion in the first trimester is 15%. Approximately 50–60% of these abortions have chromosome abnormalities. (28) This suggests that a minimum of 7.5% of all human conceptions are chromosomally abnormal. The fact that only 1 in 200 newborns has a chromosome abnormality attests to the powerful selection mechanisms operating in early human gestation.

In Vitro Fertilization

A number of the in vivo protective mechanisms are not present during in vitro fertilization. The filtering effect of the cervical mucus and the uterotubal junction is not available to remove grossly abnormal sperm. In most in vitro experiments, relatively large numbers of sperm are placed in the vicinity of the egg, and this may increase the risk for penetration of the egg by more than one sperm. This appears to be the case in mice. Fraser and her co-workers found an increased incidence of triploidy in embryos derived from mouse eggs fertilized in vitro (12.8%) compared to those fertilized in vivo (2.7%). (29) Interestingly, the incidence of aneuploidy other than triploidy was not different between those two-cell mouse embryos that had been fertilized in vivo and those fertilized in vitro. Fortunately, almost all triploid embryos are aborted spontaneously, and additional protection could be derived by doing karyotypes on fetal cells obtained by amniocentesis in every baby conceived in vitro. Thus, an increased risk of triploidy will not be a deterrent to the use of in vitro fertilization. In a series of 4 in vitro fertilized pregnancies reported by Steptoe and Edwards, there was one triploid fetus that was aborted spontaneously. (30)

Lopata summarized the Australian and English experience with in vitro fertilization for the years 1979 and 1980 and reported that 3 of 56 (5.4%) transferred embryos had produced live births. (31) All 3 births followed spontaneous ovulation. Steptoe and Edwards had abandoned the use of induction of ovulation because of failure to achieve a normal pregnancy. Instead, during spontaneous cycles they measured the level of LH in the urine every 3 hours around ovulation time and scheduled their laparoscopies approximately 20 hours after the LH surge. Timing is crucial. Eggs removed from the follicle too early cannot be fertilized normally. If laparoscopy is delayed, it is more likely that the egg will have been ovulated and, therefore, not retrievable.

The accumulated worldwide experience now has demonstrated quite conclusively that success is greater if ovulation inducing drugs are used to accomplish both better timing and the development of more than one egg. Jones and colleagues (32) used injections of Pergonal (human menopausal gonadotropin, HMG) and followed follicular development with both ultrasound and estradiol assays to determine the proper time to administer the human chorionic gonadotropin (HCG) that triggers ovulation. Once the eggs are retrieved by laparoscopy, rigorous culture techniques are employed and attention to details such as the use of triple distilled water is crucial. Results continue to improve and Jones and co-workers have reported success in 20–25% of their cases. (32) Preliminary results indicate that the chances for pregnancy increase when two or three eggs are fertilized and placed in the uterus. This increases the risk of multiple births, but the risk appears to be small.

The relatively low percentage of pregnancies achieved with in vitro fertilization to date is explainable to some extent by the high rate of embryo loss associated even with in vivo fertilization. This alone, however, does not completely account for the current results. Many of the losses result following transfer of embryos, and in some animals this process is associated with a 50% embryo mortality. With increased experience the results should improve. It is clear, however, that there is a need for further understanding of the fertilization process and of implantation, before we can feel confident that the in vitro environment is as physiologic as possible.

Implantation

Implantation is defined as the process by which an embryo attaches to the uterine wall and penetrates first the epithelium and then the circulatory system of the mother. It is a process that is limited in both time and space. Implantation begins 2–3 days after the fertilized egg enters the uterus, and is marked initially by apposition of the blastocyst to the uterine epithelium. A prerequisite for this contact is a loss of the zona pellucida, which, in vitro, can be ruptured by contractions and expansions of the blastocyst. In vivo this activity is less critical, as the zona can be lysed by components of the uterine fluid. The exact nature and function of these components and related proteins which are thought to mediate the implantation process (implantation-initiating factor, uteroglobin and blastokinin) are uncertain. Their production is, however, known to be dependent upon secretion of ovarian steroid hormones. Even if the hormonal milieu and protein composition of the uterine fluid are hospitable to implantation, it may not occur if the embryo is not at the proper stage of development. It has been inferred from this information that there must be developmental maturation of the surface of the embryo before it is able to achieve attachment and implantation.

Reports on changes in the surface charge of preimplantation embryos differ in their findings. Nilsson et al. showed that blastocysts activated for implantation had a lower affinity for positively charged iron oxide than did inactive blastocysts. (34) This suggests that there is a decrease in negative surface charge just prior to implantation. Others, however, have found evidence for an increase in negative charge at the same stage. (35) In either case, it is unlikely that changes in surface charge are solely responsible for adherence of the embryo to the surface of epithelial cells. Binding of the lectin concanavalin A to the embryo also changes during the preimplantation period, an indication that the surface glycoproteins of the embryo are in transition. (36) It is reasonable to assume that these changes in configuration on the surface occur in order to enhance the ability of the embryo to adhere to the maternal surface.

As the embryo comes into close contact with the endometrium, the microvilli on the surface flatten and interdigitate with those on the luminal surface of the epithelial cells. A stage is reached where the cell membranes are in very close contact and junctional complexes are formed. The embryo can no longer be dislodged from the surface of the epithelial cells by flushing the uterus with physiological solutions. Schlafke and Enders described three types of subsequent interactions between the implanting trophoblast and the uterine epithelium. (37) In the first, trophoblast cells intrude between uterine epithelial cells on their path to the basement membrane. In the second type of interaction, the epithelial cells lift off the basement membrane, an action which allows the trophoblast to insinuate itself underneath the epithelium. Lastly, fusion of trophoblast with individual uterine epithelial cells has been identified by electron microscopy in the rabbit. (38) This latter method of gaining entry into the epithelial layer raises interesting questions concerning the immunologic consequences of mixing embryonic and maternal cytoplasm.

Trophoblast has the ability to phagocytose a variety of cells, but in vivo this activity seems largely confined to removal of dead endometrial cells, or cells that have been sloughed from the uterine wall. Similarly, despite the invasive nature of the trophoblast, destruction of maternal cells by enzymes secreted by the embryo does not seem to play a major role in implantation. The embryo does secrete a variety of enzymes, and these may be important for digesting the intercellular matrix that holds the epithelial cells together. Studies in vitro have demonstrated the presence of plasminogen activator in mouse embryos, and its activity is important in the attachment and early outgrowth stages of implantation. (39)

The embryo at a somewhat later stage of implantation can digest, in vitro, a complex matrix composed of glycoproteins, elastin and collagen, all of which are components of the normal intercellular matrix. (40) Additional studies in vitro have shown that cells move away from trophoblast in a process called "contact inhibition." (41) Trophoblast then spreads to fill the spaces vacated by the co-cultured cells. Once the intracellular matrix has been lysed, this movement of epithelial cells away from trophoblast would allow space for the implanting embryo to move through the epithelial layer. Trophoblast movement is aided by the fact that only parts of its surface are adhesive, and the major portion of the surface is nonadhesive to other cells.

Invasion by the trophoblast is limited by the formation of the decidual cell layer in the uterus. Fibroblast-like cells in the stroma are transformed into glycogen and lipoid-rich cells. In the human, decidual cells surround blood vessels late in the nonpregnant cycle, but extensive decidualization does not occur until pregnancy is established. Ovarian steroids govern decidualization, and in the human a combination of estrogen and progesterone is critical. In animals, implantation is preceded by an increase in uterine stromal capillary permeability at the site where the blastocyst will attach. The increase in capillary permeability is noted following injection of macromolecular dyes (Pontamine blue, Evans blue) into the animal. Within a short time the dye is seen collecting in the areas of the increased permeability. The localized nature of this reaction and of decidualization in rodents raised the possibility that a signal from the embryo might be an important triggering stimulus. Thus, maternal recognition of and preparation for pregnancy may depend upon receiving signals released by the embryo.

Boving suggested that the release of CO_2 by the embryo in the form of bicarbonate raises the pH of the embryo surface, which, in turn, increases its stickiness. (42) CO_2 may also act as a signal to induce a decidual response in the mother.

Another role for the embryo in initiating implantation has been demonstrated in pigs. (43) The pig blastocyst synthesizes estrogen starting on day 12 of pregnancy, which is 6 days before definitive attachment to the uterine wall occurs. The estrogen can feedback on the pituitary to promote LH secretion, which is essential for maintenance of the corpus luteum.

The human conceptus produces HCG about the time of implantation on day 6 of pregnancy. The exact timing of the release in terms of whether it begins before or after the embryo enters the epithelium is uncertain. Function of the corpus luteum is crucial during the first 7–9 weeks of pregnancy, and lutectomy early in pregnancy can precipitate abortion. (44) Similarly, early pregnancy loss in primates can be induced by injections of anti-HCG serum. (45).

In rodents, implantation can be interrupted by injection of prostaglandin inhibitors. Kennedy showed that indomethacin prevented the increase in endometrial vascular permeability normally seen just prior to implantation. (46) Additional evidence for a role by prostaglandins in the earliest stages of implantation is the finding of increased concentrations of the drug at prospective implantation sites. The source or sources of the prostaglandins is not known. Rabbit blastocysts contain prostaglandins, but there is no evidence of significant prostaglandin production by rat blastocysts in vitro. The endometrial cells are a likely source of prostaglandin, and its synthesis may be stimulated by the tissue damage that accompanies implantation.

Shelesnyak suggested that histamine initiated the decidual response. (47) He found that antihistamines given systemically or directly into the uterus prevented the decidual response in rats. This was disputed when other workers found that systemic antihistamines were not effective in preventing the decidual response. More recently, however, it has been shown that there are two different receptors for histamines, H1 and H2. These are not blocked by the same agents, and early experiments demonstrating a lack of effect of antihistamines may have utilized only a block to one receptor. Brandon and Wallis blocked both receptors in rats and found a decrease in the number of implantation sites. (48) Mast cells in the uterus are a major source of histamine, but it is possible that the embryo can also synthesize histamine. (49) This would explain why the increase in capillary permeability and decidualization in the endometrium is localized to areas near the implanting embryo.

One of the great mysteries associated with implantation is the mechanism by which the mother rejects a genetically abnormal embryo or fetus. It is possible that the abnormal embryo cannot produce a signal in early pregnancy that can be recognized by the mother.

The embryonic signals will be effective only in a proper hormone milieu. Much of the knowledge concerning the hormone requirements for implantation in animals has been gained from studies of animals in delayed implantation. In a number of species, preimplantation embryos normally lie dormant in the uterus for periods of time which may extend for as long as 15 months before implantation is initiated. In other species, delayed implantation can be imposed by postpartum suckling or by performing ovariectomy on day

461

3 of pregnancy. This produces a marked decrease in synthesis of DNA and protein by the blastocyst. The embryo can be maintained at the blastocyst stage by injecting the mother with progesterone. Using this model, hormonal requirements for implantation have been determined. In mice there is a requirement for estrogen and progesterone followed by estrogen, which initiates implantation. In other species the nidatory stimulus of estrogen is not required, and progesterone alone is sufficient.

Although it is known that the hormone milieu of delayed implantation renders the embryo quiescent, it is not known whether this represents a direct effect on the embryo or whether there is a metabolic inhibitor present in uterine secretions that acts upon the embryo. Removal of the embryo from the uterus in delay to culture dishes allows rapid resumption of normal metabolism, suggesting that there has, in fact, been a release from the inhibitory effects of a uterine product. (50)

Unanswered Questions

Why is gamete production so wasteful? Billions of sperm are produced, but only a few are ever successful in fertilizing an egg. Does it relate to early forms of reproduction—for example, those in fish, where the sperm are released into the sea and large numbers are needed to assure that a few reach the egg? Does the overpopulation of sperm allow selection processes to take place ensuring that the more abnormal sperm are filtered out before the tube is reached? In the female approximately 350 ova are ovulated during a woman's life, yet the ovaries contain over a million eggs at birth.

What is the purpose of capacitation? Is it needed to overcome the protective mechanisms that have been built into the sperm, specifically those that prevent premature release of acrosomal enzymes. Penetration by sperm of the egg is desirable, but invasion of other maternal cells might trigger immunologic reactions against sperm.

It is known that there is selection against morphologically abnormal sperm in the female. There is also suggestive evidence that sperm that reach the tube may have superior fertilizing ability compared with those recovered from the uterus. What governs this mechanism of selection?

Why are there so many abnormal embryos? Current estimates are that 50% of embryos do not survive to term. Why is there a high rate of embryo loss, and, specifically, why is there a high selection against abnormal embryos? Is it because of intrinsic programming defects within the embryo, or to an inability of the embryo to produce a signal recognized by the mother; or does the maternal organism in some way recognize abnormality and react against it?

Why has embryo transfer in the human following in vitro fertilization resulted in a low number of takes? Can the uterine environment be manipulated in such a way as to increase successful implantation of in vitro fertilized eggs?

462

References

1. **Sobrero AJ, MacLeod J,** The immediate postcoital test, Fertil Steril 13:184, 1962.

2. **Bedford JM,** The rate of sperm passage into the cervix after coitus in the rabbit, J Reprod Fertil 25:211, 1971.

3. **Settlage DSF, Motoshima M, Tredway DR,** Sperm transport from the external cervical os to the fallopian tubes in women: a time and quantitation study, Fertil Steril 24:655, 1973.

4. **Overstreet JW, Cooper GW,** Rabbit sperm do not survive rapid transport through the female reproductive tract, abstract presented at the Ninth Annual Meeting of the Society for the study of Reproduction, Philadelphia, August 10–13, 1976.

5. **Ahlgren M,** Sperm transport to and survival in the human fallopian tube, Gynecol Invest 6:206, 1975.

6. **Williams WL,** Biochemistry of capacitation of spermatozoa, in *Biology of Mammalian Fertilization and Implantation,* Moghissi KS and Hafez ESE, eds, Charles C Thomas, Springfield, Ill., 1972.

7. **Bedford JM,** Sperm capacitation and fertilization in mammals, Biol Reprod Suppl 2:128, 1970.

8. **Edwards RG, Steptoe PC, Purdy JM,** Fertilization and cleavage in vitro of preovulatory human oocytes, Nature 227:1307, 1970.

9. **Clewe TH, Mastroianni L,** Mechanisms of ovum pickup: I. Functional capacity of rabbit oviducts ligated near the fimbriae, Fertil Steril 9:13, 1958.

10. **Halbert SA, Tam PY, Blandau RJ,** Egg transport in the rabbit oviduct: the roles of cilia and muscle, Science 191:1052, 1976.

11. **Eddy CA, Flores JJ, Archer DR, Pauerstein CJ,** The role of cilia in infertility: an evaluation by selective microsurgical modification of the rabbit oviduct, Am J Obstet Gynecol 132:814, 1978.

12. **Jean Y, Langlais J, Roberts KD, Chapdelaine A, Bleau G,** Fertility of a woman with nonfunctional ciliated cells in the fallopian tubes, Fertil Steril 31:349, 1979.

13. **Croxatto HB, Ortiz MS,** Egg transport in the fallopian tube, Gynecol Invest 6:215, 1975.

14. **Pauerstein CJ, Eddy CA,** The role of the oviduct in reproduction; Our knowledge and our ignorance, J Reprod Fertil 55:223, 1979.

15. **Tompkins P,** Letter to the editor, Fertil Steril 31:696, 1979.

463

16. **Novy MJ,** Reversal of Kroener fimbriectomy sterilization, Am J Obstet Gynecol 137:198, 1980.

17. **Glass RH,** Fate of rabbit eggs fertilized in the uterus, J Reprod Fertil 31:139, 1972.

18. **Adams CE,** Consequences of accelerated ovum transport, including a re-evaluation of Estes' operation, J Reprod Fertil 55:239, 1979.

19. **Ikle FA,** Pregnancy after implantation of the ovary into the uterus, Gynaecologia 151:95, 1961.

20. **Hartmann JF, Gwatkin RBL,** Alteration of sites on the mammalian sperm surface following capacitation, Nature 234:479, 1971.

21. **Zaneveld LJD, Polakoski KL, Williams WL,** Properties of a proteolytic enzyme from rabbit sperm acrosomes, Biol Reprod 6:30, 1972.

22. **Barros C, Yanagimachi R,** Induction of zona reaction in golden hamster eggs by cortical granule material, Nature 233:2368, 1971.

23. **Hurst PR, Jefferies K, Eckstein P, Wheeler AG,** Recovery of uterine embryos in rhesus monkeys, Biol Reprod 15:429, 1976.

24. **Hendrickx AG, Kraemer DC,** Preimplantation stages of baboon embryos, Anat Rec 162:111, 1968.

25. **Hertig AT, Rock J, Adams EC, Menkin MC,** Thirty-four fertilized ova, good, bad and indifferent from 210 women of known fertility, Pediatrics 23:202, 1959.

26. **Krzanowska H,** The passage of abnormal spermatozoa through the uterotubal junction of the mouse, J Reprod Fertil 38:81, 1974.

27. **Bell P, Glass RH,** Development of the mouse blastocyst after actinomycin D treatment, Fertil Steril 26:449, 1975.

28. **Short RV,** When a conception fails to become a pregnancy, in *Maternal Recognition of Pregnancy*, Whelan J, ed, *Ciba Foundation Symposium 64* (NS), Excerpta Medica, Amsterdam, 1979.

29. **Fraser L, Zanellotti HM, Paton GR, Drury LM,** Increased incidence of triploidy in embryos derived from mouse eggs fertilized in vitro, Nature 260:39, 1976.

30. **Steptoe PC, Edwards RG,** Pregnancies following implantation of human embryos grown in culture, presented at the Scientific Meeting, Royal College of Obstetricians and Gynaecologists, London, January 26, 1979.

31. **Lopata A,** Successes and failures in human in vitro fertilization, Nature 288:642, 1980.

32. **Jones HW Jr, Jones GS, Andrews MC, Acosta A, Bundren C, Garcia J, Sandow B, Veeck L, Wilkes C, Witmyer J, Wortham JE, Wright G,** The program for in vitro fertilization at Norfolk, Fertil Steril 38:14, 1982.

33. **Beier HM, Mootz U,** Significance of Maternal Uterine Proteins in the Establishment of Pregnancy, in *Material Recognition of Pregnancy*, Whelan J, ed, *Ciba Foundation Symposium 64* (NS), Excerpta Medica, Amsterdam, 1979.

34. **Nilsson O, Lindquist I, Ronquist G,** Decreased surface charge of mouse blastocysts at implantation, Exp Cell Res 83:421, 1974.

35. **Holmes PV, Dickson AD,** Estrogen induced surface coat and enzyme changes in the implanting mouse blastocyst, J Embryol Exp Morphol 29:639, 1973.

36. **Sobel JS, Nebel L,** Changes in concanavalin A agglutinability during development of the inner cell mass and trophoblast of mouse blastocyst in vitro, J Reprod Fertil 52:239, 1978.

37. **Schlafke S, Enders AC,** Cellular basis of interaction between trophoblast and uterus at implantation, Biol Reprod 12:41, 1975.

38. **Larsen JF,** Electron microscopy of the implantation site in the rabbit, Am J Anat 109:319, 1961.

39. **Strickland S, Reich E, Sherman MI,** Plasminogen activator in early embryogenesis: enzyme production by trophoblast and parietal endoderm, Cell 9:231, 1976.

40. **Glass RH, Spindle AI, Aggeler J, Pedersen RA, Werb Z,** Digestion of extracellular matrices—a model for embryo implantation, Society for Gynecologic Investigation, 28th Annual Meeting, Abstract 91, St. Louis, March 18–21, 1981.

41. **Glass RH, Spindle AI, Pedersen RA,** Mouse embryo attachment to substratum and the interaction of trophoblast with cultured cells, J Exp Zool 203:327, 1979.

42. **Boving BG,** Implantation, Ann NY Acad Sci 75:700, 1959.

43. **Heap RB, Flint AP, Gadsby JE,** Embryonic signals that establish pregnancy, Br Med Bull 35:129, 1979.

44. **Csapo AI, Pulkkinen MO, Wiest WO,** Effects of luteectomy and progesterone replacement therapy in early pregnant patients, Am J Obstet Gynecol 115:759, 1973.

45. **Stevens VC,** Potential control of fertility in women by immunization with HCG, Res Reprod 7:1, 1975.

46. **Kennedy TG,** Evidence for a role for prostaglandins in the initiation of blastocyst implantation in the rat, J Biol Reprod 16:286, 1977.

47. **Shelesnyak MC,** Inhibition of decidual cell formation in the pseudopregnant rat by histamine antagonists, Am J Physiol 170:522, 1952.

48. **Brandon JM, Wallis RM,** Effect of mepyramine, a histamine H_1-, and burimamide, a histamine H_2-receptor antagonist, on ovum implantation in the rat, J Reprod Fertil 50:251, 1977.

49. **Dey SK, Johnson DC, Santos JG,** Is histamine production by the blastocyst required for implantation in the rabbit? Biol Reprod 21:1169, 1979.

50. **Psychoyos A,** Hormonal requirements for egg implantation, in *Advances in the Biosciences 4*, Raspe G, ed, Pergamon Press, Oxford, 1970.

17

Investigation of the Infertile Couple

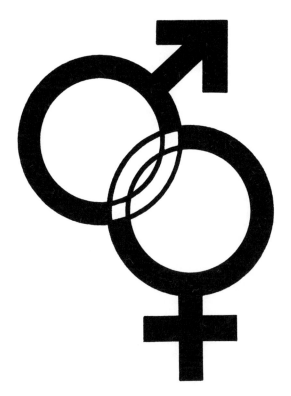

Infertility is defined as 1 year of unprotected coitus without conception. It affects approximately 10% of couples, which makes it one of the more common problems for which people seek medical aid. In response to this need physicians should have four goals in mind:

1. The first is to seek out and to correct the causes of infertility. With proper evaluation and therapy, approximately 50% of the women attending an infertility clinic will become pregnant.

2. The second goal is to provide accurate information for the couple and to dispel the misinformation commonly gained from friends and mass media. A few of the myths concerning infertility are detailed at the end of this chapter.

3. The third goal is to provide emotional support for the couple during a trying period. The inability to conceive generates a feeling in many couples that they have lost control over a very significant segment of their lives. That burden is aggravated by the additional impositions generated by the manipulations that couples have to undergo during the infertility investigation, including the need to have intercourse on schedule. Couples need to have an opportunity to ventilate their concerns and dispel some of their fears. A valuable adjunct to the efforts of the physician are support groups for infertile couples such as those organized by RESOLVE:

    RESOLVE, Inc.
    P.O. Box 474
    Belmont, MA 02178

    Meeting in groups allows individuals to realize that their problem is not unique, and it enables them to obtain information on how others cope with infertility. It must be emphasized that, while severe anxieties can interfere with ovulation and frequency of intercourse, there is no evidence that infertility is caused by the usual anxieties besetting a couple trying to conceive. Debner pointed out that the available information does not provide any solid ground for incriminating personality factors as a cause for female infertility. (1)

4. An often neglected goal is that of counseling a couple concerning the proper time to discontinue investigation and treatment. This is especially important in the 10% of couples with no known cause for their infertility. Despite the absence of pathology, couples with 4 years or more of infertility have a poor prognosis. If the couples are receptive, it is appropriate to provide advice about adoption.

    People who turn to social agencies involved with adoption may be afforded a bleak picture of their prospects. This can compound the depression the individuals already may feel from their inability to conceive. An alternative is private adoption, which may provide babies more rapidly, at reasonable cost, and without resorting to foreign countries. Patients should be encouraged to spread the word that they are interested in adoption. In addition, letters can be directed to obstetricians throughout the country describing the couple and their desire for adoption. Consultation with a lawyer is advisable to obtain information on the adoption laws in effect in the individual states. California law spells out the fees that the adoptive couples are allowed to pay. In this state lawyers should receive only their usual hourly fee, and the woman giving up the baby can receive money from the adoptive couple only for her medical expenses and reasonable living expenses. The woman cannot be paid a large sum of money for giving up the baby. In other words, private, or independent, adoption is not black market adoption. An excellent review of adoption in general, and private adoption in particular, is the book by Cynthia Martin called

Beating the Adoption Game, Oak Tree Publications, La Jolla, California. Anyone interested in adoption should read this book as a first step.

When local resources have been explored and a scarcity of available children requires a long waiting period, international adoptions may be investigated through the following agency:

> Holt International Children's Services
> P.O. Box 2880
> Eugene, OR 97402

The Infertility Investigation

There are advantages to having the male present during the initial interview. He may contribute valuable historical information. It also gives the physician the opportunity to emphasize that both partners are involved in the infertility investigation. A male who has been acquainted at its inception with the physician's treatment of the infertility problem will be less reluctant, as time progresses, to ask for clarification of any aspect of the testing. This can prevent misunderstandings engendered when the male's only source of information is the woman. Early in the physician-couple interaction, frequency of coitus and possible sexual problems should be ascertained.

The examination of the semen should be the first diagnostic step of the investigation (see Chapter 19). If the male, upon examination of the semen, is thought to have a reasonable potential for fertility, attention is directed to the woman. Failure to ovulate is the major problem in 40% of women with infertility, another 30–50% have tubal pathology, and 10% or less have a cervical barrier to fertility. Tests for all of these factors need to be scheduled at specific times in the menstrual cycle. It is estimated that the male factor accounts for 40% of infertility problems.

Postcoital Test

The postcoital test provides information both as to the receptivity of cervical mucus and the ability of sperm to reach and survive in the mucus. The test is scheduled for the anticipated day of ovulation and the scheduling is aided by prior basal body temperature charts, length of prior cycles, and/or the woman's perception of heightened vaginal moisture. At ovulation time the mucus contains 95–98% water and should be watery, thin, clear, acellular, and abundant. When dried on a slide it should form a distinct fern pattern. These characteristics contrast with the thick and viscid nature of mucus found prior to, and starting 24–48 hours after ovulation. The length of time the mucus is optimum is usually 2–3 days, but this will vary from one person to another, and the range may be from 1 to 5 days or even more. The woman is examined within 8 hours of intercourse, following 48 hours of abstinence, and the cervical mucus removed with a nasal polyp forceps. The stretchability (spinnbarkeit) of the mucus at ovulation time should be 8–10 cm or more. This characteristic can be assessed as the mucus is pulled from the cervix, or alternatively, by placing the mucus on a slide, covering it with a coverslip, and then lifting the coverslip. The gross clarity and the quantity of the mucus are assessed. The mucus is viewed under the microscope with a 10× objective without a coverslip, and then under a coverslip with a 10× and a 40× objective. If the mucus is thick, rather than thin, opaque instead of clear, the proximity of the test to ovulation should be determined by the onset of the next period (or by the temperature chart, for one should be taken during that cycle). If the poor mucus quality of the postcoital test is related to inaccurate timing, the test should be repeated during the subsequent cycle.

Fern Pattern

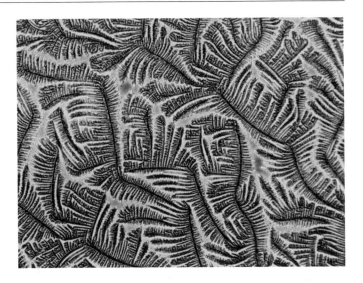

Lack of Fern

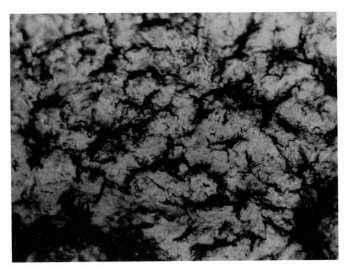

Improvement of a poor postcoital test can be attempted by giving low dose estrogen prior to ovulation. Conjugated estrogen 0.3 mg, or diethylstilbestrol 0.1 mg is given daily between days 5 and 13 of a 28-day cycle. If the mucus fails to improve, the dose of estrogen can be increased to 0.625 mg/day and then to 1.25 mg/day if the lower dose does not work. It is prudent to advise the woman that even these low doses of estrogen may cause prolongation of the proliferative phase of the menstrual cycle and thus may raise false expectations of pregnancy when the cycle is long.

Poor mucus is not an absolute barrier to fertility, but it does lower the possibility of conception. Additional treatment should be pursued if estrogen does not work. If there is evidence of chronic cervicitis, culture of cervical secretions and antibiotic therapy can be tried. Chlamydia has been implicated as a cause of cervicitis, but it has not yet been proven to be a cause of infertility. On occasion, cervicitis is treated with cryosurgery or electrocautery. Care must be taken not to destroy the entire mucus-producing endocervical canal.

Another tactic to overcome the barrier of thick cervical mucus is intrauterine insemination of sperm. (2) This is accomplished using a tuberculin syringe and a No. 16 intracath, which is threaded through the cervix into the uterine cavity. Normally after intercourse only sperm enter the uterine cavity and semen remains in the vagina. Intrauterine inseminations of even small amounts of semen may stimulate strong uterine contractions and produce an anaphylactic type of reaction. For this reason, no more than 0.3 ml should be injected into the uterus, and the sperm can be washed. Washing can be accomplished by diluting the semen with an equal volume of a sterile physiological solution such as Tyrode's and centrifuging for 3–5 minutes. The supernatant is discarded and the sperm pellet is resuspended in 0.3 ml of Tyrode's solution. Usually the sperm motility improves following the washing, centrifugation and resuspension. As a balance to this advantage, the intrauterine method of insemination allows direct introduction of bacteria into the uterus, and a few cases of tubal infection have been reported from the procedure.

If the woman has no cervical mucus, possibly because of removal of all of the glandular tissue from a previous cone biopsy, donor mucus, which has been stored frozen, can be used. The mucus is held in a polyethylene tube, one end of which is placed in a reservoir of semen. Sperm swim into the mucus column which is then deposited into the cervix.

Although a majority of viewers would agree on the assessment of the quality of a given mucus sample, there is no such agreement as to what constitutes a normal number of sperm in the postcoital test. The estimates in various books and journals range from 1 to over 20 sperm per high power field (HPF). Almost all the estimates have been arbitrarily chosen and have no scientific basis. The way to derive meaningful "normals" is to compare results with the occurrence of subsequent pregnancies. There is only limited information on this prognostic value of the postcoital test. If there are over 20 motile sperm/HPF, the sperm count will be above 20 million/ml and the pregnancy rate will be higher than if there are less than that number. The pregnancy rate is approximately 50% even with less than 20 sperm per HPF, and for that reason we do not designate these results as abnormal. (3) In one study there was no significant difference in subsequent pregnancy rates whether there were 1–5 sperm/HPF or 11–20 sperm/HPF. (3) For that reason it is our feeling that even 1 or 2 motile sperm/HPF can be considered a "normal" postcoital test, and it is not worthwhile to subject the couple to numerous postcoital tests in the hope of finding one with higher numbers. This view has been strengthened by the results of a study of postcoital tests in *fertile* couples. (4) Twenty percent in this fertile group had either no sperm or less than 1 sperm/HPF. As further evidence of the imprecision of the postcoital test, Asch performed laparoscopic aspiration of peritoneal fluid in 8 women with repeated postcoital tests showing no sperm. Six of these 8 women had sperm in the peritoneal cavity. (5)

If the postcoital test is so imprecise, what useful information can be obtained from it? Finding sperm in mucus provides reassurance of adequacy of coital technique and obviates useless advice such as staying in bed for 30 minutes or more after intercourse, or flexing the thighs after ejaculation. The couple should be told that normally there is a loss of semen from the vagina, and that a normal postcoital test indicates that the vital element, sperm, is reaching the cervix. If the mucus is clear and abundant, with good spinnbarkeit, the patient has a better chance for pregnancy than if it is thick and sparse. If there are more than 20 sperm/HPF, the male, in all likelihood, has a normal count, and the couple has a significantly better chance of achieving pregnancy than if the postcoital test contains less than 20 sperm/HPF. If there are no sperm, or only nonmotile sperm on repeated tests, the prognosis is poorer than if live sperm are found.

One of the most difficult problems in infertility is the couple who have postcoital tests which repeatedly show only dead sperm, or absence of sperm, despite good mucus and a normal semen analysis. The couple should be cautioned that lubricants such as KY Jelly and Surgilube have a spermicidal effect when tested in vitro and should not be used by infertile couples. (6) Vegetable oils or glycerin can be substituted because they do not interfere with sperm motility. Low dose estrogen can be tried. The pH of midcycle mucus should be determined. Ansari et al. reported that when a poor postcoital test was found in association with a cervical mucus pH of 7 (measured by pHydrion paper), a douche of 1 tablespoon of $NaHCO_3$ and 1 quart of water 30–60 minutes prior to intercourse markedly improved results. (7) Artificial insemination of sperm followed by a postcoital test 2 hours later can indicate whether negative postcoital tests after intercourse are due to faulty coital technique.

In vitro testing utilizing donor or bovine mucus and donor sperm can help to determine whether the poor postcoital test is due to factors in the mucus or to intrinsic defects in the sperm. A drop of the consort's sperm and a drop of donor sperm are placed next to the patient's mucus on a slide, with the borders touching. A similar test is performed with donor mucus. Penetration and survival of different sperm specimens are evaluated under the microscope.

Sperm antibody testing should be done in cases where there are no sperm or mostly nonmotile sperm without explanation. In addition, sperm antibody testing is mandatory when, on the postcoital test, the sperm are found shaking in place but not moving progressively. This shaking movement is a common finding in immunologic infertility.

Attempts have been made to refine the postcoital test either by doing intrauterine aspirations or by doing fractional postcoital tests. (8) The latter technique, which utilizes a polyethylene catheter, is thought to give a better assessment of sperm number at the uppermost portion of the endocervix. Evidence of the value of sampling selectively this particular area versus the entire cervical canal has never been forthcoming. In addition, Drake et al. have shown that sperm distribution is uniform throughout the cervical canal and that selective sampling at the level of the internal os is not necessary. (9)

The need for scheduling the postcoital test at precise times in the cycle may produce problems for the couple who cannot have sex on demand. This may further burden a couple already troubled by the need to cope with their infertility and the loss of control involved in the fertility investigation. A physician must be sympathetic to this problem and, on occasion, precise timing must be sacrificed and the woman told to come into the office following unscheduled intercourse.

Tests of Tubal Patency

A history of pelvic inflammatory disease, septic abortion, intrauterine device (IUD) use, ruptured appendix, or ectopic pregnancy alerts the physician to the possibility of tubal damage. One-half of patients who are eventually found to have tubal damage and/or pelvic adhesions, however, have no history of antecedent disease. There have been a few reports of damaged tubes showing histologic evidence suggestive of viral infection which could explain the absence of traditional causes of tubal damage. In cases of tubal damage of unknown etiology, we have found it both honest and helpful for the patient's peace of mind to suggest that a viral infection in childhood may have caused the problem.

The convenience of performing a Rubin's test with CO_2 in the office and the avoidance of radiation are outweighed by the discomfort of the test and the high percentage of false readings which suggest tubal occlusion. This may result from tubal spasm initiated by the gas.

In our practice, hysterosalpingography (HSG) has replaced the Rubin's. The x-ray study is performed 3–6 days after cessation of the menstrual flow. If there is a history suggestive of pelvic inflammatory disease, a sedimentation rate is first obtained and, if elevated, antibiotic therapy is given. The procedure is scheduled for 2–3 months following treatment, and, shortly before, a repeat sedimentation rate is obtained. If there is a documented history of pelvic inflammatory disease, the risk of a serious infection following HSG is too high, and it should be replaced by laparoscopy. If an HSG is done on a patient who is a questionable risk for infection, a water-soluble rather than an oil-base dye should be used. The antibiotics commonly given as prophylaxis such as tetracyclines and ampicillin are relatively ineffective because they do not eliminate the anaerobic bacteria which are a major cause of the severe infections that can follow an HSG. The overall risk of severe infection with HSG is probably less than 1%, although in a high-risk population it is approximately 3%. (10)

Pelvic examination should always precede the HSG, and if masses or tenderness are found, the HSG should be bypassed in favor of a laparoscopy.

HSG should be done under image intensification fluoroscopy and a minimum number of films taken. Too often multiple oblique views are obtained to delineate minimal defects of the uterus which have no clinical significance. In our experience the oblique films are of little help in diagnosing tubal patency. Only 3 films are usually required—a preliminary film before dye is injected, a film showing spill of dye from one or both tubes, and a delayed film to show the spread of dye through the peritoneal cavity. It is advantageous if the gynecologist does the injection of the dye, but in many instances this is now done by a radiologist. Dye can be injected using a classic Jarcho cannula aided by a single-tooth tenaculum to stabilize the cervix. Alternatively, a suction apparatus can be appended to the cervix and dye injected through a contained cannula. The third technique, and the one we prefer, involves threading a No. 8 pediatric Foley catheter with a deflated 3-ml balloon into the uterus. A drawback is that the balloon, following inflation, may, on occasion, obscure the view of the uterine cavity. There is usually no need to premedicate the patient although some patients benefit from taking codeine or an inhibitor of prostaglandin synthesis just prior to the procedure. An enema is not required. In short, the patient needs little or no preparation, and she certainly does not require an anesthetic.

The dye should be injected slowly so that abnormalities of the uterine cavity are not missed. This is of special importance in diethylstilbestrol (DES) daughters, many of whom have abnormalities of the uterine contour. There is preliminary evidence that DES daughters may have a higher incidence of infertility problems than women who were not exposed to the drug. Usually no more than 3–6 ml of dye are required to fill the uterus and tubes. If the patient complains of cramping, the injection of dye should be stopped for a few minutes and fluoroscopy discontinued temporarily. Spasm is rare with Ethiodol, an oil dye which is our preferred medium. If it does occur, small injections with pauses may be helpful. The droplets which are seen coming from the end of the tube are the result of mixing of the oil dye and peritoneal fluid. On occasion, injection of dye into a hydrosalpinx will produce a similar pattern. The delayed (2–24 hours) film is crucial in differentiating this condition from normal spill. If dye does not pass from the cornua into the tubes, changing the woman to a prone position will sometimes facilitate the passage of dye. (11) If dye goes through one tube rapidly and fails to enter the other tube, it usually means that the dye-containing tube presents the path of least resistance. In this situation the nonfilling tube is usually normal. When both tubes were patent on x-ray, the pregnancy rate in our own series was only slightly higher (58%) than when there was unilateral patency and no fill of the second tube (50%). (12) The proximal portion of the tube should be carefully assessed. A speckled appearance of dye at this point is suggestive of salpingitis isthmica nodosa.

While the diagnostic usefulness of HSG is generally unquestioned, its value as a therapeutic procedure in infertility is the subject of some controversy. While some have found no increase in the pregnancy rate following HSG, Palmer reported that 75% of patients having an HSG showing tubal patency, and whose husbands had normal sperm counts, became pregnant within 1 year of the procedure. (13, 14) This was 3 times the pregnancy rate found by the same author among patients who had not had an HSG. Speculation concerning the precise mode of therapeutic action of HSG has included the following: 1) It may effect a mechanical lavage of the tubes, dislodging mucus plugs. 2) It may straighten the tubes and thus break down peritoneal adhesions. 3) It may provide a stimulatory effect on the cilia of the tube. 4) It may improve the cervical mucus. 5) The iodine may exert a bacteriostatic effect on the mucous membranes.

If HSG does enhance fertility, is the effect seen with both oil- and water-soluble dye? Gillespie reported a conception rate of 41.3% within 1 year with oil medium, whereas the rate was only 27.3% when water-soluble agents were employed. (15) This is similar to our experience. Fertility was enhanced in the 6–7 months following an x-ray done with Ethiodol. (12) A recent study by DeCherney and co-workers confirmed the therapeutic value of Ethiodol. (16) Within 4 months of an HSG with this oil dye, 29% of patients were pregnant. The result was 13% when water-soluble dye was used. In addition to its value in enhancing fertility, Ethiodol produces a better film image than the water-soluble dye, and there is a lower incidence of pain upon injection. The use of an oil medium has been criticized on the grounds that it is only slowly absorbed and may cause granuloma formation in the peritoneum. This is very rare. An additional fear with oil dye is embolization. Bateman et al. reported that there were 13 cases of dye intravasation in 533 HSGs performed with Ethiodol. (17) Six of these women had embolization of the dye, but there were no symptoms, and no morbidity was noted. The authors emphasized that, when fluoroscopy is used, venous or lymphatic intravasation can be detected immediately and injection of dye halted. Intravasation appears initially as a fine network adjacent to the uterine cavity. This is followed by streak-like opacities extending toward the pelvic sidewalls and then moving in a cephalad direction. Siegler, in his book on HSG, reported 9 deaths attributable to the procedure. (18) Lipiodol, an oil medium which is more viscid than Ethiodol, was used in 6 of these cases, the last occurring in 1947. Since that time there has been only 1 fatality reported; it occurred in 1959 after embolization of a water-soluble dye.

Disorders of Ovulation

Disorders of ovulation account for 10–15% of all infertility problems. These may be either anovulation or severe oligoovulation. In the latter cases, even though ovulation does occur, its relative infrequency diminishes the woman's chances for pregnancy. If a woman has periods only every 3 or 4 months, for practical purposes it matters little whether these are ovulatory or anovulatory. She should be treated with clomiphene to increase the frequency of, or to initiate, ovulation (see Chapter 20), and this can be started immediately, even before other areas have been investigated.

Basal Body Temperature

Women who have menstrual periods at monthly intervals marked by premenstrual symptoms and dysmenorrhea are almost always ovulatory. Indirect confirmatory evidence of ovulation is obtained by use of basal body temperature (BBT) charts. The temperature can be taken either orally or rectally with a regular thermometer or with special instruments that show a range of only a few degrees and thus are easier to read. It is worth emphasizing that the temperature is best taken immediately upon awakening and before any activity. The woman may be surprised to find that the basal temperatures are substantially lower than the usual 98.6°F. Characteristically, prior to ovulation they are in the 97.2–97.4°F range, and after ovulation the basal temperature is over 98°F. Use of the BBT chart has been criticized because a small percentage of women who ovulate have monophasic graphs, and there is often disagreement among physicians concerning the interpretation of individual charts. We find the charts helpful when they are clearly

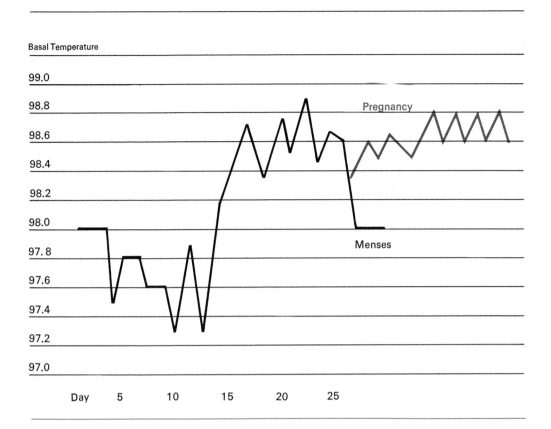

Basal Temperature

99.0
98.8
98.6
98.4
98.2
98.0
97.8
97.6
97.4
97.2
97.0

Pregnancy

Menses

Day   5   10   15   20   25

biphasic, and seek confirmatory evidence when the BBT is unclear. An important clinical point is that a slow rise in a biphasic chart is not an indication of a hormone abnormality. Days when intercourse takes place should be noted on the chart, and this may give the physician an indication that coital frequency is a problem.

Even using temperature charts, no one can pinpoint the exact day of ovulation. A significant increase in temperature is not noted until 2 days after the luteinizing hormone (LH) peak, which coincides with a rise in peripheral levels of progesterone to greater than 4 ng/ml. (19) Physical release of the ovum probably occurs on the day prior to the time of the first temperature elevation. This may or may not be marked by a dip in the temperature to the lowest level of the cycle. The temperature rise should be sustained for 11–16 days and it will then drop at the time of the subsequent menstrual period. If an approximate time of ovulation can be determined by temperature charts, a sensible schedule for coitus is every 36–48 hours in a period encompassed by 3–4 days prior to, and including 2–3 days after, expected ovulation. Although this timing would be ideal, it is unwise to demand rigid adherence to a schedule. This may produce psychologic stress sufficient to inhibit sexual relations.

In discussing coital timing, the patient will usually want to know the fertilizable life of the sperm and the egg. The information on human gametes is speculative. Cases have been reported where isolated coitus even up to 7 days prior to the rise in BBT has resulted in pregnancy, but this probably represents the limits of biologic variation. Estimates have been made that sperm usually retain their ability to fertilize for 24–48 hours, and that the human egg is fertilizable for 12–24 hours.

Endometrial Biopsy

Biopsy is performed 2–3 days prior to the expected period and the histology is read by the criteria outlined by Noyes et al. (20) While premenstrual biopsy may present the possibility of interrupting a pregnancy if performed in a conception cycle, the danger is minimal. Buxton and Olson, in their study of biopsies done during the conception cycle, found that only 2 of 26 patients aborted. (21) The alternative of taking the biopsy on the first day of menses has three disadvantages: 1) inconvenient time for patient and physician, 2) the tissue is disrupted and often more difficult to interpret, and 3) a slight amount of bleeding may occur at the time of the expected period even if the patient has become pregnant. We have found the Meig's curette (Codman and Shurtleff, Inc.) very suitable for obtaining a small strip of tissue from high on the anterior wall.

Progesterone

A serum progesterone value of 3–4 ng/ml or greater is indicative of ovulation. However, values at the midluteal phase, just at the midpoint between ovulation and the onset of the subsequent menstrual period, should be 10 ng/ml or more. Lower levels at this time can indicate insufficient hormone production by the corpus luteum.

Inadequate Luteal Phase

An inadequate luteal phase is due to a relative deficiency in secretion of progesterone by the corpus luteum. The term has been applied to both a short interval (less than 11 days) between ovulation and menstruation, with relatively normal peak values of progesterone, and more commonly, to a luteal phase of normal length with lower than normal progesterone levels. Both result in inadequate stimulation of the endometrium. A related, but rare, condition is caused by the absence of progesterone receptors in the endometrium. An inadequate luteal phase can be found in isolated cycles of normal women, and only if the defect is found repetitively is it thought to be a significant factor in infertility. Approximately 3–4% of infertile women will be diagnosed as having an inadequate luteal phase; the incidence may be higher in women with a history of habitual abortion. (22)

Although an inadequate luteal phase is a direct result of decreased hormone production by the corpus luteum, the underlying causes of this dysfunction can be multiple. Decreased levels of follicle-stimulating hormone (FSH) in the follicular phase of the cycle, and decreased levels of

FSH and LH at the time of ovulation have been implicated. More recently it has been shown that elevated prolactin levels may be associated with an inadequate luteal phase. (23)

The diagnosis should be considered in women with normal cycles and unexplained infertility, in women with a short luteal phase as demonstrated by basal temperature charts, and in women with a history of habitual abortion. The diagnosis can be approached in a number of ways. The BBT chart may be biphasic but the duration of the rise may be less than 11 days. A diagnosis made on the basis of basal temperature charts should be corroborated by endometrial biopsy taken from high on the fundus of the uterus. Even with a normal temperature chart, an endometrial biopsy taken 2–3 days prior to menstruation can indicate that the development of the endometrium lags behind the cycle day (in relation to the onset of the subsequent menstrual period) by more than 2 days. The lag must be more than 2 days. Tredway et al., using the LH surge to pinpoint ovulation, found 5 of 11 normally ovulating women had biopsies 2 days out of synchrony with the day of onset of the subsequent menstrual cycle. (24) This is a crucial point. Some physicians have suggested that a biopsy found to be 2 days out of phase makes the diagnosis of inadequate luteal phase. Many normal women will be inaccurately categorized as having hormone deficiency if the 2-day criterion is used.

There may be difficulties in establishing a diagnosis based on the histologic criteria. There can be differences in interpretation by different observers. The endometrial sample can show varying patterns, and there may be discrepancies between the maturation of the glands and that of the stroma. Despite these drawbacks, endometrial biopsy remains the classical way to diagnose an inadequate luteal phase.

Because of the discomfort and expense associated with endometrial biopsy, attention has turned to direct measurements of serum progesterone levels as a means of diagnosing the adequacy of the luteal phase. The exact values of progesterone that are needed to rule out an inadequate luteal phase are in dispute. Radwanska et al. have claimed that a single value of 10 ng/ml or more 5–10 days prior to the next period effectively rules out an inadequate luteal phase. (25) More recently, however, she also treated women with values between 10 and 15 ng/ml. (26) It is uncertain, therefore, whether Radwanska believes that 10 or 15 ng/ml is the true lower limit of normal. Proponents of use of the biopsy cite cases of women who have progesterone levels above these values, but who, on biopsy, are found to have an endometrium with the characteristic lag of an inadequate luteal phase. (27, 28)

Admittedly based upon limited information, our feeling is that if the basal temperature chart shows a normal luteal phase length, and if 2 serum progesterones taken near the midluteal phase in one cycle are both above 10 ng/ml, it is unlikely that the patient is infertile because of luteal phase inadequacy. Furthermore, based upon 1) the experience that only 3–4% of infertile women have an inadequate luteal phase, 2) the requirement that the diagnosis be based upon positive findings in 2 cycles, 3) the fact that 30% of women will have an occasional inadequate luteal phase on biopsy which is not repetitive and therefore they are not candidates for therapy, and 4) that treatment with progesterone is associated with a 50% pregnancy rate, it can be calculated that somewhere between 72 and 88 endometrial biopsies must be done to achieve one pregnancy. Remember, too, that successful pregnancies have occurred without treatment in women who were diagnosed as having an inadequate luteal phase. (29) In addition, it is somewhat disappointing to note that, despite the numerous articles that have been written during the past 30 years about the inadequate luteal phase, there are *no controlled studies* which conclusively establish either its role as a cause for infertility, or the value of therapy. Information on the usefulness of treatment must be obtained from clinical reports in the literature, as well as through physician observations.

Based upon findings that some cases of inadequate luteal phase are due to low FSH values, it would seem reasonable, in selected cases, to use human menopausal gonadotropins (HMG, Pergonal) or clomiphene citrate. A rational explanation for the mechanism of inadequate luteal function is found in the sequence of receptor formation and action in the growing follicle. The key is to achieve an adequate number of LH receptors on the granulosa cells. This is accomplished by adequate FSH stimulation, and therefore, it is not surprising that increasing FSH levels is an effective therapeutic approach. Because of its potential for causing hyperstimulation of the ovaries and multiple births, Pergonal is a poor choice. Clomiphene has been used in treating inadequate luteal phase, with some claiming good success, and it is our first choice. (30) Its risks are small (see Chapter 20). The usual starting dose is 50 mg daily for 5 days starting on the 5th day of the cycle.

Because there is a deficiency of progesterone in the inadequate luteal phase, replacement by exogenous progesterone has been utilized. Progesterone is not active by mouth, and Jones has pioneered the use of progesterone vaginal suppositories. (27) A suppository containing 25 mg of progesterone is inserted twice a day starting approximately 3 days after ovulation. Treatment is maintained until menstruation occurs or until pregnancy is diagnosed. Once the pregnancy test is positive, a switch is made to 17-hydroxyprogesterone caproate, 250 mg i.m. weekly through week 12 of pregnancy. Using this therapy, success rates of approximately 50% have been achieved.

The progesterone suppositories are not available commercially and they must be compounded by a pharmacist from the following formula: Progesterone powder, 44 gm; polyethylene glycol 400, 2096 gm; polyethylene glycol 6000, 1392 gm. This makes 1760 suppositories of 25 mg each. Another method of treatment, but one that is more troublesome to administer, is the use of progesterone in oil 12.5 mg daily by injection.

Progesterone replaces the missing hormone. An alternative treatment, human chorionic gonadotropin (HCG) 2500 IU by intramuscular injection every 3 days starting 3 days after ovulation and continuing for 4 doses, has been advocated to stimulate the corpus luteum to produce more progesterone. The patient should be warned that this therapy may delay the onset of menses without the occurrence of pregnancy. Because the mechanism of the inadequate luteal phase is probably a deficiency of LH receptors, HCG treatment should not be effective, and we do not recommend its use.

Medroxyprogesterone acetate has been a popular drug for treatment of an inadequate luteal phase. However, in doses higher than those commonly used, it has been found to have a luteolytic effect, and this may interfere with the goals of the therapy. (31) In addition, there is evidence that synthetic steroids given during pregnancy may increase the risk of fetal malformation. We conclude that the use of medroxyprogesterone acetate in treatment of the inadequate luteal phase is both unwise and potentially hazardous.

The Food and Drug Administration has also raised questions concerning possible teratogenic effects of progesterone. At the time of this writing the issue has not been resolved; but it seems unlikely that use of natural progesterone involves a significant risk.

Bromocriptine (Parlodel) has been reported to correct luteal phase defects associated with hyperprolactinemia. In our practice it is the drug of choice in the presence of galactorrhea or an elevated prolactin. However, its value in women with normal prolactin levels has not been demonstrated, especially in controlled studies. (32).

Mycoplasma

Mycoplasma, a pleuropneumonia-like organism, has been implicated as a possible cause of habitual abortion, and also salpingitis and other sexually transmitted diseases. Gnarpe and Friberg reported that infertile couples had a markedly higher prevalence of T-mycoplasma (now called *Ureaplasma urealyticum*) in cervical mucus and semen than did a group of fertile women and men. (33) Treatment with doxycycline decreased the numbers of couples with mycoplasma and also was associated with pregnancy in 15 of 52 couples (29%), all of whom had had primary infertility for at least 5 years. However, a series of reports from England agreed with these findings in only one respect. (34, 35) They confirmed that treatment with doxycycline could eliminate mycoplasma from the genital tract of the majority of indi-

481

viduals. In these studies, however, there were no differences in the frequency of either T-strain or *Mycoplasma hominis* between infertile and fertile couples. In a double blind study, treatment with doxycycline for 28 days had no effect on the rate of conception, and the English group suggested that culturing for mycoplasma in the routine investigation of infertility was unrewarding. (35) A number of other studies also have failed to show infection with mycoplasma as a cause for infertility. At present, there is no rationale for the empiric treatment of infertile couples with doxycycline or any other tetracyclines. Similarly, although chlamydia may be a causative agent in tubal infection and cervicitis, there is no evidence that it is a cause for infertility in couples who have a normal workup.

Sperm Allergy

This is the most troublesome area of the infertility investigation because of the lack of controlled studies which offer clear guidance to the clinician. Most studies have concerned themselves with the role of agglutinating antibodies found in the serum. In men there is a good correlation between the titer of agglutinating antibodies and the prognosis for future fertility. (36) In women, a clear correlation is not found. For example, the prognosis for pregnancy does not appear to be influenced by the presence or absence of agglutinating antibodies in the woman's serum, and many fertile women have positive reactions. In addition, agglutinating antibodies can be found in nonimmunologic components of the serum. (37)

A complement-dependent sperm immobilization test is a more precise method of determining immunologic infertility in women. It is positive in 5–10% of women with unexplained infertility and is almost never positive in fertile controls. (38) Jones has suggested that sperm immobilization tests be performed on both serum and cervical mucus, because antibodies to sperm have been found in the mucus in individuals who do not have circulating antibodies. (39, 40) Working with mucus is a more logical approach, but it may be difficult for a clinical laboratory. Testing of mucus may be suitable only in laboratories with a special interest in the field. Use of a fluorescent antibody test or radiolabeled testing has not been shown at this time to be an advantage.

A crucial, but unresolved question, is whether all couples with unexplained infertility should be tested for sperm antibodies or whether it should be restricted to only those couples with poor postcoital tests. Our current practice, which is admittedly controversial, is to test only when repetitive postcoital tests show mostly immobilized sperm, sperm with shaking tails but no progressive motility, or no sperm despite a normal semen analysis and adequate coital technique. We also test if the semen shows massive agglutination of sperm on repetitive tests.

Treatment has also been the subject of controversy. Occlusive condom therapy has been used in the presence of agglutinating antibodies in women. Results, however, are uncertain. In addition, there is no evidence that the pregnancy rate is increased when occlusive therapy is used to treat immobilizing antibodies. The use of high dose corticosteroids (methylprednisolone 96 mg/day for 7 days) has been suggested, but side effects and the potential risks (one individual suffered bilateral aseptic necrosis of the femoral heads following steroid treatment for sperm antibodies) seem to outweigh any current evidence of success. (41) A few women have been treated with intrauterine inseminations of washed sperm in order to remove antigens and to bypass antibodies localized in the cervix. (41) The cases reported to date are too few to provide an estimate of the efficacy of this approach. It holds scant theoretical promise because most antigens adhere tightly to the sperm membrane and are unlikely to be washed free; or they are intrinsic constituents of the sperm membrane. In addition, if there are antibodies in the cervix there is a good possibility that they are also present in the uterus. In males with positive antibody tests, treatment of genitourinary infection, if present, is worthwhile. Use of high doses of corticosteroid for males is open to the same reservations expressed above. (42) In addition, evidence for its success is currently lacking despite claims to the contrary.

In summary, it is our impression that there are only a few men and women who are infertile on the basis of an immunologic reaction. It is worthwhile to try to diagnose these cases by testing both the male and the female for agglutinating and immobilizing antibodies. We test for sperm antibodies when there is a poor postcoital test with no explanation or when the semen shows massive agglutination of the sperm on repeated examinations.

Endoscopy

Laparoscopy is the final diagnostic procedure of any infertility investigation. If the HSG is normal, the endoscopic procedure is done after an interval of 6 months from the x-ray. This allows time for the fertility-enhancing effect of the x-ray procedure. Because of the possible benefit from the HSG, we disagree with physicians who bypass it and go directly to laparoscopy. An exception is the individual who is at high risk for pelvic infection. Obviously, if the HSG shows tubal occlusion or other major abnormalities, we do not hold to the 6-month delay. The findings at laparoscopy agree with those of HSG in approximately two thirds of the cases. The major area of disagreement is the failure of the HSG to detect pelvic adhesions. Approximately 50% of patients undergoing laparoscopy will have pelvic pathology, usually endometriosis or pelvic adhesions. With due care in selection of cases, some of these abnormalities can be treated through the laparoscope either by lysis of thin adhesions or fulguration of implants of endometriosis if pain is a problem. If manipulation through the laparoscope is not possible, alternative approaches include laparotomy or hormone therapy. For techniques of infertility surgery, the reader is referred to the monograph by Kistner and Patton, and the volume on *Microsurgery* by Silber. (43, 44)

When findings at laparoscopy are combined with those of the other test procedures, the majority of couples with an undiagnosed infertility problem will be discovered to have a cause for their inability to conceive. Still there will be approximately 10% of couples in whom no abnormality is found.

Hormonal Treatment for Habitual Abortion in the First Trimester

Abortion is defined as the termination of pregnancy before 20 weeks of gestation or below a fetal weight of 500 gm. Approximately 15% of all pregnancies between 4–20 weeks of gestation will undergo spontaneous abortion. The true abortion rate is closer to 50% because of the high rate of abortion in the 1–4 weeks immediately following conception. The majority of these cases are caused by chromosomal abnormalities in the sperm or the egg.

Habitual abortion classically has been defined as 3 or more consecutive abortions. In 1938, Malpas, using theoretical calculations, stated that a woman with a history of 3 consecutive abortions had a 73% chance of aborting in the next pregnancy. (45) In 1946 Eastman presented statistical calculations indicating that after 3 abortions the risk was 83.6%. (46) These early papers, based primarily upon intuition rather than clinical studies, established the notion that the chance for a subsequent abortion increases dramatically with each successive abortion and that after 3 abortions the chances for a successful pregnancy are very low. Studies on the efficacy of many types of treatments used these pessimistic figures for comparison rather than containing their own controls. If treatment increased the salvage rate to 70% it was considered curative. However, clinical studies have indicated that the risk of abortion after 3 successive abortions is in fact only 30–55%. (47–49) The projections by Malpas and Eastman were theoretical exercises which were not confirmed when appropriate data were collected. Thus, it is not surprising that treatment with a wide range of approaches, including vitamins and psychotherapy, produced successful pregnancies in a reasonable percentage of women with habitual abortion. These cures were not due to the therapy but, rather, the claims for success were based on a comparison with the discredited statistics of Malpas and Eastman.

Despite the knowledge that the spontaneous salvage rate is 45–70%, it is still worth trying to uncover causes for repetitive first trimester pregnancy losses. A recognized cause for the problem is a genetic abnormality, and karyotyping of couples will reveal that 8% have some abnormality, most frequently a translocation. (50) Karyotyping is especially vital if the couple have had a malformed infant or fetus in addition to abortions. It is important to emphasize that karyotyping uncovers only a percentage of those pregnancies lost due to genetic abnormalities. There may be single gene defects which are not manifested by chromosomal abnormalities, and it is very likely that a percentage of those patients now considered to have unexplained repetitive pregnancy loss have this type of genetic defect. In addition, karyotyping of blood cells misses abnormalities of meiosis, which can be found in sperm cell lines. If the karyotype is abnormal, nothing can be done to lessen the chances for another abortion. Amniocentesis should be offered, however, in any pregnancy that goes beyond the first trimester, because of the risk of an abnormal child.

Approximately 12–15% of women with habitual abortion have a uterine malformation, and this can be diagnosed by HSG. Surgical repair of these defects is rewarded with salvage rates in the 70–80% range.

Study of the role of hormonal deficiency as a cause of habitual abortion has largely focused on deficiencies of progesterone or its metabolites. Attempts to implicate low pregnanediol levels in early pregnancy as a cause for abortion, and, as a corollary, to treat with exogenous progesterone or progestins, have been shown to be fruitless. (51) A second approach has been to diagnose an inadequate luteal phase during the nonpregnant state and to initiate treatment with progesterone a few days after each ovulation. Jones claimed that 30% of women with pregnancy wastage had an inadequate luteal phase, whereas Tho et al. found that 23% of the women in their group of 100 couples with recurrent abortion had an inadequate luteal phase. (50, 52) In this latter study it was unclear whether the diagnosis was made on the basis of only one endometrial biopsy. If this were so, their report overdiagnoses the frequency of inadequate luteal phase. Botella-Llusia found that 38% of women with 3 or more consecutive abortions had poorly developed secretory endometrium compared with only 6% of infertile women. (53)

Two studies dealt with serum progesterone levels of women who had had 3 consecutive abortions. One study indicated that 10 such women had abnormally low levels of progesterone during the luteal phase, and all 10 women subsequently aborted again. (54) The authors neglected to indicate how the women were selected for the study, although all were said to have progestational deficiency on biopsy. The second study found that 6 habitual aborters had a midluteal serum progesterone concentration of greater than 4 ng/ml and 5 had full-term pregnancies. (55) The fate of the 6th woman was not specified. Four other women did not become pregnant again. Three of them had progesterone values below 4 ng/ml. Interestingly, there were no subsequent abortions in this latter study. Hensleigh and Fainstat treated women, who had a history of recurrent abortion and a serum progesterone level below 10 ng/ml, with progesterone suppositories. (56) In addition, they treated women with a similar history who had serum progesterones below 15 ng/ml during the first trimester of pregnancy. While their results were good in terms of pregnancy outcome, the study contained no controls, and for that reason can be judged only as an interesting observation.

The uncertainty that plagues physicians in dealing with the inadequate luteal phase in infertility is also apparent when considering habitual abortion. If repetitive endometrial biopsies or progesterones are abnormal or if the BBT chart shows a luteal phase of less than 11 days, it is reasonable to treat with clomiphene or progesterone suppositories as described in the section on the inadequate luteal phase. Progesterone should be used only if these criteria are met; it should not be used empirically. Placebo treatment may be useful in maintaining a physician/patient relationship in which the patient derives needed psychologic sustenance. It seems to us, however, that the use of a hormonal substance for placebo effect on the basis of no known harmful effect denies the important lesson learned in the discovery of the relationship between DES treatment and vaginal neoplasia. Reputed harmlessness is a potentially dangerous approach based on negative data. It must be remembered that there is a reasonable cure rate in unexplained habitual abortion, even without treatment.

Other causes of pregnancy loss include lack of blocking antibodies, infections with herpesvirus, and lupus erythematosus. (57) It has been reported, but disputed, that some women with recurrent abortions have a significantly increased frequency of sharing HLA antigens with their spouses. There have been attempts to treat habitual abortion by injecting the female with white blood cells from the spouse, but the number of cases treated is so small that it precludes any evaluation of efficacy.

The patient with recurrent abortions usually presents as an anxious, frustrated individual on the verge of despair. Evaluation should be spaced over several visits, allowing the physician to establish communication and rapport with the patient. The emotional support that the physician can bring to this interaction will be most useful, and in some cases may be therapeutic. (58)

Infertility and Age

Because many women are delaying attempts to become pregnant until they are in their late 30s or even their early 40s, there is a great deal of interest in the decline of fertility with age. Some of the best information comes from a study of Hutterite women published by Dr. Christopher Tietze. (59) The Hutterites are a religious sect who live on communal farms in Montana and neighboring areas in the United States and Canada. Their fertility rate is high and the use of contraception is proscribed by their religion. Only 5 of the 209 women studied by Tietze had never had any children. Eleven percent of the Hutterite women bore no children after age 34, 33% were infertile by age 40, and 87% had no children after age 44. A study reported from France on pregnancy following donor insemination (AID) also

486

indicated a decline in fertility associated with age, but the magnitude of the decline has been disputed. (60) The attractiveness of the AID study is that it eliminates coital frequency as a variable. In the French study, which looked at conception occurring over 1 year's time, the pregnancy rate was approximately 74% before age 31, whereas it was 61.5% between the ages of 31 and 35, and 53.6% for those women older than 35. The study was criticized because it was felt that the 1-year cutoff was too soon, and that optimum fertility is not achieved with AID. Despite these reservations that the French figures are too low, it is reasonable to conclude that there is a decline of fertility with age, but this decline is not precipitous until the woman enters her 40s. Overall, the information should be reassuring to those who desire postponing pregnancy beyond their 20s.

Myths

It is important for physicians and other health care professionals to dispel some of the myths that are associated with infertility. We suggested earlier in this chapter that women should not be told that they are infertile because they are too nervous. Physicians who tell patients that if they relax they will become pregnant are perpetuating an old wive's tale and are doing a disservice to their patients.

It is now quite clear that, despite many anecdotes to the contrary, adoption does not increase a couple's fertility. (61) The treatment of euthyroid infertile women with thyroid has been repeatedly shown to be worthless. We see no advantage in doing a dilatation and curettage (D and C), because it neither enhances fertility nor provides information that cannot be picked up in a routine infertility investigation and subjects the woman to the risks and expense of anesthesia. By the same token we have seen no improvement in fertility following dilatation of the cervical canal.

It is important when doing a pelvic examination not to make comments suggesting that the uterus is small. The woman may interpret this to mean that she cannot become pregnant. The uterus has a tremendous capacity for expansion given the proper stimulus, and this holds true for every size uterus. Therefore, we do not believe that the so-called infantile or hypoplastic uterus should ever be blamed for infertility.

Although almost every physician who writes about the use of clomiphene suggests that its proper place is for induction of ovulation, or for regulation of ovulation time in the cycle, there is no doubt that the drug is widely prescribed for fertile women who have perfectly regular and normal ovulatory function. This reflects both a demand by patients who refer to it as a "fertility pill," thinking that it has a nonspecific effect of enhancing fertility, and the response by physicians who want to do something positive for their patients. This is understandable although not desirable. If couples are informed of the risks of multiple births, the rare ovarian cysts caused by clomiphene, and the small risk of unrecognized future hazards (see Chapter 20), we do not condemn its use even though there is no evidence that it improves fertility. An argument in favor of clomiphene use in ovulatory cycles, although strictly theoretical, is that it can cause ovulation of more than one egg, and this may increase the chance for at least one egg to be fertilized during a given cycle. On the other hand, Trounson and colleagues have shown by in vitro fertilization of human eggs that many cases of unexplained infertility are caused by failure of sperm to penetrate the egg. (62) This has important implications because it would mean that manipulations, such as giving clomiphene or using artificial insemination, when there is no indication for their use, hold very little promise of enhancing fertility.

On balance it would be better if physicians could avoid the philosophy of "try it, it just might work." There are many disillusioned couples who, without any indication, have been given clomiphene, Provera, low dose estrogen, thyroid, and then have been treated with husband inseminations. The goals of the practitioner should be to accomplish a thorough investigation, to treat any abnormalities that are uncovered, to educate the couple to the workings of the reproductive system, to give the couple some estimate of their fertility potential, to counsel for adoption when appropriate, and to provide emotional support. If these goals are achieved by a sympathetic and understanding physician, they will satisfy most couples who suffer from infertility.

References

1. **Debner HCB,** Psychiatric aspects of infertility, J Reprod Med 20:23, 1978.

2. **White RM, Glass RH,** Intrauterine insemination of husband's sperm, Obstet Gynecol 47:119, 1976.

3. **Jette NT, Glass RH,** Prognostic value of the postcoital test, Fertil Steril 23:29, 1972.

4. **Kovacs GT, Newman GB, Henson GL,** The postcoital test: what is normal? Br Med J 1:818, 1978.

5. **Asch RH,** Laparoscopic recovery of sperm from peritoneal fluid in patients with negative or poor Sims-Huhner test, Fertil Steril 27:1111, 1976.

6. **Goldenberg R, White R,** The effect of vaginal lubricants on sperm motility in vitro, Fertil Steril 26:872, 1975.

7. **Ansari AH, Gould KG, Ansari VM,** Sodium bicarbonate douching for improvement of the postcoital test, Fertil Steril 33:608, 1980.

8. **Moran J, Davajan V, Nakamura R,** Comparison of the fractional post coital test with the Sims-Huhner post coital test, Int J Fertil 19:93, 1974.

9. **Drake TS, Tredway DR, Buchanan GC,** A reassessment of the fractional postcoital test, Am J Obstet Gynecol 133:382 1979.

10. **Stumpf PG, March CM,** Febrile morbidity following hysterosalpingography: identification of risk factors and recommendations for prophylaxis, Fertil Steril 33:487, 1980.

11. **Spring D,** Prone hysterosalpingography, Radiology 136:235, 1980.

12. **Mackey RA, Glass RH, Olson LE, Vaidya RA,** Pregnancy following hysterosalpingography with oil and water soluble dye, Fertil Steril 22:504, 1971.

13. **Whitelaw MJ, Foster TN, Graham WH,** Hysterosalpingography and insufflation, J Reprod Med 4:56, 1970.

14. **Palmer A,** Ethiodol hysterosalpingography for the treatment of infertility, Fertil Steril 11:311, 1960.

15. **Gillespie HW,** The therapeutic aspect of hysterosalpingography, Br J Radiol 38:301, 1965.

16. **DeCherney AH, Kort H, Barner JB, DeVore GR,** Increased pregnancy rate with oil soluble hysterosalpingography dye, Fertil Steril 33:407, 1980.

17. **Bateman BG, Nunley WC Jr, Kitchin JD,** Intravasation during hysterosalpingography using oil-base contrast media, Fertil Steril 34:439, 1980.

18. **Siegler AM,** *Hysterosalpingography*, Medcon Press, New York, 1974.

19. **Moghissi KS, Syner FN, Evans TN,** A composite picture of the menstrual cycle, Am J Obstet Gynecol 114:405, 1972.

20. **Noyes RW, Hertig AT, Rock J,** Dating the endometrial biopsy, Fertil Steril 1:3, 1950.

21. **Buxton CL, Olson LE,** Endometrial biopsy inadvertently taken during conception cycle, Am J Obstet Gynecol 105:702, 1969.

22. **Murthy YS, Arronet GH, Parekh MC,** Luteal phase inadequacy, Obstet Gynecol 36:758, 1970.

23. **Del Pozo E, Wyss H, Tolis G, Alcaniz J, Campana A, Naftolin F,** Prolactin and deficient luteal function, Obstet Gynecol 53:282, 1979.

24. **Tredway DR, Mishell DR Jr, Moyer DL,** Correlation of endometrial dating with luteinizing hormone peak, Am J Obstet Gynecol 117:1030, 1973.

25. **Radwanska E, McGarrigle HHG, Swyer GIM,** Plasma progesterone and oestradiol estimations in the diagnosis and treatment of luteal insufficiency in menstruating infertile women, Acta Eur Infertil 7:39, 1976.

26. **Radwanska E, Hammond MJ, Smith P,** Single midluteal progesterone assay in the management of ovulatory infertility, J Reprod Med 26:85, 1981.

27. **Jones GE, Aksel S, Wentz AC,** Serum progesterone values in the luteal phase defects: effect of chorionic gonadotropin, Obstet Gynecol 56:26, 1974.

28. **Rosenfeld DL, Chudow S, Bronson RA,** Diagnosis of luteal phase insufficiency, Obstet Gynecol 56:193, 1980.

29. **Driessen F, Holwerda PJ, Putte SCJ, Kremer J,** The significance of dating an endometrial biopsy for the prognosis of the infertile couple, Int J Fertil 25:112, 1980.

30. **Quagliarello J, Weiss G,** Clomiphene citrate in the management of infertility associated with shortened luteal phase, Fertil Steril 31:373, 1979.

31. **Johansson EDB,** Depression of the progesterone levels in women treated with synthetic gestagens after ovulation, Acta Endocrinol 68:779, 1971.

32. **Saunders DM, Hunter JC, Haase HR, Wilson GR,** Treatment of luteal phase inadequacy with bromocriptine, Obstet Gynecol 53:287, 1979.

33. **Gnarpe H, Friberg J,** T-mycoplasmas as a possible cause for reproductive failure, Nature (Lond) 242:120, 1973.

34. **de Louvois J, Blades M, Harrison RF, Hurley R, Stanley VC,** Frequency of mycoplasma in fertile and infertile couples, Lancet 1:1073, 1974.

35. **Harrison RF, de Louvois J, Blades M, Hurley R,** Doxycycline treatment and human infertility, Lancet 1:605, 1975.

36. **Rumke P, Van Amstel N, Messer EN, Bezemer PD,** Prognosis of fertility of men with sperm agglutins in the serum, Fertil Steril 25:393, 1974.

37. **Boettcher B, Kay DJ,** Agglutination of spermatozoa by human sera with added steroids, Andrologie 5:265, 1973.

38. **Isojima S, Li T, Ashitaka Y,** Immunologic analysis of sperm immobilizing factor found in sera of women with unexplained infertility, Am J Obstet Gynecol 101:677, 1968.

39. **Jones WR,** Immunological infertility, fact or fiction? Fertil Steril 33:577, 1980.

40. **Parish WE, Caron-Brown JA, Richards CB,** The detection of antibodies to spermatozoa and the blood group antigens in cervical mucus, J Reprod Fertil 13:469, 1967.

41. **Shulman S, Harlin B, Davis P, Reyniak JV,** Immune infertility and new approaches to treatment, Fertil Steril 29:309, 1978.

42. **Shulman S,** Treatment of immune male infertility with methylprednisolone, Lancet 2:1243, 1976.

43. **Kistner RW, Patton GW Jr,** *Atlas of Infertility Surgery,* Little Brown, Boston, 1975.

44. **Silber S,** *Microsurgery,* Williams & Wilkins, Baltimore, 1979.

45. **Malpas P,** A study of abortion sequence, J Obstet Gynaecol Br Emp 45:932, 1938.

46. **Eastman NJ,** Habitual abortion, in *Progress in Gynecology, Vol. I,* Meigs JV, Sturgis S, eds, Grune & Stratton, New York, 1946.

47. **Warburton D, Fraser FC,** Spontaneous abortion risks in man: data from reproductive histories collected in a medical genetics unit, Am J Hum Genet 16:1, 1964.

48. **James WH,** Notes toward an epidemiology of spontaneous abortion, Am J Hum Genet 15:223, 1963.

49. **Poland BJ, Miller JR, Jones DC, Trimble BK,** Reproductive counseling in patients who have had a spontaneous abortion, Am J Obstet Gynecol 127:685, 1977.

50. **Tho PT, Byrd JR, McDonough PG,** Etiologies and subsequent reproductive performance of 100 couples with recurrent abortion, Fertil Steril 32:389, 1978.

51. **Shearman RP, Garrett WJ,** Double blind study of effect of 17-hydroxyprogesterone caproate on abortion rate, Br Med J 1:292, 1963.

52. **Jones GES, Delfs E,** Endocrine patterns in term pregnancies following abortion, JAMA 146:1212, 1951.

53. **Botella-Llusia J,** The endometrium in repeated abortion, Int J Fertil 7:147, 1962.

54. **Hernandez Horta JL, Gordillo Fernandez J, Soto de Leon B, Cortes-Gallegos V,** Direct evidence of luteal insufficiency in women with habitual abortion, Obstet Gynecol 49:705, 1977.

55. **Yip SK, Sung ML,** Plasma progesterone in women with a history of recurrent early abortions, Fertil Steril 28:151, 1977.

56. **Hensleigh PA, Fainstat T,** Corpus luteum dysfunction: serum progesterone levels in diagnosis and assessment of therapy for recurrent and threatened abortion, Fertil Steril 32:396, 1979.

57. **Glass RH, Golbus MS,** Habitual abortion, Fertil Steril 29:257, 1978.

58. **Tupper C, Weil RJ,** The problem of spontaneous abortion: IX. The treatment of habitual aborters by psychotherapy, Am J Obstet Gynecol 83:421, 1962.

59. **Tietze C,** Reproductive span and rate of reproduction among Hutterite women, Fertil Steril 8:89, 1957.

60. **Federation CECOS, Schwartz D, Mayaux MJ,** Female fecundity as a function of age, N Engl J Med 306:404, 1982.

61. **Rock J, Tietze C, McLaughlin MB,** Effect of adoption on infertility, Fertil Steril 16:305, 1965.

62. **Trounson AO, Leeton JF, Wood C, Webb J, Kovacs G,** The investigation of idiopathic infertility by in vitro fertilization, Fertil Steril 34:431, 1980.

18 Endometriosis and Infertility

Very few problems in infertility have as many unresolved questions as does endometriosis. Does minimal endometriosis cause infertility? What is the proper treatment of endometriosis—surgery or drugs? If a drug is used, should it be the birth control pill or danazol? What is the minimum effective dose of danazol? If surgery is performed, should it be accompanied by preoperative or postoperative use of danazol or birth control pills?

The introduction of danazol for the treatment of endometriosis stimulated renewed interest in the disease. As a result, studies are providing information that can allow the clinician to provide educated answers to some of the perplexing problems involved in the management of endometriosis. Before considering the more recent information, it is worthwhile to review what is known about the etiology and pathophysiology of endometriosis.

Endometriosis was described in the medical literature in the 1800s, but it was not until this century that its common occurrence was appreciated. Based on clinical observation and examination of histopathologic specimens, Dr. John Sampson of Albany, in 1921, suggested that peritoneal endometriosis in the pelvis arose from seedings from ovarian endometriosis. Subsequently, in 1927, he published his classic paper, "Peritoneal Endometriosis Due to Menstrual Dissemination of Endometrial Tissue into the Peritoneal Cavity," which established retrograde flow of endometrial tissue through the Fallopian tubes and into the abdominal

493

cavity as the primary cause of the disease. (1) The conclusions of Sampson have been validated by the following observations.

1. During laparoscopy, flow of blood from the fimbriated end of the tube has been noted in some menstruating women.

2. Endometriosis is most commonly found in dependent portions of the pelvis.

3. Endometrial fragments from the menstrual flow can grow both in tissue culture and following injection beneath the abdominal skin.

4. When the cervix of monkeys was transposed so that menstruation occurred into the peritoneal cavity, endometriosis developed. (2)

Because endometriosis has been found at sites distant from the abdominal cavity—for example, lung and nasal mucosa—and there are even case reports of its occurrence in men who received treatment with estrogen, there must be alternatives to retrograde flow as an explanation for the disease. (3) Endometriosis at sites distant from the pelvis may be due to vascular or lymphatic transport of endometrial fragments. Another possible cause of endometriosis is the transformation of coelomic epithelium into endometrial-type glands as a result of unspecified stimuli. (4)

There may be both genetic and immunologic factors that influence the susceptibility of a woman to endometriosis. Simpson and co-workers reported 6.9% of first-degree relatives of patients with endometriosis were found to have the disease, compared to 1.0% in a control group. (5) Dmowski and co-workers demonstrated that monkeys with endometriosis had decreased cellular immunity to endometrial tissue, suggesting that specific immunologic defects can render some individuals susceptible to endometriosis. (6)

Widely varying figures for the prevalence of endometriosis have been published, and a rough estimate is that 25–50% of infertile women have endometriosis. The common perceptions that endometriosis occurs only in women over the age of 30 and is not found often in black women, have now been discredited. Whereas endometriosis does not occur before menarche, there are increasing reports of its occurrence in the teen years. (7) A number of these cases involve anatomic abnormalities that intercept the outflow tract. Endometriosis is not confined to nulliparous women, and physicians should be alert to the presence of endometriosis in cases of secondary infertility.

Diagnosis of Endometriosis

Symptoms and Signs

Endometriosis should be suspected in any woman complaining of infertility. Suspicion is heightened when there are also complaints of dysmenorrhea and dyspareunia.

Dysmenorrhea is even more suggestive of endometriosis if it begins after years of relatively pain-free menses. It should be recognized, however, that many women who have endometriosis are asymptomatic. A common observation is that some women with extensive endometriosis have little or no pain, whereas others with only minimal endometriosis complain of severe pain. Pain can be diffuse in the pelvis or it can be more localized, often in the area of the rectum. Symptoms also can arise from rectal or bladder involvement with endometriosis, and may be present throughout the month. Low back pain, too, may be due to endometriosis. An association of endometriosis and premenstrual spotting has been reported, but in most cases menstrual dysfunction is not increased with endometriosis.

Examination

The uterus is often in fixed retroversion and the ovaries may be enlarged. Nodularity of the uterosacral ligaments and cul de sac can be found in one third of patients with endometriosis. The diagnosis usually should be confirmed by laparoscopy before treatment is initiated. Minimal findings such as slight beading of the uterosacral ligaments in the young, asymptomatic patient can be treated by observation or by cyclic use of birth control pills.

Because both treatment and prognosis are determined to some extent by the severity of the disease, it is desirable to have a uniform system of classification that takes into account both the extent and severity of the disease. A uniform classification is also crucial for comparing the results of different treatments. The American Fertility Society has developed a classification system, and forms are available from the Society. (8)

Endometriosis and Infertility

When endometriosis involves the ovaries and causes adhesions that block tubal motility and pickup of the egg from the ovarian surface, there is no question of its role in causing mechanical interference with fertility. Less secure is our information on the role of peritoneal endometriosis on fertility. Most physicians believe that even minimal endometriosis on the peritoneal surface can cause infertility. A mediator of this effect could be production of prostaglandins by the implants, which could, in turn, affect tubal motility or folliculogenesis and corpus luteum function. Meldrum et al. noted increased levels of prostaglandin $F_{2\alpha}$ in the peritoneal fluid of patients with endometriosis. (9) Drake and co-workers found that patients with endometriosis had an increase in both the volume of peritoneal fluid and in the concentration of thromboxane B_2 and 6-keto-prostaglandin $F_{1\alpha}$ in the fluid. (10, 11) Rock et al., however, found neither an increase in peritoneal fluid nor an increase in concentration of peritoneal fluid prostaglandin E_2, prostaglandin $F_{2\alpha}$, 15-keto-13,14-dihydroprostaglandin $F_{2\alpha}$, and thromboxane B_2. (12) Further studies are needed to resolve these contradictory findings.

495

American Fertility Society Classification of Endometriosis

Patient's name _____

Stage I	(Mild)	1-5
Stage II	(Moderate)	6-15
Stage III	(Severe)	16-30
Stage IV	(Extensive)	31-40

Total _____

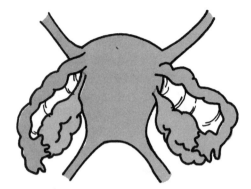

			< 1 cm	1-3 cm	> 3 cm
Peritoneum	Endometriosis		< 1 cm	1-3 cm	> 3 cm
			1	2	3
	Adhesions		filmy	dense with partial cul-de-sac obliteration	dense with complete cul-de-sac obliteration
			1	2	3
Ovary	Endometriosis		< 1 cm	1-3 cm	> 3 cm or ruptured endometrioma
		R	2	4	6
		L	2	4	6
	Adhesions		filmy	dense with partial ovarian enclosure	dense with complete ovarian enclosure
		R	2	4	6
		L	2	4	6
Tube	Endometriosis		< 1 cm	> 1 cm	tubal occlusion
		R	2	4	6
		L	2	4	6
	Adhesions		filmy	dense with tubal distortion	dense with tubal enclosure
		R	2	4	6
		L	2	4	6

Associated Pathology :

The role of minimal endometriosis in infertility has been called into question by three studies that found that women with untreated peritoneal endometriosis have pregnancy rates equal to those of women who have received treatment for the endometriosis. Garcia and David reported that 11 of 17 (64.7%) women with mild endometriosis became pregnant without treatment within 2 years of laparoscopy. (13) These 17 women had had a mean duration of infertility of 3.3 years. Schenken and Malinak found that 12 of 16 (75%) patients with mild endometriosis conceived within a year without treatment compared with a conception rate of 72.4% (21 of 29) in women with similar disease who had conservative surgery. (14) In a prospective study, Seibel et al. reported 13 of 19 (68%) women with minimal endometriosis became pregnant during 1 year of observation. (15) This compared with 5 pregnancies in 13 women (38%) with minimal endometriosis who were treated with danazol for 6 months and then observed for 6 months. Although the control group had 6 months longer to achieve a pregnancy than the danazol group, the success obtained without treatment is impressive.

These reports force us to reassess our thinking concerning the role of minimal endometriosis in infertility. Specifically, should peritoneal implants be treated if the only complaint is infertility? Whereas the studies cited above suggest that medical or surgical treatment of minimal peritoneal endometriosis is not worthwhile, there are those who champion fulguration treatment under laparoscopic visualization. (16, 17) Because of lack of proof of its efficacy, the occasional report of ureteral injury occurring during fulguration of endometrial implants on the uterosacral ligaments, and the suspicion of some clinicians that burned areas may become a nidus for adhesion formation, we would reserve laparoscopic fulguration of endometrial implants for those patients who have significant pelvic pain. (18)

Not everyone would agree with this hands-off approach. Buttram and Betts noted that in a group of 56 women with mild endometriosis and an average duration of infertility of 37 months, 73.2% were pregnant within 15 months of conservative surgery *by laparotomy*. Of those who conceived 36.6% did so in 3 months and 55.7% within 6 months. (19)

Surgical Treatment of Endometriosis

In contrast to the dispute over the proper treatment of minimal endometriosis, there is little doubt that adhesive disease associated with endometriosis and large (>1 cm) endometriomas are best treated by surgery. The object of surgery should be to restore normal anatomical relationships and to excise or fulgurate as much of the endometriosis as possible. A moderate approach that emphasizes avoiding the creation of large areas that cannot be reperitonealized and not risking damage to blood vessels and vital organs, has been rewarded with a higher pregnancy rate in women with moderate or severe endometriosis than an aggressive approach attempting to remove every vestige of the disease. (20) Similarly, removal of a severely diseased adnexa, when the other side is more normal, has produced better results than attempts to do major repairs. (20)

Because of the propensity for adhesion formation at the site of ovarian surgery, great care must be given to approximating the edges of the ovary if an endometrioma is removed. A fine running suture of 6-0 Dexon, or Vicryl of similar size should be used. As a further protection against formation of adhesions, approximately 200 ml of 32% dextran 70 should be instilled and left in the peritoneal cavity following conservative surgery for endometriosis. (21) Suspension of a retroverted uterus also may be a useful adjunct to prevent further adhesion formation by preventing the ovaries from adhering to raw areas in the cul de sac. Plication of the uterosacral ligaments following excision of endometrial implants will aid in keeping the uterus in an anterior position. (19) Covering the raw areas in the pelvis can be achieved with the use of free peritoneal or omental grafts to prevent adhesions. Presacral neurectomy has not been shown to enhance fertility, although many surgeons advocate it to alleviate dysmenorrhea. (19) This may be a less compelling reason, now that prostaglandin inhibitors are available to accomplish the same purpose.

The success of surgery in relieving infertility is directly related to the severity of endometriosis. Patients with moderate disease can expect a pregnancy success of approximately 60%, whereas the comparable figure is 35% in those with severe disease. (19) There is increasing support for selective use of danazol for 2–3 months following laparoscopy and prior to conservative surgery. Preoperative treatment for 6–8 weeks aids surgery by softening endometrial implants. Postoperative use of hormones has been the subject of greater controversy. The highest pregnancy rates following conservative surgery occur in the first year after surgery, and most physicians have been reluctant to use hormones that prevent pregnancy even for a few months. Wheeler and Malinak, however, treated 19 women with 400–800 mg/day of danazol for 3–6 months following surgery for *severe* endometriosis. (22) All became amenorrheic for at least 3 months. Fifteen (79%) of these women conceived. By contrast, only 36 of 199 (30%) women with severe endometriosis treated by surgery alone conceived. On the basis of this report, danazol appears to be a useful postoperative adjunct to surgery for severe endometriosis.

If pregnancy does not occur within 2 years of surgery for endometriosis, the chances are poor that it will ever occur. The recurrence rates reported for endometriosis after surgery are usually below 20%, but when it does recur, second surgeries to aid fertility have only a small chance for success.

The type of surgery that we have been discussing has been labeled "conservative" to indicate that reproductive function is maintained. When endometriomas are removed a vigorous attempt should be made to leave behind any normal ovarian tissue. Even 1/10 of an ovary can be enough to preserve function and fertility.

"Conservative" surgery is in contradistinction to "radical" surgery, which involves hysterectomy and bilateral salpingo-oophorectomy. When radical surgery is performed, an uninvolved ovary can be preserved in some cases of endometriosis if all of the endometriosis is removed by fulguration or excision. This does provide a risk for recurrent disease, but the risk seems to be small.

Hormonal Treatment of Endometriosis

Implants of endometriosis react to steroid hormones in a manner similar to normally stimulated endometrium. Thus, estrogen stimulates growth of the implants. Hormone therapy is designed to interrupt the cycle of stimulation and bleeding of the implants. An early approach was the use of massive doses of diethylstilbestrol (DES), which, because of variable success, the risk of affecting a female fetus, and severe side effects of bleeding and nausea, is now of only historical interest. Treatment with androgens (methyltestosterone linguets 5–10 mg/day) can provide temporary relief of the pain of endometriosis, but its effect on infertility appears to be negligible. In addition, ovulation can occur while on treatment, and there is at least a theoretical risk of exposure of the fetus to the androgen.

Until the late 1970s the most important alternative to conservative surgery was the use of combination birth control pills taken in a continuous fashion. (23) It seemed to matter little which preparation was used to accomplish the conversion of endometrial implants into decidualized cells associated with a few inactive endometrial glands. The usual dose is one pill per day continuously for 6–12 months. The addition of estrogen (Premarin 2.5 mg daily for 1 week), is used if breakthrough bleeding occurs. The treatment with birth control pills was called pseudopregnancy because of the amenorrhea and the decidualization of the endometrial tissue induced by the estrogen-progestin combination. It also reflected the commonly held belief that pregnancy can improve endometriosis, a belief that has been disputed. The side effects of treatment are those associated with birth control pills (Chapter 15), but some—e.g., weight gain—are more common with continuous as opposed to cyclic use. Pregnancy rates after stopping medication are reported to be in the 40–50% range. Whereas published recurrence rates are not excessive, this therapy, as with all hormone treatment for endometriosis, must be viewed as suppressive rather than curative.

In distinction to the pseudopregnancy induced by birth control pills, danazol produces what has been termed a pseudomenopause. Danazol is an isoxazole derivative of the synthetic steroid 17α-ethinyltestosterone. (24) It originally was thought to exert its effect solely by inhibition of pituitary gonadotropins. Although danazol can decrease follicle stimulating hormone (FSH) and luteinizing hormone (LH) in castrated individuals, it does not alter basal gonadotropin concentrations in premenopausal women. It does, however, eliminate the midcycle surge of FSH and LH. Asch et al. demonstrated a shortening of the luteal phase in monkeys treated with danazol, an effect that was not reversed by injections of human chorionic gonadotropin (HCG), suggesting a direct effect on the ovary. (25) Similarly, danazol inhibits steroidogenesis in the human corpus luteum. (26) In a comprehensive review of the actions of danazol, Barbieri and Ryan pointed out the multiplicity of actions of the drug. (27) Their list included:

1. Prevention of the midcycle surge of FSH and LH, but not significant suppression of basal FSH or LH in gonadally intact human beings.

2. Prevention of the compensatory rise in LH and FSH in castrated animals.

3. Binding to androgen, progesterone, and glucocorticoid receptors.

4. Translocation of the danazol-androgen receptor into the nucleus with initiation of androgen-specific RNA synthesis. On the other hand, the danazol-progesterone receptor translocates poorly.

5. No binding to intracellular estrogen receptors.

6. Binding to sex-hormone-binding globulin and to corticosteroid-binding globulin.

7. Increase in metabolic clearance rate of progesterone.

8. Inhibition of cholesterol cleavage enzyme, 3β-hydroxysteroid dehydrogenase, 17β-hydroxysteroid dehydrogenase, 17,20-lyase, 17α-hydroxylase, 11β-hydroxylase, and 21-hydroxylase. Danazol does not inhibit aromatase.

The multiple effects of danazol produce a hypoestrogenic, hypoprogestational environment that does not support the growth of endometriosis, and the amenorrhea that is produced prevents new seeding from the uterus into the peritoneal cavity.

The side effects of danazol are related both to the hypoestrogenic environment it creates and to its androgenic properties. The most common side effects are weight gain, fluid retention, fatigue, decreased breast size, acne, oily skin, deepening of the voice, growth of facial hair, atrophic vaginitis, hot flushes, muscle cramps, and emotional lability. Some of these side effects occur in approximately 80% of women who are taking danazol, but less than 10% find the side effects sufficiently troublesome to warrant discontinuation of the drug. Because danazol has been associated with the development in utero of female pseudohermaphroditism, it should not be given if there is the possibility of pregnancy. (28) Danazol is metabolized largely in the liver,

500

and in some patients it causes hepatocellular damage. Its use, therefore, is contraindicated in women with liver disease. The fluid retention that is often associated with danazol makes it dangerous to use when there is severe hypertension, congestive heart failure, or impaired renal function. There is one report of increased cholesterol levels and decreased high density lipoproteins in women taking danazol. (29) It is uncertain how this should influence use of danazol.

Danazol is used to relieve the pain and to treat the infertility due to endometriosis, and to prevent progression of the disease. The original dose was two 200-mg tablets twice a day (although some claim that spacing the drug at 6-hour intervals may be more effective) for 6 months. Dmowski and Cohen reported on 99 women who completed danazol treatment for a period of 3–18 months (average 6 months) and who were reevaluated an average of 37 months later. (30) During the course of treatment all the patients had symptomatic improvement and the majority (85%) were clinically improved. At the time of the reevaluation, however, approximately one third were symptomatic and had clinical findings suggestive of recurrent endometriosis. In the majority of patients, the symptoms recurred within the first year after discontinuation of the drug. Of the 84 patients who desired pregnancy after treatment with danazol, 39 (46.5%) conceived. The authors claimed that if couples with other causes of infertility, in addition to endometriosis, were excluded, the corrected pregnancy rate was 72.2%. The success of danazol treatment seems greatest in cases of peritoneal endometriosis or those with small lesions of the ovary. Endometriomas larger than 1.0 cm are less likely to respond to danazol, although quite surprising regression of endometriomas larger than 1.0 cm is sometimes seen.

Because of the significant side effects encountered with danazol, and its cost (approximately $150 per month), there has been a trend toward the use of lower doses. Dmowski et al. feel, however, that doses below 800 mg might be less effective. (31) They also imply that the occurrence of amenorrhea is correlated with improved outcome and that this is more consistently obtained at the 800-mg level. Others, however, do not believe that amenorrhea is an important consideration because many of the patients will bleed from an atrophic endometrium.

Biberoglu and Behrman compared women receiving 100, 200, or 600 mg daily of danazol. (32) Patients receiving 100 mg of danazol required 2 months to gain considerable relief of symptoms, whereas relief came in the 1st month for those using higher doses. By the 6th month of treatment, the percentages of patients with amenorrhea were 29% with 100 mg, 38% with 200 mg, 86% with 400 mg, and 88% with 600 mg. These figures correlated roughly with laparoscopically determined freedom from endometriosis, which was 14.2% with 100 mg, 62.5% with 200 mg, 57.1% with 400 mg, and

87.5% with 600 mg. These latter figures do not take into consideration endometriomas, because the authors believe that ovarian endometriomas greater than 1.0 cm are relatively unresponsive to danazol. The numbers of pregnancies were too small to compare for the different groups.

Gambrell and Greenblatt reported on a double blind study that utilized daily doses of 0.2, 6.25, 25 and 100 mg of danazol in 27 infertile women with laparoscopically proven endometriosis. (33) The results were compared with 37 women treated with either 400 or 800 mg of danazol. Amenorrhea occurred in all 41 patients treated with the two higher doses but only 3 (11.1%) of those treated with doses below 400 mg. When patients with other infertility factors were eliminated from consideration, pregnancy rates were 69.2% when 0.2–100 mg of danazol were used, compared to 81.8% in those women treated with 400–800 mg of danazol. One drawback to the use of very low doses of danazol is that pregnancy may occur while the patient is taking the medication, entailing a risk of genitourinary abnormalities in the fetus.

There is growing evidence that the higher doses of danazol (600–800 mg/day) are necessary for optimal therapy. Archer recommends 200–400 mg per day for treatment of peritoneal implants. (34) When endometriomas of 1–3 cm in diameter are present, he begins with 600 mg per day and reduces it if symptoms improve over 6–8 weeks. With severe endometriosis he prescribes 800 mg/day. The usual length of treatment is 6 months, although there is no specific contraindication to longer therapy. Prolonged treatment may be very appropriate for symptomatic, recurrent endometriosis.

There is a general perception, but only limited experimental evidence, that danazol is more effective than birth control pills for the treatment of endometriosis. (35) Noble and Letchworth compared danazol with mestranol (75 µg)-norethynodrel (5 mg). (36) The dose of both danazol and the birth control pill was increased until the patients became amenorrheic. One of 25 patients taking danazol could not complete 5 months of treatment, whereas 7 of 17 (41%) of the group taking birth control pills dropped out because of side effects. Danazol was more effective than mestranol-norethynodrel in relieving symptoms, and laparoscopic assessment showed much better results with danazol. Seven of 12 danazol-treated patients became pregnant compared with 4 of the 10 women who had taken birth control pills.

Both oral Provera (medroxyprogesterone acetate) (30 mg/day) and injectable Depo-Provera have been used to treat endometriosis. (37) Breakthrough bleeding is a common problem although it is usually cleared by short-term (7 days) administration of ethinyl estradiol, 20 µg, or Premarin 2.5 mg. The usefulness of Depo-Provera in infertile patients

502

is limited by the varying length of time it takes for ovulation to resume after discontinuation of therapy.

Recently, a long-acting gonadotropin releasing hormone (GnRH) agonist has been used to create a pseudomenopause for the treatment of endometriosis. (38) At the end of 28 days of daily subcutaneous administration of the agonist, estrogen levels decreased to levels similar to those found in oophorectomized women. Thus, the "medical oophorectomy" caused by the continuous use of a GnRH agonist could add a new approach to the treatment of endometriosis. As with all other drug therapies of endometriosis, it would provide suppression rather than cure of the disease.

Definitive surgery for severe endometriosis, which includes abdominal hysterectomy and bilateral salpingoophorectomy as well as resection of all endometriosis, is the only cure for the disease. If oophorectomy is performed, estrogen replacement can be used with only a small risk of inciting growth of residual endometriosis.

Long-Term Hormonal Therapy

Long-term hormonal therapy without surgery is useful in patients with severe symptoms but with little in the way of palpable findings. Before undertaking prolonged therapy, diagnosis should be established by laparoscopy. Prolonged therapy is also indicated if symptoms recur after conservative surgery.

Prevention of Infertility

A common clinical problem is the finding at surgery of endometriosis in a young woman who has no immediate interest in pregnancy. Cyclic birth control pills to prevent further growth and further shedding are appropriate treatment for very mild disease, for example a few implants in the cul de sac. More advanced disease should be treated with 6 months of danazol or Provera, followed by cyclic birth control pills to decrease the risks of further seeding and preserve future fertility.

References

1. **Sampson JA,** Peritoneal endometriosis due to the menstrual dissemination of endometrial tissue into the peritoneal cavity. Am J Obstet Gynecol 14:422, 1927.

2. **Scott RB, TeLinde RW, Wharton LR Jr,** Further studies on experimental endometriosis, Am J Obstet Gynecol 66:1082, 1953.

3. **Oliker AJ, Harris AE,** Endometriosis of the bladder in a male patient, J Urol 106:858, 1971.

4. **Merrill JA,** Endometrial induction of endometriosis across millipore filters, Am J Obstet Gynecol 94:780, 1966.

5. **Simpson JL, Elias S, Malinak LR, Buttram VC Jr,** Heritable aspects of endometriosis: I. Genetic studies, Am J Obstet Gynecol 137:327, 1980.

6. **Dmowski WP, Steele RW, Baker GF,** Deficient cellular immunity in endometriosis. Am J Obstet Gynecol 141:377, 1981.

7. **Schifrin BS, Erez S, Moore JG,** Teen-age endometriosis, Am J Obstet Gynecol 116:973, 1973.

8. **The American Fertility Society,** Classification of endometriosis, Fertil Steril 32:633, 1979.

9. **Meldrum DR, Shamonki IM, Clark KE,** Prostaglandin content of ascitic fluid in endometriosis: a preliminary report, Program, Twenty-Fifth Annual Meeting, Pacific Coast Fertility Society, October 1977.

10. **Drake TS, Metz SA, Grunert GM, O'Brien WF,** Peritoneal fluid volume in endometriosis, Fertil Steril 34:280, 1980.

11. **Drake TS, O'Brien WF, Ramwell PW, Metz SA,** Peritoneal fluid thromboxane B_2 and 6-keto-prostaglandin $F_1\alpha$ in endometriosis, Am J Obstet Gynecol 1:401, 1981.

12. **Rock JA, Dubin NH, Ghodgaonkar RB, Berquist CA, Erozan YS, Kimball AW Jr,** Cul de sac fluid in women with endometriosis: fluid volume and prostanoid concentration during the proliferative phase of the cycle-days 8 to 12, Fertil Steril 37:747, 1982.

13. **Garcia CR, David SS,** Pelvic endometriosis: infertility and pelvic pain, Am J Obstet Gynecol 129:740, 1977.

14. **Schenken RS, Malinak LR,** Conservative surgery versus expectant management for the infertile patient with mild endometriosis, Fertil Steril 37:183, 1982.

15. **Seibel M, Berger MJ, Weinstein FG, Taymor ML,** The effectiveness of danazol on subsequent fertility in minimal endometriosis (abstr), Fertil Steril 37:310, 1982.

16. **Hasson HM,** Electrocoagulation of pelvic endometriotic lesions with laparoscopic control, Am J Obstet Gynecol 135:115, 1979.

17. **Sulewski JM, Curcio FD, Bronitsky C, Stenger VG,** The treatment of endometriosis at laparoscopy for infertility, Am J Obstet Gynecol 138:128, 1980.

18. **Cheng YS,** Ureteral injury resulting from laparoscopic fulguration of endometriotic implant. Am J Obstet Gynecol 126:1045, 1976.

19. **Buttram VC Jr, Betts JW,** Endometriosis, Curr Probl Obstet Gynecol 11: No. 11, 1979.

20. **Buttram VC Jr,** Surgical treatment of endometriosis in the infertile female: a modified approach, Fertil Steril 32:635, 1979.

21. **diZerega G, Utian W,** Efficacy of 32% Dextran-70 in the prevention of peritoneal adhesions and the utility of second-look laparoscopy in infertility surgery (abstr), Fertil Steril 37:291, 1982.

22. **Wheeler JM, Malinak LR,** Postoperative danazol therapy in infertility patients with severe endometriosis, Fertil Steril 36:460, 1981.

23. **Kistner RW,** Management of endometriosis in the infertile patient, Fertil Steril 26:1151, 1975.

24. **Dmowski WP,** Endocrine properties and clinical application of danazol, Fertil Steril 31:237, 1979.

25. **Asch RH, Fernandez EO, Siler-Khodr TM, Bartke A, Pauerstein CJ,** Mechanism of induction of luteal phase defects by danazol, Am J Obstet Gynecol 136:932, 1980.

26. **Barbieri RL, Osathanondh R, Ryan KJ,** Danazol inhibition of steroidogenesis in the human corpus luteum, Obstet Gynecol 57:722, 1981.

27. **Barbieri RL, Ryan KL,** Danazol: endocrine pharmacology and therapeutic applications, Am J Obstet Gynecol 141:453, 1981.

28. **Duck SC, Katayama KP,** Danazol may cause female pseudohermaphroditism, Fertil Steril 35:230, 1981.

29. **Fraser IS, Allen JK,** Danazol and cholesterol metabolism, Lancet 1:931, 1979.

30. **Dmowski WP, Cohen MR,** Antigonadotropin (danazol) in the treatment of endometriosis: evaluation of post-treatment fertility and three-year follow-up data, Am J Obstet Gynecol 130:41, 1978.

31. **Dmowski WP, Kapetanakis E, Scommegna A,** Variable effects of danazol on endometriosis at 4 low-dose levels, Obstet Gynecol 59:408, 1982.

32. **Biberoglu KO, Behrman SJ,** Dosage aspects of danazol therapy in endometriosis: short-term and long-term effectiveness, Am J Obstet Gynecol 139:645, 1981.

33. **Gambrell RD Jr, Greenblatt RB,** Treatment of infertility due to endometriosis with low dosages of danazol (abstr), Fertil Steril 37:304, 1982.

34. **Archer DF,** Treating endometriosis with low dose danazol, Contemp Obstet Gynecol 19:47, 1982.

35. **Barbieri RL, Evans S, Kistner RW,** Danazol in the treatment of endometriosis: analysis of 100 cases with a 4-year follow-up, Fertil Steril 37:737, 1982.

505

36. **Noble AD, Letchworth AT,** Medical treatment of endometriosis: a comparative trial, Postgrad Med J 55 (Suppl 5):37, 1979.

37. **Moghissi KS, Boyce CR,** Management of endometriosis with oral medroxyprogesterone acetate, Obstet Gynecol 47:265, 1976.

38. **Meldrum D, Chang J, Lu J, Vale W, Rivier J, Judd H,** "Medical oophorectomy" using a long-acting GnRH agonist—a new approach to the treatment of endometriosis, Program, Twenty-Ninth Annual Meeting, Society for Gynecologic Investigation, March 1982.

19 Male Infertility

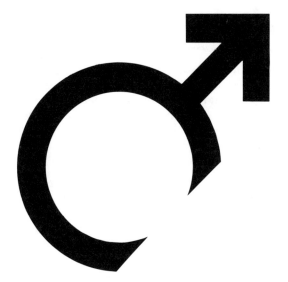

The perception of the degree of male involvement in infertility has undergone a number of revisions during the past 40 years. Initially, infertility was considered primarily a female problem. This notion gave way to the realization that 40–50% of infertility is wholly or in part due to a male factor. More recently, there have been attempts to redefine, in a downward direction, the lower limit of "normal" for a sperm count. Thus, many men who in the past would have been categorized as subfertile now are considered normal, and the focus has turned to their female partners. Despite these recent changes, there is no doubt that a substantial percentage of infertility is due to deficiencies in the semen. For that reason it is important for the gynecologist to be knowledgeable concerning male infertility. After the initial semen analysis, it is our responsibility to determine whether urologic consultation is required. *This chapter will consider the analysis of semen, indicate factors responsible for abnormalities in the semen, and consider available treatment for problems of male infertility, including artificial insemination.*

507

Regulation of the Testis

Testicular function is regulated by secretion of the pituitary follicle-stimulating hormone (FSH) and luteinizing hormone (LH). The primary effect of LH is to stimulate the synthesis and secretion of testosterone by Leydig cells, an effect that is enhanced by FSH which increases the number of LH receptors on the cells. Increasing levels of testosterone, in turn, inhibit LH secretion.

FSH, in conjunction with testosterone, acts on the seminiferous tubules to stimulate spermatogenesis. This effect may be mediated by activation of Sertoli cell function. In contrast to the effects of testosterone on LH, steroid hormones at physiologic levels do not suppress FSH secretion. Orchiectomy is followed, however, by a rise in FSH levels. This phenomenon led to the discovery of inhibin, a polypeptide that specifically inhibits FSH secretion. Inhibin has been found in seminal fluid, spermatozoa, testes and Sertoli cells.

Prolactin at normal levels stimulates testosterone secretion, wheras hypersecretion of prolactin leads to reduced testosterone secretion. A role for prolactin, however, has not been established for normal testicular function.

Semen Analysis

A semen analysis should be obtained as the first step in the investigation of infertility. This is true even if the male has fathered children in the past. There are specific guidelines for the collection and analysis of semen. The specimen should be collected by masturbation into a clean container, protected from cold, and brought to the laboratory within 1 hour of collection. Abstinence of 48–72 hours prior to ejaculation is recommended. The specimen should not be collected by withdrawal, because the sperm-rich fraction may be lost, nor should it be collected in a condom. The latter contain spermicidal agents. If the male cannot collect a specimen by masturbation, he can be supplied with a special sheath manufactured by the Milex Company that does not contain a spermicide.

Interpretation of the semen analysis often is hampered by two factors. The first is the variability in semen characteristics over time in the same male, and the second is the erroneous range for "normal" printed on the data sheets of many laboratories. Sherins et al. observed the variability in sequential semen specimens over a 6-month period and concluded that if the first semen specimen had a good count (>20,000,000/ml), or a poor count (<10,000,000/ml), subsequent counts tended to remain in the same category. (1) If the initial semen specimen had a count between 10,000,-000 and 19,900,000/ml, there was greater variability in subsequent counts, and at least 3 semen analyses were required to provide confidence in the evaluation of the male. If the initial specimen showed good motility (defined as 60%), or equivocal motility (40–60%), subsequent specimens often had motilities in different ranges. If the initial specimen had poor motility (<40%), however, the motility tended to remain in the poor category. The most stable characteristic from one specimen to another in the same individual was the percentage of normal forms. The variability between specimens of counts and motilities demonstrates the importance of doing at least 2 or 3 semen analyses during the course of the investigation. Because it takes 74 days for germ cells to become mature sperm, an interval of at least this length is appropriate between the first and the last analysis. In this way, transient injuries to the germ cell, as opposed to permanent injuries, can be demonstrated.

It is still common to see laboratories quote the lower limits of normal as 60,000,000/ml, 80,000,000/ml, or even 100,-000,000/ml. The work of MacLeod established that the percentage of pregnancies decreases when the sperm count drops below 20,000,000/ml, and this is the currently accepted lower limit of normal. (2) Some believe that this figure is too high and that 10,000,000/ml should be used as the lower limit of normal. It should be pointed out that pregnancies do occur even with counts below 20,000,000/ml, and this has been emphasized by reports of sperm counts in fertile males prior to vasectomy. (3) Of 386 men undergoing elective vasectomy, all of whom had at least one child, 20% had sperm counts less than 20,000,000/ml. (4)

The sperm count usually is performed by placing a diluted aliquot of semen on a hemocytometer chamber. A simpler method which does not involve dilution utilizes the Makler counting chamber produced by Israel Electrooptical Industry Ltd., Rehovot, Israel. Sperm motility determination can be performed in any office equipped with a microscope and glass slides. A drop of semen is placed on the slide and looked at initially without a coverslip at 100× magnification, and then at 400× with a coverslip in place. A rough estimate is made of both the percentage of motile sperm and the percentage of sperm that show *progressive* motility across the field. At least 50% of sperm should show progressive motility 2 hours after ejaculation. To compare specimens, it should be standard procedure to evaluate motility 1–2 hours after ejaculation; there is no current evidence that checking in vitro motility at more prolonged intervals (e.g., 24 hours) gives any useful information concerning the male's fertility potential. Over 60% of sperm should have normal morphology. There is a wide range of interpretations concerning what constitutes normal sperm morphology. For this reason, the clinician can have only limited confidence in reports from clinical laboratories.

The usual ejaculate volume is between 3 and 5 ml (range of 1–7 ml), and it is influenced by the frequency of ejaculation. Low volumes, in association with absence of sperm in the postcoital test, suggest the possible need for artificial insemination with the husband's sperm. Higher than normal volumes, associated with a low concentration of sperm, can be treated by the use of split ejaculate inseminations, a technique that will be discussed later in this chapter.

Other abnormalities in the semen that can contribute to infertility are:

1. Infection, manifested by the presence of white blood cells. Almost all semen specimens contain some of these cells, and it is important for each laboratory to establish its own range for a normal reading.

2. Failure of the semen to liquefy. If a thick, viscid specimen is associated with a poor postcoital test, the semen can be liquefied by running it back and forth through a No. 19 hypodermic needle and then using it for insemination. Enzyme digestion of semen also has been used to overcome this problem. (5) Splitting the ejaculate by collection in two jars also may produce a less viscid specimen in the first jar. A viscid specimen in conjunction with a normal postcoital test is not a significant infertility factor.

3. Agglutination of sperm. This occurs on occasion in most males, but if present in repeated specimens, it may represent an autoimmune reaction or signal the presence of infection.

Abnormal Semen Follow-up

If the semen characteristics are abnormal on successive specimens, inquiry is made concerning the presence of the following factors, any of which can produce abnormal sperm quality and quantity:

1. History of testicular injury, surgery, mumps, or venereal disease.

2. Heat. A small rise in scrotal temperature can adversely affect spermatogenesis, and a febrile illness may produce striking changes in sperm count and motility. The effect of the illness can still be seen in the sperm count and motility 2–3 months later. This reflects the 74 days required for a spermatozoon to be generated from a primary germ cell. Environmental sources of heat—such as the use of jockey shorts instead of boxer shorts, excessively hot baths, frequent use of a sauna, steam bath or hot tub, or occupations that require long hours of sitting, as in long-distance trucking—can all diminish fertility. Cooling of the testes has been used in a few cases as a treatment for infertility.

3. Severe allergic reactions with systemic effects.

4. Exposure to radiation.

5. Use of certain drugs such as Furadantin, sulfasalazine, or chemotherapeutic agents. Spermatogenesis may return in a few cases many years after the chemotherapy. The effect of marijuana on spermatogenesis is still uncertain, although heavy use suppresses gonadotropin releasing hormone (GnRH) leading to decreased gonadotropins and testosterone, and this may be associated with oligospermia.

6. Coital frequency and timing. Counts at the lower levels of the normal range may be depressed to below normal levels by ejaculations occurring daily or more frequently. Conversely, abstinence for 7 days or more "to save up sperm" is counterproductive, because the minimal gain in numbers is offset by the increased proportion of older sperm cells. For most couples, coitus every 36–48 hours around the time of ovulation gives the optimum chance for pregnancy.

7. Cigarettes, alcohol and hard work. All three have been cited as causes of abnormal semen, but only heavy use of tobacco has been shown to have a deleterious effect on sperm. Nicotine can inhibit both the quantity and quality of spermatogenesis. Sperm motility is decreased in association with more than one pack per day. Excessive working hours and alcohol are certainly of importance in infertility as causes of impotence or decreased libido. Alcohol can also lower circulating levels of testosterone.

8. Exposure to diethylstilbestrol in utero has been suggested, but not proved, as a cause of male infertility.

Urologic Evaluation

If none of these problems pertains to the couple under investigation, then referral is made to a urologist in order to look for an anatomic abnormality, an infection, a varicocele, or an endocrine disorder.

Examination may reveal a physical impairment such as cryptorchidism, or a marked hypospadias that can cause sperm to be deposited outside the vagina. In rare cases of diabetes, in neurologic disease, or following prostatectomy, there can be retrograde ejaculation into the bladder. Pregnancies have been reported after insemination of sperm obtained by catheterization of the bladder or by post-ejaculation voiding. (6) Therapy utilizing ephedrine or Ornade has been used with limited success in cases of retrograde ejaculation, as has ejaculating with a full bladder. Retrograde ejaculation may be only partial, and some men with this condition may have small amounts of ejaculate emitted from the urethra.

Small testes are commonly found in men with Klinefelter's syndrome. A small percentage of males with azoospermia or severe oligospermia will have chromosomal abnormalities, and the majority of these men have Klinefelter's syndrome. Others will have androgen insensitivity, a defect in androgen receptors.

Causes of Male Infertility	**Chromosomal Abnormalities**
	Cryptorchidism
	Decreased Semen Volume (<1.0 ml)
	Drugs (anti-cancer)
	Ductal Obstruction
	Endocrine Disorders
	Ejaculatory Disorders
	Failure of Sperm Maturation
	Immunologic Reactions
	Increased Heat
	Increased Viscosity of Semen
	Infection
	Sexual Problems
	Ultrastructural Defects
	—Absence of dynein arms
	—Absence of acrosome
	Varicocele

If the physical examination of the male does not uncover an abnormality, testicular biopsy may reveal the cause of the infertility. This procedure is usually reserved for males who have azoospermia or very severe oligospermia. Azoospermia associated with normal spermatogenesis indicates ductal obstruction. If the ducts are congenitally absent, fructose will not be found in the semen because it is normally produced in the seminal vesicles. If the biopsy reveals complete hyalinization and fibrosis of the seminiferous tubules, there is no chance for fertility. Some who feel that hormonal therapy of male infertility is of value use testicular biopsy as a means of selecting those men who have the greatest chance of responding to drugs.

If the urologist finds infection in the genitourinary tract, it can be cleared with antibiotics and possibly prostatic massage. The role of chlamydia and mycoplasma in male infertility is unknown. Routinely treating with tetracyclines without doing urethral cultures is unwarranted.

Hormonal Therapy

Endocrine disorders are an uncommon cause of male infertility. It may be worthwhile, however, to test for abnormalities of thyroid, FSH, LH, and testosterone. FSH levels are elevated with germ cell aplasia, whereas testosterone levels are decreased in men who are hypogonadotropic. Hyperprolactinemia is uncommon in the male as compared to the female, but when present is usually associated with such low testosterone levels that impotence is a problem.

At the present time, there seems to be no reason to use hormonal therapy unless there is evidence of deficiency. This viewpoint is contrary to common urologic practice. Cytomel is still frequently prescribed, even when evidence of thyroid dysfunction is lacking. This treatment continues despite its condemnation by those urologists with the greatest experience in problems of male infertility.

512

Treatment of men with low sperm counts with clomiphene has, on occasion, raised sperm numbers. One report indicated a marked increase in sperm counts when clomiphene was given at a dose of 25 mg a day for 25 days of each month. The improvement was transient and only 2 pregnancies were achieved by the 22 males who were treated. (7) In another series reported by Paulson, the results were better when therapy was restricted to males classified as having pregerminal hypofertility. (8) Unfortunately, this success was not duplicated in a study by Charny. (9) The results to date suggest that clomiphene is only of marginal, if any, value in male infertility.

Disappointing results have been found after therapy with human menopausal gonadotropins in men with normal levels of FSH and LH. (10) Injections of human chorionic gonadotropin (HCG) have been reported, in a few cases, to increase sperm motility. The usual dosage is 2500–3000 international units (IU) intramuscularly every 5 days. Substantial evidence is lacking for its clinical usefulness. A use for HCG following varicocele repair is described in the next section of this chapter.

Testosterone rebound therapy has a long history. Two to three months of testosterone, usually by injection, results in a marked depression of sperm count. In successful cases, 2–3 months after therapy is discontinued the sperm count is elevated above the pretreatment level. Urologic literature would suggest that these successes are few. Two additional drawbacks are the often short duration of the improved sperm count and the occasional cases in which the oligospermic male becomes permanently azospermic as a result of therapy.

Infusion of GnRH can stimulate secretion of gonadotropins. There have been isolated reports of its usefulness in male infertility. Because the evidence is, at the moment, equivocal, GnRH should be used only in investigational studies.

Arginine, an amino acid, once touted as a cure for male infertility, is of no value.

In a review of the management of male infertility, de Kretser pointed out that many different medications have been claimed to exert a beneficial effect on sperm, but that in the majority of cases claims have not been substantiated. (11) He condemned empirical therapy with vitamins and thyroid.

A fundamental problem is that most studies of the efficacy of drug therapy of male infertility do not include a control group for comparison. The investigators make the assumption that the spontaneous cure rate of male infertility is zero and that any pregnancies that occur are due solely to treatment. A number of studies have attested, however, to the spontaneous cure rate of male infertility. In addition, Rodrigues-Rigau et al. reported that approximately one third of males with counts below 10,000,000/ml, who were not treated, successfully impregnated their partners. (12) The importance of control groups was illustrated by a survey of the psychiatric literature. (13) Eighty-three percent of studies that did not use control groups found their treatment to be effective. In contrast, when control groups were used, only 20% of the studies found that the treatment was beneficial. Any article purporting to show benefits from a treatment should be viewed with suspicion if control groups are not included.

Varicocele

In the Second Edition of this text it was stated that one of the most striking advances in the field of male infertility was the discovery of the importance of varicocele in influencing semen quality and quantity. This appraisal was based on the information that 25% of infertile males will have a varicocele of the left internal spermatic vein and that ligation of this vein results in a 50% pregnancy rate. The enthusiasm for ascribing a prominent role for varicocele in male infertility has been dampened somewhat by a recent report in which groups of men, with counts both below and above 10,000,000/ml, had essentially the same pregnancy rates whether they did or did not have a varicocele. (12) In addition, varicocelectomy did not appear to change the pregnancy rate.

Dubin and Amelar reported that in a study of 331 men who had sperm counts over 10,000,000/ml and had a varicocelectomy, a 68% pregnancy rate was achieved. (14) If the preoperative sperm count was below 10,000,000/ml, the pregnancy rate was 23%. In a subgroup of 50 males who had preoperative counts of less than 10,000,000/ml, 22 (44%) achieved fertility when they were treated postoperatively with a total of 80,000 IU of HCG given over a period of 10 weeks.

Every infertile male requires a careful examination. Even a small varicocele could affect semen quality. A varicocele may empty in the recumbent position, and the urologist must be alert to the need to examine the patient in the upright position, and to have the patient perform a Valsalva maneuver. The varicocele may exert its effect by raising testicular temperature. It should be noted that varicocele is found in 10–15% of males in the general population, and about one half of these will have poor semen characteristics. A clue to the presence of a varicocele (or other insult to the testes) is the finding of long tapering sperm heads when sperm morphology is evaluated.

At the present time the influence of varicocele, and its repair, in infertility remains to be proven by controlled studies. The weight of current work suggests that it still should be sought for and treated in infertile males. There is no evidence, however, that males with normal semen characteristics, even if a varicocele is present, need treatment other than observation.

The Sperm Penetration Assay

The sperm penetration assay determines the capacity of human sperm to penetrate hamster ova from which the zona pellucida has been removed. The test involves the use of sperm capacitated in vitro and ova from superovulated hamsters. The cumulus mass and zona pellucida are removed from the eggs by proteolytic enzymes. After incubation of sperm and eggs, the presence of a sperm head within the egg is considered a sign of penetration. The test is relatively difficult to perform with consistency and accuracy, and therefore comparisons between laboratories may not be meaningful. In addition, it is relatively expensive (several hundreds of dollars). Until its clinical indications and correlations are clearly delineated, we recommend that it not be obtained routinely in all cases.

Because this laboratory assay is a functional test of the fertilizing ability of spermatozoa, it is not surprising that the results do not always correlate with the semen analysis or the postcoital test. The hamster penetration test should be performed when no cause of infertility can be detected, with persistently poor postcoital tests, and as an indication of the fertilization ability when sperm number and sperm motility are abnormal. The most reliable result is given as percent of hamster ova penetrated. A percentage below 10% is consistent with an inability to achieve fertilization. The answer, however, may not be absolute. We recommend a time period of 6 months to 1 year (when the semen analysis is otherwise normal) before moving to the only alternative remaining, artificial insemination with a donor specimen.

There has been a suggestion that the presence of white cells in the semen is associated with a poor penetration test that is reversible. Treatment with antibotics may restore the fertilizing ability of the spermatozoa and pregnancy may follow.

Artificial Insemination of Husband's Sperm (AIH)

If the urologist is unable to find an anatomic abnormality, an infection, a varicocele, or an endocrine deficiency, we prefer to work on the ejaculate rather than subject the male to nonspecific endocrine therapy.

Two questions that often arise in cases where the male has poor sperm quality concern the use of husband insemination and/or the possibility of freezing the husband's ejaculate and pooling a number of samples. While a priori it would seem logical to insert sperm with poor motility or specimens with a low count into the cervical os or uterus and save them part of their journey, this tactic has not been

515

a successful one. The pregnancy rates achieved with artificial insemination of husband's sperm are in the 18–20% range. (15) This is similar to the spontaneous pregnancy rate reported when oligospermia or poor motility is not treated. (16) It also closely approximates the pregnancy rate (14%) following normal intercourse in those couples who discontinue AIH. (15) While insemination of whole ejaculates are seldom helpful in these cases, husband inseminations using whole ejaculates are of value in refractory premature ejaculation, retrograde ejaculation, severe hypospadias, and cases where the male cannot ejaculate in the vagina but can give a specimen by masturbation. (See also Chapter 17 for use of husband insemination for treatment of poor postcoital tests.)

Freezing and thawing depress, to some extent, sperm motility. If a man has a low count with excellent motility, there may be some rationale for freezing and pooling his specimens for later insemination. Unfortunately, poor counts are most often associated with poor motility. In these cases freezing would be detrimental.

It is evident that in some males seminal fluid may be harmful to sperm. The first portion of the ejaculate contains the sperm-rich fraction and prostatic fluid. The remainder of the ejaculate originates in the seminal vesicles. Separating the two fractions by use of a split ejaculate can provide a specimen with a greater concentration of sperm and improved motility. In this technique, the first few drops of the ejaculate are collected in one jar and the rest in a second jar. Collection can be facilitated by taping the two jars together. Both must be checked, for, whereas the first jar contains the superior specimen in 90% of cases, the second is better in 5%. In 5% there is no difference between the two. If one of the specimens is not substantially better than the whole ejaculate, there is no reason for using the split ejaculate for inseminations.

Amelar and Hotchkiss reported a series of couples in whom split ejaculates were used and 22 of 39 (56%) achieved pregnancies. (17) Males with very poor counts were largely excluded, however, and some of the treated couples had counts and motilities in the whole ejaculates that now would be considered within the normal range. The technique seems to benefit men with poor motility, whereas oligospermia usually does not respond. In cases where split ejaculates are advisable, the couple may also use an in vivo technique: The husband withdraws as soon as he feels that ejaculation is starting. Amelar and Dubin have reported 33 pregnancies in couples using this method. (18)

Whatever mode of insemination is used, there is a high dropout rate; if the couple can persist with the treatment, a 6-month trial is a reasonable one.

Ericsson and co-workers (19) layered sperm on columns of liquid albumin as a means of separating out Y-bearing sperm. The albumin column also allows separation of the most vigorous sperm from the dead and poorly moving sperm. The vigorously moving sperm, suspended in physiologic solutions, can be used for intrauterine inseminations. This technique is under study in a number of clinics in the United States and Europe. In our experience, the technique provided a specimen with enhanced motility, but, surprisingly, pregnancies did not occur. (20) Others have reported a few successes.

The Ericsson method is in clinical use for sex preselection and the results to date indicate that it increases the male to female ratio from 1:1 to 2.5:1. Interestingly, results with a small number of couples show an *increase in females* when the Ericsson method is used in conjunction with ovulation induction with clomiphene. Methods of sex preselection that depend on timing of coitus in the menstrual cycle or adjustments of vaginal pH are of no proven value. pH has no differential effect on the X- or Y-chromosome bearing sperm. (21)

There have been a few reports of a transient increase in sperm motility following incubation in vitro with caffeine. (22, 23) Caffeine is mutagenic in bacteria, and therefore its use to treat sperm seems questionable. More importantly, a study by Harrison showed that the addition of caffeine to semen did not increase the pregnancy rate. (24)

Artificial Insemination with Donor Sperm (AID)

The combined problems of male infertility and decreased availability of adoptive babies have increased the interest and demand for AID. Thousands of babies are born each year in the country as a result of AID.

The procedure raises emotional, ethical and legal questions. The husband may feel that he is devalued and his virility questioned. In a few cases a woman's ovulation may become abnormal in the cycle when inseminations have been planned. For obvious reasons the physician must never do inseminations without the consent of both husband and wife. Both must be in favor of the procedure, and the stability of their marriage as well as their emotional maturity should be assessed by the physician. It is not only couples that are using AID. It is our perception that there is an increasing interest in AID among single women. In many areas physician resistance to inseminating single women has largely disappeared, and stable, well motivated women are using AID to achieve single parenthood.

Three points are worth emphasizing to the couple:

1. Donor inseminations do not guarantee pregnancy. The success rate with fresh semen is about 70%. The use of frozen semen lowers the success rate to 50%, although some claim to find no difference between fresh and frozen semen.

517

2. The couple should give some thought to their feelings should the child be born with a congenital anomaly. This will occur in perhaps 4–5% of all pregnancies, irrespective of whether they follow normal intercourse or artificial insemination.

3. It is a wise precaution to have both the man and the woman sign a consent form. An example can be found in an article by Kleegman. (25) The procedure is covered by law in less than 20 states. In California and Oregon, once the husband signs the consent forms, he is the legal father of the baby conceived through AID. In other areas, it would be worthwhile for the physician to know the legal status of AID in the state so that correct information can be conveyed to patients.

In general, the donor should be unknown to the couple. His health and fertility must be unimpeachable, and there should be no family history of genetic diseases. A survey of physicians performing AID has revealed a wide range of criteria for screening donors. (26) The usual genetic screening consisted of a superficial family history and only a rare biochemical test. As the compilers of the survey point out, such screening depends on both the awareness of family medical history and the honesty of the donor. Two recent reports detail the transmission of serious genetic disease through donor inseminations. (27, 28) In one case the same donor was used for two affected children in one family, and the authors suggest that a donor be discontinued if an affected child is born following AID. Certainly all donors should be questioned for family history of reproduction, genetic diseases and their own drug and teratogen exposure. There should also be carrier testing of prospective donors at high risk for Tay Sachs disease, sickle cell anemia and thalassemia. It is unlikely, however, that karyotyping of donors would be cost effective. The couple must always be informed of possible genetic risks associated with AID.

Among the other problems that can occur with donor insemination are the transmission of venereal disease from donor to recipient, and the possibility that one donor may provide the sperm for two children who will, in later life, marry one another. The former problem can be avoided by culturing each specimen and treating the recipient if it is positive for gonorrhea. We have not followed this practice although we do warn recipients of the potential risks of infection. The chance of inbreeding following AID is thought to be small. It is probably less than the inbreeding that occurs continuously throughout the population. A number of studies of selected newborn populations have indicated that over 10% of the infants could not be the offspring of the putative fathers on the basis of blood typing.

The donor will not be a mirror image of the husband, but an attempt should be made to match physical characteristics. Use of RhoGAM makes Rh compatability between the donor and the woman a less crucial issue today, although we still advise Rh negative sperm donors for Rh negative women. AID is a private matter between the physician and the couple. Discussions with friends or relatives should be discouraged. Use of friends or relatives as donors raises the potential for emotional problems in the future, although we have used a relative when it was requested by a stable, intelligent couple who understood the long-term implications. Requests to mix the husband's sperm with the donor's signifies that the couple may not have made the emotional adjustment to the thought of donor insemination. The husband's semen may also be deleterious to the donor's sperm, although this idea is in dispute.

Donor inseminations are useful in azoospermia, severe oligospermia or necrospermia refractory to treatment. They are also useful if the woman has a long history of fetal loss due to Rh sensitization. Here an Rh negative donor would be used. Genetic diseases may, on occasion, be an indication for donor insemination.

The basal body temperature chart and perception by the woman of increased vaginal wetness are useful guides to the approximate time of ovulation. Initially, an attempt is made to inseminate on the day just before (or 2 days before) the temperature rise based on reviewing 2 months of charts. Usually 1–3 inseminations are done each month. In approximately 50% of the successful cases, pregnancy will occur within the first 2 months. If pregnancy has not occurred by that time, a hysterosalpingogram is performed. Approximately 90% of pregnancies that will occur happen within 6 months.

Inseminations can be placed in the uterus, cervix or vagina. A cervical cap, used by some physicians, does not appear to enhance the success rate. Intrauterine inseminations run the potential risks of infection and of severe pain due to uterine cramping. For these reasons, intrauterine insemination with donor semen should not be performed routinely.

We prefer to inject at the entrance to the cervical canal by means of a polyethylene catheter. The major portion of the semen overflows into the posterior fornix. The overflow collects on the posterior blade of the speculum, and the cervical os is allowed to dip into the pool while the woman rests for 20 minutes with her hips elevated.

References

1. **Sherins RJ, Brightwell D, Sternthal PM,** Longitudinal analysis of semen of fertile and infertile men, in *The Testis in Normal and Infertile Men,* Troen P, Nankin HR, eds, Raven Press, New York, 1977.

2. **Macleod J,** Human male infertility, Obstet Gynecol Surv 26:335, 1971.

3. **Derrick FC, Johnson J,** Reexamination of "normal" sperm count, Urologie 3:99, 1974.

4. **Nelson CMK, Bunge RG,** Semen analysis: evidence for changing parameters of male fertility potential, Fertil Steril 25:503, 1974.

5. **Amelar RD,** Coagulation, liquefaction and viscosity of human semen, J Urol 87:187, 1962.

6. **Bourne RB, Kretzchmer WA, Esser JH,** Successful artificial insemination in a diabetic with retrograde ejaculation, Fertil Steril 22:275, 1971.

7. **Paulson DF, Wacksman J, Hammond CB, Wiebe HR,** Hypofertility and clomiphene citrate therapy, Fertil Steril 226:982, 1975.

8. **Paulson DF,** Clomiphene citrate in the management of male hypofertility: predictors for treatment selection, Fertil Steril 28:1226, 1977.

9. **Charny CW,** Clomiphene therapy in male infertility: a negative report, Fertil Steril 32:551, 1979.

10. **Sherins RJ,** Clinical aspects of treatment of male infertility with gonadotropins: testicular response of some men given HCG with and without Pergonal, in *Male Fertility and Sterility,* Mancini RE, Martini L, eds, Academic Press, New York, 1974.

11. **de Kretser DM,** The management of the infertile male, Clin Obstet Gynaecol 1:409, 1974.

12. **Rodriguez-Rigau LJ, Smith DK, Steinberger E,** Relationship of varicocele to sperm output and fertility of male partners in infertile couples, Urology 120:691, 1978.

13. **Foulds GA,** Clinical research in psychiatry, J Ment Sci 104:259, 1958.

14. **Dubin L, Amelar RA,** Varicocelectomy as therapy in male infertility: a study of 504 cases, Fertil Steril 26:217, 1975.

15. **Nachtigall RD, Faure N, Glass RH,** Artificial insemination of husband's sperm, Fertil Steril 32:141, 1979.

16. **Glass RH, Ericsson RJ,** Spontaneous cure of male infertility, Fertil Steril 31:305, 1979.

17. **Amelar RD, Hotchkiss RS,** The split ejaculate, Fertil Steril 16:46, 1965.

18. **Amelar RD, Dubin L,** A new method of promoting fertility, Obstet Gynecol 45:56, 1975.

19. **Ericsson RJ, Langevin CH, Nishino M,** Isolation of fractions rich in human Y sperm, Nature 246:421, 1973.

20. **Glass RH, Ericsson RJ,** Intrauterine insemination of isolated motile sperm, Fertil Steril 29:535, 1978.

21. **Glass RH,** Sex preselection, Obstet Gynecol 49:122, 1977.

22. **Bunge RG,** Caffeine stimulation of human ejaculated spermatozoa, Urologie 1:371, 1973.

23. **Schoenfeld C, Amelar RD, Dubin L,** Stimulation of ejaculated human spermatozoa by caffeine, Fertil Steril 26:158, 1975.

24. **Harrison RF,** Insemination of husband's semen with and without the addition of caffeine, Fertil Steril 29:532, 1978.

25. **Kleegman SJ,** Therapeutic donor insemination, Fertil Steril 5:7, 1954.

26. **Curie-Cohen M, Luttrell L, Shapiro S,** Current practice of artificial insemination by donor in the United States, N Engl J Med 300:585, 1979.

27. **Johnson WG, Schwartz RC, Chutorian AM,** Artificial insemination by donors: the need for genetic screening, N Engl J Med 30:755, 1981.

28. **Shapiro DN, Hutchinson RJ,** Familial histiocytosis in offspring of two pregnancies after artificial insemination, N Engl J Med 304:757, 1981.

20 Induction of Ovulation

In the past, a woman with an ovulatory dysfunction had little hope of achieving a pregnancy. The successful therapy of this problem is one of the most dramatic advances in gynecologic endocrinology. Today, if lack of ovulation is the only problem causing infertility, a persistent couple can expect their chances of conceiving to almost match the rate found in the general population.

The physician has available for general clinical use three pharmacologic preparations for the induction of ovulation, clomiphene citrate, bromocriptine (Parlodel), and human menopausal gonadotropins (Pergonal). The programs of clomiphene and Pergonal administration described in this chapter have evolved over the past 2 decades. These methods have reduced side effects to a clinically acceptable frequency and retained a high success rate in terms of induced pregnancies. Bromocriptine is only a recent addition to our armamentarium, and an understanding of its use is still evolving. *This chapter will review the principles which guide the use of clomiphene, Pergonal, and bromocriptine, and consider the results and complications of the medical induction of ovulation. In addition, ovarian wedge resection will be examined, and mention will be made of the use of gonadotropin releasing hormone (GnRH).*

Despite the specificity of the therapy and the promise of successful results, it is incumbent upon the practitioner to perform the appropriate medical evaluation to ensure that a contraindication to therapy is not overlooked. The reader is referred to Chapter 6 and Chapter 7 for a consideration of anovulation and hirsutism, Chapter 5 and Chapter 9 for the evaluation of amenorrhea and galactorrhea.

Clomiphene Citrate

Clomiphene citrate is an orally active nonsteroidal agent distantly related to diethystilbestrol. Its chemical name is 2-[*p*-(2-chloro-1,2-diphenylvinyl)phenoxy]triethylamine dihydrogen citrate. Clomiphene is available in 50-mg tablets under the trade names of Clomid and Serophene. In some countries, the preparation is available in its *cis* form as a 10-mg tablet which is approximately equivalent to the 50-mg tablet sold in the United States.

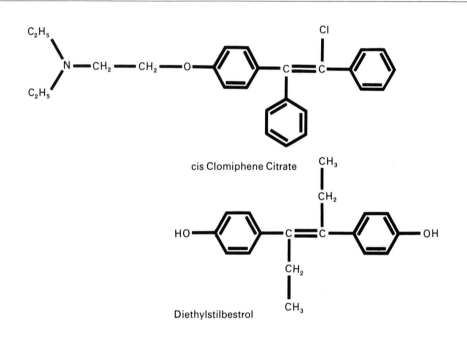

cis Clomiphene Citrate

Diethylstilbestrol

The similarity of its structure to an estrogenic substance is the clue to its mechanism of action. Clomiphene exerts only a very weak biologic estrogenic effect. The structural similarity to estrogen is sufficient to achieve uptake and binding by estrogen receptors. Clomiphene, however, does not competitively inhibit the action of estrogen at the receptor level, but rather it modifies hypothalamic activity by affecting the concentration of the intracellular estrogen receptors. Specifically, the concentration of cytoplasmic estrogen receptors is reduced by inhibition of the process of receptor replenishment. (1) Therefore, the hypothalamic-pituitary axis cannot perceive or act upon the true endogenous estrogen level in the circulation. Thinking that the estrogen level in the circulation is low because perception is obscured, the neuroendocrine mechanism is activated. In view of the newly appreciated primary role for the pituitary as discussed in Chapter 2, it is not certain whether clomiphene acts principally in the hypothalamus, on the pituitary, or at both sites. During the period of clomiphene administration, peripheral serum levels of follicle stimulating hormone (FSH) and luteinizing hormone (LH) rise. The subsequent ovulation which occurs after clomiphene therapy is then a manifestation of the hormonal and morphologic changes produced by the growing follicles. Clomiphene therapy does not directly stimulate ovulation, but it supports a sequence of events that are the physiologic features of a normal cycle. The effectiveness of the drug is restricted to its ability to cause an appropriate FSH discharge.

Clomiphene has no progestational, androgenic, or antiandrogenic effects. Clomiphene does not interfere with adrenal or thyroid function. In rats and rabbits, a dose-dependent increase in the incidence of fetal malformations is seen when clomiphene is given during the period of organogenesis. Extremely high doses inhibit fetal development. Although clomiphene therapy should be withheld if there is any possibility of pregnancy, there is no good evidence that clomiphene is teratogenic in humans. Furthermore, infant survival and performance after delivery are normal.

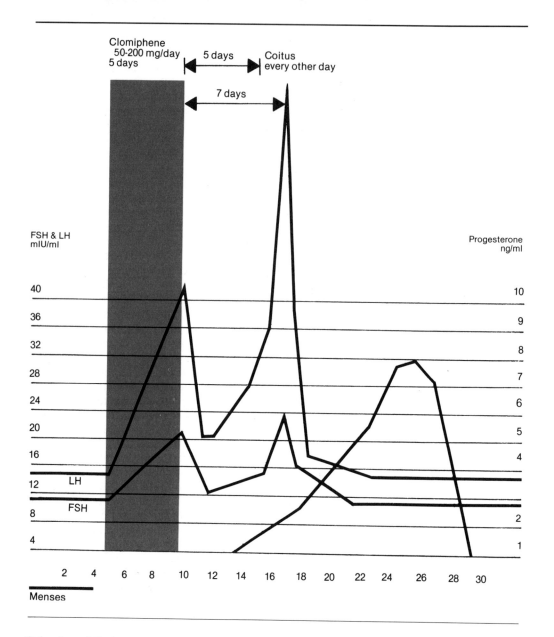

Selection of Patients

Absent or infrequent ovulation is the chief indication for clomiphene therapy. It is the physician's responsibility to rule out nonreproductive disorders of pituitary, adrenal, and thyroid origin requiring specific treatment before initiating clomiphene therapy. A complete history and physical examination are mandatory, but only a minimum of laboratory procedures is necessary. The vast majority of patients are healthy women suffering only from infertility secondary to oligo-ovulation or anovulation.

While the effect of the drug is brief, only 51% of the oral dose is excreted after 5 days, and radioactivity from labeled clomiphene appears in the feces up to 6 weeks after administration. If history and physical examination findings suggest liver disease, liver function evaluation should precede clomiphene therapy.

If periods are infrequent, it is not absolutely necessary to document infrequent or absent ovulation by basal body temperature records and endometrial biopsy. An endometrial biopsy is a wise precaution in a patient who has been anovulatory for a long period of time because of the tendency for these patients to develop adenomatous hyperplasia and even carcinoma of the endometrium. It is also wise to precede therapy with an evaluation of the semen, to avoid an unnecessary waste of time and effort in the presence of azoospermia. A dedicated effort must be made to detect galactorrhea, and the prolactin level must be measured. Galactorrhea or hyperprolactinemia dictate a different therapeutic approach: bromocriptine. The remainder of the infertility workup in a patient with no previous medical or surgical problems is deferred until after a trial of clomiphene therapy. Because approximately 75% of pregnancies occur during the first 3 treatment cycles, the infertility workup is pursued only after the patient has responded with 3 months of ovulatory cycles and has not become pregnant. (2) Despite the antiestrogen action of clomiphene the incidence of poor cervical mucus on the postcoital test is only 15%. (3)

Cases of ovarian failure are unresponsive to any form of ovulation induction. Therefore, the presence of ovarian tissue capable of responding to gonadotropins must be documented. This is only a problem in the patient with amenorrhea, since the presence of menstrual bleeding confirms the function (although perhaps limited) of the hypothalamic-pituitary-ovarian axis. The patient with amenorrhea who fails to produce a withdrawal bleed after a course of a progestational agent (Provera, 10 mg daily for 5 days) must be further evaluated (see Chapter 5). A case has been made by others for the usefulness of an ovarian biopsy, perhaps via the laparoscope, to establish the presence of competent ovarian tissue. It is our practice, however, to rely on the radioimmunoassay of gonadotropin levels and the response to Provera, thus avoiding unnecessary surgical and anesthetic risks, to accurately rule out hypergonadotropic hypogonadism (ovarian failure). Attempts at medical induction of ovulation in these patients would be a waste of time and money except in a few very rare cases of primary ovarian failure as discussed in Chapter 5.

The patients most likely to respond to clomiphene display some evidence of pituitary-ovarian activity as expressed in the biologic presence of estrogen (spontaneous or withdrawal menstrual bleeding). These are anovulatory women who have gonadotropin and estrogen production, but do not cycle. The patient who is deficient in gonadotropin secretion and, as a result, is hypoestrogenic, cannot be expected to respond to a further lowering of the estrogen signal, and thus should not respond to clomiphene. However, this principle is not completely applicable to clinical practice. An occasional patient who is, by every criteria, hypoestrogenic, will respond. Therefore, any otherwise medically uncomplicated patient with infertility secondary to lack of ovulation is a candidate for clomiphene therapy unless galactorrhea or hyperprolactinemia is present. In addition, treatment is indicated in order to improve the timing and frequency of ovulation to enhance the possibilities of conception in the patient who ovulates only occasionally.

To our knowledge, the use of drugs for induction of ovulation does not improve the quality of the ovum, and the chance of pregnancy is not improved in women who ovulate regularly and spontaneously. There is one special instance where this restriction may not apply. Certain religious requirements, such as in orthodox Judaism, interfere with the normal reproductive process. In the devout orthodox Jewish couple, intercourse is prohibited in the presence of menstrual flow and for 7 days following its conclusion. In some women menstrual flow is prolonged or the follicular phase is shortened, so that coitus cannot take place until after ovulation. Clomiphene therapy can be utilized to defer ovulation. In the usual mode of treatment, medication is begun on day 5 of the cycle. Ovulation can be delayed to a more appropriate time by starting clomiphene later, usually on day 7 or 8 of the cycle. Ovulation can be expected in the interval 5–10 days after the last day of medication. This manipulation has its limitations. Administration too late in the cycle, beyond day 9, may have no effect. It is appropriate to use clomiphene to achieve an increased frequency and regularity of ovulation in patients with oligoovulation. Clomiphene is also useful to regulate the timing of ovulation in women undergoing donor insemination.

The question is often asked whether the indications for clomiphene therapy should be extended to include the initiation of cyclicity in the oligoamenorrheic patient who does not seek fertility. In our opinion, this is an inappropriate use of clomiphene for several reasons: 1) the effectiveness of clomiphene is restricted to the cycle in which it is used and it should not be expected to induce cyclicity following the conclusion of treatment, 2) the use of clomiphene may aggravate the clinical problems of acne and hirsutism during the treatment cycle by increasing LH stimulation of ovarian steroid production, and 3) the inability to induce cyclicity can be so discouraging to the patient that her acceptance of the drug will be impaired at some future date when it is legitimately offered as a fertility agent for the induction of ovulation.

How to Use Clomiphene

A program of clomiphene therapy is begun on the 5th day of a cycle following either spontaneous or induced bleeding. The initial dose is 50 mg daily for 5 days. There is no advantage to beginning with a higher dose for the following two reasons: 1) In a random distribution of our patients begun with initial doses of either 50 mg or 100 mg daily, the pregnancy rate was identical; and 2) the highest incidence of side effects in our experience occurs at the 50-mg dose and at 100 mg patients may develop more serious reactions.

Beginning clomiphene on the 5th day is a method arrived at empirically, however, we can now offer a rational explanation based on current physiology. The clomiphene-induced increase in gonadotropins during days 5–9 occurs at a time when, in most cases, the dominant follicle has already been selected. Beginning clomiphene earlier can be expected to stimulate multiple follicular maturation resulting in a greater incidence of multiple gestation. Indeed, clomiphene is administered earlier in in vitro fertilization programs in order to obtain more than one oocyte.

If ovulation is not achieved in the very first cycle of treatment, dosage is increased to 100 mg. Thereafter, if ovulation is not achieved in any cycle, dosage is increased in a staircase fashion by 50-mg increments to a maximum of 200–250 mg daily for 5 days. The highest dose is pursued for 3–4 months before considering the patient to be a clomiphene failure. The quantity of drug and the number of cycles go beyond those recommended by the manufacturer. However, in our experience those recommendations are inappropriately limiting. We have achieved a 15% pregnancy rate at the 150-mg and 200-mg dose levels. (2)

There is a significant correlation between body weight and the dose of clomiphene required for ovulation. (4, 5) One must adhere to the usual regimen, however, because the weight cannot be used to predict prospectively the correct ovulatory dose. In other words some obese women ovulate at the same low dose which achieves ovulation in thin women. Clomiphene is not stored in adipose tissue, and the increased dose often necessary in obese women is more likely due to a more intense anovulatory state with higher androgen levels producing a more resistant hypothalamic-pituitary-ovarian axis.

At the present time there is no clinical or laboratory parameter which can predict the dose of clomiphene necessary to achieve ovulation. Androgen and estrogen levels do not show any correlation with the dose of clomiphene which proves successful. (5)

Following the 5-day course of clomiphene, the ovulatory surge of gonadotropins may occur anywhere from 5 to 10 days after the last day of clomiphene administration. The patient is advised to have intercourse every other day for 1 week beginning 5 days after the last day of medication. In view of the role prostaglandins play in the physical expulsion of an oocyte, it is prudent to advise patients involved in programs of ovulation induction to avoid the use of agents which inhibit prostaglandin synthesis.

After the first treatment cycle the patient is evaluated for side effects, residual ovarian enlargement, and basal body temperature changes. In recent years we have found it unnecessary to perform a pelvic examination every month because significant ovarian enlargement is encountered infrequently and it is usually symptomatic. It is more economical, for both patient and physician, to mail the temperature chart to the office and several days later plan by telephone for the following month.

A basal body temperature record is necessary to follow the response. If an inadequate luteal phase is evident, (temperature elevation less than 11 days' duration) the amount of clomiphene is increased to the next dose level. If the patient is already at the maximum level, human chorionic gonadotropin (HCG) is added as discussed below. Biphasic changes are taken as an indication of ovulation and success. Maintenance of the temperature elevation beyond the expected time of menses is the earliest practical indication of success and pregnancy.

Care should be taken to review with the patient and her husband the pathophysiology of her condition, the principles of treatment, the prolonged course of therapy which may be necessary, and possible complications. Repeated failures accumulate frustration and despair in the couple, making each successive cycle of treatment more difficult. The anxiety and stress may hinder coital performance, and it is not uncommon for a couple to have difficulty performing scheduled intercourse.

The additional use of HCG is limited to those cases in which there is a failure to ovulate at the maximum dose level or, when at that level, a short luteal phase is demonstrated. The rationale is to improve on the midcycle LH surge; therefore 10,000 IU of HCG are given as a single intramuscular dose on the 7th day after clomiphene when follicular maturation is at its peak. Premature HCG administration may interfere with normal ovulation by down-regulating LH receptors. Accurate timing, however, requires either measurement of the blood estradiol level or estimation of follicular size by sonography. If HCG is administered in the morning intercourse is advised for that night and for the next 2 days.

Results

In properly selected patients, 80% can be expected to ovulate, and approximately 40% become pregnant. The percent of pregnancies per induced ovulatory cycle is about 15%. The multiple pregnancy rate is approximately 5%, almost entirely twins; there have been rare cases of quintuplet and sextuplet births. In our own experience in recent years, with standardization of therapy, the incidence of twins has decreased.

The abortion rate is not increased. Most importantly, the incidence of congenital malformations is not increased, and infant survival and performance after delivery are no different from normal. (3, 6) The discrepancy between ovulation rates and pregnancy rates is mainly due to two factors, the presence of other causes of infertility and a lack of persistence. In those patients with no other cause of infertility, the conception rate approaches 80–90%. (3) The pregnancy rate in 70 of our patients who received therapy sufficient to ovulate in at least 3 cycles was 55.7%, the same pregnancy rate after 3 months of exposure in the general population. (2) With additional treatment cycles, the pregnancy rate decreases although the ovulatory rate remains high. Approximately 15% of patients treated with the higher doses of 150–250 mg will become pregnant. (2) If all factors are corrected, and conception has not occurred in 6 months, prognosis is poor. In one large series, only 7.8% of those who had one or more factors in addition to anovulation became pregnant. (3)

Complications

Side effects do not appear to be dose-related, occurring more frequently at the 50-mg dose. Patients requiring the high doses are probably less sensitive to the drug. The most common problems are vasomotor flushes (10%), abdominal distention, bloating, pain, or soreness (5.5%), breast discomfort (2%), nausea and vomiting (2.2%), visual symptoms (1.5%), headache (1.3%), and dryness or loss of hair (0.3%).

Visual symptoms include blurring of vision, scotoma (visual spots or flashes), or abnormal perception. The cause of these symptoms is unknown, but in every case studied thus far, the visual symptoms have disappeared upon discontinuation of the medication, and no permanent effects have been reported. Usually these symptoms disappear within a few days, but may take 1 or 2 weeks.

Significant ovarian enlargement is associated with longer periods of treatment, and is infrequent (5%) with the usual 5-day course. Maximal enlargement of the ovary usually occurs several days after discontinuing the clomiphene (in response to the increase in gonadotropins). If the patient is symptomatic, pelvic examination, intercourse, and undue physical exercise should be avoided because the enlarged ovaries are very fragile. Ovarian enlargement dissipates rapidly and only rarely is a subsequent treatment cycle delayed. Of course, if ovarian enlargement is encountered, clomiphene therapy should be withheld until normal size returns.

There are several options available for the 10–20% of women who fail to become pregnant with clomiphene up to the highest dose with added HCG. These include the addition of dexamethasone, extending the duration of clomiphene treatment, considering the empiric use of bromocriptine, and finally, going on to the use of human menopausal gonadotropins (Pergonal).

First, make sure galactorrhea has not been overlooked and a prolactin level has been obtained. The good results with bromocriptine make it essential that this cause of anovulation be detected.

Approximately 30% of patients who have evidence of ovulation with clomiphene but fail to achieve pregnancy do become pregnant when treated with Pergonal. After 6–9 months of clomiphene therapy, and in the absence of any other infertility factors, we proceed to one of the available options.

The Addition of Dexamethasone to Clomiphene. Despite the fact that the ovulatory dose of clomiphene does not correlate with androgen levels (5), patients with hirsutism and high circulating androgen concentrations are more resistent to clomiphene. Dexamethasone, 0.5 mg at bedtime to blunt the night time peak of ACTH, is added to decrease the adrenal contribution to circulating androgens, and thus diminish the androgen level in the microenvironment of the ovarian follicles. While this is a rational maneuver to increase sensitivity to clomiphene, we have been disappointed in the overall success rate, and limit this approach to the patient with obvious evidence of significant androgen levels. The dexamethasone is maintained daily until pregnancy is apparent. The dose of clomiphene is returned to the starting point of 50 mg, and increased in incremental fashion as needed.

Extended Clomiphene Treatment. Two approaches have been reported for extending clomiphene treatment. We have very little experience with either. In the first, 250 mg of clomiphene are given for 8 days, followed by 10,000 IU HCG 6 days later. Three pregnancies were achieved out of 25 treatment cycles. (7) In another series, the clomiphene dose was increased every 5 days, with some patients receiving up to 25 days of consecutive treatment, the last 5 days at 250 mg daily. (8) Eight of 21 patients conceived and, in those patients who responded, measurement of gonadotropins revealed sustained elevations in FSH. This latter approach requires estrogen monitoring with discontinuation of the clomiphene when an increase in estrogen is detected. No patient ovulated after more than 21 days of treatment.

The Addition of Bromocriptine to Clomiphene. While the use of bromocriptine to induce ovulation is clearly indicated in the presence of galactorrhea or hyperprolactinemia, its use in the clomiphene failure patient with a normal prolactin and no galactorrhea is controversial. Anovulatory patients with normal levels of prolactin do respond to bromocriptine, but the effectiveness of this treatment has not been established by controlled studies. Nevertheless, the clinical response has been impressive.

Bromocriptine (Parlodel)

Elevated prolactin levels interfere with the normal function of the menstrual cycle by suppressing the pulsatile secretion of GnRH. This is manifested clinically by a spectrum, ranging from a subtle inadequate luteal phase to total suppression and hypoestrogenic amenorrhea. Regardless of the prolactin level, we interpret the presence of galactorrhea to indicate excessive prolactin stimulation. We screen all patients with galactorrhea or any ovulatory disorder with an assessment of the prolactin level. After a consideration of the problems of amenorrhea, galactorrhea, and the pituitary adenoma (as discussed in Chapter 5 and Chapter 9), bromocriptine emerges as the drug of choice for the induction of ovulation in these patients.

Bromocriptine is examined in detail in Chapter 5, but it would be helpful to review pertinent details here. Bromocriptine is a dopamine agonist, directly inhibiting pituitary secretion of prolactin. (9) Suppression of prolactin levels restores CNS-pituitary gonadotropin function and also appears to increase ovarian responsiveness. The increase in ovarian responsiveness is seen in patients with normal prolactin levels and no galactorrhea, the apparent mechanism for an increase in sensitivity to clomiphene when bromocriptine is added to the therapeutic regimen.

The gastrointestinal and cardiovascular systems react to the dopaminergic action of bromocriptine, and, therefore, the side effects are mainly nausea, diarrhea, dizziness, headache, and fatigue. Side effects can be minimized by slowly building tolerance toward the usual dose, 2.5 mg b.i.d. We start treatment with an initial dose of 2.5 mg at bedtime. If intolerance occurs, the tablet can be cut in half and a slower program, developed by the patient, can be followed to work up to the standard dose. Usually, the second dose is added after 1 week, at breakfast or at lunch.

The usual regimen is to administer bromocriptine daily until it is apparent the patient is pregnant, as usually determined by the basal body temperature chart. Although there has been no evidence of any harmful effects on the fetus, (10) some patients and physicians prefer to avoid taking bromocriptine in the luteal phase, and, therefore, during early pregnancy. The drug is stopped when a temperature rise occurs, and resumed when menses begins.

533

Ovulatory menses and pregnancy are achieved in 80% of patients with galactorrhea and hyperprolactinemia. (11, 12) Response is rapid, and, therefore, if there is no indication of ovulation (a rise in the basal body temperature) within 2 months, clomiphene is added to the regimen. The starting dose of clomiphene is 50 mg daily for 5 days, given and increased in the usual fashion.

As discussed in Chapter 5, once pregnant, the majority of women with a pituitary prolactin-secreting adenoma remain asymptomatic. Women with both microadenomas and macroadenomas may undergo uneventful pregnancies. It is extremely rare for a patient to develop a problem which results in perinatal damage or serious maternal sequelae. Surveillance during pregnancy need only consist of an awareness for the development of symptoms, headaches and visual disturbances. Assessment of visual fields, prolactin assay, and the sella turcica changes by limited CT scanning can await the onset of suspicious symptoms. Tumor expansion (and its symptoms) promptly regress with bromocriptine treatment. No adverse effects of bromocriptine on the pregnancy or the newborn have been reported.

Resolution of galactorrhea or hyperprolactinemia may occur spontaneously after a pregnancy. (12) Perhaps a tumor can undergo infarction in response to the expansion and shrinkage during and after pregnancy, or the condition was associated with dysfunction of the hypothalamus, now corrected.

Bromocriptine for Euprolactinemic Women. There has been a growing clinical experience indicating successful induction of ovulation and achievement of pregnancy with bromocriptine in the absence of galactorrhea and with a normal prolactin level. Until this practice is either established or discredited based upon controlled study, we offer bromocriptine to clomiphene failure patients, prior to embarking upon a complicated course of gonadotropin therapy. The mechanism of action may be an increase in follicular responsiveness either due to suppression of prolactin or suppression of LH (a known action of dopamine). A decrease in LH may alter local follicular steroidogenesis in such a way to create a more favorable microenvironment. The method of administration is the same as above. If, after 2 months of treatment, there is no response, clomiphene is reinitiated, working up again from the starting dose of 50 mg daily. While it is our impression that this is successful in a significant number of patients, it is clear that bromocriptine has nothing to offer for ovulatory women with unexplained infertility. (13)

534

| Human Menopausal Gonadotropins (Pergonal) | Pergonal (human menopausal gonadotropins) is a purified preparation of gonadotropins extracted from the urine of postmenopausal women. The commercial preparation contains 75 units of FSH and 75 units of LH. The potency is expressed in terms of international units based on an international reference preparation. A significant factor in the use of Pergonal is its high cost, approximately $20–$30/ampule. Treatment may cost from $500 to $1000/cycle for the drug alone. Pergonal is inactive orally and, therefore, must be given by intramuscular injection. |

Human Menopausal Gonadotropins (Pergonal)

Pergonal (human menopausal gonadotropins) is a purified preparation of gonadotropins extracted from the urine of postmenopausal women. The commercial preparation contains 75 units of FSH and 75 units of LH. The potency is expressed in terms of international units based on an international reference preparation. A significant factor in the use of Pergonal is its high cost, approximately $20–$30/ampule. Treatment may cost from $500 to $1000/cycle for the drug alone. Pergonal is inactive orally and, therefore, must be given by intramuscular injection.

Selection of Patients

Not only because of its expense, but because of its greater complication rate, patients should not receive Pergonal without a very careful evaluation. An absolute requirement is the demonstration of ovarian competence. Abnormally high serum gonadotropins with a failure to demonstrate withdrawal bleeding indicate ovarian failure and preclude induction of ovulation except in those special cases of primary ovarian failure as discussed in Chapter 5.

A thorough infertility investigation must be performed. In addition to the demonstration of ovarian competence, tubal and uterine pathology should be ruled out, anovulation documented, and semen analysis obtained. Nongynecologic endocrine problems must be treated. Hypogonadotropic function (low serum gonadotropins), including galactorrhea syndromes, requires evaluation for an intracranial lesion, with a sella turcica x-ray and measurement of prolactin levels. It is imperative to take all steps necessary to exclude treatable pathology to which anovulation is secondary.

In our practice we first offer a course of clomiphene, not only because of the cost and complications associated with Pergonal, but also because some apparently hypogonadotropic patients will unpredictably respond to clomiphene.

How to Use Pergonal

In the past there were two commonly used techniques of Pergonal administration, the variable and the fixed dosage methods. Pregnancy rates with the fixed dosage method are unacceptably low, and the variable dosage method should be used to achieve follicular growth and maturation. Follicle stimulation is achieved by 7–14 days of continuous Pergonal, beginning with 2 ampules daily. Response is judged by the degree of estrogen produced by the growing follicles. Clinically, the quantity and quality of the cervical mucus are used as indicators of estrogen production. In addition, the patient is monitored periodically with the measurement of the 24-hour urinary excretion of total estrogens or the plasma estradiol level. The patient is seen on the 7th day of treatment and a decision is made to continue or increase the dose. After the 7th day, the patient is seen anywhere from daily to every 3rd day.

Pergonal comes as a dry powder in a sealed glass ampule, along with a second ampule containing 2 ml of diluent. One ampule of Pergonal requires 1 ml of diluent. When 2 ampules are to be administered, solution with 1 ml is accomplished in the first vial of Pergonal, and the solution is then deposited in the second vial. Thus, when giving 2 ampules of Pergonal the contents of 2 vials are dissolved in a total of 1 ml of diluent. When 4 ampules are given, a total of 2 ml of diluent are used. Should 6 ampules of Pergonal be required, 3 ampules are dissolved in 1.5 ml of diluent and two injections are administered, each in the upper outer quadrant of each buttock. The HCG injection comes as a vial containing 10,000 units as a dry powder. One milliliter of the accompanying diluent is used for administration.

It cannot be emphasized too strongly that dosage administration and the judicious use of estrogen measurements depend upon the experience of the physician administering Pergonal. Clinically, when the cervical os opens and when cervical mucus changes (clarity, quantity, spinnbarkeit) comparable to a normal midcycle are achieved, the patient is ready to receive the ovulatory stimulus, 10,000 units of HCG given as a single dose intramuscularly. Because of its structural and biologic similarity to LH, HCG, readily available from human pregnancy urine and placental tissue, is used to simulate the midcycle LH ovulatory surge. The patient is advised to have intercourse the day of the HCG injection and for the next 2 days. In view of the fragility of hyperstimulated ovaries, further intercourse as well as strenuous physical exercise should be avoided.

The use of estrogen measurements is necessary to choose the correct moment for administering the ovulatory dose of HCG in order to prevent hyperstimulation. The cervical mucus begins to change rapidly when estrogen levels begin to rise. After a moderate rise in estrogen, however, there are no additional significant changes in the mucus. In addition, the response of the cervical glands varies considerably among individuals. The cervical assessment can therefore alert the clinician to an estrogen change, but it cannot be relied on for precise timing to avoid excessive stimulation. On day 7 of the therapeutic cycle the patient is examined and urine or blood is assayed for estrogen. Depending on the findings, the dosage of Pergonal is individualized for the duration of the cycle. With experience, the physician can avoid daily estrogen measurements although sometimes this is necessary.

What should the urinary estrogen level be? Below 100 μg/24 hours, a significant but not maximal pregnancy rate may be achieved. Over 200 μg/24 hours, a significant rate of hyperstimulation is encountered. Between 100 and 200 μg/24 hours, hyperstimulation or multiple ovulation may be encountered, but also the maximal pregnancy rate is achieved. To project dosage requirements, a useful fact to keep in mind is that once the phase of rapidly increasing estrogen production is reached, the urinary estrogen level will approximately double each day.

What should the blood estrogen level be? Because the blood estradiol is determined on a single sample of blood, the timing of the sampling with relationship to the previous injection of Pergonal becomes a significant variable. When Pergonal injections are given between 5 and 8 P.M., and blood samples are obtained first thing in the morning, an estradiol window of 1000–1500 pg/ml is optimum. (14) The risk of hyperstimulation is significant from 1500 to 2000 pg/ml, and over 2000 pg/ml, HCG should not be given, and the ovarian follicles should be allowed to regress.

As with the use of urinary estrogen, attempting to reproduce the normal midcycle levels of estrogen does not achieve a maximal pregnancy rate and higher levels are required. The relative safety of this approach was seen in our series, where only 2 of 24 patients with estradiol levels over 1000 pg/ml developed hyperstimulation and it was moderate in both cases. (14) When a patient nears ovulation on the weekend and estrogen monitoring is unavailable, timing of the HCG administration can be predicted fairly accurately by plotting the estradiol values on semilogarithmic paper. The rate of increase in estradiol is the same in spontaneous and induced cycles, and does not differ in cycles which result in multiple gestation. (15) The level which is reached at the time of HCG administration is more critical than the slope of increase.

In some individuals, pregnancy will be achieved with the administration of 2 ampules/day for 7–12 days. In other individuals, presumably with extremely hyposensitive ovaries, adequate follicular stimulation requires doses up to 4, 6, and more ampules/day. In this group of amenorrheic women massive doses of gonadotropins are necessary, and with proper monitoring, pregnancy can be safely achieved. The range between the dose which does not induce ovulation and the dose which results in hyperstimulation is narrow. The situation is made even more difficult because the ovaries may react differently to essentially similar doses from month to month. Close supervision and experience in the use of Pergonal are necessary to avoid difficulties.

Instruction and counseling of the couple are essential. A thorough understanding of the need for daily treatment and frequent observation is necessary prior to initiating therapy. As part of this instruction, the husband may be taught to administer injections. Daily recording of the basal body temperature and body weight is important for proper management. The couple should be told about the need for scheduled intercourse, the possibility that more than one course of treatment may be necessary, and the expense of the treatment. Above all, the patient must be prepared for the anguish that accompanies failure. Because this is a pressure-packed situation, unexpected impotence is occasionally encountered on the days of scheduled intercourse.

Results

The most significant aspect of this method of treatment is that it does achieve pregnancy in an otherwise untreatable situation. In general, more than 90% of patients with competent ovaries will ovulate in response to Pergonal and a pregnancy rate of approximately 50–70% may be achieved. As with clomiphene, there is a normal incidence of congenital malformations, and the children born have a normal postnatal development. (16, 17)

HCG disappears from the blood with an initial component having a half-life of about 6 hours and a second, slower, component with a half-life of about 24 hours. (18) It is this relatively slow half-life which enables a single injection of 10,000 IU to maintain the corpus luteum until pregnancy takes over. The HCG concentration after the ovulating injection should be less than 100 mIU/ml by day 16 after the injection. A β-subunit assay of HCG at this time or one of the urine assays performed 2–4 weeks after the HCG injection are reliable tests for pregnancy.

The multiple pregnancy rate has been reported as approximately 30% (triplets or more, 5%). The multiple pregnancies are secondary to multiple ovulations, and therefore the siblings are not identical. The rate of spontaneous occurrence of twins is only about 1% and that of triplets 0.010–0.017% of the pregnant population. Monozygotic twinning rate is about 0.3–0.4%, fairly constant, and uninfluenced by heredity. Dizygotic twinning varies among different populations and is inherited through the mother. It is not known whether the multiple pregnancy rate with Pergonal is significantly affected by a maternal history of twinning.

Fetal loss due to prematurity in the multiple pregnancies has been a serious problem. In addition, the abortion rate with Pergonal is somewhat higher, probably a combination of the effect of multiple pregnancies and recognition of early abortions. With the use of estrogen monitoring, some have reported a significant reduction in the multiple pregnancy rate, while others have found no correlation between estrogen levels and the incidence of multiple pregnancy. (19) Currently, the multiple pregnancy rate with careful monitoring is probably closer to 10%.

Therapeutic abortion in the case of triplets or more is an option, but it would be surprising if patient and physician would choose this solution. Attention has turned, therefore, to ultrasonography in the attempt to further reduce the multiple pregnancy rate.

The most useful predictor of ovulation is the reaching of a follicular diameter of 20 mm. (20) Unfortunately, there is no correlation between multiple gestation and the visualization of multiple follicles. In addition, there is no strict correlation between the size and number of follicles and the estrogen level. (21) Unless this approach is further refined, it cannot replace our present methods, and its expense argues against its routine use.

The likelihood of ovulation is dose related, and complications are likewise dose related. In general, 2–5 therapeutic cycles are required to achieve pregnancy. The rate of serious hyperstimulation has been 1%, but proper estrogen monitoring has reduced this complication to a rare happening. After at least one Pergonal-induced pregnancy the spontaneous pregnancy rate reaches 30% after 5 years. (22) Most of the pregnancies occur within 3 years of the Pergonal pregnancy.

Clomiphene-Pergonal Sequence

The combination of both clomiphene and Pergonal was explored in order to minimize the cost of Pergonal alone. As long as treatment is monitored with estrogen levels the side effects and complications should not be dissimilar to those with Pergonal alone. It has not been demonstrated that patients unresponsive to Pergonal alone would respond to the sequence method, and there is no logical reason to assume that this would be true.

The usual method of treatment is to administer clomiphene 100 mg for 5–7 days, then to immediately proceed with Pergonal beginning with 2 ampules per day. Estrogen levels are monitored as usual. This method may decrease the amount of Pergonal required by approximately 50%; however, the same risks of multiple pregnancy and hyperstimulation can be expected. This reduced requirement for Pergonal is found only in those patients who demonstrate a positive withdrawal bleed following progestin medication or who have spontaneous menses. (23)

Hyperstimulation Syndrome

Ovarian hyperstimulation may be life threatening. In mild cases the syndrome includes ovarian enlargement, abdominal distension, and weight gain. In severe cases, a critical condition develops with ascites, pleural effusion, electrolyte imbalance, and hypovolemia with hypotension and oliguria. (24) The ovaries are tremendously enlarged with multiple follicle cysts, stromal edema, and many corpora lutea.

The basic disturbance is a shift of fluid from the intravascular space into the abdominal cavity creating a massive third space. The resulting hypovolemia leads to circulatory and excretory problems. The genesis of the ascites is unclear. The very high level of estrogen secretion by the ovaries may be the primary factor, inducing increased local capillary permeability and leakage of fluid from the ovaries. The leakage of fluid is also critically related to the mass, volume, and surface area of the ovaries. Therefore, the larger the ovaries and the greater the steroid production, the more severe the condition. Experiments in animals have implicated a role for histamine and prostaglandins.

The loss of fluid and protein into the abdominal cavity accounts for the hypovolemia and hemoconcentration. This in turn results in low blood pressure and decreased central venous pressure. The major clinical complications are increased coagulability and decreased renal perfusion. Blood loss as the cause of the clinical picture can be easily ruled out since a hematocrit will reveal hemoconcentration. The decreased renal perfusion leads to increased salt and water reabsorption in the proximal tubule producing oliguria and low urinary sodium excretion. With less sodium being presented to the distal tubule, there is a decrease in the exchange of hydrogen and potassium for sodium, resulting in hyperkalemic acidosis. A rise in the blood urea nitrogen is due to decreased perfusion and increased urea reabsorption. Because it is only filtered, creatinine does not increase as much as the blood urea nitrogen (BUN). Thus, the patient is hypovolemic, azotemic, and hyperkalemic.

Treatment is conservative and empiric. Although both antihistamines and indomethacin have been demonstrated to ameliorate the hyperstimulation in animal studies, their efficacy and safety in early human pregnancy are unknown. When a patient displays excessive weight gain (usually 20 or more pounds), hemoconcentration (hematocrit over 50%), oliguria, dyspnea, or postural hypotension, she should be hospitalizied. Pelvic and abdominal examination are contraindicated in view of the extreme fragility of the enlarged ovaries. Ovarian rupture and hemorrhage are easily precipitated.

Upon admission, the patient is put on bed rest, with daily body weights, strict monitoring of intake and output, and frequent vital signs. Serial studies of the following are obtained: hematocrit, BUN, creatinine, electrolytes, total proteins with albumin-globulin ratio, coagulation studies, and urinary sodium and potassium. The electrocardiogram is utilized to follow and evaluate hyperkalemia. Fluid and salt are rigidly restricted because of the third spacing effect. As long as the BUN remains stable, an abnormally low urine output can be tolerated. (25) Potassium exchange resins may be necessary. Diuretics are without effect and, indeed, may be disadvantageous. The fluid in the abdominal cavity is not responsive to diuretic treatment, and diuresis may further contract the intravascular volume and produce hypovolemic shock or thrombosis. Arterial thrombosis has been reported.

The possibility of ovarian rupture should always be considered, and serial hematocrits may be the only clue to intraperitoneal hemorrhage. Of course, a falling hematocrit accompanied by diuresis is an indication of resolution, not hemorrhage. Laparotomy should be avoided in these precarious patients. If surgery is necessary, only hemostatic measures should be undertaken and the ovaries should be conserved if possible, since a return to normal size is inevitable.

The key point is that the hyperstimulation syndrome will undergo gradual resolution with time. In a patient who is not pregnant, the syndrome will cover a period of approximately 7 days. In a patient who is pregnant and in whom the ovaries are restimulated by the emerging endogenous HCG production, the syndrome will last 10–30 days.

The syndrome will not develop unless the ovulatory dose of HCG is given. Thus, the major emphasis in recent years has been to utilize estrogen monitoring to avoid hyperstimulation. A 24-hour urinary excretion of more than 200 μg estrogen or a blood estradiol level greater than 2000 pg/ml makes the development of the syndrome a good possibility, and the ovulatory dose of HCG should be withheld. Current methodology permits urinary or blood estrogen measurement within 6 hours, and hence daily therapeutic projections are possible. A severe case of hyperstimulation is not encountered unless the patient has ovulated.

The relationship between estrogen levels and hyperstimulation is not a perfect one. Hyperstimulation has been found with relatively low estrogen levels, and high estrogen is not necessarily followed by hyperstimulation. Nevertheless, this is the only available deterrent to a potentially life-threatening situation.

What to Do with the Pergonal Failure

If funds and emotional reserves are sufficient, a repeat course of therapy is permissible after a review of the etiologic basis for infertility. The effectiveness of treatment does not diminish with repeated cycles. Conception rates remain about the same. (17) If a couple can handle it, they should persist if no other infertility problems are present. Guidance to adoption services and emotional support continue to be part of the physician's obligation.

Gonadotropin Releasing Hormone (GnRH)

The advantage in the utilization of GnRH lies in the impossibility of producing hyperstimulation. An excessive amount of GnRH, as in the studies discussed in Chapter 2, results in down regulation of its own receptor. In addition, the multiple pregnancy rate with GnRH should be identical to the normal rate. Because GnRH serves largely a permissive role, the internal feedback mechanisms between the ovary and pituitary should be operative, yielding follicular growth and development similar to a normal menstrual cycle in response to the "turning on" of the system by GnRH.

In order to achieve follicular growth and ovulation, the normal GnRH pattern of pulsatile secretion must be approximated. We and others have successfully used an automatic pump to deliver 5 μg of GnRH intravenously every 90 minutes. (26) HCG is administered to support the corpus luteum, 1500 IU every 3 days for 3 doses, beginning at the time of the temperature rise, which also is the signal to discontinue the pump. The success rate and the problems with this method remain to be determined.

The inconvenience and mechanical problems of the pump may be overcome in the future by the utilization of a long-acting GnRH analog which may be administered intranasally several times a day. The potential safety and simplicity of GnRH administration are powerful attractions.

Ovarian Wedge Resection

The purpose of wedge resection of the ovaries is to remove a significant amount of steroid-producing tissue. Documentation of hormonal changes following wedge resection indicates that the only important change is a sustained reduction in testosterone levels. (27) This suggests that the barrier to ovulation is the intraovarian, atresia-promoting effects of the high testosterone production. Removal of androgen-producing tissue effectively lowers this barrier, and ovulatory cycles may ensue.

The response to ovarian wedge resection is variable. Some patients resume ovulation permanently. However, most patients return to their anovulatory state. Some patients fail to respond at all. Furthermore, the surgical procedure carries with it the potential problem of postoperative adhesion formation.

The operative risk, the variable response, and the possibility of postoperative adhesion formation are the liabilities of wedge resection. These must be weighed against the excellent results obtained with medical induction of ovulation (approximating the normal conception rate when anovulation is the only fertility problem present). It should truly be a rare patient in whom wedge resection of the ovaries is necessary.

References

1. **Clark JH, Peck EJ, Anderson JN,** Estrogen receptors and antagonism of steroid hormone action, Nature 251:446, 1974.

2. **Gorlitsky GA, Kase NG, Speroff L,** Ovulation and pregnancy rates with clomiphene citrate, Obstet Gynecol 51:265, 1978.

3. **Gysler M, March CM, Mishell DR Jr, Bailey EJ,** A decade's experience with an individualized clomiphene treatment regimen including its effect on the postcoital test, Fertil Steril 37:161, 1982.

4. **Shepard MK, Balmaceda JP, Leija CG,** Relationship of weight to successful induction of ovulation with clomiphene citrate, Fertil Steril 32:641, 1979.

5. **Lobo RA, Gysler M, March CM, Goebelsmann U, Mishell DR Jr,** Clinical and laboratory predictors of clomiphene response, Fertil Steril 37:168, 1982.

6. **Hack M, Brish M, Serr DM, Insler V, Salomy M, Lunenfeld B,** Outcome of pregnancy after induced ovulation: follow-up of pregnancies and children born after clomiphene therapy, JAMA 220:1329, 1972.

7. **Lobo RA, Granger LR, Davajan V, Mishell DR Jr,** An extended regimen of clomiphene citrate in women unresponsive to standard therapy, Fertil Steril 37:762, 1982.

8. **O'Herlihy C, Pepperell RJ, Brown JB, Smith MA, Sandri L, McBain JC,** Incremental clomiphene therapy: a new method for treating persistent anovulation, Obstet Gynecol 58:535, 1981.

9. **Parkes D,** Bromocriptine, N Engl J Med 301:873, 1979.

10. **Griffith RW, Turkalj I, Braun P,** Outcome of pregnancy in mothers given bromocriptine, Br J Clin Pharm 5:227, 1978.

11. **Cuellar FG,** Bromocriptine mesylate (Parlodel) in the management of amenorrhea/galactorrhea associated with hyperprolactinemia, Obstet Gynecol 55:278, 1980.

12. **Crosignani PG, Ferrari C, Scarduelli C, Picciotti MC, Caldara R, Malinverni A,** Spontaneous and induced pregnancies in hyperprolactinemic women, Obstet Gynecol 58:708, 1981.

13. **Weight CS, Steele SJ, Jacobs JS,** Value of bromocriptine in unexplained primary infertility: a double-blind controlled trial, Br Med J 1:1037, 1979.

14. **Haning RV Jr, Levin RM, Behrman HR, Kase NG, Speroff L,** Plasma estradiol window and urinary estriol glucouronide determination for monitoring menotropin induction of ovulation, Obstet Gynecol 54:442, 1979.

15. **Wilson EA, Jawad MJ, Hayden TL,** Rates of exponential increase of serum estradiol concentrations in normal and human menopausal gonadotropin-induced cycles, Fertil Steril 37:46, 1982.

16. **Hack M, Brish M, Serr DM, Insler V, Salomy M, Lunenfeld B,** Outcome of pregnancy after induced ovulation: follow-up of pregnancies and children born after gonadotropin therapy, JAMA 211:791, 1970.

17. **Schwartz M, Jewelewicz R,** The use of gonadotropins for induction of ovulation, Fertil Steril 35:3, 1981.

18. **Rizkallah T, Gurpide E, Vande Wiele RL,** Metabolism of HCG in man, J Clin Endocrinol Metab 29:92, 1969.

19. **Schenker JG, Yarkoni S, Granat M,** Multiple pregnancies following induction of ovulation, Fertil Steril 35:105, 1981.

20. **Bryce RL, Shuter B, Sinosich MJ, Stiel JN, Picker RH, Saunders DM,** The value of ultrasound, gonadotropin and estradiol measurements for precise ovulation prediction, Fertil Steril 37:42, 1982.

21. **Seibel MM, McArdle CR, Thompson IE, Berger MJ, Taymor ML,** The role of ultrasound in ovulation induction: a critical appraisal, Fertil Steril 36:573, 1981.

22. **Ben-Rafael Z, Mashiach S, Oelsner G, Farine D, Lunenfeld B, Serr DM,** Spontaneous pregnancy and its outcome after human menopausal gonadotropin/human chorionic gonadotropin-induced pregnancy, Fertil Steril 36:560, 1981.

23. **March CM, Tredway DR, Mishell DR Jr,** Effect of clomiphene citrate upon amount and duration of human menopausal gonadotropin therapy, Am J Obst Gynecol 125:699, 1976.

24. **Engel T, Jewelewicz R, Dyrenfurth I, Speroff L, Vande Wiele RL,** Ovarian hyperstimulation syndrome: report of a case with notes on pathogenesis and treatment, Am J Obstet Gynecol 112:1052, 1972.

25. **Shapiro AG, Thomas T, Epstein M,** Management of hyperstimulation syndrome, Fertil Steril 28:237, 1977.

26. **Reid RL, Leopold GR, Yen SSC,** Induction of ovulation and pregnancy with pulsatile luteinizing hormone releasing factor: dosage and mode of delivery, Fertil Steril 36:553, 1981.

27. **Judd HL, Rigg LA, Anderson DC, Yen SSC,** The effects of ovarian wedge resection on circulating gonadotropin and ovarian steroid levels in patients with polycystic ovary syndrome, J Clin Endocrinol Metab 43:347, 1976.

21 Clinical Assays

The purpose of this chapter is to review the laboratory assays which are commonly used in clinical gynecologic endocrinology. With this information, the clinician will have confidence in the selection of specific laboratory tests, and will be secure in the personal interpretation of the data.

Classically, hormones were measured in blood by bioassays, i.e. dose-response measurements based upon organ responses in animals. Some of the principles fundamental to endocrinology were established by such methods. However, bioassay methods, although adequate for qualitative statements, are relatively imprecise, nonspecific, time-consuming, expensive, and require too large an amount of the biologic sample in order to meet the quantitative requirements of modern research and clinical practice. Assays with far greater sensitivity and precision have been developed. These new methods depend upon the use of radioactive tracers and the delicate measurement of radioactivity. The most recent and popular techniques are the methods of saturation analysis.

Saturation Analysis (Radioimmunoassay, Competitive Protein Binding)

$$R \begin{array}{l} + \, S \rightarrow RS \\ + \, S^* \rightarrow RS^* \end{array}$$

Free   Bound

Basic Principles

The methods of saturation analysis yield greater simplicity, sensitivity, and precision. Reactions in saturation analysis follow the law of mass action. A protein or antibody (R) is mixed with a substance (S) for which it has specific binding sites, forming a complex, RS. The radioactive form of the substance (S*) also forms a complex, RS*. Since the number of binding sites on the protein or antibody are limited, the labeled and unlabeled compound, S and S*, will compete for binding sites in proportion to their concentrations. Since the binding reagent, R (protein or antibody), is kept constant, increasing the unlabeled compound, S, will displace more and more labeled tracer, S*. Plotting the change in either bound or unbound (free) tracer, S*, against the amount of unlabeled compound, S, added will produce a standard curve. The amount of radioactivity bound or free in the presence of an unknown level of compound will reveal the concentration of the compound when compared to the standard curve. The requirements for saturation analysis are, therefore, either a suitable binding protein, or an antibody, and a labeled pure form of the compound to be measured.

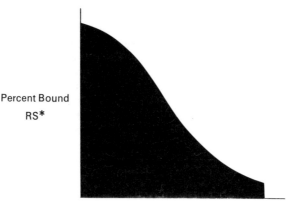

Percent Bound
RS*

S

Methodology   A purified, labeled amount of the substance to be measured is added to the biologic sample (e.g. plasma) to be assayed. The radioactive tracer equilibrates with the unlabeled and unknown amount of compound in the sample. The sample is now mixed with an appropriate solvent to extract the desired compound and tracer. The extraction process usually removes several compounds which may interfere with the assay, and separation (purification) of the desired substance is frequently necessary. A chromatographic separation utilizing thin layer chromatography or column chromatography is used for most steroid assays.

The next step is to mix the extracted compound with a specific reagent. In the case of radioimmunoassay, this reagent is an antiserum, and in the case of competitive protein binding, this reagent is a protein which has affinity for the compound to be measured. The combination of the compound with this reagent (antiserum or specific protein) is called binding. Since the compound is in equilibrium with a small amount of labeled compound, the labeled compound will bind to the reagent in proportion to the amount of unlabeled compound present. This is the fundamental principle: the distribution of bound and unbound radioactivity is dependent upon the total concentration of the compound in the system. Measurement of the radioactivity, therefore, can be utilized to calculate the unknown amount of compound in the system.

In the case of polypeptide hormones (gonadotropins), radioimmunoassay techniques are based upon the use of antibodies prepared by injecting the protein hormone of one species into another. The protein hormones vary in their physicochemical characteristics and amino acid composition from species to species, and, therefore, antibodies for use in radioimmunoassay are formed when protein hormones are administered cross-species. A highly specific antiserum can be produced to be utilized as the binding reagent. This specificity may make chromatographic separation that ordinarily follows extraction unnecessary.

Since steroid compounds are not antigenic, the production of a specific antiserum depends upon the linkage of a steroid to a large protein molecule. The protein molecule is antigenic in itself, but when combined with a steroid, the steroid-protein complex (hapten) stimulates a variety of antibodies, some of which recognize and are specific for the steroid. Thus, when the steroid-protein complex is injected into an animal the antiserum formed may be utilized as a reagent (R) for measurement of the steroid (S) in the technique of saturation analysis.

547

For example, a testosterone-bovine albumin conjugate can be formed by covalently linking testosterone to albumin at the 3 position via an oxime linkage to *o*-carboxymethyl hydroxylamine.

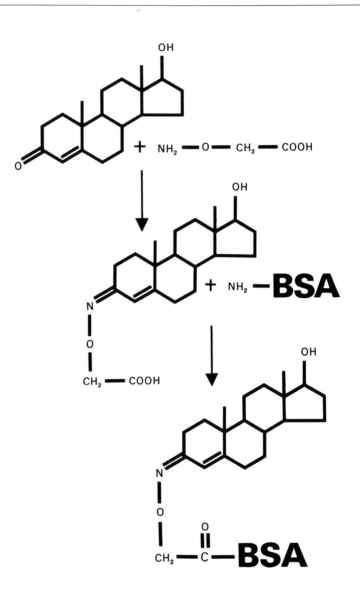

The cross-reactions to the antiserum produced with the above conjugate vary, and this antiserum may be used to measure testosterone and dihydrotestosterone, but the testosterone and dihydrotestosterone must be separated by some chromatographic means.

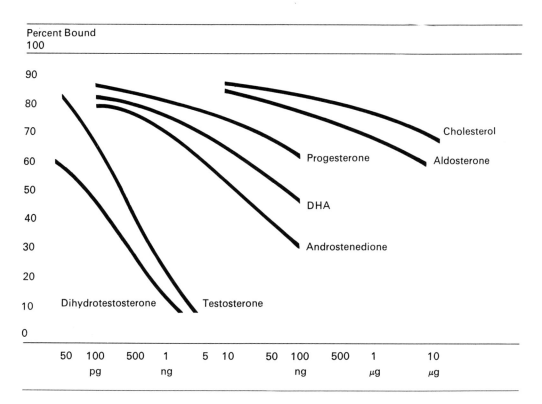

Competitive Protein Binding. In competitive protein binding, the antiserum is replaced with a protein which has a high affinity for the steroid to be measured. For example, corticosteroid-binding globulin may be utilized to measure progesterone, with the corticosteroids separated by chromatography. Pregnancy plasma or estrogen-treated plasma is the source for this protein. Competitive protein-binding assays have been replaced by radioimmunoassays.

Problems. These methods are not without problems. Utmost precision and care in technique are necessary. An unknown variation in technique may completely disrupt an assay. The periodic appearance of the well-known laboratory "gremlin" may be traced to a simple thing like the water supply or a change in glassware-washing routine. The accuracy of the results depends upon:

1. Specificity of the antibody or protein for the hormone to be measured.

2. Purity and specificity of the radiolabeled tracer.

3. Purity and availability of the standard reference hormone.

4. Sensitivity and precision of the assay.

5. Intra-assay and inter-assay experimental error.

If cross-reaction of the binding protein exists for other hormones, these cross-reacting substances must be removed. The radiolabeled tracer must have a high specific radioactivity, and purity is essential to ensure that it behaves identically as the substance being measured. Experimental error between assays as well as within an assay is an important determinant of assay reliability. A coefficient of variation of less than 15% for each is considered acceptable.

Measurement of Pituitary Gonadotropins

Pituitary gonadotropins can be measured by bioassay or by radioimmunoassay. The bioassay measures gonadotropins following injection of a kaolin extract of a 24-hour urine sample into an immature mouse. The increase in the weight of the uterus is taken as the end point. This assay has commonly, but erroneously, been referred to as urinary follicle-stimulating hormone (FSH). It should be called a total urinary gonadotropin assay since uterine growth is the result of both FSH and luteinizing hormone (LH) stimulation of the ovaries and the resulting estrogen production. The greatest dilution of a 24-hour urine extract which will produce a 100% increase in uterine weight is the titer of gonadotropins, and is expressed as mouse uterine units per 24 hours (muu/24 hours). The normal adult level is 6–50 muu/24 hours. A prepubertal level and an adult hypogonadotropic level is less than 6 muu/24 hours. A castrate and postmenopausal level is greater than 200 muu/24 hours. It should be emphasized that the bioassay of total gonadotropins is notoriously unreliable and is rarely used today.

Normal serum levels for pituitary gonadotropins during the normal menstrual cycle are illustrated:

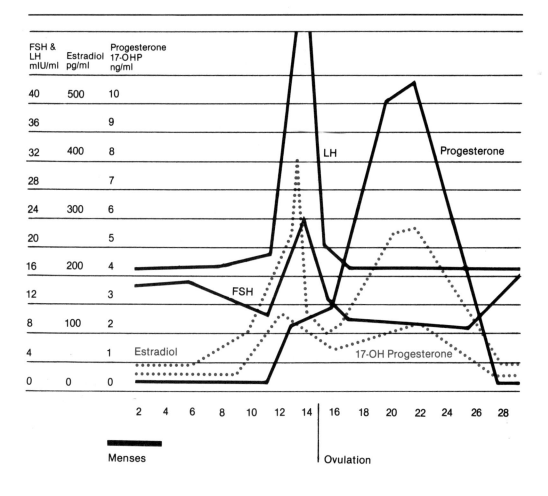

FSH & LH mIU/ml	Estradiol pg/ml	Progesterone 17-OHP ng/ml
40	500	10
36		9
32	400	8
28		7
24	300	6
20		5
16	200	4
12		3
8	100	2
4		1
0	0	0

2 4 6 8 10 12 14 | 16 18 20 22 24 26 28

Menses

Ovulation

For clinical purposes, the following ranges are useful:

Clinical State	Serum FSH	Serum LH
Normal adult female	5–20 mIU/ml, with the ovulatory midcycle peak about 2 times the base level	5–20 mIU/ml with the ovulatory midcycle peak about 3 times the base level
Hypogonadotropic state: Prepubertal, hypothalamic and pituitary dysfunction	Less than 5 mIU/ml	Less than 5 mIU/ml
Hypergonadotropic state: Postmenopausal, castrate and ovarian failure	Greater than 40 mIU/ml	Greater than 25 mIU/ml

| | **Measurement of Gonadal Steroids** | The normal levels for total plasma estrogens or estradiol, and plasma progesterone during the normal menstrual cycle have been illustrated. Variation is seen from individual to individual, however, and the following ranges in gonadal steroids are normally reported: |

Measurement of Gonadal Steroids

The normal levels for total plasma estrogens or estradiol, and plasma progesterone during the normal menstrual cycle have been illustrated. Variation is seen from individual to individual, however, and the following ranges in gonadal steroids are normally reported:

	Estradiol	Progesterone	Testosterone
Follicular phase	25–75 pg/ml	Less than 1 ng/ml	20–80 ng/dl
Midcycle peak	200–600 pg/ml		20–80 ng/dl
Luteal phase	100–300 pg/ml	5–20 ng/ml	20–80 ng/dl
Pregnancy: 1st trimester	1–5 ng/ml	20–30 ng/ml	
Pregnancy: 2nd trimester	5–15 ng/ml	50–100 ng/ml	
Pregnancy: 3rd trimester	10–40 ng/ml	100–400 ng/ml	
Postmenopause	5–25 pg/ml	Less than 1 ng/ml	10–40 ng/dl

The radioimmunoassay of 17-hydroxyprogesterone has replaced measurement of the urinary pregnanetriol level for the diagnosis of adrenal enzyme deficiency. Dramatic differences exist between normal individuals and patients with adrenal hyperplasia. Levels from 5 to 2000 times greater than normal have been observed.

17-Hydroxyprogesterone	
Children	3–90 ng/dl

Adult females
  Follicular phase
  Luteal phase
	15–70 ng/dl
	35–290 ng/dl

Urinary Steroid Assays

The measurement of estrogen in a 24-hour urine collection can be utilized during administration of human menopausal gonadotropins (Pergonal).

Total Urinary Estrogen	
Prepubertal	0–5 μg/24 hr
Follicular phase	10–25 μg/24 hr
Midcycle peak	35–100 μg/24 hr
Luteal phase	25–75 μg/24 hr
Postmenopausal	5–15 μg/24 hr

Pregnanediol is the main urinary metabolite of progesterone, although it accounts for only 7–20% of total progesterone production. Measurement of pregnanediol in a 24-hour urine sample has been used in the past to document pregnancy and epecially the well-being of an early pregnancy. However, with the advent of the measurement of plasma progesterone, the use of urinary pregnanediol has waned.

Urinary Pregnanediol	
Follicular phase	Less than 1 mg/24 hr
Luteal phase	2–5 mg/24 hr
Pregnancy: 20 weeks	40 mg/24 hr
Pregnancy: 30 weeks	80 mg/24 hr
Pregnancy: 40 weeks	100 mg/24 hr

Pregnanetriol is the urinary metabolite of 17-hydroxyprogesterone, and was used for the diagnosis of adrenal hyperplasia (the adrenogenital syndrome). Very little pregnanetriol is found in the urine of normal adults, but with the increased production of 17-hydroxyprogesterone due to an enzyme deficiency in the adrenal gland (adrenogenital syndrome), increased urinary excretion of pregnanetriol will occur.

Urinary Pregnanetriol	
Children	Less than 0.5 mg/24 hr
Adults	0.2 to 2–4 mg/24 hr, the upper limit varying among laboratories

553

Measurement of Human Chorionic Gonadotropin

Secretion of human chorionic gonadotropin (HCG) by the syncytiotrophoblast cells of the placenta is predominantly into the maternal circulation. The assay of HCG in maternal urine has been the basis of pregnancy tests for many years. Aschheim and Zondek originated the bioassay pregnancy test in immature mice (the A-Z test) in the late 1920s.

The biologic tests for HCG depended upon the response of ovaries or testes in immature animals. This response was due to the gonadotropic properties of HCG and was measured either in terms of increased gonadal weight or hyperemia, or the secondary response in sex organs due to the increased gonadal steroidogenesis induced by the HCG. The expulsion of ova or sperm in amphibia was widely utilized as an end point for HCG. These biologic assays have now been succeeded by immunoassays for HCG in urine and blood.

There are three general types of immunologic assays for HCG, utilizing specific antisera. The three are: hemagglutination-inhibition, complement-fixation, and radioimmunoassay. In the hemagglutination-inhibition reaction, the presence of HCG in maternal urine will inhibit an agglutination reaction between HCG-coated red cells and the antisera. This is the basic reaction in most commercial methods, with latex particles replacing the red cells in some methods. The rapid slide tests utilize latex particles and take 2 minutes to perform. The usual 2-hour test performed in a test tube is more sensitive and reliable. A first morning voided specimen is more concentrated than a random sample and this increases the chances of detecting HCG.

HCG is similar to LH in its structure and thus antibodies to one cross-react with the other. The sensitivity of most commercial assays is limited in order to avoid false positive tests due to cross-reactivity with LH. Assays utilizing highly specific receptors for HCG have a greater sensitivity, but also respond to LH. The greatest sensitivity and specificity is found with the radioimmunoassay for the β subunit of HCG.

β-HCG can be detected in the blood 9–11 days after the LH peak, 7–9 days after ovulation. A concentration of 100 mIU/ml is reached about 2 days after the date of expected menses (day 30 in an ideal cycle). Most radioimmunoassays for the β subunit of HCG have a lower sensitivity of 2–5 mIU/ml. The commercially available receptor assays have a lower sensitivity of 200 mIU/ml, a level reached on day 32 from the onset of the last menstrual period (LMP). The 2-hour urinary pregnancy tests (tube tests) are reliably positive approximately 36 days after the LMP, and the 2-minute slide tests, approximately 41 days after the LMP. Because of the various sensitivities, negative pregnancy tests may be due to an insufficient HCG titer, depending upon the time of gestation. A positive test is almost always reliable. Do not forget that most cycles have something

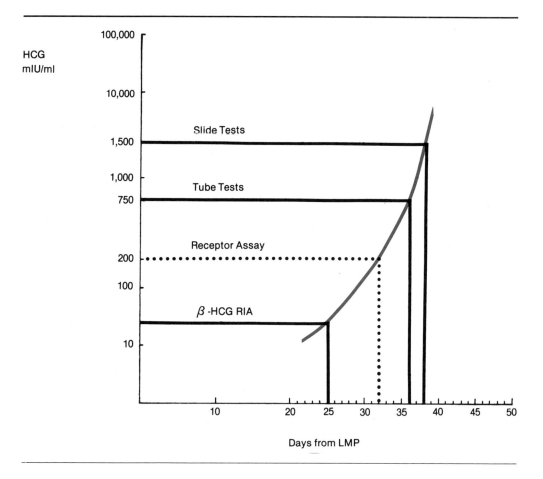

HCG
mIU/ml

Slide Tests

Tube Tests

Receptor Assay

β -HCG RIA

Days from LMP

other than a 14-day follicular phase, and, therefore, the timing of HCG levels compared to an ideal 28-day cycle may not apply.

Peak levels of HCG (approximately 100,000 mIU/ml) occur at 10 weeks of gestation, declining and remaining at approximately 10,000–20,000 mIU/ml by 12–14 weeks. Evaluation of a patient following a spontaneous or therapeutic abortion is occasionally a difficult problem. The urinary pregnancy test will be negative 3 weeks after abortion.

There are two clinical conditions in which blood HCG titers are very helpful, trophoblastic disease and ectopic pregnancies. Following molar pregnancies, in patients without persistent disease, the HCG titer should fall to a nondetectable level by 15 weeks. Patients with trophoblastic disease show an abnormal curve (a titer greater than 500 mIU/ml) frequently by 3 weeks and usually by 6 weeks.

Virtually 100% of patients suspected of an ectopic pregnancy, but not having the condition, will have a negative blood HCG assay. A positive test can also be utilized in diagnosis. The HCG level increases at different rates in normal and ectopic pregnancies. In a normal pregnancy, the HCG should approximately double every 2 days. An HCG above 6000 mIU/ml is almost always associated with an intrauterine pregnancy. When the HCG titer is below 6000 mIU/ml and ultrasound examination fails to identify an intrauterine pregnancy, a patient may be managed expectantly if the HCG titer doubles in 2 days. If the titer does not double, laparoscopy is indicated. Laparoscopy is also indicated when the titer is above 6000 mIU/ml and ultrasound shows no evidence of an intrauterine pregnancy.

Measurement of 17-Ketosteroids, 17-Ketogenic Steroids, and 17-Hydroxycortico-steroids

These assays provide essential clinical information, yet misunderstanding of their meaning and limitations is still common. A basic appreciation for the methods and what they measure is necessary for the proper interpretation of these urinary assays.

A 24-hour urine specimen is required to avoid the variations in steroid excretion which occur throughout a day. Refrigeration is essential to avoid degradation of metabolites. It is wise to obtain a urinary creatinine as a check of the validity of the 24-hour collection. Urinary creatinine excretion is a reflection of body muscle mass and remains relatively constant, approximately 1000 mg/24 hours.

The name "17-ketosteroids" is descriptive, designating compounds with a ketone group at the 17 position (C-17). The 17-KS are composed of the major urinary androgenic metabolites, but testosterone itself is not a 17-KS, and significant levels of testosterone may be associated with normal levels of 17-KS.

17-keto group

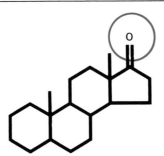

The commonly measured 17-ketosteroids are also known as the neutral 17-KS. Other compounds have a ketone group in the 17 position, but are not "neutral," for example, estrone. Estrone, due to its phenolic structure in ring A, is acidic, and therefore is removed from the urinary extract when washed with alkali in the procedure.

The 17-KS are divided into two groups: the major part being 11-deoxy-17-KS produced by the gonads and adrenal cortex, and the 11-oxy-17-KS, produced *only* by the adrenal cortex.

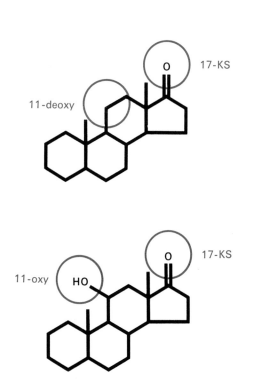

The three major urinary 11-deoxy 17 KS, and therefore, the three major urinary metabolites of androgens are: dehydroepiandrosterne (DHA), etiocholanolone, and androsterone. Note that the only difference between etiocholanolone and androsterone is the stereochemistry at the 5 position: alpha (α) in androsterone and beta (β) in etiocholanolone.

Dehydroepiandrosterone
(DHA)

Etiocholanolone

Androsterone

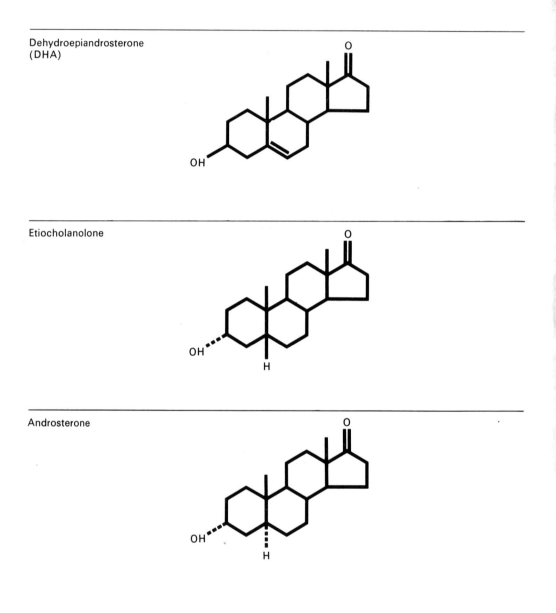

The major 11-oxy-17KS are of adrenal origin: 11-hydroxyetiocholanolone and 11-ketoetiocholanolone (metabolites of corticosteroids), and 11β-hydroxyandrosterone (metabolite of 11β-hydroxyandrostenedione).

11β-Hydroxyandrosterone

11-Hydroxyetiocholanolone

11-Ketoetiocholanolone

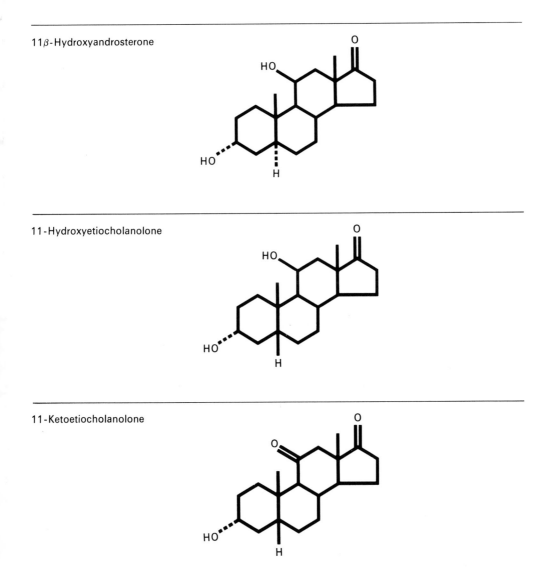

The majority of methods in clinical use for the assay of 17-KS include five major steps:

1. Hydrolysis of the 17-KS conjugates by acid to liberate the free steroids for extraction.

2. Extraction with organic solvents.

3. Removal of acidic material by washing with alkali.

4. Development of color, usually by the Zimmermann reaction (17-KS will give a purple color when treated with dinitrobenzene in the presence of alkali).

5. Measurement by colorimetric methods.

Normal 17-KS

The normal level of 17-ketosteroid excretion in a female is 10 ± 3 mg/24 hours. It should be kept in mind that excretion of 17-KS in the urine changes with age. This can be especially important in the evaluation of an elderly woman.

17-KS
mg/24 hrs

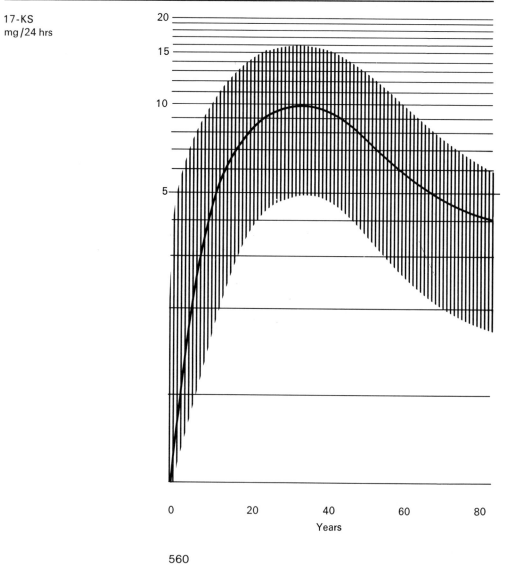

Years

As stated above, the urinary 17-KS arise from precursors secreted by the adrenal cortex and the ovaries. In addition, a certain minimum of nonspecific pigments is present in every urine sample. The composition of normal 17-KS excretion is illustrated.

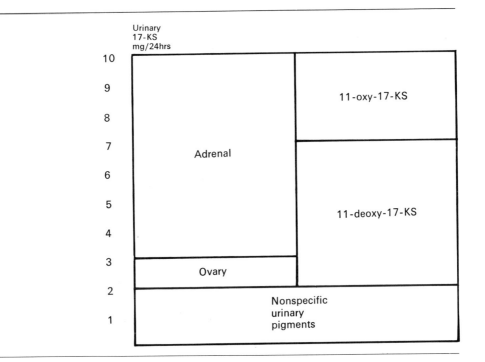

17-Ketogenic Steroids and 17-Hydroxycorticosteroids

17-Ketogenic steroid and 17-hydroxycorticosteroid (17-OHC) determinations measure urinary metabolites of glucocorticoids. There are significant differences in the two tests because more metabolites are measured by the 17-KG test.

The 17-KG and 17-OHC assays require the presence of a 17α-hydroxyl group. The mineralocorticoids (deoxycorticosterone (DOC), corticosterone (B), and aldosterone) do not have a 17-hydroxyl group, and therefore are not measured in 17-KG and 17-OHC assays.

17-hydroxyl group

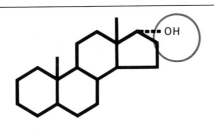

561

Desoxycorticosterone
(DOC)

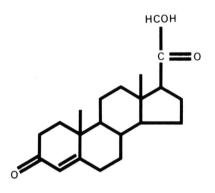

Corticosterone
(B)

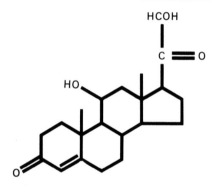

Aldosterone

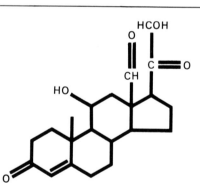

The principal glucocorticoid in the human is cortisol (hydrocortisone, Compound F). Cortisone (Compound E) is a metabolite of cortisol in the human.

Cortisol

Cortisone

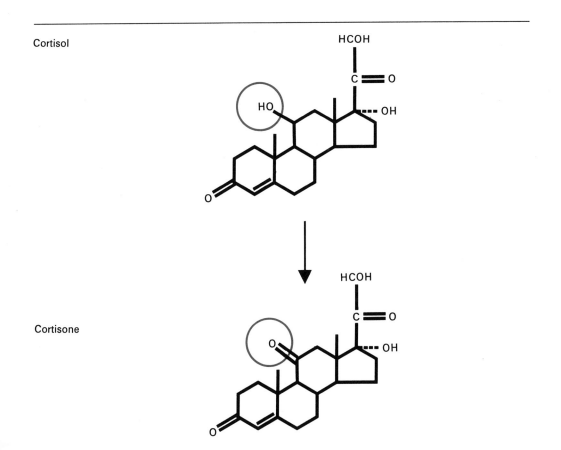

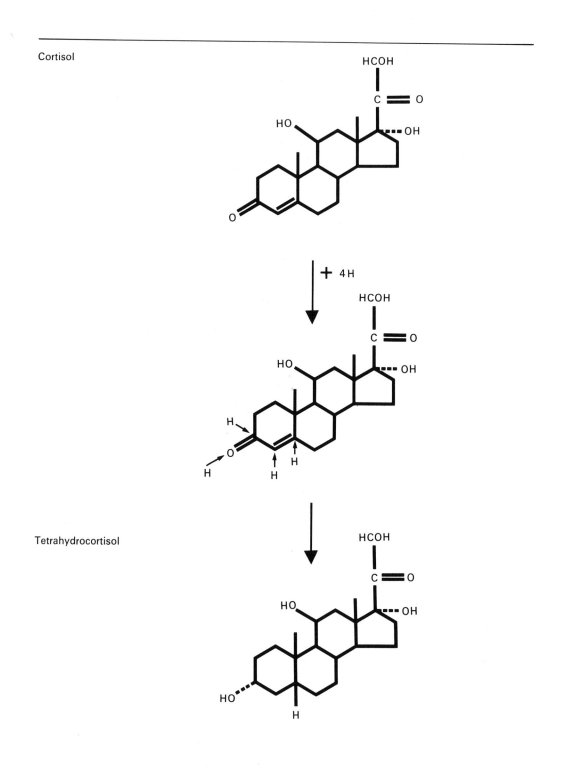

Cortisol

+ 4 H

Tetrahydrocortisol

A similar reduction sequence applies to cortisone, yielding tetrahydrocortisone. Further reduction of tetrahydrocortisol and tetrahydrocortisone involves the ketone at the carbon-20 position, yielding cortol and cortolone.

Tetrahydrocortisol

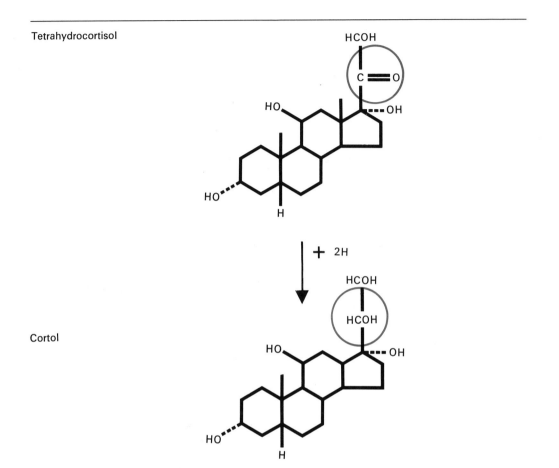

Cortol

The Porter-Silber reaction produces a color with phenylhydrazine and sulfuric acid. The reaction requires an alpha ketolic group plus the 17-hydroxyl group. Therefore, a hydroxyl group must be at C-21 and C-17, and a ketone must be present at C-20. This reaction measures the 17-hydroxycorticosteroids, abbreviated as 17-OHC.

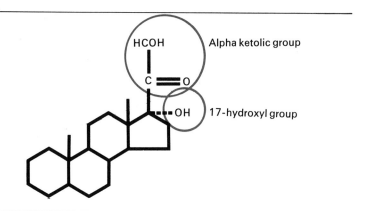

The 17-OHC assay, therefore, cannot measure cortol and cortolone, the further reduction products of tetrahydrocortisol and tetrahydrocortisone, because the C-20 group is reduced and is not a ketone. Nor can the 17-OHC assay measure pregnanetriol since the α-ketolic group is not present.

Pregnanetriol

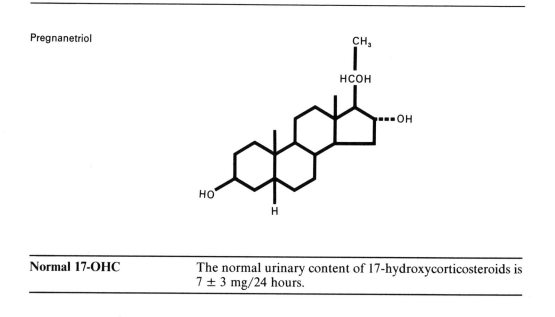

Normal 17-OHC

The normal urinary content of 17-hydroxycorticosteroids is 7 ± 3 mg/24 hours.

The 17-ketogenic (17-KG) steroids are compounds which, when oxidized with sodium bismuthate ($NaBiO_3$), give rise to 17-ketosteroids (17-KS), which can then be measured by the Zimmermann reaction. The initial measurement of 17-KS is subtracted and the difference represents the 17-KG steroids. The requirement is a 17-hydroxyl group and a second hydroxyl group on either the C-20 or the C-21 position.

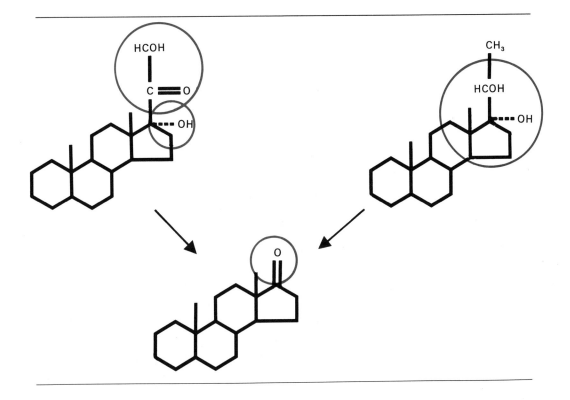

Therefore, the following compounds are measured: tetrahydrocortisol, tetrahydrocortisone, cortol, cortolone, and pregnanetriol (the latter three compounds are not measured in the 17-OHC assay). The compounds missing a 17-hydroxyl group, mainly mineralocorticoids (DOC, corticosterone, and aldosterone) will not be measured by either 17-OHC or 17-KG procedures.

Normal 17-KG

The normal urinary content of 17-KG is 10 ± 3 mg/24 hours. The measurement of additional steroids, when compared to the 17-OHC assay, may be troublesome in the adrenogenital syndrome where pregnanetriol excretion is elevated. Therefore, the 17-KG in the adrenogenital syndrome may be high, while the 17-OHC will be normal.

One should also keep in mind that values change with age.

17-OHC
mg/24hrs

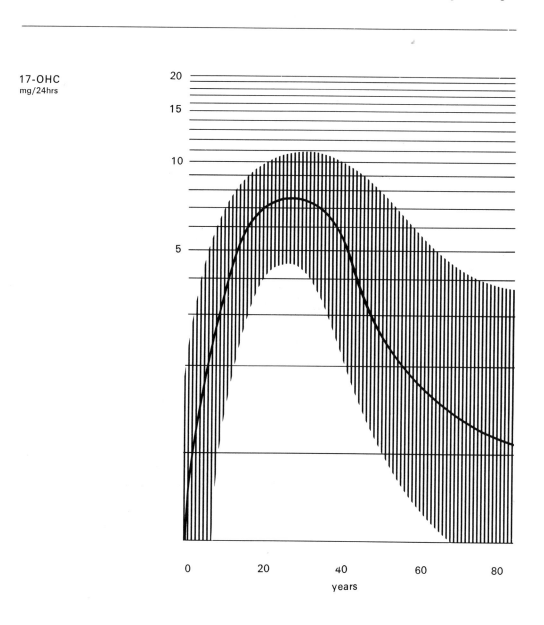

years

Adrenal Tests

The 24-Hour Urinary Free Cortisol. This measurement accurately reflects the daily production rate and the amount of cortisol which is free and active in the circulation. The normal value ranges from 20 to 90 μg/24 hours.

The Blood Cortisol Level. ACTH is secreted in a pulsatile fashion with the pulses being more frequent and of greater magnitude in the early morning hours, shortly before waking. A nadir in secretion is reached in the evening. Blood levels of ACTH and cortisol are highest in the early morning and lowest in the evening. When the sleep-awake cycle is altered, the diurnal rhythm shifts over about a week's time to resume the same sleep-awake pattern. At 8 A.M., the normal plasma cortisol concentration ranges from 10 to 25 μg/dl. At 8 P.M., the level is about half the morning concentration, and at 10 P.M. the level is usually less than 12 μg/dl.

The ACTH Infusion Test. This is a test for adrenal reserve. Adrenal glands not exposed to ACTH over a long period of time will not have a normal response. Synthetic ACTH is injected in a bolus of 0.25 mg. The plasma cortisol should increase 2–3 times over baseline at 30 and 60 minutes.

The Metyrapone Test. This is a test for hypothalamic-pituitary-adrenal function (a test of ACTH reserve). Metyrapone blocks 11β-hydroxylase enzyme activity in the adrenal gland, thus interfering with cortisol production. After a baseline 24-hour urinary 17-hydroxycorticosteroid or plasma 11-deoxycortisol is obtained, metryapone is given orally, 750 mg every 4 hours for 6 doses. The 17-OHC should at least double during the 24 hours of metryapone administration or the next day. A plasma 11-deoxycortisol at 8 A.M., 4 hours after the last dose of metyrapone, should exceed 10 μg/dl.

Thyroid Gland

Thyroid hormone synthesis depends in large part upon an adequate supply of iodine in the diet. In the small intestine iodine is absorbed as iodide, and is transported to the thyroid gland. Plasma iodide enters the thyroid under the influence of thyroid stimulating hormone (TSH), the anterior pituitary thyrotropin hormone. Within the thyroid gland, iodide is oxidized and bound to tyrosine. Monoiodotyrosine and diiodotyrosine combine to form thyroxine (T_4) and triiodothyronine (T_3). These iodinated compounds are part of the thyroglobulin molecule, the colloid which serves as a storage depot for thyroid hormone. TSH induces a proteolytic process which results in the release of iodothyronines into the bloodstream as thyroid hormone. In the blood, thyroid hormone is tightly associated with a group of proteins chiefly thyroxine-binding globulin (TBG). Estrogen produces a rise in thyroxine-binding globulin capacity, and, therefore, thyroid function tests are affected by pregnancy and estrogen-containing medication. With the increase in TBG capacity, the maintenance of an euthyroid state depends upon the concept that free thyroxine concentration (unbound and metabolically active thyroid hormone) is within the normal range.

569

Although T_4 is secreted at 8–10 times the rate of T_3, it is T_3 which is responsible for most if not all of the thyroid action in the body. T_3 is 3–4 times more potent than T_4. About one third of the T_4 secreted each day is converted in peripheral tissues, largely liver and kidney, to T_3, and about 40% is converted to the inactive, reverse T_3.

There are at least two reasons why T_3 is more active than T_4. The cellular nuclear receptor for thyroid hormone has about a 10-fold higher affinity for T_3 than T_4, and blood proteins which restrict the entry of thyroid hormone into cells bind T_4 more tightly than T_3.

One would think that measurement of T_3, therefore, would be the most accurate appraisal of thyroid function. Because of the peripheral source of T_3, however, it is not a direct reflection of thyroid secretion. In addition T_3 levels may be normal despite the presence of a goiter with elevated TSH and depressed T_4 concentrations. T_4 plays the instrumental role in TSH regulation. Thyroid hormones regulate TSH by both suppressing thyroid releasing hormone (TRH) secretion and affecting the pituitary sensitivity to TRH (by reducing the number of TRH receptors). While some tissues depend mainly on the blood T_3 for their intracellular T_3, the brain and the pituitary depend on their own intracellular conversion of T_4. The measurement of T_4 and TSH, therefore, provides the most accurate assessment of thyroid function.

The modern assessment of thyroid function is relatively easy. The confusing array of tests previously available (protein-bound iodine, T_3 uptake, free thyroxine index) has been replaced by the radioimmunoassay of free T_4, TSH, and T_3. The free T_4 level has a different range of normal values from laboratory to laboratory. The serum TSH ranges from nondetectable to 12 μU/ml. The radioimmunoassay of T_3 is unnecessary on a routine basis, but important for the occasional case of hyperthyroidism due to excessive production of T_3 with normal T_4 levels (T_3 toxicosis). The normal range for serum T_3 is 80–180 ng/dl.

Drugs taken orally for cholecystograms inhibit the peripheral conversion of T_4 to T_3, and can disrupt normal thyroid levels (giving an elevated T_4). This effect can last 30 days after administration. In early hypothyroidism, with undetectable symptoms or signs, a compensated state can be detected by an elevated TSH and normal T_4. With progressive deterioration, a progressively lower T_4 is apparent.

In hypothyroidism, the therapeutic decision is easy: replacement thyroid medication should be prescribed to return TSH levels to normal, even though T_4 levels are already normal. This avoids the appearance of a goiter and the progressive development of clinical hypothyroidism. The best preparation for hormone replacement is T_4. Mixtures of T_4 and T_3, such as desiccated thyroid, provide T_3 in excess of normal thyroid secretion. It is better to provide T_4 and allow the peripheral conversion process to provide the T_3. Likewise, for suppression of TSH after treatment of thyroid carcinoma or nodular thyroid disease, the drug of choice is T_4, thyroxine. Both TSH and T_4 should be measured when monitoring treatment because TSH alone cannot detect overdosage.

Index

Note: *f* = graphs and charts, *Illus.* = drawings and illustrations

586